FELINE CLINICAL PARASITOLOGY

FELINE CLINICAL PARASITOLOGY

Dwight D. Bowman

Charles M. Hendrix

David S. Lindsay

Stephen C. Barr

Iowa State University Press

A Blackwell Science Company

Dwight D. Bowman, MS, PhD, is an Associate Professor of Parasitology in the Department of Microbiology and Immunology at the College of Veterinary Medicine, Cornell University, Ithaca, New York.

Charles M. Hendrix, DVM, is a Professor of Parasitology in the Department of Pathobiology at the College of Veterinary Medicine, Auburn University, Auburn, Alabama.

David S. Lindsay, PhD, is an Associate Professor in the Department of Biomedical Sciences and Pathobiology at the Center for Molecular Medicine and Infectious Diseases, Virginia-Maryland Regional College of Veterinary Medicine, Virginia Tech, Blacksburg, Virginia.

Stephen C. Barr, BVSc MVS, PhD, is a Diplomate of the American College of Veterinary Internal Medicine and an Associate Professor of Medicine in the Department of Clinical Sciences at the College of Veterinary Medicine, Cornell University, Ithaca, New York.

Iowa State University Press
2121 South State Avenue, Ames, Iowa 50014

Orders: 1-800-862-6657
Office: 1-515-292-0140
Fax: 1-515-292-3348
Web site: www.isupress.com

∞ Printed on acid-free paper in the United States of America

First edition, 2002

Library of Congress Cataloging-in-Publication Data

Bowman, Dwight D.
Feline clinical parasitology / Dwight D. Bowman . . . [et al.]—1st ed.
p. cm.
Includes bibliographical references and index (p.).
ISBN 0-8138-0333-0 (alk. paper)
1. Cats—Parasites. 2. Veterinary clinical parasitology. I. Bowman, Dwight D. II. Title.
SF986.P37 F46 2001
636.8'089696—dc21

2001003565

The last digit is the print number: 9 8 7 6 5 4 3 2 1

CONTENTS

PREFACE

In 1998 the number of cats in the United States was estimated to be approximately 70.9 million; cats were found in 34 percent of the 100 million U.S. households. This figure now surpasses the number of dogs in the United States, approximately 57.6 million in 38.1 percent of households (www.petfood-institute.org, Pet Food Institute, Washington, D.C.). For 1985 in Canada, the number of cats was approximately 4,134,200 and also surpassed the number of dogs, 3,028,100. Nearly 23 percent of households in the United Kingdom have at least one cat, and in Australia about 35 percent of the households each have one cat or more. This love for the cat, however, is not restricted to predominantly English-speaking countries. Between 1980 and 1990, the cat populations of almost all European nations increased—in some cases dramatically—to the extent that cat populations are currently level with those of the dog. Among Europeans, the Swiss are dedicated cat lovers, preferring to own cats rather than dogs. The French and the Belgians are well-known for their love of both cats and dogs. Among nations surveyed regarding the presence of cats in households, the Japanese have the least number, with a little over 5 percent with cats in 1990. However, there are more and more households with cats all the time in Southeast Asia, especially in countries such as Taiwan and Malaysia. Regardless of national boundary, with the ever-increasing limitations of time, money, and space, the cat is rapidly becoming the cosmopolitan pet of the twenty-first century.

Awareness of cats as something other than "small dogs" has also emerged among cat owners and veterinarians as is evidenced by the increasing number of established specialized feline veterinary practices in the United States and Europe. For 1999, the number of members in the American Association of Feline Practitioners and the Academy of Medicine was 1,550, of which 33.5 percent (520) dealt exclusively with cats (Kristi Kruse Thomson, American Association of Feline Practitioners, Nashville, Tennessee). One way in which cats differ from dogs is in their parasitic infections and infestations. Although dogs and cats do share a few parasites, the vast majority of the parasites of these pets are actually specific to either dogs or cats, not to both. Also, even those parasites that are shared between cats and dogs will often cause different host responses when parasitizing the cat and often require different treatment regimens.

The purpose of this book is to offer an in-depth examination of feline parasites. Topics discussed include parasite identification, history, geographic distribution, pathogenesis, epizootiology, zoonosis if applicable, diagnosis, treatment, control, and prevention. The authors have attempted to produce a book that is international in scope due to the immense worldwide popularity of cats and due to the amount of travel undertaken by cats and their owners. Also, it was felt that this text would prove useful to veterinarians in other countries.

It is hoped that this book will be useful to both the veterinarian and the veterinary parasitologist. It includes concise and in-depth knowledge that is useful to both groups. Overall, the ultimate goal of this book is to improve the health of cats around the world by providing a ready reference text that can be used to assist (1) in diagnosing parasitic infections or infestations and (2) in treating cats and kittens that host these parasites.

The parasites of the cats fall into four major groups: the common cosmopolitan parasites, the parasites that are important in only certain geographic areas, those that are rare and show up in rather large numbers in certain countries or certain foci, and those that tend to be rare or incidental findings where cats are serving as atypical hosts of some adult form that is usually found in the local wildlife. We have tried to include all these parasites in the text with the hope that it would help practitioners develop a better understanding of the scope of parasites around the world. Thus, there are a lot of species in the text that have appeared only once in cats or only in very limited geographical areas. Also, we are aware that we are also dealing with a number of parasites with which we do not actually have first-hand knowledge. We do believe, however, that the book will serve to stimulate individuals to consider the parasites of cats in more detail so that new information and corrections can be added to future editions.

There are many individuals that need to be thanked in the production of this text. Dr. J. Ralph Lichtenfels and Patricia A. Pilitt at the U.S. National Parasite Collection, U.S. Department of Agriculture, Agricultural Research Service, Biosystematics and National Parasite Collection Unit, require special thanks for their assistance in making the specimens of myriad trematodes from cats available for photography. There have been many individuals that have helped in the collection of the numerous references that were used to produce the text, with special thanks going to Dr. Megan Williams. Michael Porch assisted with many of the photographs of trematodes. Elizabeth A. Fogarty is thanked for her able assistance with all aspects of the book's final assembly, help with the generation of the final digitized images, and the production of the maps detailing geographic distribution. Vanessa Nicolle Bowman was a great help when the format for all the maps had to be changed for the final generation of the text. The line drawings of the life cycle of the cat flea and the life cycle of *Cuterebra* were generated by Dr. Laurie Duffield. The book has been a long time coming, and thanks go out to the original editor, Caroll C. Cann, who has since retired. The editor who helped with the actual rendition of the book that has gone to press is Lynne Bishop, and without her help this text may never have been completed. Colleagues who have been especially helpful in the generation of the text include Dr. de Lahunta, who has kept us honest relative to the neurology sections of the text, Dr. Robert Foley, who has always been helpful with practical information relative to mite infestations in cats, and Dr. William Hornbuckle for his assistance with day-to-day answers to questions.

FELINE CLINICAL PARASITOLOGY

1 THE PROTOZOA

Protozoan parasites of animals are typically single-celled organisms. Protozoa differ from bacteria in that the protozoan cell contains a discrete nucleus with a nuclear membrane. Also, undulipodia (flagella), when present on the protozoan cell, have a structure that is distinct from the flagellum of bacteria but not unlike that of the cilium of mammals and other animals. The protozoa differ from fungi in that fungal cells do not have undulipodia and typically are binucleate organisms. Protozoa differ from plants and animals by the fact that both plants and animals develop from an embryo, a developmental stage lacking from all protozoan forms.

Although the protozoal kingdom contains somewhere around 35 phyla and myriad species of organisms (Margulis et al., 1990), only 4 phyla are implicated as pathogens of the cat. Protozoa within these phyla differ markedly in their biology, which is an indication of their widely divergent relationships. Certain aspects of the biology of protozoa, the ability to form resistant stages, utilization of vectors, and genetic exchange of material through sexual union, are important in a general understanding of these parasites because they are directly related to the transmission of these pathogens between feline hosts.

Protozoan parasites are typically transmitted between cats in one of four different ways (Table 1.1). First, direct contact is the means of transmission used by *Trichomonas felistomae,* a parasite of the mouth of the cat. In this form of transmission, the stage of the parasite is not resistant to environmental extremes and will die rapidly if deposited by the cat in drinking water or on skin by licking. Second, exposure to resistant stages in the environment is the means by which cats are infected with *Giardia felis, Cryptosporidium felis, Isospora* species, and on some occasions *Toxoplasma gondii.* These parasites all have a resistant stage that is protected by a thick protective wall, and once these stages enter a favorable environment, they are capable of persisting for months to years. A third means of transmission is via the ingestion of other hosts containing resistant stages; this type of transmission occurs with *Sarcocystis* species, *Hammondia hammondi, Toxoplasma gondii,* and occasionally with species of *Isospora.* In this case, the host eaten by the cat has become infected by the ingestion of a resistant stage shed into the environment in the cat's feces; with the notable exception being that there can be vertical transmission in the nonfeline host in the case of toxoplasmosis. The host protects the protozoan from environmental extremes, and the parasite is capable of persisting within the host for months to years. Fourth, there is transmission by a blood-feeding arthropod vector, which is the means by which cats typically become infected with *Leishmania* species, species of *Trypanosoma,* and the apicomplexan genera *Cytauxzoon* and *Babesia.* For the most part, the arthropod is required to increase the quantity of infectious agents ingested when the arthropod bites to a quantity sufficient for the infection of the next host. The arthropod also serves to protect the parasite from environmental extremes as it moves from host to host. Other, less frequent forms of transmission of protozoa between cats do occur, but in general, these four modes of transmission are the most typical.

Some protozoan parasites of the cat are rare or only occasionally seen, while others are very common (Table 1.2). Factors that affect the prevalence of these parasites include such things as the geographic range of the parasite or its vector, local conditions of housing or environment, and age of the cats being surveyed. For instance, *Trypanosoma cruzi* is restricted to the Americas, mainly south of Mexico. The reason for the restriction of this parasite is in part due to vectors,

TABLE 1.1—Transmission of the protozoan parasites of the cat

Phylum of parasite genus	Resistant stage	Intermediate host	Paratenic host	Vector
APICOMPLEXA				
Cryptosporidium	Oocyst	–	–	–
Isospora	Oocyst	–	Sometimes	–
Besnoitia	Oocyst	+	–	–
Hammondia	Oocyst	+	–	–
Sarcocystis	Sporocyst	+	–	–
Toxoplasma	Oocyst	–	Sometimes	–
Hepatozoon	–	–	–	Tick[1]
Cytauxzoon	–	–	–	Tick
Babesia	–	–	–	Tick
SARCOMASTIGOPHORA				
Trichomonas	–	–	–	–
Giardia	Cyst	–	–	–
Trypanosoma (Old World)	–	–	–	Fly
Trypanosoma (New World)	–	–	–	Bug
Leishmania	–	–	–	Sandfly
RHIZOPODA				
Entamoeba	Cyst	–	–	–
MICROSPORA				
Encephalitozoon	Spore	–	–	–

1. In the case of *Hepatozoon canis,* the cat is infected by eating the tick rather than by the bite of the tick.

TABLE 1.2—General prevalence and geographical distribution of the protozoan parasites of the cat

Phylum of parasite genus	General prevalence	Geographic distribution
APICOMPLEXA		
Cryptosporidium	Uncommon	Global
Isospora	Very common	Global
Besnoitia	Uncommon	Global
Hammondia	Uncommon	Global
Sarcocystis	Uncommon	Global
Toxoplasma	Very common	Global
Hepatozoon	Uncommon	Africa and Asia
Cytauxzoon	Rare	Southeast United States
Babesia	Uncommon	South Africa and Asia
SARCOMASTIGOPHORA		
Trichomonas	Common	Global
Giardia	Common	Global
Trypanosoma (Old World)	Uncommon	Africa and Asia
Trypanosoma (New World)	Sporadic	Americas
Leishmania (Old World)	Sporadic	Africa and Asia
Leishmania (New World)	Sporadic	Americas
RHIZOPODA		
Entamoeba	Potential	Tropics
MICROSPORA		
Encephalitozoon	Rare	Global

triatomid bugs, that are adapted to human dwellings in that part of the world; typically these bugs are found mainly in the wild. Local conditions can have a great effect on the prevalence of parasites in a cat population. If the cats are hunters and spend a good deal of time outdoors, they will develop parasite infections different from those of the indoor cat (e.g., the indoor cat would be free from tick bites under most circumstances). If one looks at kittens, the prevalence of protozoan parasites in this population is much different than in adult cats. Kittens are more likely to be shedding large number of oocysts than adult cats. Of course, the truly rare parasites are probably rare because they are not typically parasites of the domestic cat.

The stages involved with the transmission of protozoan parasites are often, but not always, the same as those involved with diagnosis (Table 1.1). In those cases where the resistant stage is shed in the cat's feces, it can often be recovered using routine methodologies of flotation. However, in cases with severe diarrhea and rapid intestinal motility, the resistant stages may not form, making diagnosis more difficult. In the case of *Giardia felis,* it becomes necessary to examine the feces in a manner that will allow the diagnosis of trophozoite stages. This would also be the case in a cat with amebic dysentery and perhaps in one with severe coccidiosis. The protozoan parasites of the cat that produce stages that are found in blood or tissue samples are typically those transmitted by biting arthropods. However, it would not be uncommon for the number of circulating organisms to be at such low levels that they may not be diagnosed by a routine blood smear or biopsy specimen. Thus, other forms of diagnosis might be required.

REFERENCES

Margulis L, Corliss JO, Melkonian M, Chapman DJ (eds.). 1990. Handbook of Protoctista. Boston, Mass: Jones and Bartlett Publishers. 914 pp.

COCCIDIA: THE PHYLUM APICOMPLEXA

All members of the phylum Apicomplexa are obligatory parasites. The phylum contains the coccidial parasites and important blood parasites of cats. Two of the parasites, *Toxoplasma gondii* and *Cryptosporidium parvum,* are of public health importance because they are zoonotic agents. The phylum obtains its name from the assemblage of organelles that are present in the anterior end of invasive stages and collectively form the apical complex (Current et al., 1990). The apical complex is involved in the entrance of parasites in to host cells. Cats are definitive hosts for several apicomplexan parasites including the genera *Isospora, Toxoplasma, Hammondia, Besnoitia, Sarcocystis, Cryptosporidium, Babesia,* and *Cytauxzoon* (*Theileria* syn.). *Isospora* and *Cryptosporidium* are coccidial parasites that can be associated with diarrhea. *Toxoplasma, Hammondia, Besnoitia,* and *Sarcocystis* are coccidial parasites that have a two-host life cycle and use cats as definitive hosts. Intestinal infections in cats with these species are usually asymptomatic. *Babesia* and *Cytauxzoon* species are tick-transmitted blood parasites that can cause anemia and death.

Cryptosporidium felis Iseki, 1979

Etymology

Crypto (hidden) + *sporidium* (related to the spore-like oocyst stage) and *felis* for cat.

Synonyms

None.

History

This species was described by Iseki in 1979, but it has taken some time for the separate designation of the species in the cat to be generally accepted. At this time, it is considered by many that this is a valid species of *Cryptosporidium.*

Geographic Distribution

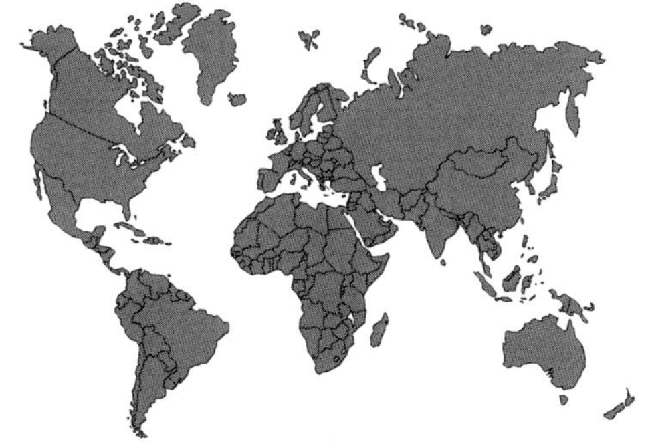

Fig. 1.1.

It is believed that this species is worldwide in distribution. There have been reports specifically identifying this species taken from cats in Japan (Iseki, 1979) and Australia (Morgan et al., 1998; Sargent et al., 1998). It has also been found in a calf in Poland (Bornay-Llinares et al., 1999).

Location in Host

Mucosal cells of the small intestine. The stages are found throughout the small intestine, but the schizont and oocysts are more common in the posterior third of the intestine. The parasites tend to be found mainly at the tips of the intestinal villi and are never found in the crypts.

Parasite Identification

The oocysts of *Cryptosporidium felis* differ from those of *Cryptosporidium parvum* in that they are smaller. The oocysts of *Cryptosporidium felis* measure 4.3 μm in diameter (3.5 to 5 μm). Those of *Cryptosporidium parvum* tend to have a mean diameter of 5 μm.

Life Cycle

Cats are infected by the ingestion of an oocyst. Each oocyst contains four sporozoites. Upon stimulation by various aspects of the digestive system of the new host, the sporozoites excyst from the oocyst and penetrate cells of the mucosa. The sporozoites, like other coccidians, induce phagocytosis; however, unlike with other coccidians, the small sporozoites appear to remain on the surface of the cell; that is, the cell membrane bulges out around the small parasite. Between the host cell and the vacuole containing the parasite develops a highly convoluted membrane-like structure that is called the "feeding organelle" or "apical organelle." Within the vacuole, the parasite undergoes schizogony to produce eight daughter merozoites. These then go on to infect other cells. The next phase of the infection is the development of sexual stages, macrogametocytes and microgametocytes. The microgametes are aflagellar but are capable of movement, and they will fuse with a macrogamete. After fusion, the macrogamete deposits an oocyst wall to become an oocyst. While still within the host, the oocyst undergoes a process of sporulation to produce oocysts that contain four infective sporozoites. Iseki (1979) described that these sporozoites were sometimes seen to be undergoing spontaneous excystation within the intestinal material he examined, and he felt that autoinfection was a distinct possibility. In experimentally infected cats, the prepatent period was 5 to 6 days, and the patent period was 7 to 10 days.

Clinical Presentation and Pathogenesis

Cryptosporidium felis has not been reported to cause disease experimentally in cats, but it is very unclear as to whether cats are routinely infected with this species or with isolates of *Cryptosporidium parvum* (See the next section on cryptosporidiosis in cats.)

Asahi et al. (1991) showed that experimentally infected cats shed oocysts for an extended period, up to 3 to 5 months. They held three of these cats for a year and then initiated prednisolone inoculations. After about a week of prednisolone treatment, these cats again shed large numbers of oocysts in their feces. None of the cats developed significant diarrhea or weight loss during the infections even though they shed large numbers of oocysts.

Treatment

Cases known to be caused by *Cryptosporidium felis* have not been treated, and there have been no attempts to treat cats experimentally infected with this species.

Epizootiology

The stage shed in the feces of cats is infective when passed in the feces. Thus, cats that are infected put other animals and their handlers at risk of infection. The fact that there have been numerous cases of zoonotic infections of *Cryptosporidium parvum* amongst veterinary students who are working with neonatal calves or foals would indicate that it is highly likely that the oocysts can be spread to people who believe they are taking proper precautions.

Hazards to Other Animals

Initially, it was felt that *Cryptosporidium felis* was fairly well restricted to the cat. Iseki (1979) tried to infect mice (three) and guinea pigs (three) with this parasite and was unsuccessful. Asahi et al. (1991) gave oocysts recovered from cats to mice, hydrocortisone-treated mice, suckling mice, guinea pigs, and dogs; none of these animals developed infection. Similarly, Mtambo et al. (1996) were unable to infect suckling mice with oocysts isolated from a cat in Scotland. Recently, however, a calf in Poland was identified that had small oocysts in its feces that were identified via molecular typing to be *Cryptosporidium felis* (Bornay-Llinares et al., 1999).

Hazards to Humans

It is unclear what the role is between *Cryptosporidium felis* and human infections. There is a report that molecular sequencing identified oocysts with the *Cryptosporidium felis* genotype in the feces of HIV-infected patients (Pieniazek et al., 1999). This would indicate that cats infected with *Cryptosporidium felis* might pose a threat to humans, perhaps only immunocompromised humans.

Control/Prevention

The oocyst is infective when passed, but it is killed by heating to over 60°C. Thus, good hygiene, the routine washing of cages, and the washing of bedding in a regular washer and drier (or drying on a line on a good sunny day) will probably destroy oocysts.

REFERENCES

Asahi H, Koyama T, Arai H, Funakoshi Y, Yamaura H, Shirasaka R, Okutomi K. 1991. Biological nature of *Cryptosporidium* sp. isolated from a cat. Parasitol Res 77:237–240.

Bornay-Llinares FJ, da Silva AJ, Moura IN, Myjak P, Pietkiewicz H, Kruminis-Lozowska W, Graczyk TK, Pieniazek NJ. 1999. Identification of *Cryptosporidium felis* in a cow by morphologic and molecular methods. Appl Environ Microbiol 65:1455–1458.

Current WL, Upton SJ, Long PL. 1990. Taxonomy and life cycles. In Coccidius of Man and Animals, ed PL Long, pp 1–16. Boca Raton, Fla: CRC Press.

Iseki M. 1979. *Cryptosporidium felis* sp. n. (Protozoa: Eimeriorina) from the domestic cat. Jap J Parasitol 28:285–307.

Morgan UM, Sargent KD, Elliot A, Thompson RCA. 1998. *Cryptosporidium* in cats–additional evidence for *C. felis*. Vet J 156:159–161.

Mtambo MMA, Wright SE, Nash AS, Blewett DA. 1996. Infectivity of a *Cryptosporidium* species isolated from a domestic cat (*Felis domestica*) in lambs and mice. Res Vet Sci 60:61–63.

Pieniazek NJ, Bornay-Llinares FJ, Slemenda SB, da Silva AJ, Moura IN, Arrowood MJ, Ditrich O, Addiss DG. 1999. New *Cryptosporidium* genotypes in HIV-infected persons. Emerg Infect Dis 5:444–449.

Sargent KD, Morgan UM, Elliot A, Thompson RCA. 1998. Morphological and genetic characterization of *Cryptosporidium* oocysts from domestic cats. Vet Parasitol 77:221–227.

Feline Cryptosporidiosis

No matter what species is involved, *Cryptosporidium felis* or *Cryptosporidium parvum,* cats do present with severe disease due to infection with this pathogen. A typical presentation of a cat with disease is one that has an underlying immunosuppressive disorder such as a feline leukemia virus infection (Monticello et al., 1987). However, there are cases where cats develop severe disease and persistent cryptosporidiosis where there is no apparent underlying condition (Lappin et al., 1997). Also, the recent development of serological tests that detect antibody in the blood of cats that have been infected would suggest that somewhere around 15 percent of cats throughout the United States have been or are currently infected with *Cryptosporidium* (Lappin et al., 1997; McReynolds et al., 1999).

The cat that presents with cryptosporidiosis will be having recurring bouts of diarrhea. The disease caused by *Cryptosporidium* infection is a water-losing diarrhea caused by the development of the parasites within the epithelial cells of the mucosa. Histologically, infection causes a blunting of the intestinal villus and crypt hyperplasia that is accompanied by an intense neutrophilic response (Tzipori et al., 1983). In AIDS patients with cryptosporidiosis, it has been found that net water, sodium, and chloride movement was the same as that in healthy controls (Kelly et al., 1996). From this work, these authors concluded that the diarrhea may be due to the secretion of electrolytes and water efflux distally to the site of infection or due to some yet undefined feature of the infection. Using monolayers of polarized colonic epithelial cells and the experimental infection of these cells with *Cryptosporidium parvum,* it has been shown that there is an increased macromolecular permeability of the monolayer, and it was felt that disruption of the epithelial cell barrier plays a role in the observed diarrhea (Adams et al., 1994). Additional work using the cell monolayer system has shown rather conclusively that the infection of the epithelial cells will ultimately result in significant changes in the host cell permeability and the permeability of the entire monolayer (Griffiths et al., 1994). Also, the infection will result in the death of the infected cells.

Treatment of cats that are undergoing infection is as difficult as treatment is in humans. The basic therapy is the relief of symptoms and increased fluids. Paromomycin has been used to treat cats with some success (Barr et al., 1994), but this therapy is not without potential complications that can include renal failure (Gookin et al., 1999).

Cats have on occasion been experimentally infected with what is thought to be *Cryptosporidium parvum* isolated from calves (Current et al., 1983; Pavlasek, 1983), but cats seem rather refractory to such infections. In a trial we performed at Cornell where two virus-free kittens were each fed 10 million oocysts, only a very few oocysts were shed in the feces of these cats, and they never developed signs of infection. Dogs have until very recently been considered to be infected with the same species, *Cryptosporidium parvum,* that occurs in calves and humans. Dogs can be experimentally infected with oocysts from calves, but the number of oocysts shed by these dogs appears to remain relatively low (Lloyd and Smith, 1997). Also, recent evidence tends to indicate that dogs may have their own phenotype as determined by DNA-sequencing methods (Pieniazek et al., 1999).

The potential transmission of *Cryptosporidium* between cats and people is currently fairly undefined. There have been reports linking feline cryptosporidiosis to human infection (Egger et al., 1990; Pieniazek et al., 1999). At the same time it would seem that many of the human isolates are neither from cats nor cattle; rather the infections are acquired from other humans. There have also been studies that have shown that pet ownership is not a risk factor for HIV-infected individuals (Glaser et al., 1998).

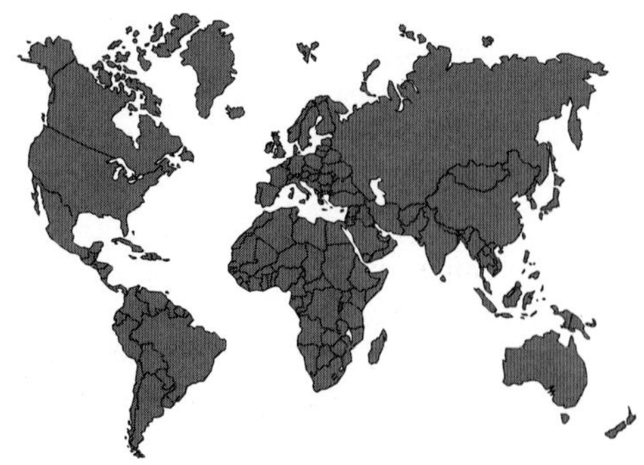

Fig.1.2. *Cryptosporidium parvum*

REFERENCES

Adams RB, Guerrant RL, Zu SX, Fang GD, Roche JK. 1994. *Cryptosporidium parvum* infection of intestinal epithelium: morphologic and functional studies in an in vitro model. J Infect Dis 169:170–177.

Barr SC, Jamrosz GF, Hornbuckle WE, Bowman DD, Fayer R. 1994. Use of paromomycin for treatment of cryptosporidiosis in a cat. JAVMA 205:1742-1743.

Current WL, Reese NC, Ernst JV, Bailey WS, Heyman MB, Weinstein WM. 1983. Human cryptosporidiosis in immunocompetent and immunodeficient persons. Studies of an outbreak and experimental transmission. N Engl J Med 308:1252–1257.

Egger M, Nguyen XM, Schaad UB, Krech T. 1990. Intestinal cryptosporidiosis acquired from a cat. Infection 18:177–178.

Glaser CA, Safrin S, Reingold A, Newman TB. 1998. Association between *Cryptosporidium* infection and animal exposures in HIV-infected individuals. J AIDS Human Retrovirol 17:79–82.

Gookin JL, Riviere JE, Gilger BC, Papich MG. 1999. Acute renal failure in four cats treated with paromomycin. JAVMA 215:1821–1823.

Griffiths JK, Moore R, Dooley S, Keusch GT, Tzipori S. 1994. *Cryptosporidium parvum* infection of Caco-2 cell monolayers induces an apical monolayer defect, selectively increases transmonolayer permeability, and causes epithelial cell death. Infect Immun 62:4506–4514.

Kelly P, Thillainayagam AV, Smithson J, Hunt JB, Forbes A, Gazzard BG, Farthing MJG. 1996. Jejunal water and electrolyte transport in human cryptosporidiosis. Digest Dis Sci 41:2095–2099.

Lappin MR, Dowers K, Taton Allen G, Cheney J. 1997. Crytsoporidiosis and inflammatory bowel disease in a cat. Feline Pract 25:10–13.

Lloyd S, Smith J. 1997. Pattern of *Cryptosporidium parvum* oocyst excretion by experimentally infected dogs. Int J Parasitol 27:799–801.

McReynolds CA, Lappin MR, Ungar B, McReynolds LM, Bruns C, Spilker MM, Thrall MA, Reif JS. 1999. Regional seroprevalence of *Cryptosporidium parvum*-specific IgG of cats in the United States. Vet Parasitol 80:187–195.

Monticello TM, Levy MG, Bunch SE, Fairleyt RA. 1987. Cryptosporidiosis in a feline leukemia virus-positive cat. JAVMA 191:705–706.

Pavlasek I. 1983. Experimental infection of cat and chicken with *Cryptosporidium* sp. oocysts isolated from a calf. Folia Parasitol 30:121–122.

Pieniazek NJ, Bornay-Llinares FJ, Slemenda SB, da Silva AJ, Moura INS, Arrowood MJ, Ditrich O, Addiss DG. 1999. New *Cryptosporidium* genotypes in HIV-infected persons. Emerg Infect Dis 5:444–449.

Tzipori S, Smith M, Halpin C, Angus KW, Sherwood D, Campbell I. 1983. Experimental cryptosporidiosis in calves: clinical manifestations and pathological findings. Vet Rec 112:116–120.

Isospora felis Wenyon, 1923

Etymology

Isospora (*Iso* equal; *spora* spore) and *felis* for cat.

Synonyms

Diplospora bigemina of Wasielewski (1904) in part; *Isospora bigemina* of Swellengrebel (1914); *Isospora rivolta* Dobell and O'Connor, 1921; *Isospora cati* Marotel, 1921; *Lucetina felis* (Wenyon, 1923) Henry and Leblois, 1926; *Isospora felis* var. *servalis* Mackinnon and Dibb, 1938; *Levinea felis* (Wenyon, 19. 1-23) Dubey, 1977; *Cystoisospora felis* (Wenyon, 1923) Frenkel, 1977.

History

The earliest report of coccidia in cats was probably given by Finck in 1854 (Wenyon, 1923; Shah, 1970a), who described stages in the villi of cats as *corpuscles gemines.* Wenyon (1923) indicated that these stages were in the lamina propria and not in the enterocytes as were *Isospora felis* and *Isospora rivolta.* The subepithelial location would indicate that these parasites were a *Sarcocystis* spp. The oocysts of *Isospora felis* (large size) and *Isospora rivolta* (medium size) found in cats closely resemble the oocysts of *Isospora canis* (large size) and *Isospora ohioensis*-like (medium size) organisms observed in the feces of dogs (Lindsay and Blagburn, 1991). During the first half of this century dogs and cats were thought to share the same species of coccidia. Nesmeséri (1960) demonstrated that *Isospora felis* from cats was not transmissible to dogs and named the canine parasite *Isospora canis.* Shah (1970a) later confirmed these findings. Several researchers were unable to produce patent infections in dogs with *Isospora rivolta* oocysts isolated from cats (Pellérdy, 1974; Dubey et al., 1970; Dubey, 1975a) or in cats with *Isospora rivolta* oocysts isolated from dogs (Dubey, 1975a). Based on the results of these studies *Isospora rivolta* was retained for the species in cats, and the species in dogs was named *Isospora ohioensis* (Dubey, 1975a).

In the early 1970s, researchers demonstrated that oocysts of *Isospora felis* and *Isospora rivolta* would excyst in mice and the sporozoites would invade mesenteric lymph nodes and other extraintestinal sites (Frenkel and Dubey, 1972). These encysted stages are infectious when fed to cats and result in oocyst production.

Geographic Distribution

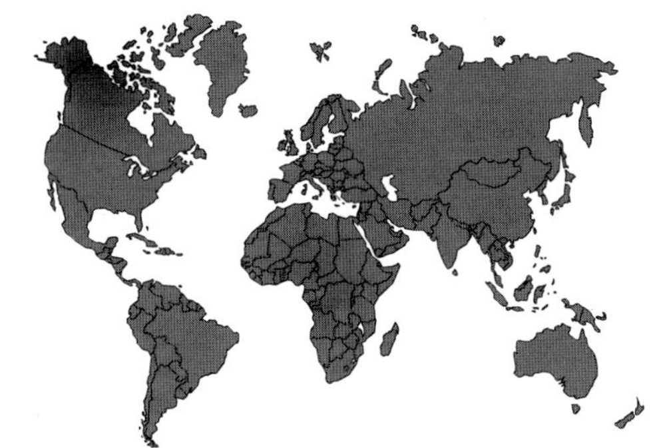

Fig. 1.3.

Isospora felis is found worldwide where cats are present.

Location in Host

Feline Definitive Hosts. Asexual and sexual multiplication occurs in enterocytes primarily in the posterior small intestine. Asexual stages are also observed in extraintestinal tissues.

Paratenic Hosts. In these hosts, sporozoites can persist within various cells in the lymphatic system of the peritoneal cavity.

Parasite Identification

Oocysts measure 38–51 by 27–39 μm (mean: 41.6 by 30.5 μm) (Shah, 1970a) (Fig. 1.4). The length to width ratio is 1.3–1.4 (mean: 1.35). The oocysts of *Isospora felis* are the largest of the coccidial oocysts observed in cats (Table 1.3). No micropyle is present. Inclusions (hazy bodies) may be observed between the sporont and oocyst wall in freshly excreted oocysts. The hazy bodies degenerate as the oocysts sporulate. No oocyst residuum is present in sporulated oocysts. Sporulated oocysts contain two sporocysts (Fig.1.5). Sporocysts measure 20–26 by 17–22 μm (mean, 22.6 by 18.4 μm) and contain a sporocyst residuum and four sporozoites but no Stieda body. The sporocyst residuum is granular and

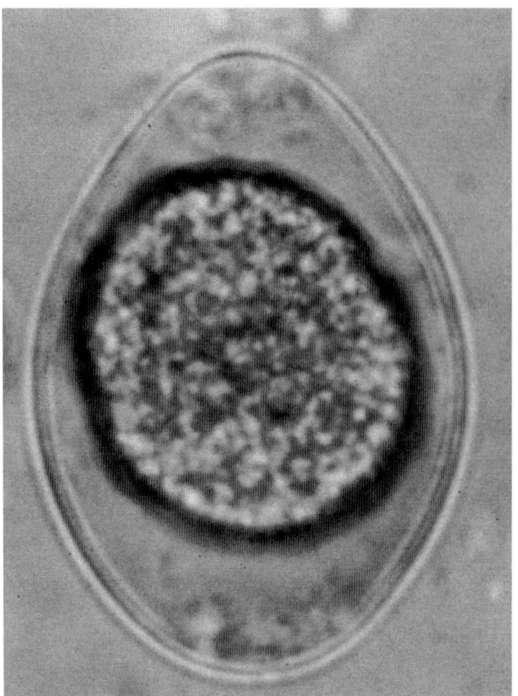

Fig. 1.4. *Isospora felis.* Oocysts passed in the feces of a naturally infected cat.

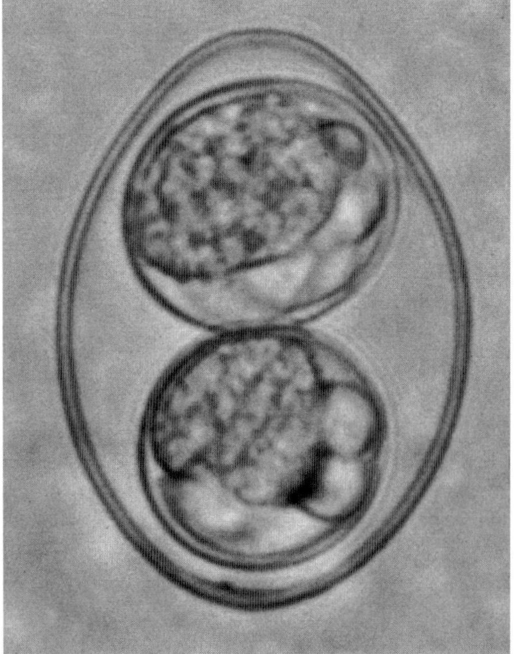

Fig. 1.5. *Isospora felis.* Sporulated oocyst.

TABLE 1.3—Comparison of measurements in micrometers of coccidial oocysts from cats

Species	Length (mean) (μm)	Width (mean) (μm)
Isospora felis	38 to 51	27 to 39
Isospora rivolta	18 to 28	16 to 23
Toxoplasma gondii	11 to 13	11 to 13
Hammondia hammondi	10 to 13	10 to 13
Hammondia pardalis	36 to 46 (40.8)	25 to 35 (28.5)
Besnoitia darlingi	11 to 13	11 to 13
Besnoitia wallacei	16 to 19 (17)	10 to 13 (11)
Cryptosporidium parvum	4 to 5	4 to 5
Sarcocystis spp.	11 to 14	7 to 9

may contain refractile globules. Sporozoites are 10–15 μm long, lie lengthwise in the sporocyst, and contain a single nucleus and a refractile globule. Occasionally a sporulated *Isospora felis* oocyst will be observed that is *Caryospora*-like, having a single sporocyst that contains eight sporozoites (Shah, 1970a).

Life Cycle

Most members of the cat family Felidae are probably suitable definitive hosts. Levine and Ivens (1981) indicated the following were suitable definitive hosts: European wild cat (*Felis silvestris*), ocelot (*Felis pardalis*), serval (*Felis serval*), tiger (*Leo tigris*), lion (*Felis leo*), jaguar (*Leo onca*), and lynx (*Lynx lynx*). Oocysts are excreted unsporulated. Oocyst sporulate in 40 hours at 20°C, 24 hours at 25°C, 12 hours at 30°C, and 8 hours at 38°C (Shah, 1970b). Sporulation does not occur at temperatures above 45°C.

Several authors have described portions of the endogenous life cycle of *Isospora felis* in cats (Wenyon, 1923; Hitchcock, 1955; Shah, 1971; Ferguson et al., 1980a, 1980b; Daly and Markus, 1981). Sporozoites excyst from *Isospora felis* oocysts in the small intestine. Developmental stages are located in enterocytes of the distal portions of the villi in the ileum, and rarely the duodenum and jejunum. The first developmental cycle is probably by endodyogeny, and at least three structural types of meronts are produced (Shah, 1971). Mature first-generation meronts of *Isospora felis* were first observed 4 days

Table 1.4—Treatment of intestinal coccidiosis and cryptosporidiosis in cats

Antiprotozoal agent	Treatment regimen
COCCIDIOSIS	
Sulfadimethoxine (SDM)	50 mg/kg for 10 days or 55 mg/kg for 1 day and 27.5 mg/kg until signs disappear
SDM plus ormetoprim (OM)	55 mg/kg SDM plus 11 mg/kg OM for up to 23 days
Sulfaguanidine	150 to 200 mg/kg for 5 days
Sulfadiazine (SD) and trimethoprim (TRI)	25 to 50 mg/kg SD plus 5 to 10 mg/kg TRI for 6 days for cats over 4 kg
	12.5 to 25 mg/kg SD plus 2.5 to 5 mg/kg TRI for 6 days for cats over 4 kg
Amprolium HCl (AMP)	300 to 400 mg/kg for 5 days
	110 to 220 mg/kg for 7 to 12 days
	20 to 40 mg/kg for 10 days (Blagburn)
AMP plus SDM	150 mg/kg AMP plus 25 mg/kg SDM for 14 days
Quinacrine	10 mg/kg for 5 days
Furazolidone	8 to 20 mg/kg once or twice daily
	Use ½ this dose if combined with sulfonamides
CRYPTOSPORIDIOSIS	
Paromomycin	165 mg/kg every 12 hours for 5 days

postinoculation (PI) and produced 16–17 merozoites. Mature second-generation meronts were first observed 5 days PI and produced about 10 merozoites. Mature third-generation meronts were first observed 6 days PI, were in the same host cell as the second-generation meronts, and produced 36 to 70 merozoites. Sexual stages were first observed 6 days PI. Oocysts were first observed 7 days PI. The prepatent period is 7–11 days, and the patent period is 10–11 days.

Mice (*Mus musculus*), Norway rats (*Rattus norvegicus*), golden hamsters (*Mesocricetus auratus*), cows (*Bos taurus*), and dogs (*Canis familiaris*) can serve as paratenic hosts (Dubey, 1975b; Dubey and Frenkel, 1972; Fayer and Frenkel, 1979; Frenkel and Dubey, 1972; Wolters et al., 1980). The sporozoites present in the tissues of these hosts are infective to cats if they are ingested.

Clinical Presentation and Pathogenesis

Experimental studies indicate that *Isospora felis* is moderately pathogenic for 6-week-old to 13-week-old kittens given 1 to 1.5 × 10^5 oocysts. Soft, mucoid, feces are observed in kittens 8 days after infection, but severe disease does not occur. Microscopic lesions in kittens examined early in infection (about 6 days after being given oocysts) are mild and consist of erosion of the superficial epithelial cells. In kittens examined later in the infection (7 to 9 days after infection) congestion, mild neutrophilic infiltration, and hypersecretion of the mucosa are observed (Shah, 1971). Additionally, epithelial hyperplasia was also noted in some kittens. *Isospora felis* is more pathogenic for younger kittens. Four-week-old kittens may develop severe disease characterized by signs of enteritis, emaciation, and death if given 1 × 10^5 oocysts (Andrews, 1926).

No signs of disease are seen in paratenic hosts.

Treatment

Coccidiosis in cats can be treated with various sulfonamides and quinacrine (Table 1.4).

Epizootiology

Cats are very commonly infected with this parasite. It is unclear whether cats are infected more commonly by oocysts or by the ingestion of paratenic hosts.

Hazards to Other Animals

None known.

Hazards to Humans

It is possible that humans could serve as paratenic hosts. No recorded cases of human infection exist.

REFERENCES

Andrews JM. 1926. Coccidiosis in mammals. Am J Hyg 6:784–798.

Daly TJM, Markus MB. 1981. Enteric multiplication of *Isospora felis* by endodyogeny. Electron Microsc Soc S Afr 11:99–100.

Dubey JP. 1975a. *Isospora ohioensis* sp. n. proposed for *I. rivolta* of the dog. J Parasitol 61:462–465.

Dubey JP. 1975b. Experimental *Isospora canis* and *Isospora felis* infection in mice, cats, and dogs. J Protozool 22:416–417.

Dubey JP, Frenkel JK. 1972. Extra-intestinal stages of *Isospora felis* and *I. rivolta* (Protozoa: Eimeriidae) in cats. J Protozool 19:89–92.

Dubey JP, Streitel RH. 1976. *Isospora felis* and *I. rivolta* infections in cats induced by mouse tissue or oocysts. Br Vet J 132:649–651.

Dubey JP, Miller NL, Frenkel JK. 1970. The *Toxoplasma gondii* oocyst from cat feces. J Exp Med 132:636–662.

Elwasila, M. 1983. A fine-structural comparison of the sporozoites of *Grellia* (*Eucoccidium*) *dinophili* in *Dinophilus gyrociliatus* and *Isospora felis* in the mouse. Z Parasitenkd 69:583–589.

Fayer R, Frenkel JK. 1979. Comparative infectivity for calves of oocysts of feline coccidia: *Besnoitia, Hammondia, Cystoisospora, Sarcocystis,* and *Toxoplasma.* J Parasitol 65:756–762.

Ferguson DJP, Birch-Anderson A, Hutchinson WM, Siim JC. 1980a. Ultrastructural observations showing enteric multiplication of *Cystoisospora* (*Isospora*) *felis* by endodyogeny. Z Parasitenkd 63:289–291.

Ferguson DJP, Birch-Anderson A, Hutchinson WM, Siim JC. 1980b. Ultrastructural observations on microgametogenesis and the structure of the microgamete of *Isospora felis.* Acta Pathol Microbiol Scand B 88:151–159.

Frenkel JK, Dubey JP. 1972. Rodents as vectors for the feline coccidia, *Isospora felis* and *Isospora rivolta.* J Infect Dis 125:69–72.

Hitchcock DJ. 1955. The life cycle of *Isospora felis* in the kitten. J Parasitol 41:383–397.

Levine ND, Ivens V. 1981. The Coccidian Parasites (Protozoa, Apicomplexa) of Carnivores. Illinois Biological Monographs 51, University of Illinois Press, Urbana. 248 pp.

Lindsay, DS, Blagburn BL. 1991. Coccidial parasites of cats and dogs. Comp Contin Educ Pract Vet 13:759–765.

Mehlhorn, H. 1976. Electron microscopy of stages of *Isospora felis* of the cat in the mesenteric lymph node of the mouse. Z Parasitenkd 51:15–24.

Nemeséri L. 1960. Beiträge zur Ätiologie der Coccidiose der Hunde I. *Isospora canis* sp. n. Acta Vet Hung 10:95–99.

Pellérdy L. 1974. Studies on the coccidia of the domestic cat. *Isospora cati* sp. n. Acta Vet Hung 24:127–131.

Shah HL. 1970a. *Isospora* species of the cat and attempted transmission of *I. felis* Wenyon, 1923 from the cat to the dog. J Protozool 17:6003–6009.

Shah HL. 1970b. Sporogony of the oocysts of *Isospora felis* Wenyon, 1923 from the cat. J Protozool 17:609–614.

Shah HL. 1971. The life cycle of *Isospora felis* Wenyon, 1923, a coccidium of the cat. J Protozool 18:3–17.

Wenyon CM. 1923. Coccidiosis of cats and dogs and the status of the *Isospora* of man. Trop Med Parasitol 17:231–288.

Wolters E, Heydorn AO, Laudahn C. 1980. Das Rind als Zwischenwirt von *CystoIsospora felis.* Berl Münch Tierärztl Wschr 93:207–210.

Isospora rivolta (Grassi, 1879) Wenyon, 1923

Etymology

Isospora (*Iso* equal; *spora* spore) and *rivolta* for Dr. Rivolta.

Synonyms

Coccidium rivolta Grassi, 1879; Diplospora bigemina of Wasielewski (1904) in part; *Isospora rivoltae* Dobell, 1919; Lucetina rivolta (Grassi, 1879) Henry and Leblois, 1926; Isospora novocati Pellerdy, 1974; *Levinea rivolta* (Grassi, 1879) Dubey, 1977; *Cystoisospora rivolta* (Grassi, 1879) Frenkel, 1977.

Geographic Distribution

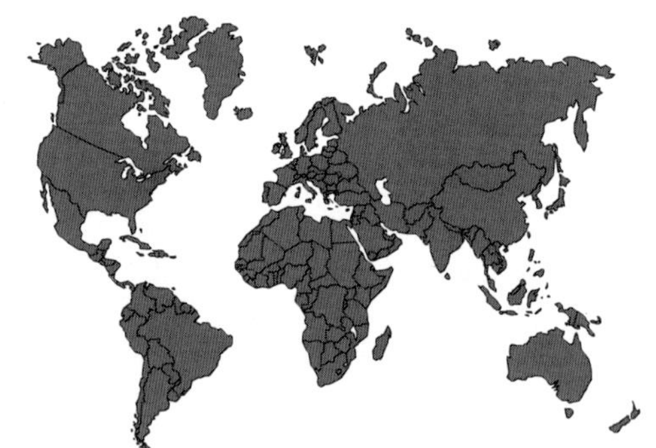

Fig. 1.6.

Isospora rivolta is found worldwide where cats are present.

Location in Host

Feline Definitive Hosts. Asexual and sexual multiplication occurs in enterocytes primarily in the posterior small intestine. Asexual stages are also observed in extraintestinal tissues.

Paratenic Hosts. In paratenic hosts, as with *Isospora felis*, sporozoites will enter and persist in cells within various lymphatic cells within the tissues of these hosts.

Parasite Identification

Sporulated oocysts measure 23–29 by 20–26 mm (mean, 25.4 by 23.4 μm). The length to width ratio is 1.08. The oocysts of *Isospora rivolta* represent the midrange of coccidial oocysts that are passed in the feces of cats (Table 1.3). No micropyle is present. Inclusions (hazy bodies) may be observed between the sporont and oocyst wall in freshly excreted oocysts. The hazy bodies degenerate as the oocysts sporulate. No oocyst residuum is present in sporulated oocysts. Sporulated oocysts contain two sporocysts. Sporocysts measure 13–21 by 10–15 μm (mean, 17.2 by 15.0 μm) and contain a sporocyst residuum and four sporozoites but no Stieda body. The sporocyst residuum is granular and may contain refractile globules. Sporozoites are 10–14 by 2.5–3 μm (mean, 12.4 by 2.8 μm) and contain a single centrally located nucleus and two refractile globules. Occasionally a sporulated *Isospora rivolta* oocyst will be observed that is *Caryospora*-like, having a single sporocyst that contains eight sporozoites.

Life Cycle

Most members of the cat family Felidae are probably suitable definitive hosts. Levine and Ivens (1981) indicated the following were suitable definitive hosts: European wild cat (*Felis silvestris*), jungle cat (*Felis chaus*), tiger (*Leo tigris*), and leopard (*Leo pardus*). Oocysts of *Isospora rivolta* are excreted unsporulated. Sporulation occurs within 24 hours at 24°C, 12 hours at 30°C, and 8 hours at 37°C.

Dubey (1979) described the endogenous development of *Isospora rivolta* in kittens. Three structural types of meronts were observed. Type 1 meronts were first observed 0.5 days PI, were divided by endodyogeny, and produced up to 8 merozoites. Type 2 meronts were first observed 2 days PI, were multinucleated and merozoite shaped, and produced an undetermined number of merozoites. Several divisional cycles probably occurred in the same parasitophorous vacuole. Type 3 meronts were first observed 3 days PI and contained 2 to 30 merozoites. Sexual stages and oocysts were first observed 5 days PI. The prepatent period is 4 to 7 days, and the patent period is greater than 2 weeks.

Mice (*Mus musculus*), Norway rats (*Rattus norvegicus*), golden hamsters (*Mesocricetus auratus*), cows (*Bos taurus*), and opossums (*Didelphis viginiana,* syn. *Didelphis marsupialis*) (Dubey and Frenkel, 1972). Rodents have been found to serve as paratenic hosts in the life cycle of *Isospora rivolta*. The developmental cycle in kittens fed mouse tissues containing *Isospora rivolta* stages was similar to that in cats given oocysts, but the appearance of the different stages was delayed 0.5 to 2 days within the cat host (Dubey and Streitel, 1976).

Clinical Presentation and Pathogenesis

Experimental studies indicate that *Isospora rivolta* is pathogenic for newborn but not weaned kittens (Dubey, 1979). Diarrhea occurs 3 to 4 days after inoculation of 1×10^5 to 1×10^6 oocysts in newborn kittens. Microscopic lesions consisting of congestion, erosion, villous atrophy, and cryptitis were seen in these kittens. No deaths occurred. No clinical signs were observed in 10- to 13-week-old kittens given 1×10^5 oocysts.

Treatment

Coccidiosis in cats can be treated with various sulfonamides and quinacrine (Table 1.4).

Epizootiology

Cats are very commonly infected with this parasite. It is unclear whether cats are infected more commonly by oocysts or by the ingestion of paratenic hosts.

Hazards to Other Animals

None known.

Hazards to Humans

It is possible that humans could serve as paratenic hosts. No recorded cases of human infection exist.

REFERENCES

Dubey JP. 1979. Life cycle of *Isospora rivolta* (Grassi 1879) in cats and mice. J Protozool 26:433–443.

Dubey JP, Frenkel JK. 1972. Extra-intestinal stages of *Isospora felis* and *I. rivolta* (Protozoa: Eimeriidae) in cats. J Protozool 19:89–92.
Dubey JP, Streitel RH. 1976. *Isospora felis* and *I. rivolta* infections in cats induced by mouse tissue or oocysts. Br Vet J 132:649–651.
Frenkel JK, Dubey JP. 1972. Rodents as vectors for the feline coccidia, *Isospora felis* and *Isospora rivolta.* J Infect Dis 125:69–72.
Levine ND, Ivens V. 1981. The Coccidian Parasites (Protozoa, Apicomplexa) of Carnivores. Illinois Biological Monographs 51, University of Illinois Press, Urbana. 248 pp.

Toxoplasma gondii (Nicolle and Manceaux, 1908)

Nicolle and Manceaux, 1909

Etymology

Toxoplasma (*Toxo* = arc shaped; *plasma* = cell) *gondii* for the type intermediate host, *Ctenodactylus gundi.*

Synonyms

Leishmania gondii Nicolle and Manceaux, 1908; several authors have described species of *Toxoplasma* from additional hosts, but they are not valid (Levine, 1977).

Type Intermediate Host

The gondi (*Ctenodactylus gundi*), a North African rodent.

Other Intermediate Hosts

Most mammals and birds are susceptible to *Toxoplasma gondii* infection. Some animal species, such as Australian marsupials, arborial monkeys, and lemurs are highly susceptible to toxoplasmosis.

Type Definitive Host

Domestic cat, *Felis catus.*

Other Definitive Hosts

Mountain lion (*Felis concolor*), ocelot (*Felis pardalis*), margay (*Felis weidii*), jaguarundi (*Felis yagouaroundi*), bobcat (*Felis rufus*), bengal tiger (*Felis bengalensis*), and Iriomote cats (*Felis iriomotensis*).

Geographic Distribution

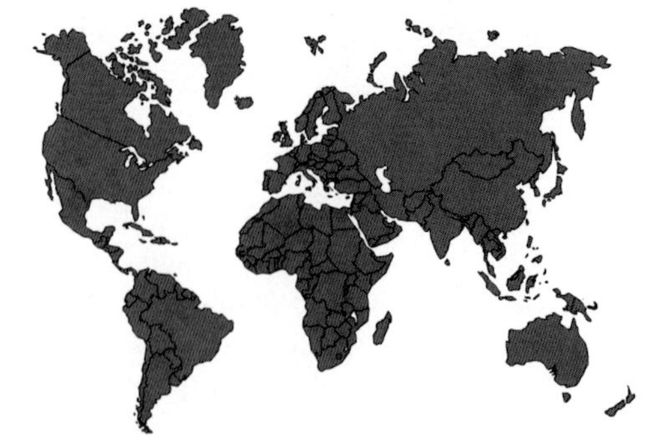

Fig. 1.7.

Distribution is worldwide.

History

The complete life cycle of *Toxoplasma gondii* was not fully described until 1970, about 62 years after its discovery in 1908. The first case of human toxoplasmosis was reported in 1923 in an 11-month-old congenitally infected infant that had hydrocephalus and microphthalmia with coloboma (Remington et al., 1995). In the late 1930s and early 1940s it became well established that toxoplasmosis is an important disease of humans and that infections in infants are acquired prenatally. The rate of congenital toxoplasmosis in humans was too low to explain the high seroprevalence of *Toxoplasma gondii* in the populations examined. Carnivorism was suggested by several researchers and conclusively proven in 1965. Ingestion of infected meat, however, did not explain *Toxoplasma gondii* infection in vegetarians or herbivores, and other modes of transmission had to be present. Hutchison first found resistant *Toxoplasma gondii* in cat feces in 1965 and thought it was enclosed in the eggs of *Toxocara cati* (Dubey and Beattie, 1988). Several studies disproved the association of *Toxoplasma gondii* with *Toxocara cati,* and in 1969–1970 several groups of researchers reported the presence of a coccidial oocyst in cat feces that was *Toxoplasma gondii* (Figs. 1.8 and 1.9). *Toxoplasma gondii* oocyst excretion has been observed in several species of felids in addition to the domestic cat (Miller et al., 1972; Jewell

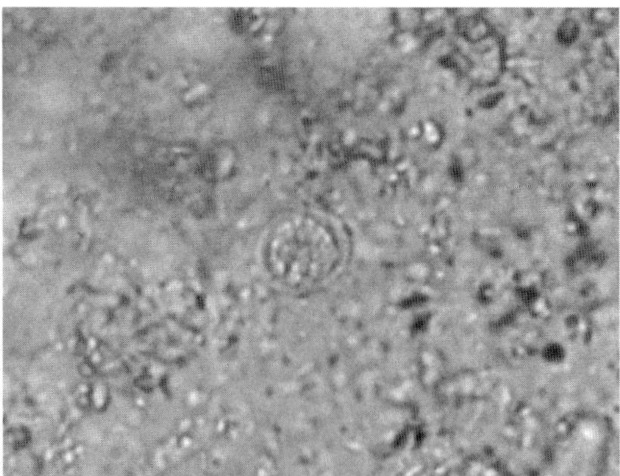

Fig. 1.8. *Toxoplasma gondii.* Oocyst passed in the feces of a cat.

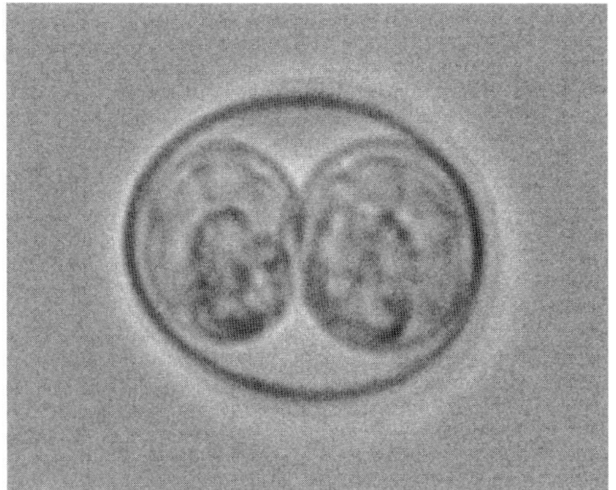

Fig. 1.9. *Toxoplasma gondii.* Sporulated oocyst.

et al., 1972). The first case of fatal toxoplasmosis in a cat was reported in 1942 (Dubey and Beattie, 1988). Fatal toxoplasmosis has been reported in wild felids in zoos and from pelt farms (Dubey et al., 1987).

Life Cycle of *Toxoplasma gondii* in Cats. The life cycle of *Toxoplasma gondii* is complex. Cats serve as both definitive and intermediate hosts for the parasite. There are two distinct types of asexual stages that are present in extraintestinal tissues of cats and other intermediate hosts (Dubey and Frenkel, 1972, 1976) These stages are intracellular except for brief periods of time when they have ruptured host cells and are actively seeking new host cells. Tachyzoites are rapidly dividing stages that cause tissue damage and disseminate the infection in host tissues. After a period of multiplication (about 3 days) some tachyzoites will begin to produce the latent tissue cyst stages that contain bradyzoites. Bradyzoites are slowly dividing stages that are found in tissue cysts. Both tachyzoites and bradyzoites divide into two by endodyogeny. Bradyzoites can transform into tachyzoites (Fig. 1.10). Bradyzoites are the only life cycle stage that can give rise to the enteroepithelial developmental cycle (oocyst-producing cycle) in the cat's intestine. Tissue cysts are present for up to 1.3 years (probably until host death) after inoculation in cats, and most tissue cysts are located in the heart (Dubey, 1977).

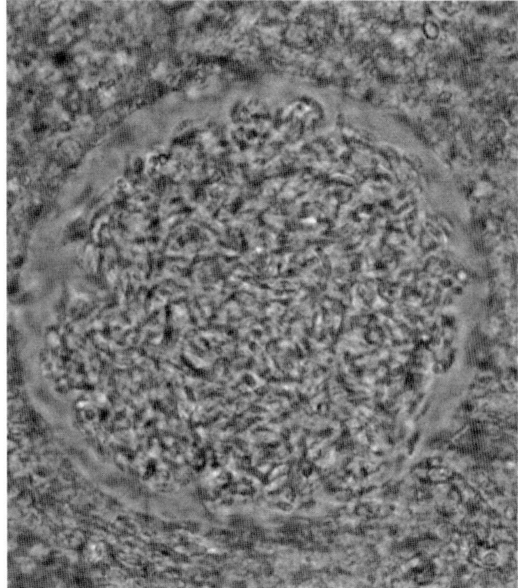

Fig. 1.10. *Toxoplasma gondii.* Cyst of strain T264 in the brain of experimentally infected mouse.

The life cycle of *Toxoplasma gondii* in the cat varies based on the developmental stage that the cat ingests (Dubey and Frenkel, 1972, 1976; Dubey, 1979; Freyre et al., 1989). When cats ingest tissue cysts, the bradyzoites are released after passage through the stomach. Some bradyzoites will penetrate enterocytes and begin the enteroepithelial cycle that will terminate in oocyst production (Dubey, 1979) (Fig. 1.11). However,

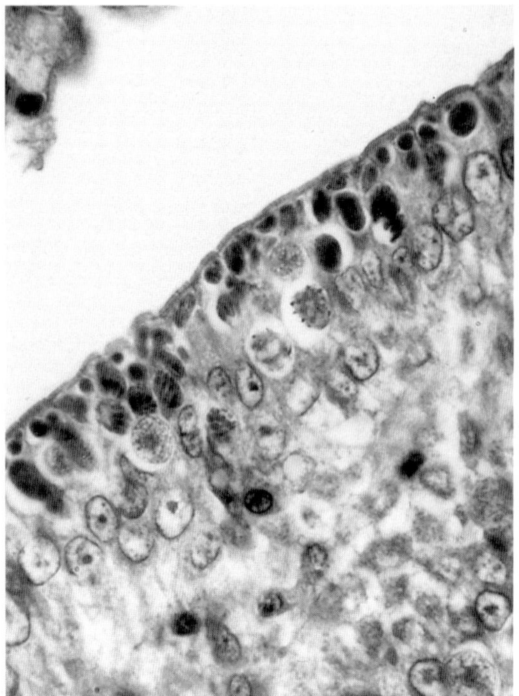

Fig. 1.11. *Toxoplasma gondii.* Gametocytes and schizonts in the epithelial cells of an experimentally infected cat. (Photo courtesy of JP Dubey)

some bradyzoites will penetrate into the intestinal lamina propria and begin development as tachyzoites. Infectious stages of *Toxoplasma gondii* are present in the liver and mesenteric lymph nodes as early as 8 hours after tissue cysts are ingested and chronic infections are produced by these stages. Five structurally distinct types of schizonts are produced in the enterocytes of the small and large intestine prior to the formation of sexual stages at 3–4 days (Dubey and Frenkel, 1972; Dubey, 1979). The prepatent period is 3 to 10 days for tissue cyst–induced infections. Oocysts are excreted in the feces for 7 to >20 days, with most being excreted between days 5 and 8.

Ingestion of sporulated *Toxoplasma gondii* oocysts or tachyzoites results in oocyst-excreting infections in only 16 to 20 percent of cats as compared with 97 percent of cats that are fed tissue cysts (Dubey and Frenkel, 1976; Freyre et al., 1989; Dubey, 1996). The prepatent period is at least 18 days in cats fed oocysts as compared with 3 to 10 days in cats that are fed tissue cysts (Dubey, 1996). The reason for the extended prepatent period is that the sporozoites or tachyzoites must first produce tissue cysts that contain bradyzoites. These bradyzoites will then find their way back to the intestine to produce the enteroepithelial cycle that results in oocyst production.

Oocyst Biology. Unsporulated *Toxoplasma gondii* oocysts are spherical to subspherical, and contain a single mass (sporont) (Fig. 1.8). Sporulation occurs in the environment and is dependent on temperature and moisture (Dubey et al., 1970a). Sporulation is asynchronous, and some oocysts will be sporulated before others. Completely infectious oocysts are present by 24 hours at 25°C (room temperature); by 5 days at 15°C, and by 21 days at 11°C (Dubey et al., 1970b). Unsporulated oocysts do not survive freezing but can remain viable at 4°C for several months and become infectious if placed under the appropriate conditions. Unsporulated oocysts die if kept at 37°C for 24 hours and are killed by 10-minute exposure to 50°C.

A small population of unsporulated oocysts can survive anaerobic conditions for 30 days and remain capable of developing. Oocysts do not sporulate in 0.3 percent formalin, 1 percent ammonium hydroxide solution, or 1 percent iodine in 20 percent ethanol but can sporulate in 5 percent sulfuric acid, 20 percent ethanol, 10 percent ethanol plus 10 percent ether, 1 percent hydrochloric acid, 1 percent phenol, and tap water (Dubey et al., 1970a, 1970b). Drying kills *Toxoplasma gondii* oocysts. Cockroaches, flies, earthworms, and other phoretic hosts can serve to distribute *Toxoplasma gondii* oocysts from the site of defecation in the soil (Dubey and Beattie, 1988).

Sporulated *Toxoplasma gondii* oocysts are subspherical to ellipsoidal, and each contains two ellipsoidal sporocysts, which enclose four sporozoites (Fig. 1.9). Sporulated oocysts are more resistant to environmental and chemical stresses than are unsporulated oocysts. Viable oocysts of *Toxoplasma gondii* have been isolated from soil samples (Ruiz et al., 1973; Coutinho et al., 1982; Frenkel et al., 1995), and experimentally they can survive for over 18 months in the soil (Frenkel et al., 1975). Sporulated oocysts cannot survive freezing or temperatures of 55°C or greater (Ito et al., 1975; Dubey, 1998). Sporulated oocysts survive for several years at 4°C in liquid medium (Dubey, 1998).

***Toxoplasma gondii* Oocyst Excretion.** All ages, sexes, and breeds of domestic cats are susceptible to *Toxoplasma gondii* infection (Dubey et al., 1977). Transplacentally or lactogenically infected kittens will excrete oocysts, but the prepatent period is usually 3 weeks or more because the kittens are infected with tachyzoites (Dubey et al., 1995b). Domestic cats under 1 year of age produce the most numbers of *Toxoplasma gondii* oocysts. Cats that are born and raised outdoors usually become infected with *Toxoplasma gondii* shortly after they are weaned and begin to hunt. *Toxoplasma gondii* naive adult domestic cats will excrete oocysts if fed tissue cysts, but they usually will excrete fewer numbers of oocysts and excrete oocysts for a shorter period of time than recently weaned kittens.

Immunity to Oocyst Excretion. Intestinal immunity to *Toxoplasma gondii* is strong in cats that have excreted oocysts (Frenkel and Smith, 1982a, 1982b, Dubey 1995). Primary *Toxoplasma gondii* infection in cats does not cause immunosuppression (Lappin et al., 1992a; Davis and Dubey, 1995). Serum antibody does not play a significant role in resistance to intestinal infection, and intestinal immunity is most likely cell mediated. Oocysts begin to be excreted in the feces before IgM, IgG, or IgA antibodies are present in the serum (Lappin et al., 1989a; Lin and Bowman, 1991; Burney et al., 1995). Partial development of the enteroepithelial stages occurs in the intestines of immune cats, but oocyst production is prevented (Davis and Dubey, 1995). Most cats that have excreted oocysts once do not re-excrete oocysts if challenged within 6 months to 1 year. Intestinal immunity will last up to 6 years in about 55 percent of cats (Dubey, 1995).

Immunosuppression with high doses of corticosteroid (10 to 80 mg/kg methylprednisolone acetate intramuscularly [IM] weekly or 10 to 80 mg/kg prednisone orally daily) will cause some chronically infected cats to re-excrete *Toxoplasma gondii* oocysts (Dubey and Frenkel, 1974). However, clinically relevant doses of 5 to 20 mg/kg corticosteroid given weekly for 4 weeks do not cause recently or chronically infected cats to re-excrete *Toxoplasma gondii* oocysts (Lappin et al., 1991). Doses of 5 mg/kg cortisone acetate for 7 days will not cause oocyst excretion in chronically infected cats (Hagiwara et al., 1981).

Cats that are chronically infected with *Toxoplasma gondii* and then undergo a primary feline immunodeficiency virus infection demonstrate an increase in *Toxoplasma gondii* antibody titers, suggesting some reactivation of encysted stages. However, experimental studies indicate that there is no reactivation of *Toxoplasma gondii* oocyst excretion or development of clinical toxoplasmosis (Lappin et al., 1992b; 1993; 1996b; Lin and Bowman, 1992; Lin et al., 1992a). Rarely has clinical disease been associated with reactivated toxoplasmosis in feline immunodeficiency virus (FIV) positive cats. Experimental feline leukemia virus infection prior to *Toxoplasma gondii* challenge does not appear to predispose cats to acute toxoplasmosis and has no effect on oocyst excretion (Patton et al., 1991).

There is an interesting relationship that exists between the intestinal coccidium *Isospora felis* and *Toxoplasma gondii* in cats (Chessum, 1972; Dubey, 1976). Cats that have previously recovered from a *Toxoplasma gondii* infection will re-excrete *Toxoplasma gondii* oocysts if they obtain a primary *Isospora felis* infection afterwards. Cats that have a primary *Isospora felis* infection followed by a primary *Toxoplasma gondii* infection develop strong immunity to *Toxoplasma gondii* and will not re-excrete *Toxoplasma gondii* oocysts if challenged with *Isospora felis* (Dubey, 1978a). The mechanism for this unusual relationship is not known.

Toxoplasmosis in Cats

Dubey and Carpenter (1993a) examined 100 cases of histologically confirmed toxoplasmosis in domestic cats and provided the definitive report on clinical toxoplasmosis in cats. Eleven of 100 cats were purebred, cats ranged in age from 2 weeks to 16 years, and 65 were male, 34 were female, and the sex of 1 was not determined. Of the 100 cats 36 had generalized, 26 had pneumonic, 16 had abdominal, 7 had neurologic, 9 had neonatal, 2 had hepatic, 2 had cutaneous, 1 had pancreatic, and 1 had cardiac toxoplasmosis (Figs. 1.12–1.16).

Fever (40 to 41.7°C) is present in many cats with toxoplasmosis. Clinical signs of dyspnea, polypnea, and icterus and signs of abdominal discomfort are frequent findings. Gross and microscopic lesions are found in many organs but are

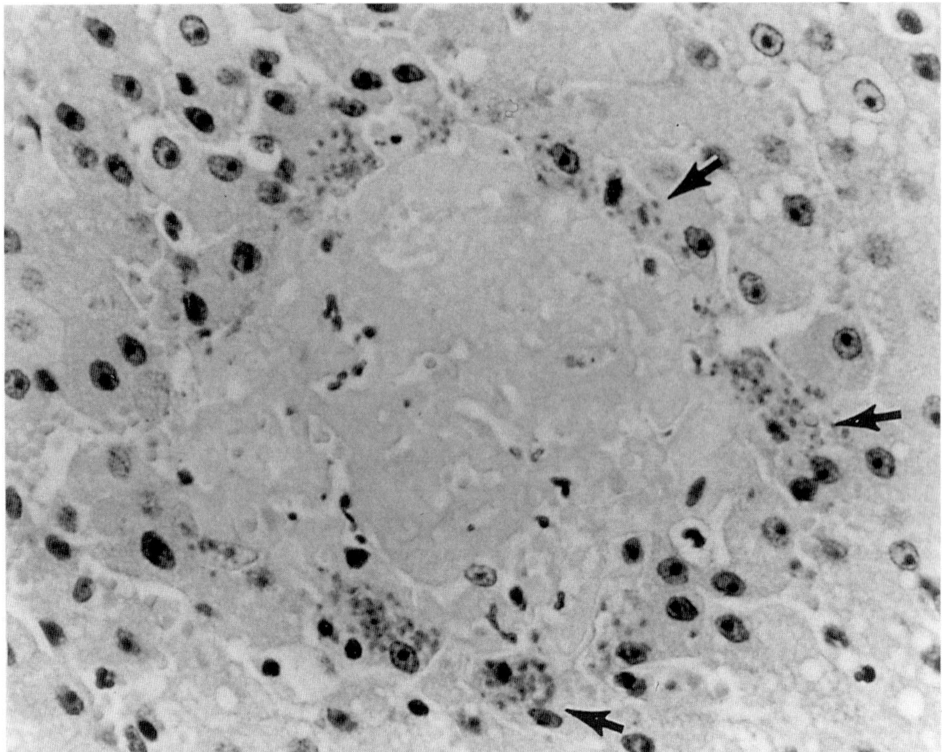

Fig. 1.12. *Toxoplasma gondii.* Focus of necrosis in a cat (H&E-stained histological section, 1000×). Note numerous tachyzoites (*arrows*) at the periphery of the lesion.

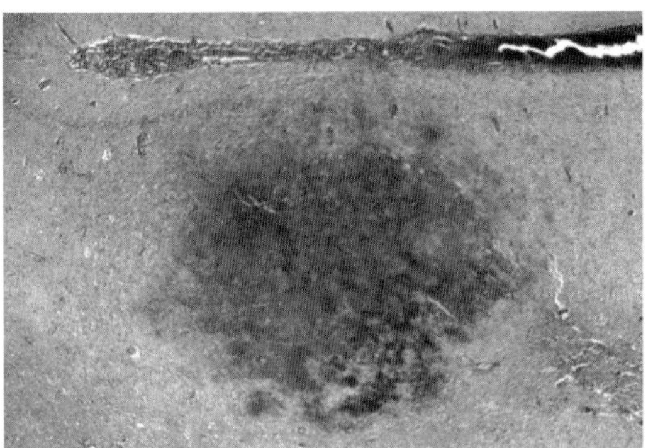

Fig. 1.13. *Toxoplasma gondii.* Necrotizing abscess in the brain of a naturally infected cat that contained numerous dividing tachyzoites.

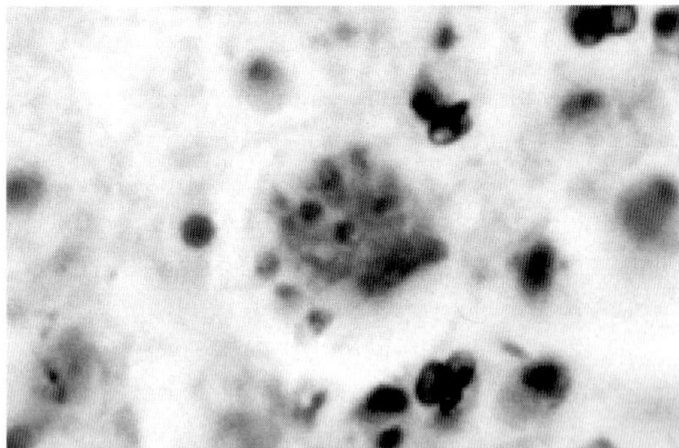

Fig. 1.14. *Toxoplasma gondii.* Higher-power view of abscess in the brain showing the organisms.

most common in the lungs. Gross lesions in the lungs consist of diffuse edema and congestion, failure to collapse, and multifocal areas of firm, white to yellow, discoloration. Pericardial and abdominal effusions may be present. The liver is the most frequently affected abdominal organ, and diffuse necrotizing hepatitis may be visible grossly. Gross lesions associated with necrosis can also be observed in the mesenteric lymph nodes and pancreas.

Ocular lesions are also common in cats, but the actual prevalence is not known. Most lesions are

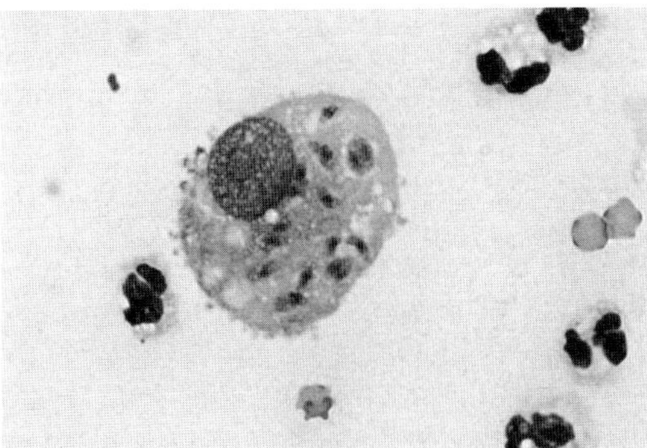

Fig. 1.15. *Toxoplasma gondii.* Macrophage from the abdominal cavity of a naturally infected cat containing numerous tachyzoites.

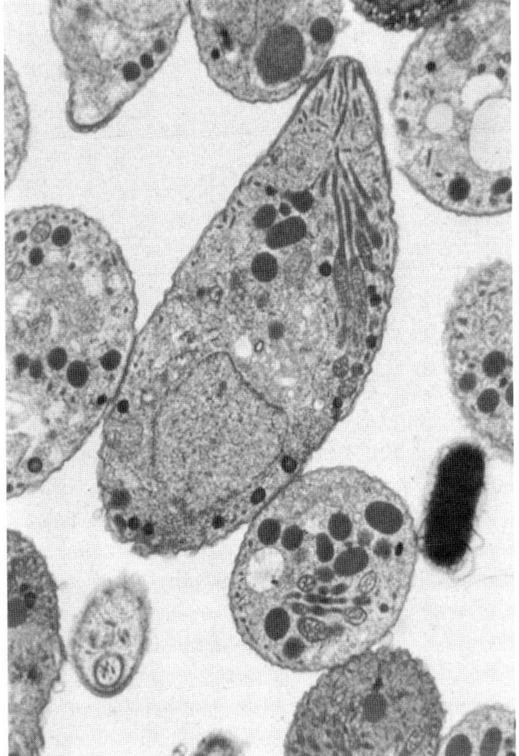

Fig. 1.16. *Toxoplasma gondii.* Electron micrograph of a tachyzoite of the RH strain showing the structures typical of this apicomplexan parasite, e.g., apical complex, rhoptries, and dense granules. (Image kindly supplied by the late Dr. John Cummings.)

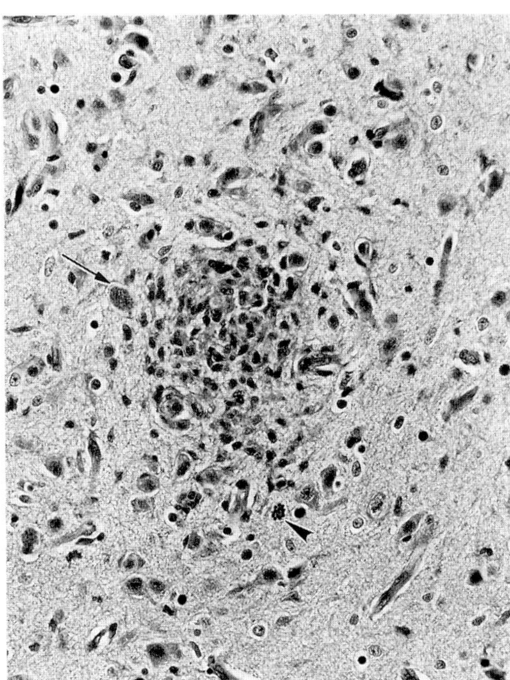

Fig. 1.17. *Toxoplasma gondii.* Glial nodule in the cerebrum of a congenitally infected kitten (H&E-stained histological section). A tissue cyst (*arrow*) and tachyzoites (*arrowhead*) are present at the periphery of the nodule.

in the anterior segment (Lappin et al., 1989c). Cats with ocular lesions have a higher seroprevalence than cats with normal eyes. Ocular findings are varied: They include aqueous flares, hyphema, velvety iris, mydriasis, anisocoria, retinal hemorrhages, retinal atrophy, retinochoriditis, and slow pupillary reflex.

Central nervous system toxoplasmosis is not common in cats. Neurological signs including hypothermia, partial or total blindness, stupor, incoordination, circling, torticollis, anisocoria, head bobbing, ear twitch, atypical crying, and increased affectionate behavior have been reported (Dubey and Carpenter, 1993a).

Congenital toxoplasmosis occurs in cats, but the frequency is not known (Dubey and Carpenter, 1993b) (Figs. 1.17 and 1.18).

Clinical Signs of Feline Toxoplasmosis. The severe central nervous system involvement observed in congenitally infected infants and AIDS patients and the tendency of tissue cysts to

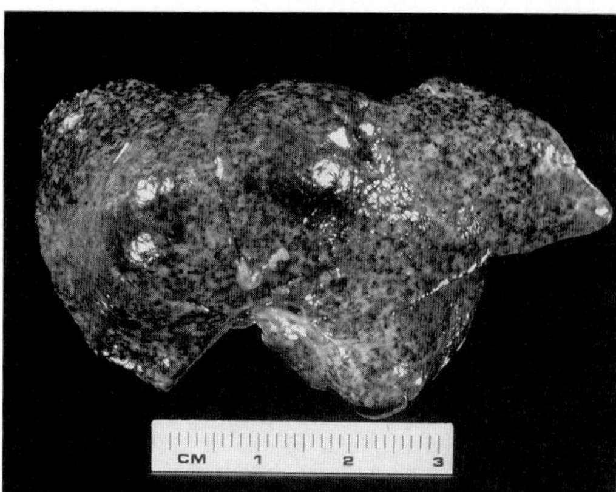

Fig. 1.18. *Toxoplasma gondii.* Liver of a congenitally infected 8-day-old kitten.

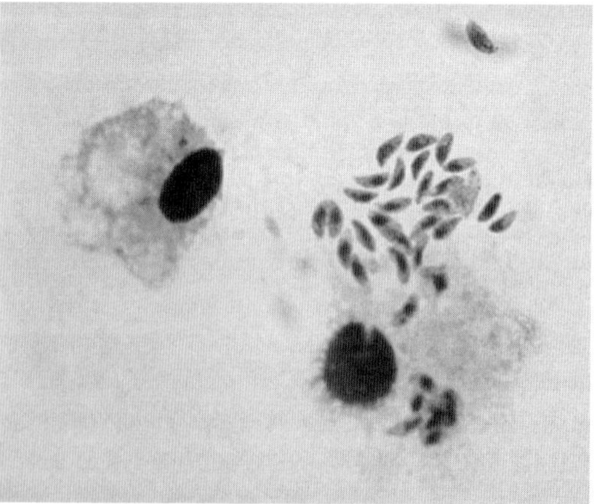

Fig. 1.19. *Toxoplasma gondii.* Alveolar macrophage of a cat with tachyzoites after 40 hours of in-vitro co-culture.

develop in the brains of humans and mice have led to the erroneous assumption by many that toxoplasmosis in all animals is a central nervous system disease. Central nervous system infections do occur in cats but neurologic signs are not the most common clinical sign of infection in cats (Dubey and Carpenter, 1993a).

Fever (40 to 41.7°C) is present in many cats with toxoplasmosis. Clinical signs of dyspnea, polypnea, and icterus and signs of abdominal discomfort were the most frequent findings in 100 cats with histologically confirmed toxoplasmosis (Dubey and Carpenter, 1993a). Uveitis and retinochoroiditis are also common clinical signs in cats with toxoplasmosis. Gross and microscopic lesions are found in many organs but are most common in the lungs. Gross lesions in the lungs consist of edema and congestion, failure to collapse, and multifocal areas of firm, white to yellow, discoloration. Pericardial and abdominal effusions may be present. The liver is the most frequently affected abdominal organ and diffuse necrotizing hepatitis may be visible grossly. Gross lesions associated with necrosis can also be observed in the mesenteric lymph nodes and pancreas.

Ocular lesions of toxoplasmosis are common in cats. The actual prevalence is not known, but antibodies to *Toxoplasma gondii* were observed in the sera of 80 percent of cats with uveitis in one study (Chavkin et al., 1992), indicating a high prevalence in infected cats. Most lesions are in the anterior segment (Lappin et al., 1992c). Ocular findings are varied: they include aqueous flare, hyphema, iritis, mydriasis, anisocoria, retinal hemorrhages, retinal atrophy, retinochoroiditis, and slow pupillary reflex.

Central nervous system toxoplasmosis is not common in cats. In one study, only 7 of 100 cases of histologically confirmed cases of toxoplasmosis had neurological signs (Dubey and Carpenter, 1993a). Neurological signs including hypothermia, partial or total blindness, stupor, incoordination, circling, torticollis, anisocoria, head bobbing, ear twitch, atypical crying, and increased affectionate behavior have been reported.

Congenital toxoplasmosis occurs in cats, but the frequency is not known. Disease in congenitally infected kittens can be severe and fatal (Dubey and Carpenter, 1993b). The most common clinical signs are anorexia, lethargy, hypothermia, and sudden death (Dubey et al., 1995b).

Diagnosis of Feline Toxoplasmosis. The diagnosis of clinical toxoplasmosis requires that three criteria be fulfilled (Lappin, 1990). The cat must have clinical signs consistent with toxoplasmosis and serological evidence of recent or active infection, and the patient must respond to anti-*Toxoplasma gondii* treatment or have *Toxoplasma gondii* demonstrated in its tissues or body fluids.

Toxoplasmosis should be suspected in cats with anterior uveitis, retinochoroiditis, fever, dyspnea, polypnea, abdominal discomfort, icterus, anorexia, seizures, ataxia, and weight loss. Fecal

Table 1.5—Serological tests for the demonstration of *Toxoplasma gondii* antibodies in cats

Test	Antibody first detected	Comments (cutoff titer)
IgG-ELISA	2 weeks	Test detects IgG, 4 fold increase in titer over 2 to 3 weeks indicates active infection (1:64)
IgM-ELISA	1–2 weeks	Test detects IgM, titer of >1:256 indicative of active infection, positive IgM with negative IgG indicates active infection. (1:64)
Modified direct agglutination	—	—
Formalin fixed (FF) antigen	2 weeks	Test detects IgG, 4 fold increase in titer over 2 to 3 weeks indicates active infection, titers remains high. (1:25)
Acetone fixed (AC) antigen	1–2 weeks	Test detects IgG, titers high during acute infection. High AC and low FF titer indicates active infection. (1:100)
Indirect hemagglutination test (IHT), latex agglutination test (LAT), IgG indirect fluorescent antibody (IgG-IFA)	2 weeks	Tests detect IgG, IHT is insensitive, 4 fold increase in titer over 2 to 3 weeks indicates active infection. (1:64)
IgM-IFA	1–2 weeks	Detects IgM, positive IgM with negative or low IgG indicates active infection. (1:64)
Sabin-Feldman dye test	1–2 weeks	Detects IgG and IgM, 4 fold increase in titer over 2 to 3 weeks indicates active infection. (1:16)

Note: Titers on paired serum samples should be examined on the same day to avoid test variability. (Adapted from Lindsay et al., 1997a.)

examination only rarely detects oocysts in cats, and most cats with clinical toxoplasmosis will not be excreting oocysts at the time of presentation. Thoracic radiographs may be helpful. Diffusely disseminated and poorly demarcated foci of increased radiodensity caused by interstitial and alveolar pneumonia are suggestive of but not definitive for *Toxoplasma gondii* in febrile cats.

Serological Tests for Active Toxoplasmosis. Several serological tests are available for the diagnosis of active toxoplasmosis in cats (Table 1.5). Titers obtained in one type of test may not correlate with titers obtained in other tests (Patton et al., 1991; Dubey and Thulliez, 1989; Lappin and Powell, 1991). Most tests rely on the detection of IgG antibodies, which do not develop until about 2 weeks postinfection and may remain at high levels for several years to the life of the cat (Dubey et al., 1995a). Therefore, diagnosis of active toxoplasmosis in cats using an IgG-based test requires that a rising titer be demonstrated (Lindsay et al., 1997a).

Diagnostic tests based on detection of IgM antibodies (Lappin et al., 1989a, 1989c; Lin and Bowman, 1991), circulating parasite antigens (AG) (Lappin et al., 1989b), or acetone-fixed (AF) tachyzoite antigens (Dubey et al., 1995a) can detect early infections at 1 to 2 weeks postexposure. The *Toxoplasma gondii*–specific IgM levels in cats peak at 3 to 6 weeks and drop to negative by 12 weeks postexposure in the IgM-ELISA test. However, some cats will have sporadic low IgM-ELISA levels for up to 1 year postexposure. Peak detection of circulating *Toxoplasma gondii* antigens occurs about 21 days postexposure, but some cats will have circulating *Toxoplasma gondii* antigens for at least 1 year in the AG-ELISA; overall, the test is not very useful in diagnosis (Lappin et al., 1989b). Reactivity to AF tachyzoites in the modified direct agglutination test (MAT, normally formalin-fixed [FF] tachyzoites are used) remains present for up to 70 months (Dubey et al., 1995a). The IgA-ELISA produces variable results in detecting serum antibodies in cats and is not used to detect early infections (Burney et al., 1995). The use of an early detection test coupled with an IgG detection test can provide valuable information on the kinetics of the *Toxoplasma gondii* infection. For example, a high IgM-ELISA titer and a negative or low IgG-ELISA titer would indicate active infection.

The reverse would be true for a chronic infection. Serology can often be difficult to interpret and should never be the sole basis for diagnosis.

Serological Tests for Ocular and CNS Toxoplasmosis. Detection of *Toxoplasma gondii* antibodies in aqueous humor has been used as an aid in the diagnosis of ocular toxoplasmosis in cats (Patton et al., 1991; Lappin et al., 1992c, 1995; Lin et al., 1992b). Calculating the Goldman-Witmer coefficient (C-value) helps correct for antibodies that may have leaked across a damaged vasculature and not been produced directly in the eye (Lappin et al., 1992c). Experimentally infected cats begin to have detectable IgA and IgG levels in aqueous humor at 4 weeks postexposure, while IgM is either not present or at levels too low to detect (Lappin et al., 1995); however, all three antibody isotypes have been found in the aqueous humor of naturally infected cats. Cats with C-values <1 are considered to have antibodies that have leaked across a damaged vasculature, while C-values of 1 to 8 are highly suggestive of clinical ocular toxoplasmosis (Lappin et al., 1992c, 1995). Cats with C-values >8 are considered to have conclusive evidence of ocular antibody production due to *Toxoplasma gondii* infection (Chavkin et al., 1994). Most cats with C-values >1 will respond to specific antitoxoplasmal treatment (Lappin et al., 1992c). Although not conclusive, a trend toward association of *Toxoplasma gondii*–specific IgA in the serum of cats with ocular disease has been reported (Burney et al., 1995).

Using the FF-MAT (Patton et al., 1991), a modified ELISA (Lin et al., 1992b), and IgG-ELISA (Muñana et al., 1995), *Toxoplasma gondii* antibodies have been demonstrated in the cerebrospinal fluid (CSF) of cats with experimental infections but no clinical signs of encephalitis. No IgM was detected in the CSF of experimentally infected cats using the IgM-ELISA. Little else is available on the diagnosis of toxoplasmic encephalitis in cats using CSF. Because *Toxoplasma gondii*–specific IgG has been observed in the CSF of clinically normal cats, it has been suggested that the diagnosis of central nervous system toxoplasmosis in cats not be based solely on detection of intrathecally synthesized *Toxoplasma gondii*–specific IgG (Muñana et al., 1995).

Serological Tests for Neonatal Toxoplasmosis. Neonatal toxoplasmosis is difficult to diagnosis antemortem because the clinical signs are vague and kittens will have nursed prior to examination. Serological indications can be inferred in some cases by comparing titers in queens with their kittens (Dubey et al., 1995b) Transplacental transfer of *Toxoplasma gondii* antibodies does not occur in cats (Dubey et al., 1995b). If the queen is seronegative, then it is unlikely that the kittens have toxoplasmosis because transplacental transmission is unlikely if the queen has acquired the infection with less than 2 weeks left in pregnancy, which is the time it takes for a detectable antibody response. If the queen has a positive IgM titer or the queen and kittens have rising IgG titers, then transplacental or lactogenic transmission is possible. Western blot analysis of serum from the queen and kitten can be helpful in diagnosing neonatal toxoplasmosis in kittens (Cannizzo et al., 1996). Antigen recognition patterns are different for congenitally infected kittens when compared with queens or kittens that have maternally acquired antibody. Serum for congenitally infected kittens will usually recognize an antigen with a molecular mass between 27 and 29 kD (Cannizzo et al., 1996).

Other Methods of Detection of *Toxoplasma gondii* Infections. Direct demonstration of *Toxoplasma gondii* stages can be used to make a method of antemortem diagnosis. Examination of brocheolavage material or material collected by abdominocentesis can be used to detect suspected cases of disseminated toxoplasmosis in cats or neonatal toxoplasmosis in kittens. Examination of CSF may also demonstrate organisms in cases of encephalitis.

The polymerase chain reaction (PCR) has been widely used in human medicine to detect *Toxoplasma gondii* in secretions and fluids, and methods are currently under development for use in cats (Stiles et al., 1996; Lappin et al., 1996b; Burney et al., 1998). The primers have been developed that amplify portions of the parasites B1 gene and used to detect tachyzoites in serum, blood, aqueous humor, and CSF. The PCR test can detect DNA from as few as 10 tachyzoites in serum, CSF, and aqueous humor (Stiles et al.,

Table 1.6—Treatment of feline toxoplasmosis

Product	Treatment regimen
Clindamycin hydrochloride	Oral, 10–2 mg/kg BID for 4 weeks
Clindamycin phosphate	IM, 12.5–25 mg/kg BID for 4 weeks
Pyrimethamine plus sulfonamide	Oral, 0.25–0.5 mg/kg combined with 30 mg/kg sulfonamide BID for 2 to 4 weeks
Trimethoprim + sulfadiazine	Oral 15 mg/kg BID for 4 weeks

1996; Lappin et al., 1996b) and DNA from as few as 100 tachyzoites in blood (Stiles et al., 1996). The use of PCR combined with traditional antibody testing may be useful in the antemortem diagnosis of toxoplasmosis in cats. Results of PCR testing alone should never be used as the sole method of diagnosis of toxoplasmosis.

Postmortem diagnosis can be made by demonstration of the parasite in tissue sections using routine methods or by supplementing histopathologic examinations with immunohistochemical staining for specific *Toxoplasma gondii*. Other methods, such as bioassays in cats or mice, can be used but are not practical.

Vaccination against Oocyst Excretion. A vaccine that prevents oocyst excretion in cats would be beneficial for both veterinary and public health reasons (Fishback and Frenkel, 1990; Frenkel et al., 1991; Freyre et al., 1993). Vaccination of cats would decrease environmental contamination with oocysts. This would aid in preventing exposure of animals and humans to oocysts and lead to a decreased prevalence of the encysted parasite in food animals.

Killed or recombinant tachyzoite–based vaccines do not stimulate intestinal immunity and are of no value in preventing oocyst excretion. Technically it is not presently possible to produce sufficient numbers of bradyzoites or enteroepithelial stages to develop killed or recombinant vaccines based on these stages.

Intestinal immunity can be induced by infecting cats with an oocyst-producing strain of *Toxoplasma gondii* and by prophylactically treating the cats for 8 to 19 days with anti–*Toxoplasma gondii* chemotherapy (Frenkel and Smith, 1982a, 1982b). Oocyst excretion can be prevented during the immunizing phase, and 80 to 85 percent of the cats become immune. Although effective, this method of vaccination is impractical for many technical and safety reasons.

The life cycle of *Toxoplasma gondii* can be manipulated by extensive passage of the parasite in mice (Frenkel et al., 1976) or in cell cultures (Lindsay et al., 1991) so that the bradyzoites lose the ability to produce oocyst excretion in cats. Unfortunately, none of these oocyst-less strains of *Toxoplasma gondii* stimulate sufficient intestinal immunity, and the cats will excrete oocysts when challenged with an oocyst-producing strain.

Vaccination of cats against intestinal *Toxoplasma gondii* infection has been successfully achieved using a chemically induced mutant strain (T-263) of the parasite (Frenkel et al., 1991; Freyre et al., 1993). Oral administration of strain T-263 bradyzoites results in intestinal infection but does not result in oocyst production in cats. These vaccinated cats do not excrete oocysts when challenged with oocyst-producing strains of *Toxoplasma gondii*. The T-263 strain is safe to use in healthy cats. It would not be recommended for use in pregnant cats or feline leukemia virus (FeLV) positive cats or immunocompromised cats (Choromanski et al., 1994, 1995). It has only limited ability to persist in the tissues of cats and cannot survive more than three back-passages in cats. No reversion to oocyst excretion or increase in virulence has been observed in over 200 inoculated cats. The T-263 strain is rapidly cleared from the mouth of inoculated cats.

Treatment of Feline Toxoplasmosis. No chemotherapeutic agents are approved for the treatment of toxoplasmosis in cats. Table 1.6 lists agents that are used to treat toxoplasmosis in cats.

Clindamycin is the drug of choice for the treatment of disseminated toxoplasmosis in cats (Lappin et al., 1989c). Clinically, the drug has been widely used with good response.

Table 1.7—Prevention of *Toxoplasma gondii* infection in cats and humans

Recommendation/Reason
Cats
1. Do not feed raw or rare meat to cats/*Prevent exposure to tissue cysts.*
2. Keep cats indoors and do not allow cats to hunt/*Prevent exposure to tissue cysts in prey animals.*
3. Vaccination (if it becomes available)/*Prevent oocyst excretion.*
Humans
1. Do not eat raw or rare meat/*Prevent ingestion of viable tissue cysts.*
2. Wash hands and food preparation surfaces with warm soapy water after handling and preparing raw meat/*Inactivate tissue cysts.*
3. Wear gloves while gardening or wash hands after gardening/*Prevent exposure to oocysts in the soil.*
4. Wash all fruits and vegetables before eating/*Remove any oocysts that may be present.*
5. Change litter box daily. Pregnant women and immunosuppressed individuals should not change litter box/*Remove oocysts before they become infective and prevent exposure of high risk individuals.*

Cats can also be treated with pyrimethamine or trimethoprim combined with a sulfonamide. Pyrimethamine is active at lower concentrations than is trimethoprim. Sulfadiazine and sulfamethoxazole are the sulfonomides most often used. Bone marrow suppression can occur with the use of pyrimethamine- or trimethoprim-sulfonamide combinations and can be corrected with the addition of folinic acid (5 mg per day) or the addition of yeast (100 mg/kg) to the cat's diet.

Prevention of *Toxoplasma gondii* Infection in Cats and Humans. Measures can be taken to prevent or lower the risk of exposure of cats and humans to *Toxoplasma gondii.* They are based on a detailed knowledge of the parasite's life cycle and are presented in Table 1.7. They are based on preventing exposure to sporulated oocysts or tissue cysts.

Pork is the most likely source of tissue cysts for people in the United States. This is because cattle are naturally resistant, and other *Toxoplasma gondii*–infected meats such as sheep and goat are not consumed in significant amounts (Dubey, 1994). Chickens are susceptible to *Toxoplasma gondii* infection, but because chicken is often frozen and seldom eaten rare, it is not considered a primary source of infection. Tissue cysts in meat are killed by cooking to temperatures of 58°C for 10 minutes or 61°C for 4 minutes (Dubey et al., 1990). Tissue cysts are believed to be killed instantaneously by exposure to –13°C; however, they will survive for up to 3 weeks at –3°C and 11 days at –6°C (Kotula et al., 1991). Gamma irradiation at an absorbed dose of 0.4 kGy is lethal for tissue cysts in meat (Dubey and Thayer, 1994).

Cutting boards, knives, and other surfaces that raw meat has contacted should be washed in warm soapy water to kill the tissue cysts and any bradyzoites that may have been liberated during handling. Hands should also be washed in warm soapy water after contact with raw meat.

Cat Ownership and the Risk of Toxoplasmosis. It is logical to assume that veterinarians, who have more exposure to cats (both sick and healthy) than the general public, would be at a greater risk for developing toxoplasmosis. However, serological studies do not confirm this assumption (Behymer et al., 1973; Sengbusch and Sengbusch, 1976; DiGiacomo et al., 1990). In one study of AIDS patients it was conclusively shown that owning cats did not increase the risk of developing toxoplasmosis (Wallace et al., 1993). However, the role of cat ownership and exposure to *Toxoplasma gondii* is not completely clear at present. Many studies have been conducted to determine the association between cat ownership or cat exposure and the prevalence of *Toxoplasma gondii* infection in humans. Many studies do not find a positive relationship (Partono and Cross, 1975; Ulmanen and Leinikki, 1975; Durfee et al., 1976; Zigas, 1976; Tizard et al., 1977; Gandahusada, 1978; Sedaghat et al., 1978; Ganley and Comstock, 1980; Stray-Pedersen and Lorentzen-Styr, 1980; Konishi and Takahashi, 1987; Arias et al., 1996; Bobic et al., 1998; Flegr et al., 1998), while many find a positive relationship (Clarke et al., 1975; Frenkel and Ruiz, 1980, 1981; Barbier et al., 1983; Martinez Sanchez et al., 1991; Ahmed, 1992; MacKnight and Robinson, 1992; Etheredge and Frenkel,

1995; del Castillo and Herruzo, 1998; Rey and Ramalho, 1999). It must be remembered that preventing exposure to cats is not the same as preventing exposure to *Toxoplasma gondii* oocysts. One study indicated that exposure to dogs was more of a risk factor than exposure to cats (Frenkel et al., 1995). If dogs are fed sporulated *Toxoplasma gondii* oocysts, many will pass out in the dogs feces and remain infectious (Lindsay et al., 1997b), and it has been suggested that dogs consume cat feces or roll in cat feces and thereby increase human contact with *Toxoplasma gondii* oocysts when they return home (Frenkel and Parker, 1996). Pregnant women or immunocompromised individuals should not change the cat's litter box. If feces are removed daily this will also help prevent exposure by removing oocysts before they can sporulate. Oocysts can survive in the soil for years and can be disseminated from the original site of deposition by erosion, other mechanical means, and phoretic vectors. Inhalation of oocysts stirred up in the dust by horses has been associated with an outbreak of human toxoplasmosis at a riding stable (Teutsch et al., 1979). Oocysts are not likely to remain in the air for extended periods of time. Washing fruits and vegetables and wearing gloves while gardening are means of preventing exposure to oocysts. Oocysts are killed by exposure to 0.25 kGy gamma irradiation, and this is a potential means of killing oocysts on contaminated fruit and vegetables (Dubey et al., 1996).

Toxoplasma gondii oocysts were not isolated from the fur of oocyst-excreting cats (Dubey, 1995). Therefore, it is unlikely that infection can be obtained by petting a cat. Tachyzoites are not likely to be present in the oral cavity of cats with active *Toxoplasma gondii* infection, and none would be in a chronic infection; therefore, it is unlikely that a cat bite would transmit *Toxoplasma gondii* infection. Cat scratches are also unlikely to transmit *Toxoplasma gondii* infection.

Important Aspects of Human Maternal Toxoplasmosis. Pregnant women and immunocompromised patients should follow the prevention guidelines in Table 1.7. Immunocompetent women with *Toxoplasma gondii* antibody titers prior to becoming pregnant are considered immune and will not transmit the parasite to the fetus if exposed during pregnancy. It is important for a pregnant woman to know her titer because it can serve as a baseline if exposure is suspected during pregnancy. About 60 percent of women infected with *Toxoplasma gondii* during pregnancy will transmit the infection to the fetus. The age at which the fetus becomes infected determines the severity of subsequent disease. Few cases of fetal infection occur when the mother is infected during weeks 1 to 10; however, severe disease occurs in the infants that do become infected (Remington et al., 1995). Pregnant women are at greatest risk of delivering a severely infected infant if infected during weeks 10 to 24 of gestation (Remington et al., 1995). If *Toxoplasma gondii* infection of the mother occurs at weeks 26 to 40, there is a low risk of delivery of a severely infected infant, but most infants will be infected and have mild symptoms (Remington et al., 1995).

REFERENCES

Ahmed MM. 1992. Seroepidemiology of *Toxoplasma* infection in Riyadh, Saudi Arabia. J Egypt Soc Parasitol 22:407–413.

Arias ML, Chinchilla M, Reyes L, Linder E. 1996. Seroepidemiology of toxoplasmosis in humans: possible transmission routes in Costa Rica. Rev Biol Trop 44:377–381.

Barbier D, Ancelle T, Martin-Bouyer G. 1983. Seroepidemiological survey of toxoplasmosis in La Guadeloupe, French West Indies. Am J Trop Med Hyg 32:935–942.

Behymer RD, Harlow DR, Behymer DE, Franti CE. 1973. Serologic diagnosis of toxoplasmosis and prevalence of *Toxoplasma gondii* antibodies in selected feline, canine, and human populations. J. Am Vet Med Assoc 162:959–963.

Bobic B, Jevremovic I, Marinkovic J, Sibalic D, Djurkovic-Djakovic O. 1998. Risk factors for *Toxoplasma* infection in a reproductive age female population in the area of Belgrade, Yugoslavia. Eur J Epidemiol 14:605–610.

Burney DP, Lappin MR, Cooper C, Spilker MM. 1995. Detection of *Toxoplasma gondii*-specific IgA in the serum of cats. Am J Vet Res 56:769–773.

Burney DP, Chavkin MJ, Dow SW, Potter TA, Lappin MR. 1998. Polymerase chain reaction for the detection of *Toxoplasma gondii* within aqueous humor of experimentally-inoculated cats. Vet Parasitol 79:181–186.

Cannizzo KL, Lappin MR, Cooper CM, Dubey JP. 1996. *Toxoplasma gondii* antigen recognition by serum immunoglobulins M, G, and A of queens and their neonatally infected kittens. Am J Vet Res 57:1327–1330.

Chavkin MJ, Lappin MR, Powell CC, et al. 1992. Seroepidemiology and clinical observations of 93 cases of uveitis in cats. Prog Vet Comp Ophthalmol 2:29–36.

Chavkin MJ, Lappin MR, Powell CC, Cooper CM, Muñana KR, Howard LH. 1994. *Toxoplasma gondii*-specific antibodies in the aqueous humor of cats with toxoplasmosis. Am J Vet Res 55:1244–1249.

Chessum BS. 1972. Reactivation of *Toxoplasma* oocyst production in the cat by infection with *Isospora felis*. Br Vet J 128:33–36.

Choromanski L, Freyre A, Brown K, Popiel I, Shibley G. 1994. Safety aspects of a vaccine for cats containing a *Toxoplasma gondii* mutant strain. J Eukaryot Microbiol 41:8S.

Choromanski L, Freyre A, Popiel R, Brown K, Grieve R, Shibley G. 1995. Safety and efficacy of modified live feline *Toxoplasma gondii* vaccine. Dev Biol Stand 84:269–281.

Clarke MD, Cross JH, Carney WP, Hadidjaja P, Joesoef A, Putrali J, Sri Oemijati. 1975. Serological study of amebiasis and toxoplasmosis in the Lindu Valley, Central Sulawesi, Indonesia. Trop Geogr Med 27:274–278.

Coutinho SG, Lobo R, Dutra G. 1982. Isolation of *Toxoplasma* from the soil during an outbreak of toxoplasmosis in a rural area in Brazil. J Parasitol 68:866–868.

Davis SW, Dubey JP. 1995. Mediation of immunity to *Toxoplasma gondii* oocyst shedding in cats. J Parasitol 81:882–886.

del Castillo F, Herruzo R. 1998. Risk factors for toxoplasmosis in children. Enferm Infecc Microbiol Clin 16:224–229.

DiGiacomo RF, Harris NV, Huber NL, Cooney MK. 1990. Animal exposures and antibodies to *Toxoplasma gondii* in a university population. Am J Epidemiol 131:729–733.

Dubey JP. 1976. Reshedding of *Toxoplasma* oocysts by chronically infected cats. Nature 262:213–214.

Dubey JP. 1977. Persistence of *Toxoplasma gondii* in the tissues of chronically infected cats. J Parasitol 63:156–157.

Dubey JP. 1978a. Effect of immunization of cats with *Isospora felis* and BCG on immunity to reexcretion of *Toxoplasma gondii* oocysts. J Protozool 25:380–382.

Dubey JP. 1978b. A comparison of cross protection between BCG, *Hammondia hammondi, Besnoitia jellisoni* and *Toxoplasma gondii* in hamsters. J Protozool 25:382–384.

Dubey JP. 1979. Direct development of enteroepithelial stages of *Toxoplasma* in the intestines of cats fed cysts. Am J Vet Res 40:1634–1637.

Dubey JP. 1994. Toxoplasmosis. JAVMA 205: 1593–1598.

Dubey JP. 1995. Duration of immunity to shedding of *Toxoplasma gondii* oocysts by cats. J Parasitol 81:410–415.

Dubey JP. 1996. Infectivity and pathogenicity of *Toxoplasma gondii* oocysts for cats. J Parasitol 82:957–961.

Dubey JP. 1998. *Toxoplasma gondii* oocyst survival under defined temperatures. J Parasitol 84: 862–865.

Dubey JP, Beattie CP. 1988. Toxoplasmosis of Animals and Man. Boca Raton, Fla: CRC Press, pp 1–40.

Dubey JP, Carpenter JL. 1993a. Neonatal toxoplasmosis in littermate cats. J Am Vet Med Assoc 203:1546–1549.

Dubey JP, Carpenter JL. 1993b. Histologically confirmed clinical toxoplasmosis in cats: 100 cases (1952–1990). J Am Vet Med Assoc 203:1556–1566.

Dubey JP, Frenkel JK. 1972. Cyst-induced toxoplasmosis in cats. J Protozool 19:155–177.

Dubey JP, Frenkel JK. 1974. Immunity to feline toxoplasmosis: modification by administration of corticosteroids. Vet Pathol 11:350–379.

Dubey JP, Frenkel JK. 1976. Feline toxoplasmosis from acutely infected mice and the development of *Toxoplasma* cysts. J Protozool 23:537–546.

Dubey JP, Thayer DW. 1994. Killing of different strains of *Toxoplasma gondii* tissue cysts by irradiation under defined conditions. J Parasitol 80:764–767.

Dubey JP, Thulliez P. 1989. Serologic diagnosis of toxoplasmosis in cats fed *Toxoplasma gondii* tissue cysts. JAVMA 194:1297–1299.

Dubey JP, Miller NL, Frenkel JK. 1970a. Characterization of the new fecal form of *Toxoplasma gondii*. J Parasitol 56:447–456.

Dubey JP, Miller NL, Frenkel JK. 1970b. The *Toxoplasma gondii* oocyst from cat feces. J Exp Med 132:636–662.

Dubey JP, Hoover EA, Walls KW. 1977. Effect of age and sex on the acquisition of immunity to toxoplasmosis in cats. J Protozool 24:184–186.

Dubey JP, Quinn WJ, Weinandy D. 1987. Fatal neonatal toxoplasmosis in a bobcat (*Lynx rufus*). J Wildl Dis 23:324–327.

Dubey JP, Kotula AW, Sharar AK, Sharar A, Andrews CD, Lindsay DS. 1990. Effect of high temperature on infectivity of *Toxoplasma gondii* tissue cysts in pork. J Parasitol 76:201–204.

Dubey JP, Lappin MR, Thulliez P. 1995a. Long-term antibody responses of cats fed *Toxoplasma gondii* tissue cysts. J Parasitol 81:887–893.

Dubey JP, Lappin MR, Thulliez P. 1995b. Diagnosis of induced toxoplasmosis in neonatal cats. JAVMA 207:179–185.

Dubey JP, Jenkins MC, Thayer DW, Kwok OC, Shen SK. 1996. Killing of *Toxoplasma gondii* oocysts by irradiation and protective immunity induced by vaccination with irradiated oocysts. J Parasitol 82:724–727.

Durfee PT, Cross JH, Rustam-Susanto. 1976. Toxoplasmosis in man and animals in South Kalimantan (Borneo), Indonesia. Am J Trop Med Hyg 25:42–47.

Etheredge GD, Frenkel JK. 1995. Human *Toxoplasma* infection in Kuna and Embera children in the Bayano and San Blas, eastern Panama. Am J Trop Med Hyg 53:448–457.

Fishback JL, Frenkel JK. 1990. Prospective vaccines to prevent feline shedding of *Toxoplasma* oocysts. Comp Cont Educ Pract Vet 12:643–651.

Flegr J, Hrda S, Tachezy J. 1998. The role of psychological factors in questionnaire-based studies on routes of human toxoplasmosis transmission. Cent Eur J Public Health 6:45–50.

Frenkel JK, Parker BB. 1996. An apparent role for dogs in the transmission of *Toxoplasma gondii:* the probable role of xenosmophilia. Ann NY Acad Sci 791:402–407.

Frenkel JK, Ruiz A. 1980. Human toxoplasmosis and cat contact in Costa Rica. Am J Trop Med Hyg 29:1167–1180.

Frenkel JK, Ruiz A. 1981. Endemicity of toxoplasmosis in Costa Rica. Am J Epidemiol 113:254–269.

Frenkel JK, Smith DD. 1982a. Immunization of cats against shedding of *Toxoplasma* oocysts. J Parasitol 68:744–748.

Frenkel JK, Smith DD. 1982b. Inhibitory effects of monensin on shedding of *Toxoplasma* oocysts by cats. J Parasitol 68:851–855.

Frenkel JK, Dubey JP, Miller NL. 1970. *Toxoplasma gondii* in cats: fecal stages identified as coccidian oocysts. Science 167:893–896.

Frenkel JK, Ruiz A, Chinchilla M. 1975. Soil survival of *Toxoplasma* oocysts in Kansas and Costa Rica. Am J Trop Med Hyg 24:439–443.

Frenkel JK, Dubey JP, Hoff RL. 1976. Loss of stages after continuous passage of *Toxoplasma gondii* and *Besnoitia jellisoni.* J Protozool 23:421–424.

Frenkel JK, Pfefferkorn ER, Smith DD, Fishback JL. 1991. Prospective vaccine prepared from a new mutant of *Toxoplasma gondii* for use in cats. Am J Vet Res 52:759–763.

Frenkel JK, Hassanein KM, Hassanein RS, Brown E, Thulliez P, Quintero-Nunez R. 1995. Transmission of *Toxoplasma gondii* in Panama City, Panama: a five-year prospective cohort study of children, cats, rodents, birds, and soil. Am J Trop Med Hyg 53:458–468.

Freyre A, Dubey JP, Smith DD, Frenkel JK. 1989. Oocyst-induced *Toxoplasma gondii* infections in cats. J Parasitol 75:750–755.

Freyre A, Choromanski L, Fishback JL, Popiel I. 1993. Immunization of cats with tissue cysts, bradyzoites, and tachyzoites of the T-263 strain of *Toxoplasma gondii.* J Parasitol 79:716–719.

Gandahusada S. 1978. Serological study for antibodies to *Toxoplasma gondii* in Jakarta, Indonesia. Southeast Asian J Trop Med Public Health 9:308–311.

Ganley JP, Comstock GW. 1980. Association of cats and toxoplasmosis. Am J Epidemiol 111:238–246.

Hagiwara T, Katsube Y, Muto T, Imaizumi K. 1981. Experimental feline toxoplasmosis. Jap J Vet Sci 43:329–336.

Ito S, Tsunoda K, Taki T, Nishikawa H, Matsui T. 1975. Destructive effect of heating against *Toxoplasma* oocysts. Natl Inst Anim Health Q (Tokyo) 15:128–310.

Jewell ML, Frenkel JK, Johnson KM, Reed V, Ruiz A. 1972. Development of *Toxoplasma* oocysts in neotropical felidae. Am J Trop Med Hyg 21:512–517.

Konishi E, Takahashi J. 1987. Some epidemiological aspects of *Toxoplasma* infections in a population of farmers in Japan. Int J Epidemiol 16:277–281.

Kotula AW, Dubey JP, Sharar AK, Andrews CD, Shen SK, Lindsay DS. 1991. Effect of freezing on infectivity of *Toxoplasma gondii* tissue cysts in pork. J Food Prot 54:687–690.

Lappin MR. 1990. Challenging cases in internal medicine: what's your diagnosis? Vet Med 84:448–455.

Lappin MR, Powell CC. 1991. Comparison of latex agglutination, indirect hemagglutination, and ELISA techniques for the detection of *Toxoplasma gondii*-specific antibodies in the serum of cats. J Vet Intern Med 5:299–301.

Lappin MR, Greene CE, Prestwood AK, Dawe DL, Tarleton RL. 1989a. Diagnosis of recent *Toxoplasma gondii* infection in cats by use of an enzyme-linked immunosorbent assay for immunoglobulin M. Am J Vet Res 50:1580–1585.

Lappin MR, Greene CE, Prestwood AK, Dawe DL, Tarleton RL. 1989b. Enzyme-linked immunosorbent assay for the detection of circulating antigens of *Toxoplasma gondii* in the serum of cats. Am J Vet Res 50:1586–1590.

Lappin MR, Greene CE, Winston S, Toll SL, Epstein ME. 1989c. Clinical feline toxoplasmosis: serological diagnosis and therapeutic management of 15 cases. J Vet Int Med 3:139–143.

Lappin MR, Dawe DL, Lindl PA, Greene CE, Prestwood AK. 1991. The effect of glucocorticoid administration on oocyst shedding, serology, and cell-mediated immune responses of cats with recent or chronic toxoplasmosis. J Am Anim Hosp Assoc 27:625–632.

Lappin MR, Dawe DL, Lindl P, Greene CE, Prestwood AK. 1992a. Mitogen and antigen-specific induction of lymphoblast transformation in cats with subclinical toxoplasmosis. Vet Immunol Immunopathol 30:207–220.

Lappin MR, Gasper PW, Rose BJ, Powell CC. 1992b. Effect of primary phase feline immunodeficiency virus infection on cats with chronic toxoplasmosis. Vet Immunol Immunopathol 35:121–131.

Lappin MR, Roberts SM, Davidson MG, Powell CC, Reif JS. 1992c. Enzyme-linked immunosorbent assays for the detection of *Toxoplasma gondii*-specific antibodies and antigens in the aqueous humor of cats. JAVMA 201:1010–1016.

Lappin MR, Marks A, Greene CE, Rose BJ, Gasper PW, Powell CC, Reif JS. 1993. Effect of feline immunodeficiency virus infection on *Toxoplasma gondii*-specific humoral and cell-mediated immune responses of cats with serologic evidence of toxoplasmosis. J Vet Intern Med 7:95–100.

Lappin MR, Burney DP, Hill SA, Chavkin A. 1995. Detection of *Toxoplasma gondii*-specific IgA in the aqueous humor of cats. Am J Vet Res 56: 774–778.

Lappin MR, Burney DP, Dow SW, Potter TA. 1996a. Polymerase chain reaction for the detection of *Toxoplasma gondii* in aqueous humor of cats. Am J Vet Res 57:1589–1593.

Lappin MR, George JW, Pedersen NC, Barlough JE, Murphy CJ, Morse LS. 1996b. Primary and secondary *Toxoplasma gondii* infections in normal and feline immunodeficiency virus infected cats. J Parasitol 82:733–742.
Levine ND. 1977. Taxonomy of *Toxoplasma*. J Protozool 24:36–41.
Lin DS, Bowman DD. 1991. Cellular responses of cats with primary toxoplasmosis. J Parasitol 77:272–279.
Lin DS, Bowman DD. 1992. Macrophage functions in cats experimentally infected with feline immunodeficiency virus and *Toxoplasma gondii*. Vet Immunol Immunopathol 33:69–78.
Lin DS, Bowman DD, Jacobson RH. 1992a. Immunological changes in cats with concurrent *Toxoplasma gondii* and feline immunodeficiency virus infections. J Clin Microbiol 30:17–24.
Lin DS, Bowman DD, Jacobson RH. 1992b. Antibody responses to *Toxoplasma gondii* antigens in aqueous and cerebrospinal fluids in cats infected with *T. gondii* and FIV. Comp Immuno Microbiol Infect Dis 15:293–299.
Lindsay DS, Dubey JP, Blagburn BL, Tovio-Kinnucan MA. 1991. Examination of tissue cyst formation by *Toxoplasma gondii* in cell cultures using bradyzoites, tachyzoites, and sporozoites. J Parasitol 77:126–132.
Lindsay DS, Dubey JP, Blagburn BL. 1997a. Feline toxoplasmosis and the importance of the *Toxoplasma gondii* oocyst. Comp Contin Educ Pract Vet 19:448–461.
Lindsay DS, Dubey JP, Butler JM, Blagburn BL. 1997b. Mechanical transmission of *Toxoplasma gondii* oocysts by dogs. Vet Parasitol 73:27–33.
MacKnight KT, Robinson HW. 1992. Epidemiologic studies on human and feline toxoplasmosis. J Hyg Epidemiol Microbiol Immunol 36:37–47.
Martinez Sanchez R, Machin Sanchez R, Fachado Carvajales A, Pividal Grana J, Cruz de la Paz R, Suarez Hernandez M. 1991. Several results of a *Toxoplasma* survey. Invest Clin 32:13–26.
Miller NL, Frenkel JK, Dubey JP. 1972. Oral infections with *Toxoplasma* cysts and oocysts in felines, other mammals, and in birds. J Parasitol 58:928–937.
Muñana KR, Lappin MR, Powell CC, et al. 1995. Sequential measurement of *Toxoplasma gondii*–specific antibodies in the cerebrospinal fluid of cats with experimentally induced toxoplasmosis. Prog Vet Neurol 6:27–31.
Partono F, Cross JH. 1975. Toxoplasma antibodies in Indonesian and Chinese medical students in Jakarta. Southeast Asian J Trop Med Public Health 6:472–476.
Patton S, Legendre AM, McGavin MD, Pelletier D. 1991. Concurrent infection with *Toxoplasma gondii* and feline leukemia virus. J Vet Intern Med 5:199–201.
Remington JS, McLeod R, Desmonts G. 1995. Toxoplasmosis. In Infectious Diseases of the Fetus and Newborn Infant, 4th ed, ed JS Remington and JO Klein, pp 140–267. Philadelphia, Pa: WB Saunders.
Rey LC, Ramalho IL. 1999. Seroprevalence of toxoplasmosis in Fortaleza, Ceara, Brazil. Rev Inst Med Trop Sao Paulo 41:171–174.
Ruiz A, Frenkel JK, Cerdas L. 1973. Isolation of *Toxoplasma* from soil. J Parasitol 59:204–206.
Sedaghat A, Ardehali SM, Sadigh M, Buxton M. 1978. The prevalence of *Toxoplasma* infection in southern Iran. J Trop Med Hyg 81:204–207.
Sengbusch HG, Sengbusch LA. 1976. *Toxoplasma* antibody prevalence in veterinary personnel and a selected population not exposed to cats. Am J Epidemiol 103:595–597.
Stiles J, Prade R, Greene C. 1996. Detection of *Toxoplasma gondii* in feline and canine biological samples by use of the polymerase chain reaction. Am J Vet Res 57:264–267.
Stray-Pedersen B, Lorentzen-Styr AM. 1980. Epidemiological aspects of *Toxoplasma* infections among women in Norway. Acta Obstet Gynecol Scand 59:323–326.
Teutsch SM, Juranek DD, Sulzer A, Dubey JP, Sikes RK. 1979. Epidemic toxoplasmosis associated with infected cats. N Engl J Med 300:695–699.
Tizard IR, Chauhan SS, Lai CH. 1977. The prevalence and epidemiology of toxoplasmosis in Ontario. J Hyg (Lond) 78:275–282.
Ulmanen I, Leinikki P. 1975. The role of pet cats in the seroepidemiology of toxoplasmosis. Scand J Infect Dis 7:67–71.
Wallace MR, Rossetti RJ, Olson PE. 1993. Cats and toxoplasmosis risk in HIV-infected adults. J Am Med Assoc 269:76–77.
Zigas V. 1976. Prevalence of *Toxoplasma* antibodies in New Britain, Papua New Guinea. P N G Med J 19:225–230.

Unclassified *Toxoplasma gondii*-Like Organism

Etymology

This organism has not been named.

History

This parasite was first reported in the early 1990s (Dubey et al., 1992; Dubey and Carpenter, 1993; Dubey and Fenner, 1993). It closely resembles *Toxoplasma gondii,* but the tissue cysts of this organism are about twice as large as those of *Toxoplasma gondii* (Figs. 1.20–1.22).

Geographic Distribution and Prevalence

Dubey and Carpenter (1993) found this organism in 3 of 103 cats examined in a retrospective study of feline toxoplasmosis. The subjects had been examined at necropsy at the Angell Memorial Animal Hospital, Boston, Massachusetts, between 1952 to 1991.

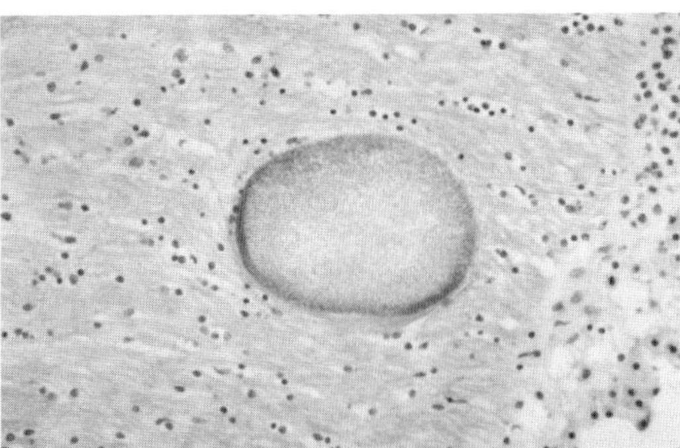

Fig. 1.20. *Toxoplasma*-like organism. Brain of a cat with a large cyst of this *Toxoplasma*-like organism. (Photo courtesy of Dr. Dave Peters)

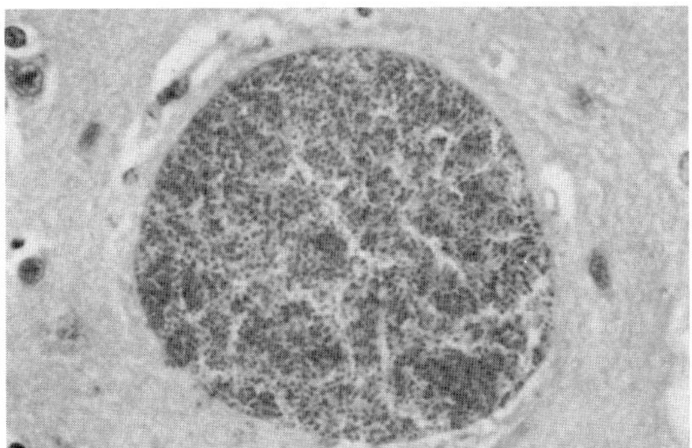

Fig. 1.21. *Toxoplasma*-like organism. Higher-power view of the cyst containing many bradyzoites. (Photo courtesy of Dr. Dave Peters)

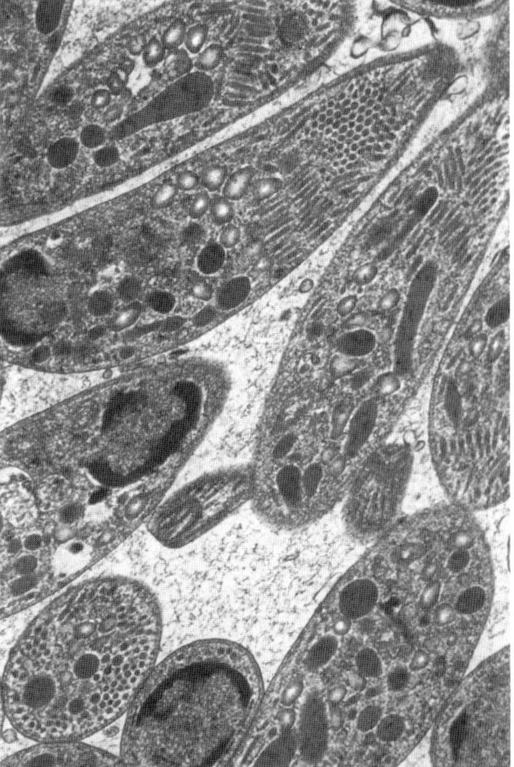

Fig. 1.22. *Toxoplasma*-like organisms. Electron micrograph of the *Toxoplasma*-like organism showing the many micronemes and rhoptries present in this organism. (Photo courtesy of Dr. Dave Peters)

Clinical Presentation and Pathogenesis

Infected cats have ranged in age from 3 to 17 years. Clinical signs attributable to parasitism have been associated with only one of six cats reported to have been infected with this organism (Dubey and Fenner, 1993). The cat was 3 years old and was presented for lameness. Neurologic and ophthalmologic abnormalities were present on physical examination. The neurologic examination indicated lesions in the spinal cord at C_6–T_2. A complete necropsy was done, and gross and microscopic lesions were confined to the spinal cord. Grossly, a focal translucent grayish area 1 × 0.3 cm extended laterally between cervical nerve roots C_5 and C_6. In addition, the spinal cord widened unilaterally from C_4 to C_6. Microscopic lesions consisted of focal granulomatous myelitis involving both gray and white matter and focal nonsuppurative meningitis including radiculoneuritis. Numerous protozoal tissue cysts were associated with the lesions.

Three of the other 5 infected cats have had concurrent lymphoid disorders and may have been suffering from varying degrees of immunosuppression. The association of this parasite and the immune status of the host needs to be better defined.

Diagnosis

A tentative diagnosis can be made on the large size of the tissue cysts. Transmission electron microscopy is needed to confirm the diagnosis. Bradyzoites of the unclassified organism have numerous micronemes that are arranged in rows, while micronemes in bradyzoites of *Toxoplasma gondii* are fewer in number and arranged randomly (Dubey et al., 1992; Dubey and Fenner,

1993). Infected cats may be *Toxoplasma gondii* antibody positive, and tissue cysts may react weakly with anti–*Toxoplasma gondii* serum in immunohistochemical tests.

REFERENCES

Dubey JP, Carpenter JL. 1993. Unidentified *Toxoplasma*-like tissue cysts in the brains of three cats. Vet Parasitol 45:319–321.

Dubey JP, Fenner WR. 1993. Clinical segmental myelitis associated with an unidentified *Toxoplasma*-like parasite in a cat. J Vet Diagn Invest 5:472–480.

Dubey JP, Peters D, Brown C. 1992. An unidentified *Toxoplasma*-like tissue cyst-forming coccidium in a cat (*Felis catus*). Parasitol Res 78:39–42.

Hammondia hammondi Frenkel 1974

Etymology

Hammondia after Dr. Datus M. Hammond and *hammondi* after Dr. D. M. Hammond.

Synonyms

Toxoplasma hammondi (Frenkel, 1974) Levine 1977; *Isospora hammondi* (Frenkel and Dubey, 1975) Tadros and Laarman, 1976. *Hammondia hammondi* was also referred to as the CR-4 strain of *Toxoplasma gondii* isolated by Frenkel and Dubey (1975a, 1975b) and the WC1170 parasite of Wallace (1973).

History

The oocysts of this parasite are structurally indistinguishable from those of *Toxoplasma gondii.* In 1971, Drs. Frenkel and Dubey isolated oocysts that were structurally similar to *Toxoplasma gondii* from a feral cat from Iowa. Dr. Wallace (1973) also isolated a similar parasite from the feces of a feral cat from Hawaii. Inoculation of mice with these oocysts produced large tissue cysts in skeletal muscles and very few tissue cysts in the brain. Both groups of researchers demonstrated that the life cycle of the parasite is heteroxenous. Dr. Frenkel first erected the genus *Hammondia* and used the name *Hammondia hammondi* in a review article on tissue cyst–forming coccidia (Frenkel, 1974). He and Dr. Dubey later fully described the life cycle of the parasite (Frenkel and Dubey, 1975a, 1975b). Because he published the name first (Frenkel, 1974), he is technically the author of the original name *Hammondia hammondi* (not he and Dr. Dubey as is frequently cited).

Geographic Distribution

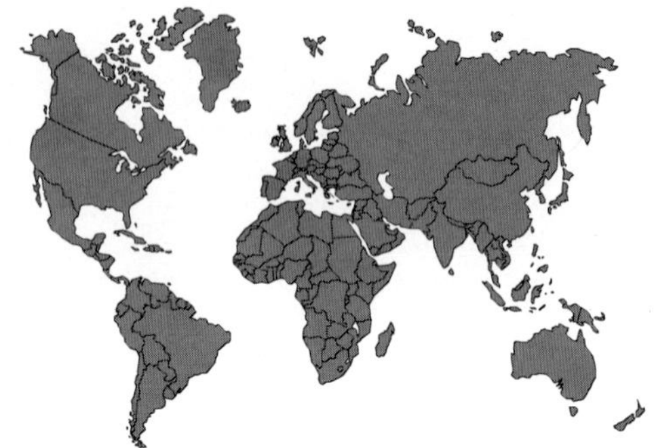

Fig. 1.23.

Probably worldwide. *Hammondia hammondi* has been found in Iowa and Hawaii in the United States (Frenkel and Dubey, 1975a, 1975b; Wallace, 1975), Germany (Rommel and Seyerl, 1975), Australia (Mason, 1978), and Japan (Shimura and Ito, 1986).

Prevalence

The prevalence of infection in cats is low. Wallace (1975) found *Hammondia hammondi* in 3 of 1,604 cats in Hawaii. Christie et al. (1977) examined the feces from 1,000 cats in Columbus, Ohio, for *Hammondia hammondi.* Nine cats were shedding oocysts that were the correct size and shape for either *Hammondia hammondi* or *Toxoplasma gondii.* Two of these proved to be *Hammondia hammondi,* and 7 were *Toxoplasma gondii* following mouse inoculation. Another isolate of *Hammondia hammondi* was obtained from a pooled sample from 175 cats by mouse inoculation.

Parasite Identification

Oocysts of *Hammondia hammondi* are excreted unsporulated in the feces. The oocysts are colorless and subspherical to spherical and measure 10.5–12.5 by 11.2–13.2 μm (mean, 10.6 by 11.4 μm). Sporulated oocysts contain two ellipsoid sporocysts each with four sporozoites.

Sporocysts measure 6–7.5 by 8–10.7 µm (mean, 6.5 by 9.8 µm), lack a Stieda body, and contain a sporocyst residuum composed of dispersed or compact granules. The sporozoites are elongate and curved within the sporocyst and have a crystalloid body. Sporulation occurs in 2 to 3 days at room temperature (22 to 26°C).

The similarity in oocyst size and structure between *Toxoplasma gondii* and *Hammondia hammondi* makes diagnosis based on oocyst structure alone impossible. Animal inoculation is needed for a definitive diagnosis to be obtained. Identification of *Hammondia hammondi* in tissues is also difficult. The tachyzoites of *Toxoplasma gondii* and *Hammondia hammondi* are indistinguishable from each other. The tissue cysts of *Hammondia hammondi* resemble those of *Toxoplasma gondii* and can be confused with sarcocysts of some thin-walled *Sarcocystis* species (Mehlhorn and Frenkel, 1980).

Life Cycle

Cats are the only know feline definitive hosts. However, other felids may be suitable definitive hosts. The life cycle is obligatorily heteroxenous. Two types of schizonts are found in a cat's small intestine 4 and 5 days after tissue cysts are ingested. The sexual stages first appear 5 days after infection. The prepatent period is 5 to 6 days, and the patent period is 12 to 28 days. Inoculation of cats with *Hammondia hammondi* oocysts does not lead to oocyst excretion or to latent infections in their tissues.

Natural intermediate hosts include rats (*Rattus rattus* and *Rattus norvegicus*), goats (*Capra hircus*), and roe deer (*Capreolus capreolus*). Experimental intermediate hosts include white mice, deer mice, long-tailed field mice, yellow-necked field mice, rats, multimammate rats, guinea pigs, hamsters, bank voles, European voles, field voles, dogs, goats, sheep, monkeys, and pigs (Dubey, 1993). Chickens cannot be infected with *Hammondia hammondi* (Dubey and Steitel, 1976). When an intermediate host ingests oocysts of *Hammondia hammondi,* the oocysts excyst in the intestine and liberate the sporozoites. The sporozoites penetrate the intestinal mucosa and multiply by endodyogeny in the lamina propria, submucosa and muscularis, Peyer's patches, and mesenteric lymph nodes for about 11 days. Tissue cysts are present in the muscles of mice by 11 days. The tissue cysts are initially small but can be over 300 µm in length in about a month. The tissue cysts remain viable for 1.3 years and probably longer. Tissue cysts are not infective for intermediate hosts. Congenital transmission of *Hammondia hammondi* does not occur in mice (Dubey and Steitel, 1976) or cats (Dubey, 1977).

Pathogenicity

Hammondia hammondi does not cause disease in cats. Mice inoculated with 10^5 to 10^6 oocysts may suffer from up to 30 percent mortality. Lesions are present in the intestinal tracts of these mice and are due to multiplication of tachyzoites. A transient myositis may be present in the skeletal muscles of infected mice.

Immunity

Immunity to *Hammondia hammondi* in cats is less stable than immunity to *Toxoplasma gondii.* About 50 percent of cats will re-excrete oocysts when challenged (Dubey, 1975). Some cats will spontaneously re-excrete small numbers of oocysts in the absence of reinfection. Immunosuppression of cats does not affect the course of a primary *Hammondia hammondi* infection in cats but does cause cats to re-excrete oocysts. Infection with *Hammondia hammondi* does not make cats immune to infection with *Toxoplasma gondii.* Cats that have recovered from a *Hammondia hammondi* infection do not develop antibodies to *Toxoplasma gondii.*

In contrast to cats, intermediate hosts that are inoculated with oocysts develop antibodies that cross-react with *Toxoplasma gondii.* This cross-reactive immunity is also protective against challenge with pathogenic strains of *Toxoplasma gondii* (Christie and Dubey, 1977; Dubey, 1978, 1981; Munday and Dubey, 1988). *Hammondia hammondi* immune serum from mice recognizes all the major surface antigens of *Toxoplasma gondii* except the 21.5 kD antigen (Araujo et al., 1984). A monoclonal antibody to the immunodominant p30 antigen of *Toxoplasma gondii* also reacts with tachyzoites of *Hammondia hammondi* (Riahi et al., 1998). Immunization of hamsters with *Hammondia hammondi* affords minimal protection against challenge with *Besnoitia jellisoni* (Dubey, 1978).

Hazards to Humans

Hammondia hammondi infection was attempted in four species of nonhuman primates (*Saguinus nigricollis, Macaca fascicularis, Macaca mulatta,* and *Cercocebus atys*) (Dubey and Wong, 1978). None of the monkeys developed clinical signs of disease, and *Hammondia hammondi* was isolated from only *Saguinus nigricollis*. It is possible that humans could serve as intermediate hosts. No recorded cases of human infection exist.

REFERENCES

Araujo FG, Dubey JP, Remington JS. 1984. Antigenic similarity between the coccidian parasites *Toxoplasma gondii* and *Hammondia hammondi*. J Protozool 31:145–147.

Christie E, Dubey JP. 1977. Cross-immunity between *Hammondia hammondi* and *Toxoplasma* infections in mice and hamsters. Infect Immunol 18:412–415.

Christie E, Dubey JP, Pappas PW. 1977. Prevalence of *Hammondia hammondi* in the feces of cats in Ohio. J Parasitol 63:929–931.

Dubey JP. 1975. Immunity to *Hammondia hammondi* infection in cats. J Am Vet Med Assoc 167:337–347.

Dubey JP. 1977. Attempted transmission of feline coccidia from chronically infected queens to their kittens. J Am Vet Med Assoc 170:541–543.

Dubey JP. 1978. A comparison of cross protection between BCG, *Hammondia hammondi, Besnoitia jellisoni* and *Toxoplasma gondii* in hamsters. J Protozool 25:382–384.

Dubey JP. 1981. Prevention of abortion and neonatal death due to toxoplasmosis by vaccination of goats with the nonpathogenic coccidium *Hammondia hammondi*. Am J Vet Res 42:2155–2157.

Dubey JP. 1993. *Toxoplasma, Neospora, Sarcocystis,* and other tissue cyst-forming coccidia of humans and animals. In Parasitic Protozoa, vol 6, ed JP Kreier and JR Baker, pp 1–158. San Diego, Calif: Academic Press.

Dubey JP, Steitel RH. 1976. Further studies on the transmission of *Hammondia hammondi* in cats. J Parasitol 62:548–551.

Dubey JP, Wong M. 1978. Experimental *Hammondia hammondi* infection in monkeys. J Parasitol 64:551–552.

Frenkel JK. 1974. Advances in the biology of sporozoa. Z Parasitenkd 45:125–162.

Frenkel JK, Dubey JP. 1975a. *Hammondia hammondi* gen. nov., sp. nov., from domestic cats, a new coccidian related to *Toxoplasma* and *Sarcocystis*. Z Parasitenkd 46:3–12.

Frenkel JK, Dubey JP. 1975b. *Hammondia hammondi:* a new coccidium of cats producing cysts in muscle of other mammals. Science 189:222–224.

Mason RW. 1978. The detection of *Hammondia hammondi* in Australia and the identification of a free-living intermediate host. Z Parasitenkd 57:101–106.

Mehlhorn H, Frenkel JK. 1980. Ultrastructural comparison of cysts and zoites of *Toxoplasma gondii, Sarcocystis muris,* and *Hammondia hammondi* in skeletal muscle of mice. J Parasitol 66:59–67.

Munday BL, Dubey JP. 1988. Prevention of *Toxoplasma gondii* abortion in goats by vaccination with oocysts of *Hammondia hammondi*. Aust Vet J 65:150–153.

Riahi H, Bouteille B, Darde ML. 1998. Antigenic similarity between *Hammondia hammondi* and *Toxoplasma gondii* tachyzoites. J Parasitol 84:651–653.

Rommel M, von Seyerl F. 1975. 1st demonstration of *Hammondia hammondi* (Frenkel and Dubey 1975) in the feces of a cat in Germany. Berl Munch Tierarztl Wochenschr 89:398–399.

Shimura K, Ito S. 1986. Isolation of *Hammondia hammondi* in Japan. Nippon Juigaku Zasshi 48:901–908.

Wallace GD. 1973. *Sarcocystis* in mice inoculated with *Toxoplasma*-like oocysts from cat feces. Science 180:1375–1377.

Wallace GD. 1975. Observations on a feline coccidium with some characteristics of *Toxoplasma* and *Sarcocystis*. Z Parasitenkd 46:167–178.

Hammondia pardalis Hendricks, Ernst, Courtney, and Speer, 1979

Etymology

Hammondia after Dr. D.M. Hammond and *pardalis* for the species name of the ocelot, *Felis pardalis*.

Synonyms

Toxoplasma pardalis (Hendricks, Ernst, Courtney, and Speer, 1979) Levine and Ivens, 1981. Oocysts of this species closely resemble those of *Isospora felis* and misidentification is possible.

History

This coccidium was first described in 1979 from the feces of an ocelot housed at the Air Force Survival School Zoo, Albrook Air Force Station, Panama Canal Zone (Hendricks et al., 1979). It has recently been isolated from domestic cats fed heart, skeletal muscles, and uterus tissues from cattle that had aborted (Abbitt et al., 1993), but this was probably a case of misinterpretation of an underlying *Hammondia pardalis* infection in the cats fed cattle tissue. The causative organism of the abortion in cattle, *Neospora caninum,* is now known to be heteroxenous, with dogs serving as the source of a *Toxoplasma gondii*–sized oocyst.

Geographic Distribution

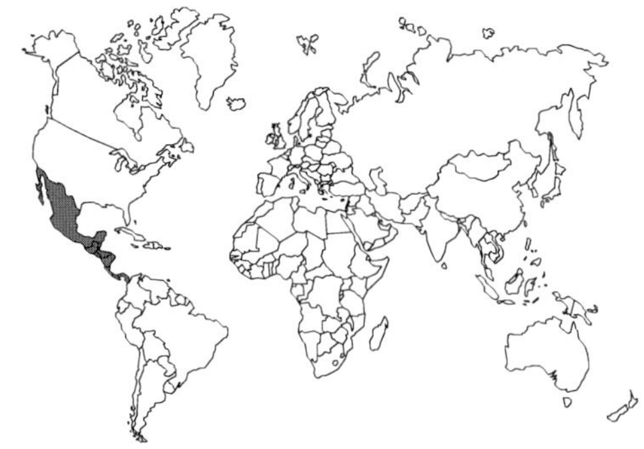

Fig. 1.24.

Panama Canal Zone, Panama; the Cockscomb Basin of Belize, Central America; and northeastern Mexico (Hendricks et al., 1979; Patton et al., 1986; Abbitt et al., 1993).

Location in Host

Feline Definitive Hosts. The number of asexual stages (if any) and location of developmental sexual stages within the feline definitive host are not known. However, it is likely that they occur within the enterocytes of the intestinal tract.

Intermediate Hosts. Asexual stages are present in the mesenteric lymph nodes, lungs, and intestinal mucosa of experimentally inoculated mice.

Parasite Identification

Oocysts are ovoid and measure 36–46 by 25–35 µm (mean, 40.8 by 28.5 µm). A micropyle is present at the small end of the oocyst, while a suture line is present in the larger end of the oocyst. A small granule is often attached to the inner portion of the oocyst wall. Sporulated oocysts contain two ellipsoid sporocysts each with four sporozoites. Sporocysts measure 19–25 by 14–19 µm (mean, 22.2 by 16.4 µm), lack a Stieda body, and contain a sporocyst residuum composed of a single refractile globule or several small globules. The sporozoites lie lengthwise within the sporocyst and have no refractile bodies.

The presence of a micropyle and suture line in the oocyst wall differentiates the oocysts of *Hammondia pardalis* from *Isospora felis,* which is similar in size but lacks these structures in its oocyst wall. The large size of *Hammondia pardalis* oocysts differentiates *Hammondia pardalis* from *Hammondia hammondi, Isospora rivolta, Toxoplasma gondii,* and *Besnoitia* species, all of which have smaller oocysts.

Identification of *Hammondia pardalis* stages in intermediate hosts is difficult. The original description of these stages was not comprehensive enough to allow for the identification of clear-cut diagnostic features. Groups of merozoites were present in the alveolar septa, mesenteric lymph nodes, and lymphoid tissue in the colon. Individual merozoites measured 6 by 3 µm.

Life Cycle

The type host is the ocelot, *Felis pardalis.* Other natural hosts are the jaguar (*Panthera onca*) and the puma (*Felis concolor*) (Patton et al., 1986). Experimental definitive hosts are the domestic cat, *Felis catus* and the jaguarundi, *Felis yagouaroundi.* Raccoons, *Procyon lotor,* are not suitable definitive hosts (Hendricks et al., 1979). The life cycle is obligatorily heteroxenous, meaning that there must be one host containing one set of stages, the sexual stages, and one host containing another set of stages, the asexual stages. Cattle are natural intermediate hosts, and mice are experimental intermediate hosts. Tissue-feeding studies indicate that infectious stages are present in the heart, skeletal muscles, and uterus of infected cows.

No life cycle stages have been identified in the cat. The prepatent period was 6 to 7 days in seven domestic cats, two ocelots, and a jaguarundi fed infective mice, and the patent period was 5 to 13 days (Hendricks et al., 1979). Sporulation occurs at room temperature within 7 days; however, no properly conducted studies have been done on this, and it is likely that sporogony is completed within 2 to 3 days. Sporulated oocysts do not produce patent infections in recipient cats. It is not known if tissues from cats fed oocysts contain stages that induce oocyst excretion in other cats. The parasite cannot be passed from mouse to mouse by the inoculation of infected tissues.

Clinical Presentation and Pathogenesis

Clinical signs of infection in cats have not been reported. Oocyst-induced infections in mice can cause clinical disease and death (Hendricks et al., 1979).

Treatment

There has been no attempt to stop the shedding of *Hammondia pardalis* oocysts by infected cats. It is possible that the shedding of oocysts might be prevented by the treatment of cats with sulfonamides or the other products used for feline coccidiosis (Table 1.4).

Epizootiology

Cats are not commonly infected with this parasite.

Hazards to Other Animals

None known.

Hazards to Humans

It is possible that humans could serve as intermediate hosts. No recorded cases of human infection exist.

REFERENCES

Abbitt B, Craig TM, Jones LP, Huey RL, Eugster AK. 1993. Protozoal abortion in a herd of cattle concurrently infected with *Hammondia pardalis*. JAVMA 203:444–448.

Hendricks LD, Ernst JV, Courtney CH, Speer CA. 1979. *Hamondia pardalis* sp. n. (Sarcocystidae) from the ocelot, *Felis pardalis*, and experimental infection of other felines. J Protozool 26:39–43.

Patton SP, Rabinowitz A, Randolph SS, Johnson SS. 1986. A coprological survey of parasites of wild neotropical felidae. J Parasitol 72:517–520.

Sarcocystis Species

Introduction and Importance

All *Sarcocystis* species have an obligatory heteroxenous life cycle. Cats are important as definitive hosts for at least 11 named species (Table 1.8) and are the intermediate host for one species. *Sarcocystis* (*Sarco* = muscle, *cystis* = cyst) was first observed in 1843 by F. Miescher in a house mouse (Dubey et al., 1989). The muscles of the mouse contained "milky white threads," which came to be known as Miescher's tubules. Later a species was found in the pig and named *Synchytrium miescherianum* by Kühn in 1865 and changed to *Sarcocystis miescheriana* by Labbé in 1899. Therefore the correct type species is *Sarcocystis miescheriana* (Kühn, 1865) Labbé 1899. It was not until the early 1970s that the two-host life cycle was described (Fayer, 1972; Rommel and Heydorn, 1972; Rommel et al., 1972).

Sarcocystis Species Life Cycle

The *Sarcocystis* life cycle is obligatorily a two-host cycle. The intermediate host becomes infected by ingestion of sporocysts from the environment. The sporozoites excyst from the sporocysts in the intestinal tract. The sporozoites leave the intestinal tract and undergo first-generation merogony in endothelial cells of arteries usually in mesenteric lymph nodes (Dubey et al., 1989). A second generation of merogony occurs in capillaries or small arteries in many tissues throughout the body. The meronts are usually most numerous in glomeruli of the kidneys. The merozoites from the last generation are released into the circulation and can occasionally be found

Table 1.8—Names and intermediate hosts of *Sarcocystis* species transmitted by cats

Species of *Sarcocystis*	Intermediate host
S. cuniculi	European rabbit (*Oryctolagus cuniculus*)
S. cymruensis	Norway rat (*Rattus norvegicus*)
S. fusiformis	Water buffalo (*Bubalus bubalis*)
S. gigantea (syn. *S. ovifelis*)	Sheep (*Ovis aries*)
S. hirsuta (syn. *S. bovifelis*)	Cow (*Bos taurus*)
S. leporum	Cottontail rabbit (*Sylvilagus floridanus, Sylvilagus nuttalli, Sylvilagus pallistris*)
S. medusiformis	Sheep (*Ovis aries*)
S. moulei (syn. *S. caprifelis*)	Goat (*Capra hircus*)
S. muris	House mouse (*Mus musculus*)
S. odoi	White-tailed deer (*Odocoileus virginianus*)
S. porcifelis	Pig (*Sus scrofa*)

intracellularly in unidentified mononuclear cells (Dubey et al., 1989). Limited multiplication may occur at this stage of infection. Eventually these merozoites will penetrate cells and develop into the sarcocyst stage that contains bradyzoites. The first- and second-generation meronts develop directly in the host cell cytoplasm, whereas the bradyzoites develop within a parasitophorous vacuole.

The developing sarcocyst contains a stage called a metrocyte that divides by endodyogeny to produce the bradyzoites. A mature sarcocyst can contain thousands of bradyzoites and be grossly visible. The presence of grossly visible sarcocysts of *Sarcocystis gigantea* in sheep and *Sarcocystis hirsuta* in cattle is a cause for condemnation of the carcass (Dubey et al., 1986; Dubey et al., 1990).

Feline *Sarcocystis* Infections

Cats are definitive hosts for about 11 species of *Sarcocystis* (Table 1.8) and intermediate hosts for one named species, *Sarcocystis felis.*

Sarcocystis felis Dubey, Hamir, Kirkpatrick, Todd, and Rupprecht, 1992

Etymology

Sarco (muscle) *cystis* (cyst) and *felis* (cat).

History

Sarcocysts of a *Sarcocystis* species have been found in a number of felids including domestic cats (Kirkpatrick et al., 1986; Everitt et al., 1987; Fiori and Lowndes, 1988; Hill et al., 1988; Edwards et al., 1988) and wild felids (Kluge, 1967; Greiner et al., 1989; Anderson et al., 1992; Dubey et al., 1992; Dubey and Bwangamoi, 1994). The ultrastructural features of sarcocysts from different feline hosts are indistinguishable, and Dubey et al. (1992) gave the name *Sarcocystis felis* to the parasite.

Hosts

The type host is the bobcat (*Felis rufus*). Other hosts include domestic cats (*Felis domesticus*), leopards (*Panthera pardus*), Florida bobcats (*Felis rufus floridanus*), Florida panthers (*Felis concolor coryi*), cougars (*Felis concolor stanleyana*), cheetahs (*Acinonyx jubatus*), and lions (*Felis leo*).

Geographic Distribution

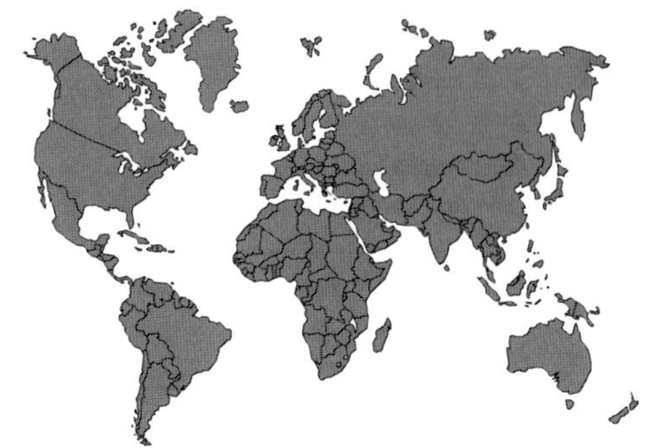

Fig. 1.25.

Geographic distribution is probably worldwide. Most current reports have been from domestic and wild felids in the United States. The prevalence in domestic cats is unknown. It is apparently common in wild felids. It has been found in four of four cougars (Greiner et al., 1989), 11 of 14 panthers (Greiner et al., 1989), four of six bobcats (Dubey et al., 1992), and 30 of 60 Florida bobcats (Anderson et al., 1992). Additionally, it was found in 7 of 10 cheetahs from a captive breeding colony in Oregon (Briggs et al., 1993). The same or a similar parasite has been observed in two lions and a leopard from zoos in India (Bhatavcdkar and Purohit, 1963; Somvanshi et al., 1987). Dubey and Bwangamoi (1994) described the parasite from a 7-year-old lioness from the Nairobi National Park in Kenya.

Parasite Identification

Tentative identification is based on observing the sarcocysts in muscle tissue. In muscle squash preparations, sarcocysts are up to 1 cm in length (Greiner et al., 1989). In tissue sections, sarcocysts can approach 2,000 μm, are septate, and have regularly spaced, finger-like projections from the tissue cyst wall. No inflammatory response is associated with the tissue cysts (Greiner et al., 1989; Briggs et al., 1993). Definitive identification of *Sarcocystis felis* is based on observation of the ultrastructural features of the tissue cyst wall (Dubey et al., 1992). The parasitophorous vacuole membrane (PVM) of the primary cyst wall is folded into hobnail-like bumps and villar projections that are 0.6–1.2 µm long by 0.3–0.4 µm wide at uneven distances. The villi lack microtubules. The PVM, including villi and hobnail bumps, is lined by a 66 nm electron dense thick layer. Ground substance is 0.7–1.0 µm thick and is composed of amorphous material and a few electron dense granules. Septa are 0.1–0.2 µm thick. Bradyzoites are 7.0–10 by 1.5–2 µm and contain micronemes that are confined to the anterior third of the bradyzoite (Fig. 1.26).

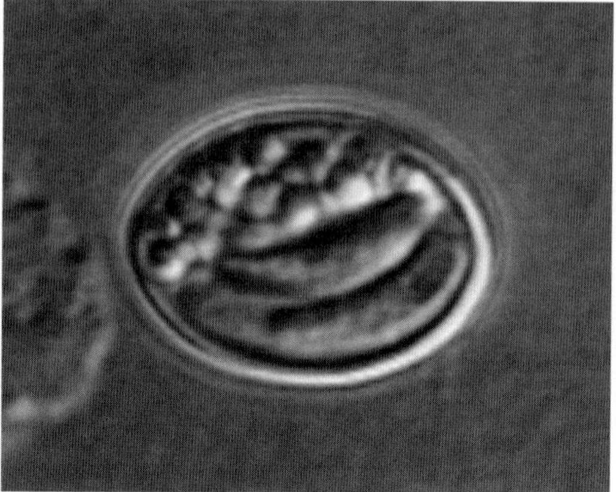

Fig. 1.26. *Sarcocystis* species. Sporulated sporocyst as it appears when passed in the feces.

Life Cycle

Sarcocysts are the only life cycle stage that has been observed (Figs. 1.27 and 1.28). Sarcocysts have been observed in heart, tongue, masseter, esophagus, diaphragm, and biceps femoris. Precystic stages probably occur in vascular endothelial cells. The definitive host is not known.

Clinical Presentation and Pathogenesis

Clinical signs of infection in cats have not been reported.

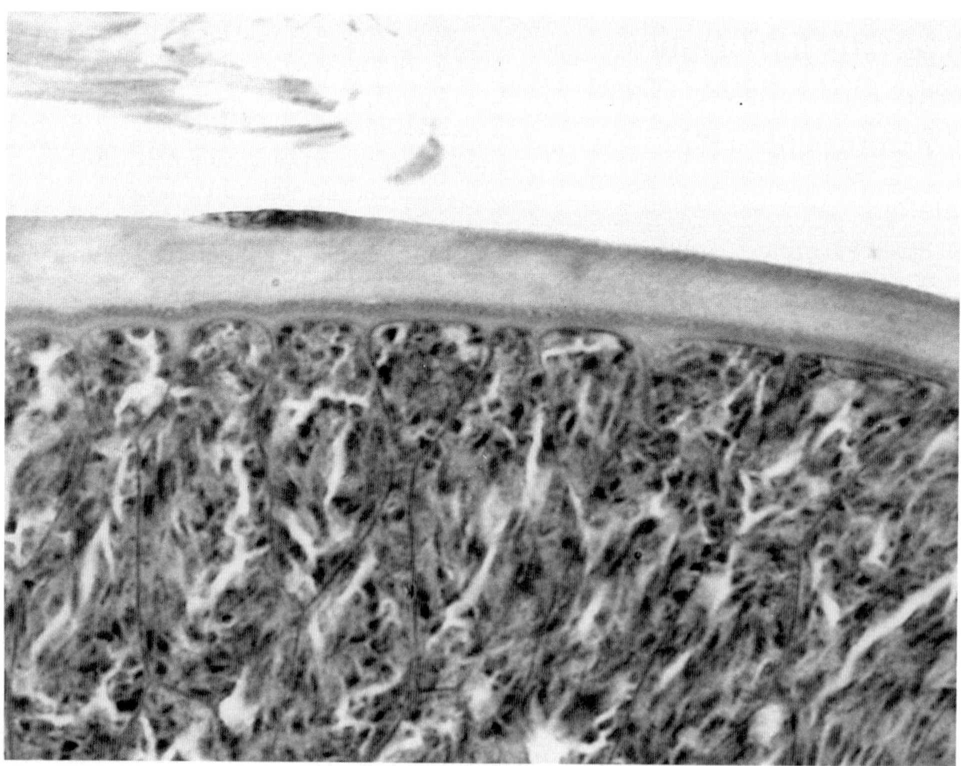

Fig. 1.27. *Sarcocystis felis.* Sarcocyst in section of skeletal muscles from an African lioness. Note villar projections on the cyst wall, septa, and bradyzoites. H&E stain. (Dubey and Bwangamoi, 1994) (Reprinted with permission, *J Helminthol Soc Wash Comp Parasitol,* 1994, Vol 61, No 1)

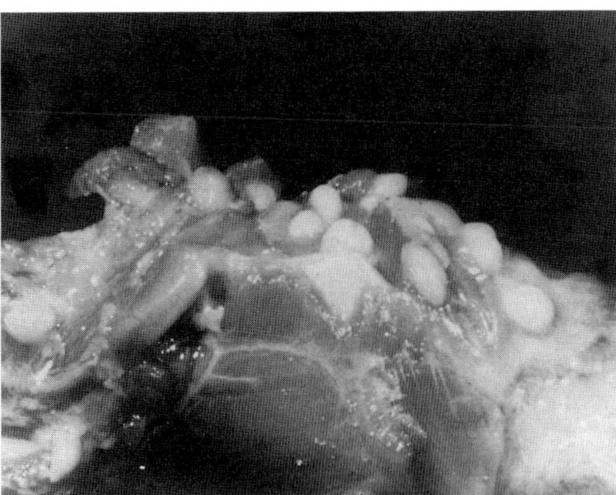

Fig. 1.28. *Sarcocystis gigantea.* Sarcocysts in laryngeal area of a naturally infected ewe. (Dubey et al., 1986)

Treatment

Sarcocystis felis infection does not cause clinical disease in cats, and no treatment is needed.

REFERENCES

Anderson AJ, Greiner EC, Atkinson CT, Roelke ME. 1992. Sarcocysts in Florida bobcats (*Felis rufus floridanus*). J Wildl Dis 28:116–120.

Bhatavedkar MY, Purohit BL. 1963. A record of sarcosporidiosis in lion. Indian Vet J 40:44–45.

Briggs MB, Leathers CW, Foreyt WJ. 1993. Sarcocystis felis in captive cheetahs (*Acinonyx jubatus*). J Helminthol Soc Wash 60:277–279.

Dubey JP, Bwangamoi O. 1994. *Sarcocystis felis* (Protozoa: Sarcocytidae) from the African lion (*Panthera leo*). J Helminthol Soc Wash 61:113–114.

Dubey JP, Leek RG, Fayer R. 1986. Prevalence, transmission, and pathogenicity of *Sarcocystis gigantea* of sheep. JAVMA 188:151–154.

Dubey JP, Speer CA, Fayer R. 1989. Sarcocystosis of Animals and Man. Boca Raton, Fla: CRC Press, pp 131–135.

Dubey JP, Udtujan RM, Cannon L, Lindsay DS. 1990. Condemnation of beef because of *Sarcocystis hirsuta* infection. JAVMA 196:1095–1096.

Dubey JP, Hamir AN, Kirkpaterick CE, Todd KS, Rupprecht CE. 1992. *Sarcocystis felis* sp. n. (Protozoa: Sarcocystidae) from the bobcat (*Felis rufus*). J Helminthol Soc Wash 59:227–229.

Edwards JF, Ficken MD, Luttgen PJ, Frey MS. 1988. Disseminated sarcocystosis in a cat with lymphosarcoma. JAVMA 193:831–832.

Everitt JE, Basgall ED, Hooser SB, Todd KS. 1987. *Sarcocystis* sp. in the striated muscle of domestic cats, *Felis catus*. Proc Helminthol Soc Wash 54:279–281.

Fayer R. 1972. Gametogeny of *Sarcocystis* in cell culture. Science 175:65–67.

Fiori MG, Lowndes HE. 1988. Histochemical study of *Sarcocystis* sp. intramuscular cysts in gastrocnemius and soleus of the cat. Parasitol Res 75:123–131.

Greiner EC, Roelke ME, Atkinson CT, Dubey JP, Wright SC. 1989. *Sarcocystis* sp. in muscles of free-ranging Florida panthers and cougars (*Felis concolor*). J Wildl Dis 25:623–628.

Hill JE, Chapman WL, Prestwood AK. 1988. Intramuscular *Sarcocystis* sp. in two cats and a dog. J Parasitol 74:724–727.

Kirkpatrick CE, Dubey JP, Goldschmidt MH, Saik JE, Schmitz JA. 1986. *Sarcocystis* sp. in muscles of domestic cats. Vet Pathol 23:88–90.

Kluge JP. 1967. Trichinosis and sarcosporidiosis in a puma. Bull Wildl Dis Assoc 3:110–111.

Rommel M, Heydorn AO. 1972. Beiträge zum Lebenszyklus der Sarkosporidien III. *Isospora hominus* (Railliet und Lucet, 1891) Wenyon, 1923, eine Dauerform der Sarkosporidien des Rindes und des Schweins. Berl Münch Tierärztl Wschr 85: 143–145.

Rommel M, Heydorn AO, Gruber F. 1972. Beiträge zum Lebenszyklus der Sarkosporidien I. Die Sporozyste von *S. tenella* in den Fäzes der Katze. Berl Münch Tierärztl Wschr 85:101–105.

Somvanshi R, Koul GL, Biswas JC. 1987. *Sarcocystis* in a leopard (*Panthera pardus*). Indian Vet Ned J 11:174–175.

Feline *Sarcocystis*-Associated Meningoencephalomyelitis

A single case of central nervous system infection of a cat with a *Sarcocystis* species has been reported. A 13-week-old Burmese kitten had clinical signs of depression and lethargy and cried as if in pain. Physical examination revealed that the kitten was depressed and afebrile and had left-sided hemiparesis. The third eyelids of both eyes were prolapsed. The kitten was euthanized and examined at necropsy. No gross lesions were present. Microscopic lesions were confined to the brain and spinal cord. The cerebral cortex and caudate nucleus were the areas of the brain most severely affected. Multifocal areas of intense inflammation associated with necrosis, widespread edema, and gemistocytic astrocytosis in the underlying subcortical white matter were present. Lesions in the spinal cord and medulla oblongata consisted of prominent perivascular cuffs of lymphocytes, plasma cells, and mononuclear cells in the gray and white matter, with mild inflammatory cell infiltrates in the neurophil. Most *Sarcocystis* stages were seen in the spinal cord and consisted of meronts and merozoites in neurons and in unidentified cells in the neurophil. The diagnosis was confirmed by immunohistochemical examination and positive reactivity with rabbit anti-*Sarcocystis* serum.

REFERENCES

Dubey JP, Higgins RJ, Barr BC, Spangler WL, Kollin B, Jorgensen LS. 1994. *Sarcocystis*-associated meningoencephalomyelitis in a cat. J Vet Diagn Invest 6:118–120.

Cats as Experimental Final Hosts of *Sarcocystis neurona*

Sarcocystis neurona Dubey, Davis, Speer, Bowman, de Lahunta, Gransrom, Topper, Hamir, Cummings, and Suter, 1991, is the agent causing equine protozoal myeloencephalitis in horses throughout the Americas (Divers et al., 2000). Horses develop schizont stages in brain tissue and associated neurologic disease but do not develop muscle cysts typical of *Sarcocystis* species. It has been known for some time that the opossum was the likely source of the sporocysts that infect horses (Fenger et al., 1997), but the intermediate host was not known. It was postulated that the intermediate host was a bird and that the parasite in horses was related to *Sarcocystis falcatula,* which uses avian hosts for the production of the muscle cyst stages. Opossums were thought to become infected with the intestinal stages of the parasite through the ingestion of the avian intermediate hosts.

Recently, it has been shown that cats can serve experimentally as suitable hosts for the development of the muscle stages of this parasite (Dubey et al., 2000). Cats were fed sporocysts from the feces of a naturally infected opossum. About 5 months after infection, it was found at necropsy that the cats had mature cysts in their muscles. When these cysts were fed to an opossum, the opossum had sporocysts present in its intestinal mucosa at necropsy 2 weeks later. The cysts present in the muscles of the cat differ from those of *Sarcocystis felis* in the structure of the cyst wall (JP Dubey, personal communication).

It is unlikely that cats are the natural source of the infective material for opossums because cats only rarely appear to have the muscle stages of *Sarcocystis* species in their tissues. Thus, the natural intermediate host is still not known, but it is now expected to be a mammalian species of some sort.

REFERENCES

Divers TJ, Bowman DD, de Lahunta A. 2000. Equine protozoa myeloencephalitis: recent advances in diagnosis and treatment. Vet Med (Feb suppl), pp 3–17.

Dubey JP, Saville WJA, Lindsay DS, Stich RW, Stanek JF, Speer CA, Rosenthal BM, Njoku CJ, Kwok OCH, Shen SK, Reed SM. 2000. Completion of the life cycle of *Sarcocystis neurona.* J Parasitol 86:1276–1280.

Fenger CK, Granstrom DE, Gajadhar AA, Williams NM, McCrillis SA, Stamper S, Langemeier JL, Dubey JP. 1997. Experimental induction of equine protozoal myeloencephalitis in horses using *Sarcocystis* sp. sporocysts from the opossum (*Didelphis virginiana*). Vet Parasitol 68:199–213.

Besnoitia Species

Introduction and Importance

The life cycle is heteroxenous. Cats are important as definitive hosts for this genus. Clinical disease is not associated with feline infections. Horses, domestic and wild ruminants, opossums, rodents, and lizards are natural intermediate hosts. Large, often grossly visible, tissues cysts are found in connective tissue cells in intermediate hosts. Severe disease has been reported in ruminants and horses. *Fibrocystis* Hadwen, 1922, is a synonym of the genus, and several authors have incorrectly referred to the genus as *Globidium,* which is a synonym for the genus *Eimeria* or *Sarcocystis,* which is a separate valid genus. *Besnoitia besnoiti* (Marotel, 1912) Henery, 1913, is the type species of this genus. *Besnoitia* species have a heteroxenous life cycle, and there are six named species (Dubey, 1993). Cats are the definitive host for two species and excrete *Toxoplasma*-like oocysts in their feces. One report (Peteshev et al., 1974) implicated cats as definitive hosts for *Besnoitia besnoitia,* but no other studies have been able to confirm these findings (Dubey, 1993).

REFERENCES

Dubey JP. 1993. *Toxoplasma, Neospora, Sarcocystis,* and other tissue cyst-forming coccidia of humans and animals. In Parasitic Protozoa, vol 6, ed JP Kreier and JR Baker, pp 1–158. San Diego, Calif: Academic Press.

Peteshev VM, Galouzo IG, Polomoshnov AP. 1974. Koshki-definitive khozyaeva besnoitii (*Besnoitia besnoiti*). Izvest Akad Nauk Kazakh SSR, Ser Biol 1:33-38

Besnoitia darlingi (Brumpt, 1913) Mandour, 1965

Etymology

Besnoitia (for Dr. C. Besnoit) *darling* (for Dr. S. T. Darling)

Synonyms

Sarcocystis darlingi Brumpt, 1913; *B. panamensis* Schneider, 1965; *Besnoitia sauriana* Garnham, 1966.

Geographic Distribution and Prevalence

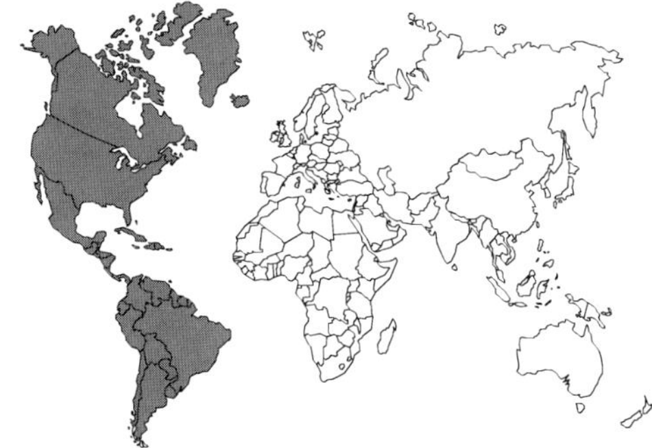

Fig. 1.29.

The prevalence of this parasite in cats is unknown. It has been described from naturally infected opossums (*Didelphis virginiana* and *Didelphis marsupialis*) in North and South America and from naturally infected lizards (basilisk lizards *Basiliscus basliscus* and *Basiliscus vittatus* and the borriguero lizard *Ameiva ameiva praesignis*) from South America. Only cyclic transmission between opossums and cats has been documented (Smith and Frenkel, 1977, 1984). Infection is apparently common in opossums in North America, ranging from 10 to 60 percent (Conti-Diaz et al., 1970; Flatt et al. 1971; Smith and Frenkel, 1977).

Parasite Identification

Oocysts measure 11.8–12.8 by 10.2–12.8 µm (mean, 12.3 by 11.9 µm). No micropyle or polar granule is present. Two elliptical sporocysts are present. Sporocysts measure 6.2–8.9 by 4.8–6.2 µm (mean, 7.9 by 5.4 µm) and do not contain Stieda bodies. Four sporozoites are present in each sporocyst and they measure approximately 5 by 2 µm.

Life Cycle

Oocysts are excreted by cats fed tissue cysts but not oocysts (Smith and Frenkel, 1984). The prepatent period is 9 to 14 days (mean, 11.5 days), and the patent period is 3 to 13 days (mean, 8 days). Oocysts are excreted unsporulated in the feces. Unsporulated oocysts sporulate in 2 to 3 days at room temperature (Smith and Frenkel, 1977). The location and structure of developmental stages in the cat intestine is not known. Extraintestinal development apparently does not occur in cats (Smith and Frenkel, 1984). Cats become immune to challenge infection but do not usually develop high antibody titers. Cats fed oocysts do not excrete oocysts, do not develop extraintestinal infections, do not develop measurable antibody titers, and do not become immune to challenge with tissue cysts (Smith and Frenkel, 1984).

It is not known if the organism named *Besnoitia darlingi* in reptiles and *Besnoitia darlingi* in opossums is the same species. Experimentally mice and hamsters can serve as intermediate hosts for *Besnoitia darlingi* isolated from opossums and cats. The tissue cysts are grossly visible and are characteristic for the genera.

Clinical Presentation and Pathogenesis

Clinical signs of infection in cats have not been reported.

Treatment

Besnoitia darlingi infection does not cause clinical disease in cats, and no treatment is needed.

REFERENCES

Conti-Diaz IA, Turner C, Tweeddale DT, Furclow ML. 1970. Besnoitiasis in the opossum (*Didelphis marsupialis*). J Parasitol 56:457–460.

Flatt RE, Nelson LR, Patton NM. 1971. *Besnoitia darlingi* in the opossum (*Didelphis marsupialis*). Lab Anim Sci 21:106–109.

Smith DD, Frenkel JK. 1977. *Besnoitia darlingi* (Protozoa: Toxoplasmatinae) cyclic transmission by cats. J Parasitol 63:1066–1071.
Smith DD, Frenkel JK. 1984. *Besnoitia darlingi* (Apicomplexa, Sarcocystidae, Toxoplasmatinae) transmission between opossums and cats. J Protozool 31:584–587.

Besnoitia wallacei (Tadros and Laarman, 1976) Dubey, 1977

Etymology

Besnoitia (for Dr. C. Besnoit) *wallacei* (for Dr. G. Wallace).

Synonyms

Isospora wallacei Tadros and Laarman, 1976.

Geographic Distribution and Prevalence

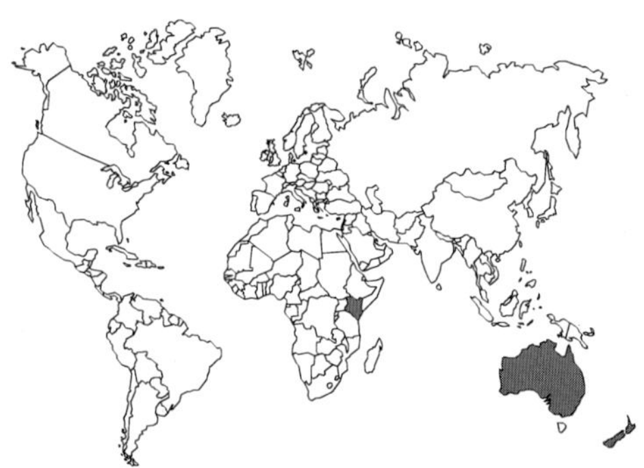

Fig. 1.30.

The prevalence of this parasite in cats is unknown. It has been reported from naturally infected cats from Oahu, Hawaii (Wallace and Frenkel, 1975), Palmerston North, New Zealand, and Kenya (Ng'ang'a et al., 1994). It has also been isolated from a cat fed naturally infected rats (*Rattus rattus, Rattus norvegicus*) collected near Launceston in Australia (Mason, 1980).

Parasite Identification

Oocysts measure 16–19 by 10–13 by μm (mean, 17 by 12 μm). No micropyle or polar granule is present. Two elliptical sporocysts are present. Sporocysts measure 11 by 7–8 μm (mean, 11 by 8 μm) and do not contain Stieda bodies. Four sporozoites are present in each sporocyst, and they measure approximately 2 by 10 μm.

Life Cycle

Only tissue cysts containing bradyzoites are infectious for cats (Wallace and Frenkel, 1975). The prepatent period is 12 to 15 days, and the patent period is 5 to 12 days. Only one asexual generation has been described, and it occurs in the lamina propria of the small intestine (Frenkel, 1977). The meronts measure between 500 and 800 μm and are found 4 to 13 days after infection. Some meronts can be found in extraintestinal tissues. Sexual stages are in goblet cells in the small intestinal epithelium. Macrogamonts are 16 to 13 μm, and microgamonts are about 11 μm. Tissue cysts do not form in the tissues of cats.

Grossly visible tissue cysts, up to 200 μm in diameter, are present in the tissues of mice 30 to 36 days after they are fed oocysts. The tissue cyst wall is up to 30 μm thick and contains numerous hypertrophic host cell nuclei.

Clinical Presentation and Pathogenesis

Clinical signs of infection in cats have not been reported.

Treatment

Besnoitia wallacei infection does not cause clinical disease in cats, and no treatment is needed.

REFERENCES

Frenkel JK. 1977. *Besnoitia wallacei* of cats and rodents: with a reclassification of other cyst-forming isosporoid coccidia. J Parasitol 63:611–628.
Mason RW. 1980. The discovery of *Besnoitia wallacei* in Australia and the identification of a free-living intermediate host. Z Parasitenkd 61:173–178.
Ng'ang'a CJ, Kanyari PW, Munyua WK. 1994. Isolation of *Besnoitia wallacei* in Kenya. Vet Parasitol 52:203–206.
Wallace GD, Frenkel JK. 1975. *Besnoitia* species (Protozoa, Sporozoa, Toxoplasmatidae): recognition of cyclic transmission by cats. Science 188: 369–371.

Haemogregarines—*Hepatozoon* Miller, 1908

A genus of apicomplexan parasites, *Hepatozoon* is occasionally found in cats. In this group of parasites, depending on the species involved, the gamonts are found within red or white blood cells of the vertebrate host; in the cat, the gamonts are found within the white blood cells. Sporogony and merogony occur within the body of the vector, a tick. Cats become infected by the ingestion of the infected tick rather than through the bite of the tick.

Hepatozoon felis Patton, 1908

Etymology

Hepato (liver) + *zoon* (animal) and *felis* for cat.

Synonyms

Haemogregarin felis-domesticae Patton, 1908; *Hepatozoon felisdomesticae* (Patton, 1908) Wenyon, 1926; *Leucocytozoon felis-domestici* (Patton, 1908) Patton, 1908. Some consider this a synonym of *Hepatozoon canis* (James, 1905) Wenyon, 1926.

History

This parasite was first described in the blood of domestic cats in India in 1908 by Patton. Since that time, there have been few other reports of *Hepatozoon* in cats. Schizonts were first reported in capillaries of cats in 1973 (Klopfer et al., 1973).

Geographic Distribution

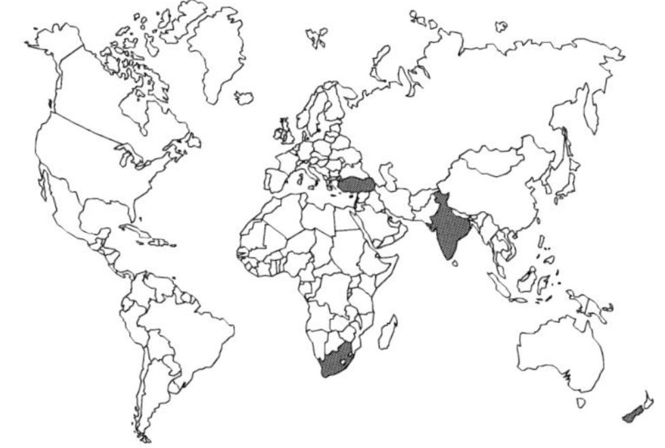

Fig. 1.31.

Patton (1908) observed *Hepatozoon felis* in cats in India. In Nigeria, *Hepatozoon* was reported from the blood of a cat that was part of a survey between 1966 and 1976 (Leeflang and Ilemobade, 1977). In Israel, stages of *Hepatozoon* have been observed at necropsy in the hearts of 30 percent of 50 cats that had been submitted for rabies examination (Klopfer et al., 1973) and in 42 percent of stray cats that were used for laboratory demonstrations (Nobel et al., 1974). *Hepatozoon* was seen in the liver of a cat that had originated from Hawaii (Ewing, 1977). The only other report has been from South Africa (van Amstel, 1979).

Location in Host

The circulating gamonts have been found in polymorphonuclear lymphocytes. In the cat, the only site in which schizont stages have been observed are in capillaries of the myocardium; however, it would be expected that other tissues would also be involved.

Parasite Identification

In the circulating neutrophils, the gamonts are elongate bodies with rounded ends, about 5 μm by 10 μm in size. There is a central compact nucleus that stains a dark red with Giemsa stain. The cytoplasm stains a light blue.

Within histological sections of the myocardium, the schizonts that have been described are of two types (Klopfer et al., 1973). In one type, the schizont appeared to be filled with individual merozoites. In the other type, the schizonts appeared to contain developing merozoites located around the periphery.

Life Cycle

The life cycle of *Hepatozoon felis* has been considered to be the same as that of *Hepatozoon canis,* which some actually consider the same parasite. Dogs can be infected by being fed a brown dog tick, *Rhipicephalus sanguineus,* that has previously been given a blood meal on a dog with circulating gametocytes (Nordgren and Craig, 1984). In the dog, two types of schizonts are formed that have been termed "microschizonts" and "macroschizonts." There has been no work on the vectors that may be involved in the transmission of this parasite between cats, and there has been very little examination of the development of different stages found within the cat.

Clinical Presentation and Pathogenesis

Clinical disease is rare, with schizonts being found in tissues of domestic cats at necropsy more frequently than clinical disease occurs. Progressive weight loss; ulcerative glossitis with hypersalivation; intermittent anorexia and pyrexia; progressive, nonresponsive anemia; and serous nasalocular discharge have been reported in one cat. Lymphadenopathy and icterus have also been reported. A progressive monocyte count with an increasing number of circulating monoblasts in peripheral blood resulting in a misdiagnosis of monocytic leukemia was made in one cat. The necrospy revealed the presence of *Hepatozoon felis* in the liver. A careful search of blood smears, bone marrow, and sections of other tissues failed to reveal any other organisms.

Treatment

There is a lack of effective treatment. Treatments tried in dogs have included oxytetracycline, chloramphenicol, sulfadimethoxine, diminazene aceturate, and dimidocarb dipropionate. The cat in South Africa treated by Van Amstel (1979) responded to treatment with oxytetracycline (50 mg/kg, BID, for 7 days) along with a single treatment of primaquine (2 mg *per os* 2 days after the initiation of oxytetracycline treatment).

Epizootiology

It is possible that the species in the cat actually represents infections with other species of *Hepatozoon,* such as *Hepatozoon canis* of the dog, *Hepatozoon procyonis,* which is common in raccoons (*Procyon lotor*) in the southern United States and in Central America, and *Hepatozoon* species of the bobcat *(Lynx rufus*), which is also common in the southern United States.

Hazards to Other Animals

Probably none, unless the cat also introduces the tick vector into the establishment. It might then be possible for the pathogen to be transmitted between animals in a boarding facility.

Hazards to Humans

None known.

Control/Prevention

Infection requires that the cat ingest an infected tick; therefore, it is important that the infestation of the cat with the tick be prevented. Unfortunately, the brown dog tick, *Rhipicephalus sanguineus,* will quite readily establish itself within a household. Thus, it may be necessary to hire exterminators to remove the tick if it has been introduced.

REFERENCES

Baneth G, Lavy E, Presentey B-Z, Shkap V. 1995. *Hepatozoon* sp. Parasitemia in a domestic cat. Feline Pract 23:10–12.

Ewing GO. 1977. Granulomatous cholangiohepatitis in a cat due to a protozoan parasite resembling *Hepatozoon canis.* Feline Pract 7:37-40.

Klopfer U, Nobel TA, Neumann F. 1973. *Hepatozoon*-like parasite (Schizonts) in the myocardium of the domestic cat. Vet Pathol 10:185–190.

Leeflang P, Ilemobade AA. 1977. Tick-borne disease of domestic animals in northern Nigeria. Trop Anim Prod 9:211–218.

Nobel TA, Neumann F, Klopfer U. 1974. Histopathology of the myocardium in 50 apparently healthy cats. Lab Anim 8:119–125.

Nordgren RM, Craig TM. 1984. Experimental transmission of the Texas strain of *Hepatozoon canis.* Vet Parasitol 16:207–214.

Patton WS. 1908. The haemogregarines of mammals and reptiles. Parasitology 1:318–321.

Van Amstel S. 1979. Hepatozoönosis in 'n kat. J S Afr Vet Assoc 10:215–216.

Wenyon CM. 1926. Protozoology. London, England: Baillere, Tindall, and Cox.

The Piroplasms: *Cytauxzoon* Neitz and Thomas, 1948, and *Babesia* Starcovici, 1893

Two genera of the phylum Apicomplexa, *Cytauxzoon* and *Babesia,* are included within a group called the piroplasms. These organisms when within the red blood cell appear very similar to malaria parasites. Individual piroplasms possess many of the typical elements of the apical complex that identify the Apicomplexa as such. The piroplasms are similar to the other apicomplexan protozoa in that there is fusion of gametes. The gametes of the piroplasms, however, cannot be morphologically distinguished from each other;

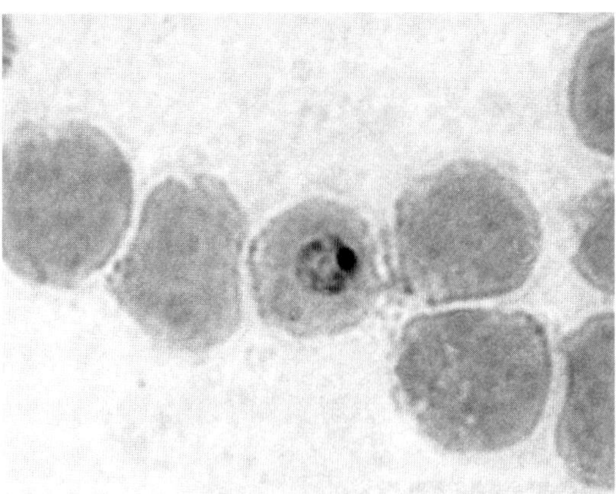

Fig. 1.32. *Babesia canis* trophozoite in a canine red blood cell. (Preparation supplied by Dr. P Conrad, College of Veterinary Medicine, University of California-Davis.) Giemsa stain.

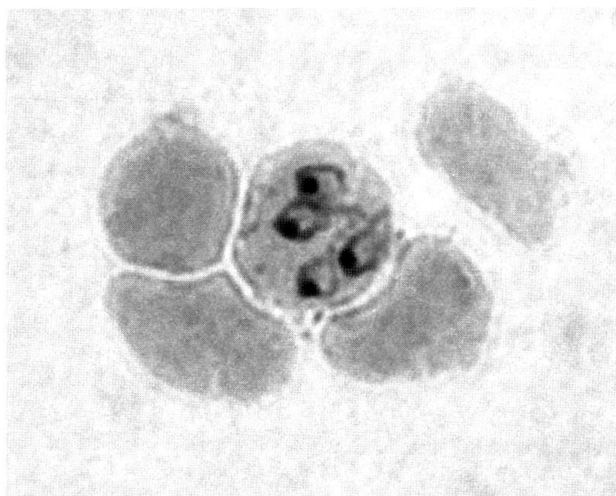

Fig. 1.33. *Babesia canis* schizont in a canine red blood cell. (Preparation supplied by Dr. P Conrad, College of Veterinary Medicine, University of California-Davis.) Giemsa stain.

that is, there is no distinguishable macrogamete and microgamete, and thus, they are termed isogamous. For the life cycles that are known, the gametes form within the stomach of the tick vector, and sporozoites that are ultimately produced from the union are found in the salivary glands of the tick. The genus *Babesia* was originally named for various blood parasites of large animals (Starcovici, 1893). *Babesia* species are also important parasites of dogs (Figs. 1.32 and 1.33). *Theileria* is a genus of piroplasm parasites that causes disease in African ungulates and other animals (Fig. 1.34); in the genus *Theileria,* schizogony

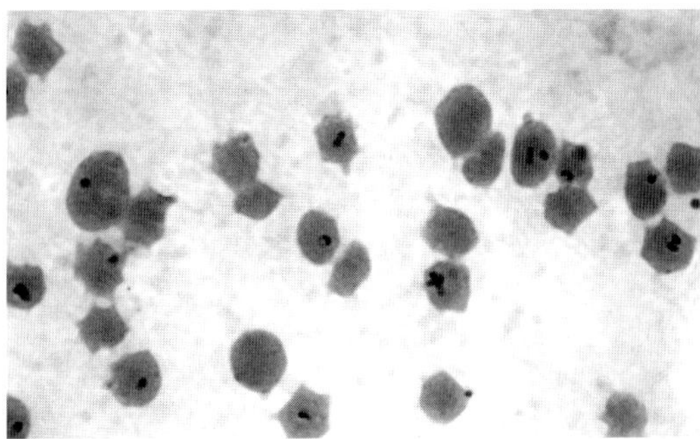

Fig. 1.34. *Theileria parva* in bovine red blood cells. Giemsa stain.

also occurs in white blood cells. The genus *Cytauxzoon* was originally named for similar blood parasites originally found in an African antelope (Neitz and Thomas, 1948). The schizonts of *Cytauxzoon* species occur in macrophages.

REFERENCES

Neitz WO, Thomas AD. 1948. *Cytauxzoon sylvicaprae* gen. nov., spec. nov., a protozoan responsible for a hitherto undescribed disease of the Duiker [*Sylvicapra grimmia* (Linné)]. Onderstep J Vet Sci Anim Ind 23:63–76.

Starcovici CG. 1893. Bemerkungen über den durch Babes entdecken Blutparasiten und die durch denselben hervorgebrachten Krankheiten, die seuchenhafte Hämoglovinurie des rindes (Babes), das Texasfieber (Th. smith) und der Carceag der Schafe (Babes). Centralblatt Bakterio 114:1–8.

Cytauxzoon felis Kier, 1979

Etymology

Kytos (cell) + *auxe* (an increase) + *zoon* (animal) and *felis* (cat).

Synonyms

Theileria felis (Kier, Wagner and Morehouse, 1982) Levine, 1982.

History

This parasite was first observed in African ungulates and described as a genus distinct from *Theileria* based on the fact that schizogony in *Cytauxzoon* occurred in histiocytes, while schizogony in *Theileria* occurs in lymphocytes. The parasite was first reported as a parasite of the domestic cat by Wagner in 1976. In 1979, Kier described in her doctoral dissertation the parasite observed in the cat as a new species, *Cytauxzoon felis*. In 1985, Levine considered *Cytauxzoon* synonymous with the genus *Theileria* and transferred the name "felis" to this genus. If one accepts the differentiation of *Cytauxzoon* and *Theileria* on the basis that schizogony occurs in histiocytes in the former and lymphocytes in the latter, then the name would be *Cytauxzoon felis*. It is possible that a species of *Babesia* observed in a blood smear from an American bobcat (*Lynx rufus*) by Wenyon and Hamerton in 1930 was *Cytauxzoon*, but it was not recognized as such.

Geographic Distribution

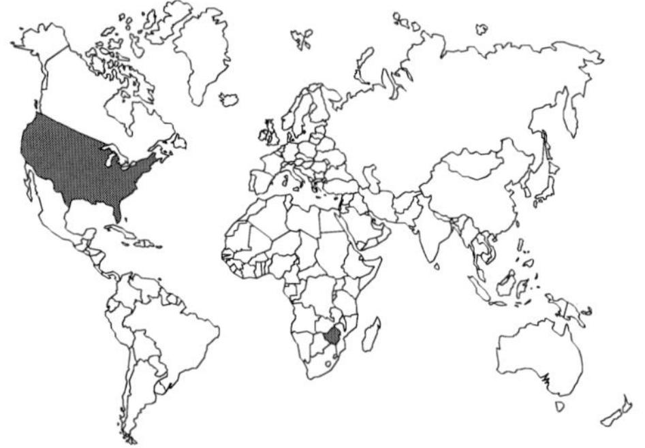

Fig. 1.35.

Most of the cases of cytauxzoonosis have been reported from the south central and southeastern United States (Motzel and Wagner, 1990). There is a single case of cytauxzoonosis-like disease reported from Zimbabwe (Foggin and Roberts, 1982), but it is difficult to ascertain the validity of this claim on the basis of the published material.

Location in Host

Merozoites can be found in erythrocytes; typical parasitemias are 1 to 4 percent of the red blood cells. Due to the fulminant course of disease in the cat, it is more typical to observe the large schizonts in the walls of the venous system in histopathologic sections. Schizonts may also be observed in bone-marrow aspirates.

Parasite Identification

In the erythrocytes, the merozoites are characterized by their small size. There is typically a single organism per red blood cell, but occasionally two to four organisms may be present. The ultrastructural morphology of the intraerythrocytic form was described by Simpson et al. (1985a).

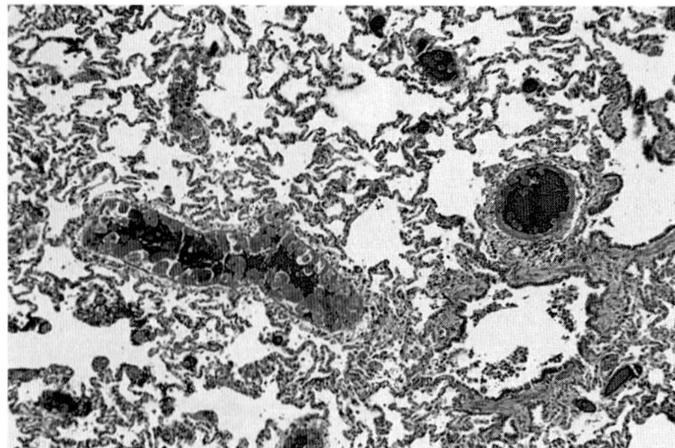

Fig. 1.36. *Cytauxzoon felis* schizonts in an H&E-stained section of the lung of a cat that died after being inoculated with the blood of a Florida panther. Schizonts can be observed lining the blood vessels in this section of lung.

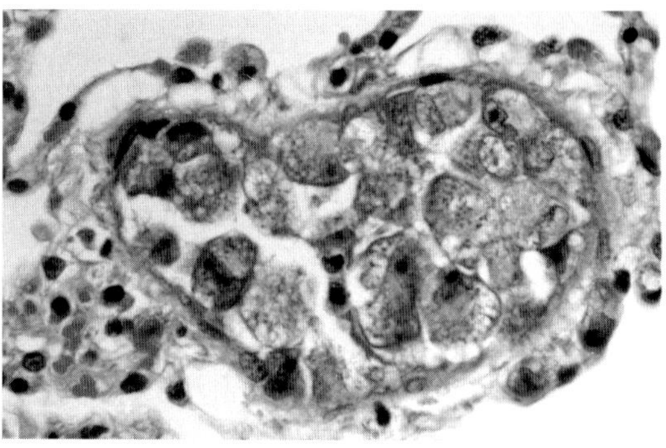

Fig. 1.37. *Cytauxzoon felis* schizonts in an H&E-stained section of the lung of a cat that died after being inoculated with the blood of a Florida panther. In this higher-power image of another blood vessel in the lung shown in Fig 1.36, the schizonts can be observed to be occluding the lumen of the blood vessel.

Schizonts may be found in veinules of the lung, liver, spleen, bone marrow, kidney, and brain (Figs. 1.36 and 1.37). The developing schizonts cause an enlargement of the infected cell, which may reach 75 μm in diameter. The ultrastructure of the schizont has been described (Simpson et al., 1985b). The morphology of schizonts within bone-marrow aspirates is much like those observed in histopathologic sections. Again, the cells become very large and contain large numbers of developing organisms.

Cytauxzoon felis has been shown to be antigenically distinct from *Babesia felis* using an indirect fluorescent antibody test (Uilenberg et al., 1987).

Life Cycle

The life cycle has been poorly described, and basically, descriptions have been developed using parallels with what is known concerning the related genus *Theileria.* In the blood of the felid, merozoites circulate within the red blood cells. (It is believed that gametogony may not occur until after the red blood cells are in the stomach of the tick.) Within the tick's stomach, it is presumed that the gametocytes undergo development and sexual fusion and ultimately produce sporozoites within the salivary glands of the tick. Once inoculated into the cat, it is not known where the sporozoites first take up residence; however, within a few days, schizonts are found within histiocytes of veins and veinules of various organs, including the liver, lungs, spleen, lymph nodes, brain, and kidneys. Within 6 to 8 days after inoculation, merozoites can be found in the peripheral blood (Franks et al., 1988). It is not known how long after the appearance of organisms in the blood that infectivity for the tick vector develops.

Clinical Presentation and Pathogenesis

Usually, by the time the cat is presented, it is severely ill. Signs include anemia and depression that may be accompanied by high fever, dehydration, icterus, splenomegaly, and hepatomegaly. Packed cell volumes decrease markedly by 6 days after infection, but the anemia is regenerative (Franks et al., 1988). Plasma appears icteric on the last day or two of life. The platelet count is decreased, but prothrombin or activated partial thromboplastin times are normal. Although there are no significant changes in total leucocyte counts or absolute neutrophil, monocyte, or basophil counts, lymphocyte and eosinophil counts are decreased markedly within 8 days after infection. Bone-marrow aspirates often contain large mononuclear cells containing schizonts. Almost all cats die within 9 to 15 days after infection. The percentage of red blood cells containing organisms is typically between 1 and 4 percent, although 25 percent of red blood cells may be infected.

Inoculation of cats with blood from bobcats containing the merozoite stage will produce persistent parasitemias in red blood cells without inducing cytauxzoonosis (Kier et al., 1982a; Blouin et al., 1984). It is believed this is due to the stage being passed being the stage that is restricted to the blood cells and that passage through the tick vector is required to produce the schizogonous stages that can typically be induced by the inoculation of splenic tissue.

Recently, cats have been identified that have survived natural infections with *Cytauxzoon felis* (Meinkoth et al., 2000). These authors described 18 cats from northwestern Arkansas and northeastern Oklahoma. Most of the cats had clinical signs, although four were without signs. Only one of the infected cats had received treatment with an antiprotozoal, and four of the surviving cats received no treatment. The authors postulated that they may have been dealing with a less virulent strain of this parasite.

Treatment

Attempts have been made to treat experimentally induced cytauxzoonosis with parvaquone (Clexon·) and buparvaquone (Butalex·); both drugs have been shown to be successful in treating theileriosis in cattle. In the regimen employed, the disease still proved fatal. Over a 24-hour period, a cat that presented with a 2-day history of lethargy and anorexia became seriously icteric and had dark brown urine (Walker and Cowell, 1995). The cat was treated with a 10-day course of enrofloxacin followed by a 5-day course of tetracycline. Organisms were present in the cat after the 10-day course of enrofloxacin but were not present in blood samples collected 6 and 15 weeks after discharge. It is not known why this cat survived; enrofloxacin is not known to be effective against protozoa. Most success in treatment has been achieved with diminizine and imidocarb. One very ill cat responded rapidly to treatment with intravenous fluids, enrofloxacin and diminizine aceturate, and heparin for prevention of disseminated intravascular clotting. Diminizine (2 mg/kg IM) was repeated weekly for two more treatments. Imidocarb dipropionate (5 mg/kg IM, twice, 2 weeks apart) has been found to produce a 50 percent cure rate (Greene et al., 1999).

Epizootiology

The life cycle appears to involve the bobcat, *Lynx rufus,* as the mammalian reservoir of infection (Glenn et al., 1982) and ticks, including *Dermacentor variabilis,* as vectors (Blouin et al., 1984). The domestic cat apparently enters the life cycle typically when it is bitten by an infected tick. After the cat is bitten by an infected tick, it will usually die of the infection in 2 weeks.

Cytauxzoon felis has also been found to be present in the blood of the Florida panther (*Felis concolor coryi*). From the infected panther, it was transmitted to a domestic cat in the buffy coat of a blood sample, and in the cat, it induced fatal disease (Butt et al., 1991). *Cytauxzoon*-like organisms have been observed in the erythrocytes of two cheetahs (*Acinonyx jubatus*) that were born and raised in the United States, in Oregon, and which had spent 2 months being trained to hunt in Namibia, Africa, as part of a release program (Zinkl et al., 1981). Inoculation of a cat with blood from one of these cheetahs produced no signs of disease or demonstrable parasitemia.

Hazards to Other Animals

The fatal disease typically induced in the cat prevents it from being an important reservoir of infection. A wide range of mammalian hosts have been inoculated with *Cytauxzoon felis* without the induction of parasitemias (Kier et al., 1982b), with sheep being the only host that appear to develop a persistent, but low, level of circulating organisms.

Hazards to Humans

Cytauxzoon felis is not known to infect humans although transmission to primates using stages from ticks have not been tried.

Control/Prevention

The only form of control is to prevent cats that share the same geographical distribution as the bobcat from being bitten by ticks. The inoculation of a cat with stages grown in tissue culture appeared to induce an immunity (Ferris, 1979), and thus, it may be possible to someday prevent the disease in cats by vaccination.

REFERENCES

Blouin EF, Kocan AA, Glenn BL, Kocan KM. 1984. Transmission of *Cytauxzoon felis* Kier, 1979 from Bobcats, *Felis rufus* (Schreber), to domestic cats by *Dermacentor variabilis* (Say). J Wildl Dis 20:241–242.

Butt MT, Bowman DD, Barr MC, Roelke ME. 1991. Iatrogenic transmission of *Cytauxzoon felis* from a Florida panther (*Felix concolor coryi*) to a domestic cat. J Wildl Dis 27:342–347.

Ferris DH. 1979. A progress report on the status of a new disease of American cats: cytauxzoonosis. Comp Immunol Microbiol Infect Dis 1:269–276.

Foggin CM, Roberts HM. 1982. A cytauxzoonosis-like disease in a cat in Zimbabwe. Zimbabwe Vet J 13:28–29.

Franks PT, Harvey JW, Shield RP, Lawman MJP. 1988. Hematological findings in experimental feline cytauxzoonosis. J Am Anim Hosp Assoc 24:395–401.

Glenn BL, Kocan AA, Blouin EF. 1982. Cytauxzoonosis in bobcats. JAVMA 183:1155–1158.

Greene CE, Latimer K, Hopper E, Shoeffler G, Lower K, Cullens F. 1999. Administration of diminazen aceturate on imidocarb dipropionate for treatment of cytauxzoonosis in cats. JAVMA 215:497–500.

Kier AB. 1979. The etiology and pathogenesis of feline cytauxzoonosis. PhD dissertation, University of Missouri, Columbia, Mo.

Kier AB, Greene CE. 1998. Cytauxzoonosis. In Infectious Diseases of the Dog and Cat, CE Greene (ed). Philadelphia, Pa: WB Saunders, pp 470–473.

Kier AB, Wagner JE, Morehouse LG. 1982a. Experimental transmission of *Cytauxzoon felis* from bobcats (*Lynx rufus*) to domestic cats (*Felis domesticus*). Am J Vet Res 43:97–101.

Kier AB, Wightman SR, Wagner JE. 1982b. Interspecies transmission of *Cytauxzoon felis*. Am J Vet Res 43:102–105.

Levine ND. 1985. Veterinary Protozoology, 2nd edition. Ames: Iowa State University Press. 414 pp.

Meinkoth J, Kocan AA, Whitworth L, Murphy G, Fox JC, Woods JP. 2000. Cats surviving natural infection with *Cytauxzoon felis:* 18 cases (1997–1998). J Vet Intern Med 14:521–525.

Motzel SL, Wagner JE. 1990. Treatment of experimentally induced cytauxzoonosis in cats with parvaquone and buparvaquone. Vet Parasitol 35:131–138.

Simpson CH, Harvey JW, Carlisle JW. 1985a. Ultrastructure of the intraerythrocytic stage of *Cytauxzoon felis*. Am J Vet Res 46:1178–1180.

Simpson CH, Harvey JW, Lawman MJP, Murray J, Kocan AA, Carlisle JW. 1985b. Ultrastructure of schizonts in the liver of cats with experimentally induced cytauxzoonosis. Am J Vet Res 46:384–390.

Uilenberg G, Franssen FFJ, Perié NM. 1987. Relationships between *Cytauxzoon felis* and African piroplasmids. Vet Parasitol 26:21–28.

Wagner, JE. 1976. A fatal cytozoonosis-like disease in cats. J Am Vet Med Assoc 168:585–588.

Walker DB, Cowell RL. 1995. Survival of a domestic cat with naturally acquired cytauxzoonosis. JAVMA 206:1363–1365.
Wenyon CM, Hamerton AE. 1930. Piroplasms of the West African civet cat (*Viverra civetta*) and the Bay lynx (*Felis rufa*) of North America. Trans Roy Soc Trop Med Hyg 24:7–8.
Zinkl JG, McDonald SE, Kier AB, Cippa SJ, Small PJ. 1981. *Cytauxzoon*-like organisms in erythrocytes of two cheetahs. JAVMA 179:1261–1262.

Babesia felis Davis, 1929

Etymology

Babesia for Dr. Babès and *felis* (cat).

Synonyms

Babesiella felis (Davis, 1929) Carpano, 1934; *Nuttallia felis* (Davis, 1929) Krylov, 1974; *Nuttallia felis* var. *domestica* Jackson and Dunning, 1937; *Nicollia felis* (Davis, 1929) Krylov, 1981.

History

Babesia felis was first described as a parasite of the domestic cat by Jackson and Dunning in 1937; these authors gave it the name *Nuttallia* (a synonym of *Babesia*) *felis* of the variety *domestica.* The variety designation was to separate it on the basis of its pathogenicity from a previously described, but morphologically indistinguishable, *Babesia felis* described by Davis in 1929 from a Sudanese wild cat (*Felis ochreata*) that was not pathogenic when inoculated into domestic cats.

Geographic Distribution

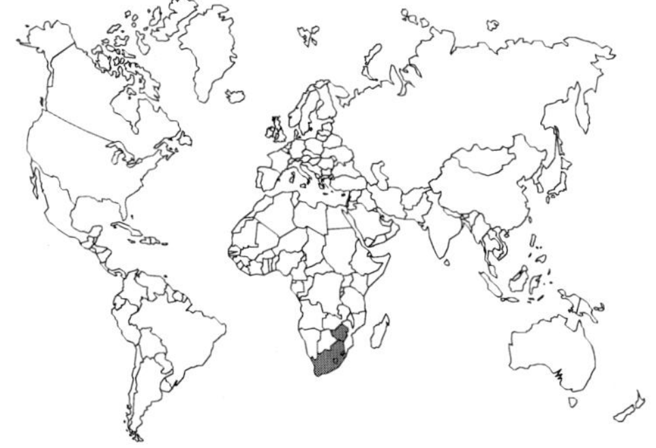

Fig. 1.38.

Reports of feline babesiosis due to *Babesia felis* are restricted almost exclusively to Zimbabwe and South Africa (Futter and Belonje, 1980a). The original isolate from a Sudanese wild cat was established experimentally in domestic cats (Davis, 1929).

Location in Host

The only cells in the body parasitized by merozoites of *Babesia* species are the red blood cells.

Parasite Identification

The merozoites of *Babesia felis* that occur within the red cell are small, faintly blue-staining organisms that have a dense chromatin granule. Many forms have a large central vacuole that gives them the appearance of being ring shaped. Single organisms measure less than 1 to 2.5 μm in diameter. Division of the organisms produces pairs and cross-shaped tetrads of organisms. The ultrastructure of *Babesia felis* was described by Dennig and Hebel (1969).

Life Cycle

The life cycle of *Babesia felis* has not been elucidated, but it is believed that ixodid ticks serve as the biological vector of the parasite. In 1937, Dr. McNeil reported that he reared larval and nymphal ticks from an adult female *Haemaphysalis leachi* that was removed from a cat with babesiosis. Neither the eggs nor the nymphs that developed transmitted the disease to cats upon which they were fed. The bottle containing the imago ticks was then broken, and the ticks escaped, and Dr. McNeil without evidence or proof was convinced that they were the source of babesiosis that developed in his own household cat. There have been no other studies on the transmission of feline babesiosis.

If, as suspected, the life cycle utilizes ixodid ticks that have fed on cats, sporozoites will develop within the salivary glands of the tick. Within the tick there is the possibility that the different stages—larvae, nymphs, and adults—may differ in their ability to transmit the infections, and further work is needed to clarify this in the case of *Babesia felis.*

Once in a cat, the merozoites infect blood cells, dividing and multiplying to form stages infecting new blood cells. In cats that have been inoculated with blood from other cats, parasites are evident within the peripheral blood within 1 to 2 days after inoculation (Futter and Belonje, 1980b). It is not known how long after the appearance of organisms in the blood that infectivity for the tick vector might develop.

Clinical Presentation and Pathogenesis

Cats are typically admitted that have a history of inappetence and lethargy and are weak or moribund. Mucous membranes may be pale, and tachycardia and tachypnea (perhaps dyspnea) consistent with profound anemia may be noted. Icterus is seldom seen, and fever does not seem to typically accompany the disease (Futter and Belonje, 1980b). In experimentally infected animals, anemia is most severe about 3 weeks after inoculation, and there are significantly lowered hematocrits, hemoglobin levels, and erythrocyte numbers (Futter et al., 1980). Erythrocytes tend to be macrocytic and hypochromic. There are no significant changes in total leukocyte counts initially. In most cases liver function, renal function, and venous blood pH will remain normal (Futter et al., 1981). Without treatment, cats are very likely to die of severe anemia. Of 70 naturally infected cats, 50 recovered, 7 died, 7 were euthanatized (3 were strays, 1 for chronic respiratory disease, 1 for aplastic anemia, and 2 for unstated reasons), and 6 were lost to follow-up (Futter and Belonje, 1980b).

Treatment

Treatment with primaquine phosphate will often lead to a rapid and successful recovery. In cases of severe anemia and prostration, it may be necessary to also give a blood transfusion followed by primaquine therapy. However, the current effective dose (0.5mg/kg, IM, once) is very close to the lethal dose in cats (1 mg/kg).

Epizootiology

It would appear that *Babesia felis* is a parasite of the cat. There may have been some initial African source of this parasite, but the parasite now seems mainly to affect its domestic host.

Hazards to Other Animals

Specimens of *Babesia* considered to be *Babesia felis* by some workers (Dennig and Brocklesby, 1972) have been found in the blood of a puma, *Felix concolor,* that had been housed in a zoo in Egypt (Carpano, 1934) and in a blood smear from an Indian leopard, *Panthera pardus fusca* (Shortt, 1940). As stated above, *Babesia felis* was first noted in the blood of a Sudanese wild cat (*Felis ocreata*). It would appear that there has been little spread of this parasite between cats and wildlife.

Hazards to Humans

Although humans have been infected with species of *Babesia,* these have been felt to be mainly of bovine and murine types. None have been considered as being due to *Babesia felis.*

Control/Prevention

The disease can be controlled by preventing tick infestations and by treatment of cats that have circulating stages in their bloodstream.

REFERENCES

Carpano M. 1934. Sur les piroplasmoses des carnassiers et wur un noveau piroplasme des félins (*Babesiella felis*) chez le puma: *Felis concor.* Bull Min Agric Egypt Tech Sci Ser No 136. 20 pp.

Davis LJ. 1929. On a piroplasm of the Sudanese Wild Cat (*Felix ocreata*). Trans Roy Soc Trop Med Hyg 22:523–534.

Dennig HK, Brocklesby DW. 1972. *Babesia pantherae* sp. nov. A piroplasm of the leopard (*Panthera pardus*). Parasitology 64:525–532.

Dennig HK, Hebel R. 1969. Licht- und elektronenmikroskopische Untersuchungen an zwei *Babesia*–Arten der Feliden. Ztschr Parasitenk 32:95–111.

Futter GJ, Belonje PC. 1980a. Studies on feline babesiosis. 1. Historical review. J S Afr Vet Assoc 50:105–106.

Futter GJ, Belonje PC. 1980b. Studies on feline babesiosis. 2. Clinical observations. J S Afr Vet Assoc 51:143–146.

Futter GJ, Belonje PC, Van Den Berg A. 1980. Studies on feline babesiosis. 3. Haematological findings. J S Afr Vet Assoc 51:272–280.

Futter GJ, Belonje PC, Van Den Berg A, Van Rijswijk AW. 1981. Studies on feline babesiosis. 4. Chemical pathology; macroscopic and microscopic *post mortem* findings. J S Afr Vet Assoc 52:5–14.

Jackson C, Dunning FJ. 1937. Biliary fever (Nuttalliosis) of the cat: a case in the Stellenbosch district. J S Afr Vet Med Assoc 8:83–87.

McNeil J. 1937. Piroplasmosis of the domestic cat. J S Afr Vet Med Assoc 8:88–90.
Shortt HE. 1940. *Babesia* sp. in the Indian leopard, *Panthera pardus fusca* (Meyer). Ind J Med Res 28:277–278.

Babesia cati Mudaliar, Achary, and Alwar, 1950

Etymology

Babesia for Dr. Babès and *cati* (cat).

Synonyms

None.

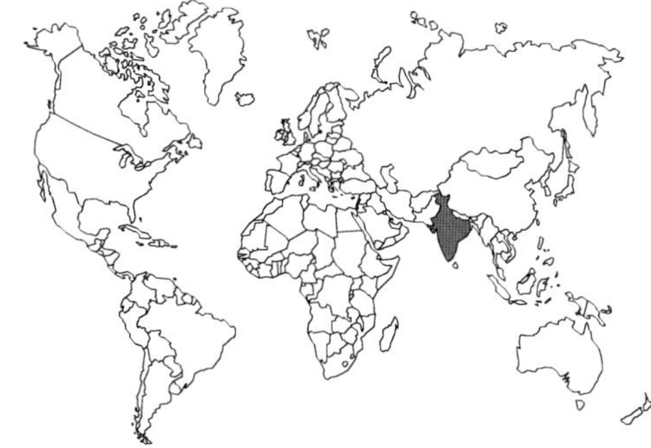

Fig. 1.39.

This parasite was described from a domestic cat in India at the Madras Veterinary College (Mudaliar, Achary, Alwar, 1950). Previously, a similar parasite had been noted in blood cells of a domestic cat necropsied in northern India (Mangrulkar, 1937). *Babesia cati,* like *Babesia felis,* is a small form of *Babesia. Babesia cati* is believed to differ from *Babesia felis* in that no cross-shaped dividing forms indicative of quaternary division within the red blood cell have been noted.

REFERENCES

Mangrulkar MY. 1937. On a piroplasm of the Indian cat (*Felis domesticus*). Ind J Vet Sci Anim Husb 7:243–246.
Mudaliar SV, Achary GR, Alwar VS. 1950. On a species of *Babesia* on an Indian wild cat (*Felis catus*). Ind Vet J 26:391–395.

Babesia herpailuri Dennig, 1967

Etymology

Babesia for Dr. Babès and *herpailuri* (genus of the jaguarundi).

Synonyms

None.

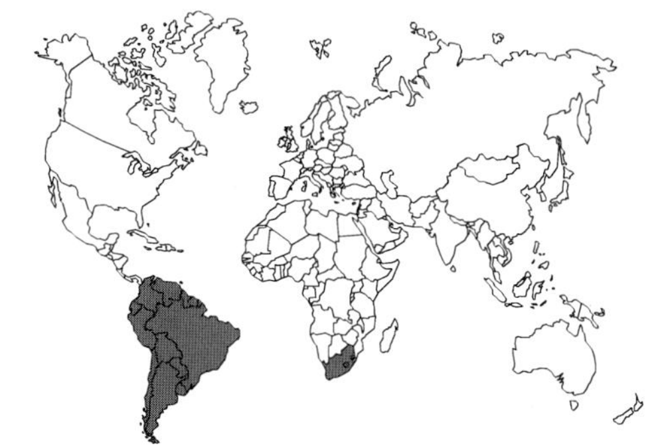

Fig. 1.40.

This parasite was originally reported from a South American jaguarundi, *Felis yagouaroundi* (syn. *Herpailurus jaguarundi*), and shown capable of persisting in domestic cats after inoculation of blood from the infected jagurundi (Dennig, 1967, 1969). A similar organism was seen again in the blood of a domestic cat with anemia in South Africa (Stewart et al., 1980). *Babesia herpailuri* represents a large form of *Babesia* that is differentiated from *Babesia felis* and *Babesia cati* by its larger size. Like *Babesia cati, Babesia herpailuri* does not form cruciform shapes typical of quaternary division within the red blood cell.

REFERENCES

Dennig HK. 1967. Eine unbekannte Babeienart beim Jaguarundi (*Herpailurus yagouarundi*). Kleintierpraxis 12:146–152.
Dennig HK. 1969. Babesieningektionen bei exotischen Katzen und die Bedeutung dieser Blutparasiten für die tierärtliche Forschung. Acta Zool Pathol Antverp 48:361–367
Stewart CG, Hackett KJW, Collett MG. 1980. An unidentified *Babesia* of the domestic cat (*Felis domesticus*). J S Afr Vet Assoc 51:219–221.

SARCOMASTIGOPHORA

The Sarcomastigophora (the flagellates) represent protozoa that have one to several large flagella. They are often grouped for the purposes of medicine on the basis of where they are found, and thus, two groups are considered: the mucosoflagellates and the flagellates of blood and tissues. The mucosoflagellates are not a "natural" grouping but rather a useful collection of parasites that live in the digestive and reproductive tracts. The blood and tissue flagellates make up a group of "related" parasites (i.e., trypanosomes and leishmanial organisms) that have morphologically similar stages as part of their life cycle.

Mucosoflagellates

There are three mucosoflagellate parasites of the cat, *Tetratrichomonas felistomae, Pentatrichomonas hominis,* and *Giardia felis.* Two of these parasites, *Tetratrichomonas felistomae* and *Pentatrichomonas hominis,* are quite similar morphologically and live in the mouth and the cecum/colon, respectively. The other mucosoflagellate, *Giardia felis,* is a parasite of the small intestine of the cat and is quite different morphologically and behaviorally from the trichomonads in that it has two nuclei in the trophozoite stage and produces a resistant cyst stage. The trichomonads have only a single nucleus and no resistant stage as part of their biology.

Tetratrichomonas felistomae (Hegner and Ratcliffe, 1927) Honigberg, 1978

Etymology

Tetra (four) + *tricho* (hair) + *monas* (body) and *felis* (cat) + *stomae* (mouth).

Synonyms

Trichomonas felistomae Hegner and Ratcliffe, 1927.

History

Tetratrichomonas felistomae was first described as a trichomonad from the mouths of cats by Hegner and Ratcliffe (1927a). Later that same year, they also described the species from the mouths of dogs, *Trichomonas canistomae* (Hegner and Ratcliffe, 1927b); thus, if the species in the dog and the cat are the same, the name for that from the cat has priority. The genus *Tetratrichomonas* was established by Honigberg in 1978 for those species of *Trichomonas* that have four anterior flagella and a trailing free flagellum. Recent work by Gothe et al. (1992) revealed that trichomonads recovered from the mouths of cats in Germany do not have a free flagellum, and it may be that this is either a different species or that the original description was in error.

Geographic Distribution

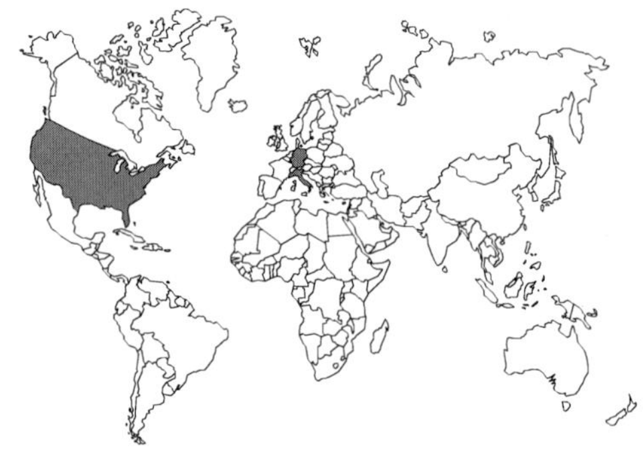

Fig. 1.41.

There is very little information on the presence of this parasite in the mouths of cats. It has been reported from the mouths of 2 of 28 cats in the United States (Hegner and Ratcliffe, 1927a) and from 21 of 110 cats from Germany and Italy (Gothe et al., 1992).

Location in Host

In the mouth, typically along the gum line.

Parasite Identification

These trophozoites have a length of about 6 to 11 μm and a width of about 3 to 4 μm. There is a marked axostyle that runs the length of the body from the base of the flagellum that appears to protrude from the posterior end. Along one side of the body is an undulating membrane that has about three undulations along its length. The original description contains a long free flagellum that is about equal in length to the portion making up the undulating membrane. Also described is a rather dense costa that runs along the cell under the site of attachment of the undulating membrane. The organism described by Gothe et al. had no free flagellum at the end of the undulating membrane. The lack of the free flagellum led these authors to postulate that this was actually a member of the genus *Trichomonas*.

Life Cycle

Trichomonads display a jerky, rapid, and erratic swimming behavior caused by the movement of the flagella. There is no cyst stage in the life cycle, and this parasite is transmitted from cat to cat by direct contact.

Clinical Presentation and Pathogenesis

Gothe et al. (1992) found trichomonads only in the mouths of cats that were FIV, FeLV, or FIP (feline infectious peritonitis virus) positive. Typically, the organisms were found only in cats that had gingivitis and that had one of these viral infections. Cats that had stomatitis due to other causes and cats that were clinically normal were not found to harbor these parasites.

Treatment

Treatment has not been tried, but it is expected that improved oral hygiene will reduce the possibility that trichomonads are present within the mouth of cats.

Epizootiology

This parasite is transmitted from cat to cat by oral contact. It appears to be more prevalent in cats that have underlying viral infections that predispose to stomatitis.

Hazards to Other Animals

It is not well understood whether this parasite is transmissible to other animals.

Hazards to Humans

It is not well understood whether this parasite is transmissible to human beings.

REFERENCES

Gothe R, Beelitz P, Schöl H, Beer B. 1992. Trichomonaden-Infektionen der Mundhöhle bei Katzen in Süddeutschland. Tierärztl Prax 20:195–198.

Hegner R, Ratcliffe H. 1927a. Trichomonads from the vagina of the monkey, from the mouth of the cat and man, and from the intestine of the monkey, opossum and prairie-dog. J Parasitol 14:27–35.

Hegner R, Ratcliffe H. 1927b. Trichomonads from the mouth of the dog. J Parasitol 14:51–53.

Honigberg BM. 1978. Trichomonads of veterinary importance. In Parasitic Protozoa, vol II, ed JP Kreier, pp 163–273. New York, NY: Academic Press.

Pentatrichomonas hominis (Davaine, 1860) Wenrich, 1931

Trichomonads have been described from the large intestine of cats (Wenrich, 1944). The species in the intestine of the cat is not the same as that found in the mouth of the cat and other animals. The parasite from the intestine of the cat has been considered a separate species by some authors (Brumpt, 1925; Cunha and Muniz, 1922); however, others have felt that it is the same species found in humans and other animals, such as the dog. The organism in the feces of humans has been shown capable of infecting cats that are orally inoculated with trophozoites (Kessel, 1926; Hegner and Eskridge, 1935). Reports of trichomoniasis from cats have been reported from the United States (Jordan, 1956; Hegner and Eskridge, 1935; Hitchcock, 1953; Visco et al., 1978), Europe (Brumpt, 1925; Simic, 1932; Wagner and Hees, 1935), South America (Cunha and Muniz, 1922), and China (Kessel, 1926, 1928).

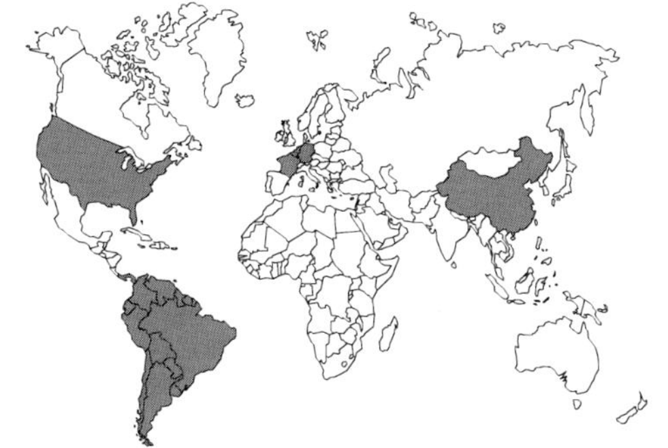

Fig. 1.42.

It does not appear that this organism causes disease in the cat; rather it is a commensal that is found in feces of cats with diarrhea due to other causes. On the other hand, Romatowski (2000) described pentatrichomoniasis in four kittens.

One cat had severe colitis that did not respond to treatment, and the trichomonads appeared in the feces after the diarrhea. A second cat had loose feces that persisted for several months after the trichomonads disappeared from the feces, but fecal consistency was normal as long as the cat received treatment with enrofloxacin. A third cat responded well to treatment with metronidazole. The fourth cat was euthanatized without treatment. All these cats were quite young, varying in age from 2 to 4 months at the time of presentation. Previously, Romatowski (1996) had presented a series of cases in three kittens. In another recent study, Gookin et al. (1999) examined the effect of pentatrichomoniasis in a large number of cases. These authors found most of the infections were in cats that were less than or equal to a year of age at the time of diagnosis. The feces of affected cats were typically malodorous and pasty to semiformed and were found to often contain fresh blood and mucus. Defecation was associated with flatulence and tenesmus. The soft stools tended to persist from days to years, but typically lasted about 5 months.

There does not seem to be a specific treatment that is highly efficacious for the removal of these protozoa from the colon of infected cats. Romatowski (2000) used both metronidazole and enroflaxacin and suggested that the long-term daily administration of enrofloxacin was a means of suppressing the soft stools associated with this infection. Gookin et al. reported that they tried paromomycin, fenbendazole, and furazolidone and in all cases had mixed success. The stools would often improve in consistency; however, the organisms often appeared to be present at low levels since they could be detected by protozoal culture of the feces even in stools that had normal consistency. Gookin et al. also reported that many of the cats they saw came to the hospital after having been treated by the referring veterinarians with a wide assortment of compounds: metronidazole, fenbendazole, albendazole, pyrantel pamoate, sulfadimethoxine, trimethoprim-sulfadiazine, furazolidone, tylosin, enrofloxacin, amoxicillin, clindamycin, and erythromycin.

The question still remains as to whether or not the organism is the cause of the associated diarrhea or another manifestation of some underlying problem. As stated by Romatowski: Diarrhea in cats infected with *P. hominis* can be difficult to treat, and disappearance of trophozoites from fecal smears does not necessarily correlate with improvement in clinical signs. Gookin et al. suggested that *P. hominis* may be a cofactor in the development of diarrhea in young kittens. The possibility still remains that there is some other cause of the underlying diarrhea and that the presence of a different microbiological flora in the colon when large quantities of fluid material are present is such that *P. hominis* multiplies in number. Arguing against this was the inability of Gookin et al. to establish cultures of organisms from normal feces of 100 random-source cats, while they did isolate it from the normal feces of cats that had been treated with fenbendazole and furazolidone.

REFERENCES

Brumpt E. 1925. Recherches morphologiques et expérimentales sur le *Trichomonas felis* da Cunha et Muniz, 1922, parasite du chat et du chien. Ann Parasitol Hum Comp 3:239–251.

Cunha AM, Muniz J. 1922. Sobre un flagellado parasito do gato. Brasil-Medico 1:285–286.

Gookin JL, Breitschwerdt EB, Levy MG, Gager RB, Benrud JG. 1999. Diarrhea associated with trichomonosis in cats. JAVMA 215(10):1450–1454.

Hegner R, Eskridge L. 1935. Absence of pathogenicity in cats infected with *Trichomonas felis* from cats and *Trichomonas hominis* from man. Am J Hyg 22:322–325.

Hitchcock DJ. 1953. Incidence of gastro-intestinal parasites in some Michigan kittens. N Am Vet 34:428–429.

Jordan HE. 1956. Trichomoniasis spp. in feline: a case report. Vet Med 51:23–24.

Kessel JF. 1926. Trichomoniasis in kittens. Proc Soc Exp Biol Med 24:200–202.

Kessel JF. 1928. Trichomoniasis in kittens. Trans R Soc Trop Med Hyg 22:61–80.

Romatowski J. 1996. An uncommon protozoan parasite (*Pentatrichomonas hominis*) associated with colitis in three cats. Feline Pract 24:10–14.

Romatowski J. 2000. *Pentatrichomonas hominis* infection in four kittens. JAVMA 216:1270–1272.

Simic T. 1932. Étude biologique et expérimentale du *Trichomonas intestinalis,* infectant spontanément l'homme, le chat et le chien. Ann Parasitol Hum Comp 10:209–224.

Visco EJ, Corwin RM, Selby LA. 1978. Effect of age and sex on the prevalence of intestinal parasitism in cats. JAVMA 172:797–800.

Wagner O, Hees E. 1935. Der kulturelle Nachweis von *Trichomonas vaginalis* und anderen Trichomonasarten. Zntralb Bakteriol 135:310–317.

Wenrich DH. 1944. Morphology of the intestinal trichomond flagellates in man and of similar forms in monkeys, cats, dogs, and rats. J Morphol 74:189–211.

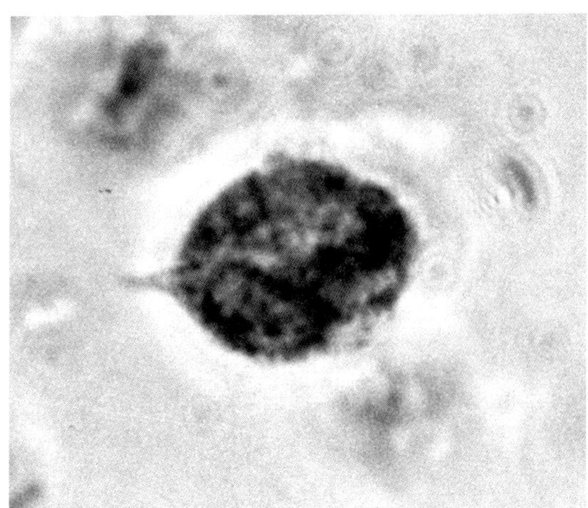

Fig. 1.43. *Pentatrichomonas hominis* trophozoite in human feces. The organism was fixed then stained with iron hematoxylin and photographed using phase microscopy. The large nucleus of the trophozoite and the undulating membrane can be seen in this photomicrograph.

Giardia felis Hegner, 1925

Etymology

Giardia for Dr. Giard (1846–1908) and *felis* for the feline host.

Synonyms

Giardia lamblia Stiles, 1915; *Giardia duodenalis* (Daviane, 1875); *Giardia cati* Deschiens, 1925.

History

The organism was discovered by Leeuwenhoek in his own stools. The parasite was first described by Lambl, who gave it the name *intestinalis.* Stiles (1915) created a new binomial for this species, *Giardia lamblia,* due to some confusion as to whether *intestinalis* was actually available as a name for this parasite. In 1925, Hegner described *Giardia felis* from domestic cats in the United States, while Deschiens (1925) described *Giardia cati* from cats in France. In 1952 Filice examined specimens of many different species of rodent *Giardia* and decided that there were two species in mammals, *Giardia duodenalis* (Daviane, 1875), originally described from rabbits, and *Giardia muris* (Grassi, 1879), from mice. If one accepts the belief of Filice that most mammals are infected with different manifestations of *Giardia duodenalis,* then this name has precedence. If there are different species of *Giardia* present in different mammalian hosts, then *Giardia felis* Hegner, 1925, would be the binomial used to describe the species typically found in the cat, and *Giardia canis* Hegner, 1922, would be the binomial used to describe the species typically found in the dog. The species found in humans would be called *Giardia lamblia* Stiles, 1915. In this scenario, the name *Giardia duodenalis* would be restricted to only those isolates from rabbits. In light of the numerous new works indicating molecular distinctions between different isolates of parasites, it would seem that the trend is once again leaning towards assigning different names to the species appearing in different hosts.

Strains, Phenotypes, and Genotypes. There has been a significant effort, using various methods, to show that there are potentially different groups of *Giardia. Giardia* isolates from humans, cattle, dogs, sheep, cats, and guinea pigs have been compared using isozymes (Andrews et al., 1989, 1998; Bertram et al., 1983; Meloni et al., 1988, 1995; Stranden et al., 1990). Overall, this work appears to be somewhat contradictory, with some groups finding a good deal of heterogeneity between isolates, while other groups seem to find the different isolates to be very similar to each other. It would appear, however, that the two major types that are found in humans also are occasionally found in dogs and cats, and some work has suggested that cats are a major source. Other work has found that the canine form is sometimes difficult to obtain in culture and that dogs may be hosts to both of the major types found in humans, as well as a third form in Western Australia that might be restricted to canine hosts (Monis et al., 1998). Using restriction endonuclease analysis of DNA from 15 *Giardia* isolates from humans, beaver, a cat, and a guinea pig, it was found that the isolates fell into two groups (Nash et al., 1985). The cat and one of the two beaver isolates were similar to the pattern produced by most of the human isolates, but the guinea pig and the other beaver isolates differed from the majority of the human isolates as did some of the other human isolates. Using DNA polymorphisms has not cleared up the continuing separation between groups although it appears that groups I and II appear to hold the majority of the genotypes so far examined (Ey et al., 1996; Morgan et al., 1993). The infection of Western Australian dogs with certain isotypes that appear to be restricted to canine hosts was supported also by examination of the ribosomal RNA sequencing of these genotypes (Hopkins et al., 1997).

Geographic Distribution

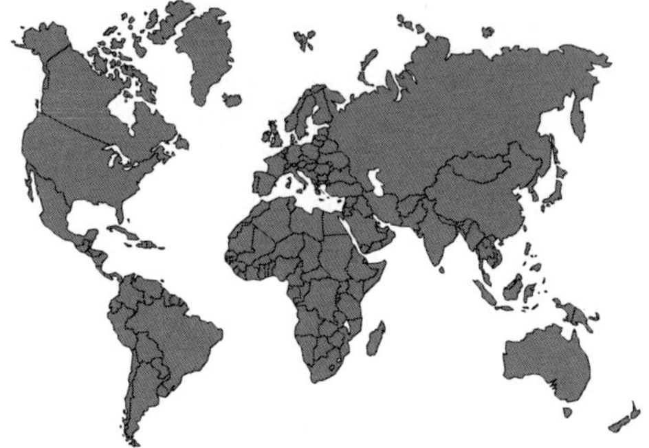

Fig. 1.44.

Giardia felis is found in cats throughout the world. Infections with *Giardia* are not uncommon in cats in the United States (Kirkpatrick, 1986). Hitchcock (1953) found *Giardia* in 57 percent of 14 cats in Michigan; Bemrick (1961) found *Giardia* in 3 percent of stools from 291 cats in Minnesota. Surveys have reported infections in 14 percent of 226 cats in Australia (Swan and Thompson, 1986) and 6.7 percent of 120 cats in New Zealand (Tonks et al., 1991). In Europe, cats have been identified as hosts of *Giardia* on numerous occasions: 5.2 percent of 94 cats in Switzerland (Seiler et al., 1983), 35 percent of 20 cats in the United Kingdom (Winsland et al., 1989), 10.8 percent of 500 cats in Belgium (Vanparijs and Thienpoint, 1973), 2.3 percent of 910 cats in Germany (Bauer and Stoye, 1984), 5.6 percent of 90 cats in Italy (Carneri and Catellino, 1963), 1.2 percent of cats in Czechoslovakia (Kucharova, 1989), and 4 percent of cats in Turkey (Burgu et al., 1985). In Iran, 7.2 percent of 97 cats have been identified as infected with *Giardia* (Anwar, 1974). In Chile, 2 percent of 50 cats were found infected (Franjola and Matzner, 1982).

Location in Host

Hitchcock and Malewitz (1956) stated that they found trophozoites of *Giardia* throughout the small intestine below the duodenum and in the cecum and large intestine. Kirkpatrick and Farrell (1984) reported that the trophozoites were concentrated in the lower portions of the jejunum, whereas lower numbers were observed in the upper portions of the jejunum and in the ileum; these authors did not find trophozoites in the large intestine. It has been shown (Tsuchiya, 1931) that the location of *Giardia* trophozoites within the intestinal tract of the dog is affected by diet, with diets rich in carbohydrates causing the majority of trophozoites to be found nearer the stomach while they were more posterior in animals fed a diet high in protein; also fewer organisms were present in the intestines of animals fed the high-protein diet.

Parasite Identification

Within cats, *Giardia* occurs as a binucleate, flagellate trophozoite (Figs. 1.45 and 1.46). The trophozoite is small (10.5 to 17.5 μm long by 5.25 to 8.75 μm in maximum width), and has eight trailing flagella. The two nuclei are just posterior to midbody; these large nuclei are about 3 μm long and 1.5 μm wide. The ventral surface of the trophozoite bears a sucking disc that occupies about one-third to one-half of the anterior surface. The trailing flagella both propel the organism and create a vacuum for the sucking disc by pumping fluid out from under it. The trophozoite moves along the surface of the intestinal epithelium.

The cyst stage is found in the large bowel as the trophozoite prepares to enter the external environment (Fig. 1.47). Cysts are about 7.4 μm wide and 10.5 μm long and have a length-to-width ratio of about 1.4. In response to an undefined stimulus, trophozoites produce the resistant cyst wall as they pass from the small to the large intestine. The trophozoite then divides, resulting in two trophozoites within the mature cyst. The cyst stage is passed in the feces.

If a cat has diarrhea and an accompanying infection with *Giardia,* a confirmatory diagnosis will often require that a direct saline examination of a small quantity of fresh feces be performed. This will allow the identification of the trophozoite stage.

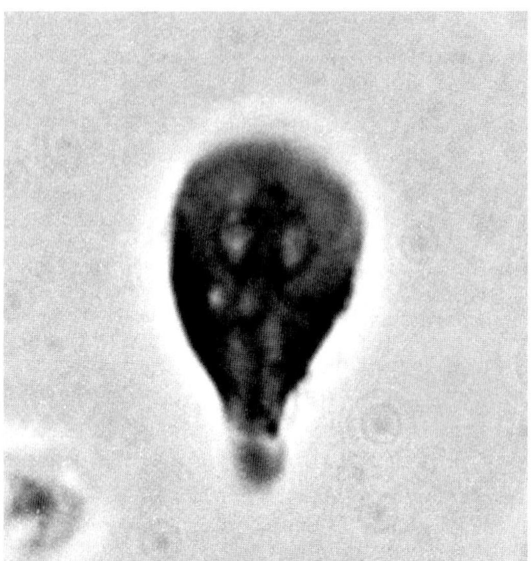

Fig. 1.45. *Giardia lamblia* trophozoite in human feces. This trophozoite was fixed then stained with iron hematoxylin and photographed using phase microscopy.

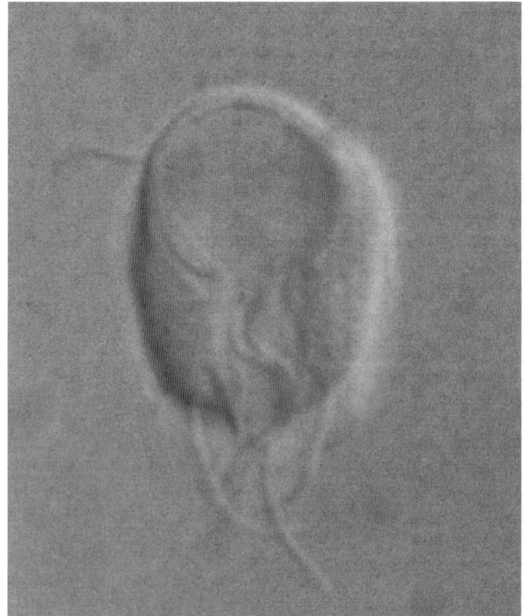

Fig. 1.46. *Giardia lamblia* trophozoite in culture. This living organism is being viewed from the bottom where it is attached to a glass coverslip in culture medium. The view gives a very clear image of the sucking disk and the trailing flagella.

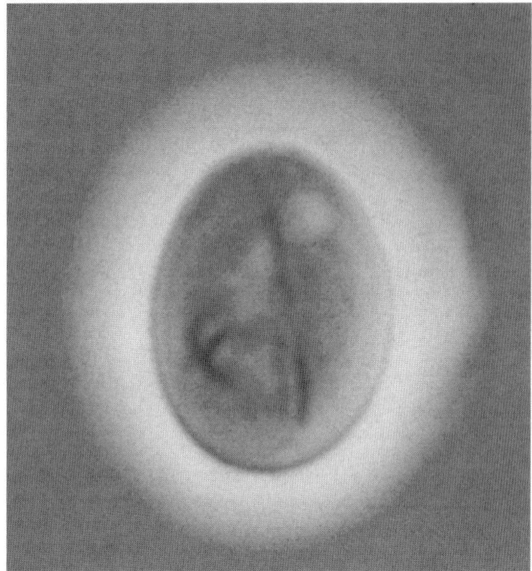

Fig. 1.47. *Giardia canis* cyst in the fresh feces of a dog photographed using phase microscopy.

Examination of diarrheic feces for cysts is often inconclusive because only trophozoites are found in stools of this type. In human medicine, fixed fecal smears are often prepared and stained with iron hematoxylin or by using a trichrome staining method for the examination of protozoa. The major reason for the examination of fixed smears of human feces is the many kinds of protozoa that must be differentiated. Few fecal protozoans are present in cats, and it is typically not necessary to perform such procedures. Fixed fecal samples do have the advantage, however, of producing a permanent slide that can be examined at a later date.

Another method now used routinely is the detection of *Giardia* in fecal smears using fluorescein-conjugated antibodies to *Giardia* and subsequent examination under a fluorescence microscope. This method increases the likelihood of finding the trophozoites and cysts because they will fluoresce when examined, but the equipment is costly, and other procedures are still required to concentrate the organisms in many samples.

A method that eliminates some of these problems is the detection of *Giardia* antigens within fecal samples. Antigen detection tests developed for use with human feces are capable of detecting infections in diarrheic fecal samples in which, due to the degeneration of nonviable trophozoites, there may be no detectable organisms. Such tests work by detecting antigens of the *Giardia* organism that are shed in the feces (Barr et al., 1992). These tests, such as ProSpecT/Giardia™ (a product of Alexon, Inc., Mountain View, Calif.), have not yet been approved for use in cats, but there are indications that they are likely to work very well. Cats should not be examined for giardiasis using the duodenal aspirate method used for dogs because the organisms may live farther posteriad in the intestine of the cat than they do in the dog.

Cysts can usually be detected by using a centrifugal flotation procedure. The zinc-sulfate method is preferred. Because cyst excretion has been shown to be sporadic (Kirkpatrick and Farrell, 1984), it may be best to examine the samples by both flotation and antigen detection. Cysts can be observed in sugar flotations of fecal matter, but the cysts will rapidly collapse. Collapsed cysts look like small crescent moons rather than the ovoid forms that are observed in direct smears or zinc-sulfate preparations soon after they are made. Antigen detection assays will also detect cysts.

Life Cycle

The cyst is passed in the feces of the host and infects a new host by direct fecal-oral contamination. Cysts may also be transmitted through contaminated drinking water to another host. When a host ingests a cyst, the trophozoites leave the cyst within the small intestine and take up residence on the intestinal mucosa. They divide repeatedly until they have populated the intestine of the new host with trophozoites. Some trophozoites periodically are carried in the fecal stream towards the anus, encysting on the way. Within five to 16 days after a cat has ingested a cyst, the cat is capable of excreting thousands of cysts into the environment.

Clinical Presentation and Pathogenesis

Cats can and do develop clinical signs from infections with *Giardia felis*. The typical sign is diarrhea (Barr and Bowman, 1994). Cats may undergo weight loss, and kittens may fail to gain weight. Cats with signs of diarrhea will usually be observed to maintain normal appetites and clinical values. Cats infected with *Giardia* will typically not undergo periods of vomiting. The diarrhea that is observed tends to be due to problems with malabsorption and steatorrhea, and for this reason, the feces tend to be soft and pale in color and to have increased levels of neutral fats. It has been shown in experimentally infected lambs that infection with *Giardia lamblia* was associated with decreased weight gain and feed efficiency when compared with uninfected controls (Olson et al., 1995).

Treatment

Several formulations of benzimidazoles have activity against *Giardia* infections (Barr and Bowman, 1994). Albendazole cleared 18 of 20 dogs that had all been shedding cysts at the beginning of therapy. A similar treatment (25 mg/kg body weight orally twice daily for 2 days) did not work. However, increasing the number of treatments (25 mg/kg body weight twice daily for 5 days) successfully cleared five dogs of the cysts they were shedding in their feces. This compound is currently not approved for use in cats or dogs, although it is used as an anthelminthic in cattle. Further, albendazole has been associated with bone marrow aplasia in one dog when used to treat *Giardia* infection (Stokol et al., 1997). Fenbendazole has been shown to stop beagles from shedding cysts in their feces at the dosage routinely applied for anthelminthic therapy (50 mg/kg body weight orally once a day for 3 days) (Barr et al., 1994). This compound is a routinely used and approved anthelminthic in dogs, but it is not approved for use in cats. Fenbendazole has been administered to cats as an anthelminthic without any apparent detrimental effects (Roberson and Burke, 1980). Febantel is approved for use in cats but has not been examined for its efficacy against *Giardia* in this species, although a compound containing febantel has been found to be effective in treating giardiasis in dogs (Barr et al., 1998.)

Drugs used to treat *Giardia* infections in cats have included quinacrine, metronidazole, and furazolidone (Kirkpatrick, 1986). Quinacrine was given orally for 12 days (2.3 mg/kg body weight once a day) to five cats, but four continued to pass cysts. Oral metronidazole at 10 or 25 mg/kg body weight given twice a day for 5 days was noted to cure cats of their infections with *Giardia*. Furazolidone given orally at 4 mg/kg body weight twice a day has also been shown to be effective.

Epizootiology

Cats are probably infected from the ingestion of the cyst in direct fecal-oral transmission or through contaminated water or fomites. The trophozoite stage passed in diarrheic feces is not considered infectious.

Due to improved sanitation, humans are no longer routinely becoming infected during childhood with constant reinfection as adults, and it has been suggested that one reason that *Giardia* is now considered a cause of diarrhea in humans when it was once thought to be a commensal is that, in the past, the immune status of humans was enhanced by constant re-exposure (Beaver et al., 1984). It would seem that as cats are prevented access to cysts through improved hygiene, they, like humans, will assume a greater risk of developing disease assignable to *Giardia* if they become infected.

Hazards to Other Animals

Giardia from cats has been transmitted experimentally to gerbils (Swabby et al., 1988). It is not known to what extent cross transmission to other animals will occur, but precautions need to be taken when animals of different species are housed in the same facilities.

Hazards to Humans

It is still unclear as to the relationship between infections in cats and in associated humans. It has been reported that cats and humans have been found to harbor genetically identical forms of *Giardia* and has been suggested that the cat is a likely reservoir of human infection (Thompson et al., 1988). A study in the United Kingdom of the potential of zoonotic transmission of *Giardia* from pets to their owners showed that cats and dogs, but especially feral dogs, were correlated with infection of humans with *Giardia* (Warburton et al., 1994). A similar study in Czechoslovakia found no correlation between infection in pets and in humans (Pospisilova and Svobodova, 1992). It has, however, been shown that cats can be infected with human and canine isolates of *Giardia* (Svovodova et al., 1990). Thus, at this time, every effort should be taken to prevent the potential transmission of cysts from cats to humans.

Control/Prevention

In catteries, infections with *Giardia* can become a chronic problem, causing periodic bouts of diarrhea in groups of animals. Typically, older cats tend to become refractory to infection, and some cats spontaneously stop shedding cysts; these manifestations have been interpreted to mean that cats may develop some form of acquired resistance to giardiasis. When *Giardia* is identified in catteries, all cats housed in contiguous cages must be treated, and particular attention given to increasing the levels of sanitation and fecal control.

The task of simultaneously clearing many animals of their infections can make disease control in a cattery very difficult. Important facts to remember in infection control are that (1) the cysts stage of the parasite tends to be waterborne; (2) the cats will not stop shedding cysts in their feces immediately after treatment, and not all will stop at the same time; and (3) if the cysts are not removed from the environment, the condition may persist through reinfection. Thus, control involves the treatment of all cats simultaneously, followed by moving the cats to clean cages. If cages cannot be steam cleaned, they should be washed with hot soapy water, rinsed, and dried thoroughly. If it is possible to dry the cages in the heat of the sun, this would be an excellent means of disinfection. If conditions are such that the cages cannot be dried completely, a disinfectant (e.g., ammonia, Lysol™, or bleach) should be added to the water. The day after the cats have received their initial treatment, they should be moved to clean cages. Following the second treatment, the cats should be moved again. This movement can be repeated a third time. If the cats cannot be moved this often, it will reduce the chances of successfully breaking the cycle of transmission.

Fecal samples to verify that the cats have been cleared of cysts should be taken 1 week after the first treatment. Because of the short prepatent period following infection, delay of more than a week after treatment in collection of fecal samples should be avoided. If such a delay occurs, a negative examination for *Giardia* will indicate clearance, but a positive result may indicate either failure to clear, or reinfection, or both.

REFERENCES

Andrews RH, Adams M, Boreham PFL, Mayrhofer G, Meloni BP. 1989. *Giardia intestinalis:* electrophoretic evidence for a species complex. Int J Parasitol 19:183–190.

Andrews RH, Monis PT, Ey PL, Mayrhofer G. 1998. Comparison of the levels of intra-specific genetic variation within *Giardia muris* and *Giardia intestinalis*. Int J Parasitol 28:1179–1185.

Anwar M. 1974. Incidence of *Giardia cati* in the stray cats in the Tehran area. J Vet Fac, University of Tehran 30:1–7.

Barr SC, Bowman DD. 1994. Giardiasis of dogs and cats. Compendium of Continuing Education for the Practicing Veterinarian 16:603–614.

Barr SC, Bowman DD, Erb HN. 1992. Evaluation of two test procedures for diagnosis of giardiasis in dogs. Am J Vet Res 53:2028–2031.

Barr SC, Bowman DD, Heller RL. 1994. Efficacy of fenbendazole against giardiasis in dogs. Am J Vet Res 55:988–990.

Barr SC, Bowman DD, Frongello MM, Joseph S. 1998. Efficacy of a drug combination of praziquantel, pyrantel pamoate, and febantel against giardiasis in dogs. Am J Vet Res 59:1134–1136.

Bauer C, Stoye M. 1984. Ergebnisse parastiologischer Kotuntersuchungen von Equiden, Hunden, Katzen un Igeln der Jahre 1974 bis 1983. Deutsche Tierartzliche Wochenschrift, 91:255–258.

Beaver PC, Jung RE, Cupp EW. 1984. Clinical Parasitology. 9th ed. Philadelphia, Pa: Lea and Febiger.

Bemrick WJ. 1961. A note on the incidence of three species of *Giardia* in Minnesota. J Parasitol 47:87–89.

Bertram MA, Meyer EA, Lile JD, Morse SA. 1983. A comparison of isozymes of five axenic *Giardia* isolates. J Parasitol 69:793–801.

Burgu A, Tinar R, Doganay A, Toparlak M. 1985. Akara'da sokak kedilerinin ekto-ve endoparazitleri uzerinde bir arastirma. Veteriner Fakultesi Dergisi, Ankara Universitesi 32:288–300.

Carneri I, Catellino S. 1963. Bassa incidenza di *Giardia cati* Deschiens 1925 e assenza di protozoi orali nei gatti a Milano. Rivista di Parassitologia 24:1–4.

Deschiens REA. 1925. *Giardia cati* (n.sp.) du chat domestique. Comptes Rendue d'Societie Biologique, Paris. 92:1271–1272.

Ey PL, Bruderer T, Wehrli C, Köhler P. 1996. Comparison of genetic groups determined by molecular and immunological analyses of *Giardia* isolated from animals and humans in Switzerland and Australia. Parasitol Res 82:52–60.

Filice FP. 1952. Studies on the cytology and life history of a *Giardia* from the laboratory rat. Univ. Calif. Publ. Zool. 57:53–146.

Franjola R, Matzner N. 1982. Prevalencia de enteroprotozoos en gatos domesticos de la ciudad de Baldivia, Chile. Zentralblatt fur Veterinarmedizin B 29:397–400.

Hegner RW. 1925. *Giardia felis* n. sp., from the domestic cat and giardias from birds. Am. J. Hyg. 4:393–400.

Hitchcock DJ. 1953. Incidence of gastro-intestinal parasites in some Michigan kittens. N Am Vet 34:428–429.

Hitchcock DJ, Malewitz TD. 1956. Habitat of *Giardia* in the kitten. J Parasitol 42:286.

Hopkins RM, Meloni BP, Groth DM, Wetherall JD, Reynoldson JA, Thompson RCA. 1997. Ribosomal RNA sequencing reveals differences between the genotypes of *Giardia* isolates recovered from humans and dogs living in the same locality. J Parasitol 83:44–51.

Kirkpatrick CE. 1986. Feline giardiasis: a review. J Small Anim Pract 27:69–80.

Kirkpatrick CE, Farrell JP. 1984. Feline giardiasis: observations on natural and induced infections. Am J Vet Res 45:2182–2188.

Kucharova M. 1989. Prehled parazitoz u psu a kocek v Praze se zamerenim a parasitarni zoonozy. Veterinarstvi 39:314–316.

Meloni BP, Lymbery AJ, Thompson RCA. 1988. Isoenzyme electrophoresis of 30 isolates of *Giardia* from humans and felines. Am J Trop Med Hyg 38:65–73.

Meloni BP, Lymbery AJ, Thompson RCA. 1995. Genetic characterization of isolates of *Giardia duodenalis* by enzyme electrophoresis: implications for reproductive biology, population structure, taxonomy, and epidemiology. J Parasitol 81:368–383.

Monis PT, Andrews RH, Mayrhofer G, Mackrill J, Kulda J, Isaac-Renton JL, Ey PL. 1998. Novel lineages of *Giardia intestinalis* identified by genetic analysis of organisms isolated from dogs in Australia. Parasitology 116:7–19.

Morgan UM, Constantine CC, Greene WK, Thompson RCA. 1993. ARAPD (random amplified polymorphic DNA) analysis of *Giardia* DNA and correlation with isoenzyme data. Trans Roy Soc Trop Med Hyg 87:702–705.

Nash TE, McCutchan T, Keister D, Dame JB, Conrad JD, Gillin FD. 1985. Restriction-endonuclease analysis of DNA from 15 *Giardia* isolates obtained from humans and animals. J Infect Dis 152:64–73.

Olson ME, Mcallister TA, Deselliers L, Cheng K-J, Mork DW. 1995. Effects of giardiasis on growth and development in the young. Proceedings of the Annual Meeting of the American Association of Veterinary Parasitologists, Abstract 202.

Pospisilova D, Svobodova V. 1992. Problematika giardiozy u chovatelu psu a kocek. Ceskoslovenska Epidemiologie, Mikrobiologie, Immunologie 41:106–108.

Roberson EL, Burke TM. 1980. Evaluation of granulated fenbendazole (22.2 percent) against induced and naturally occurring helminth infections in cats. Am J Vet Res 41:1499–1502.

Seiler M, Eckert J, Wolff K. 1983. *Giardia* und andere Darmparasiten bei Hund und Katze in der Schweiz. Schweiz Arch Tierheilk 125:137–148.

Stokol T, Randolph JF, Nachbar S, Rodi C, Barr SC. 1997. Development of bone marrow toxicosis after albendazole administration in a dog and cat. J Am Vet Med Assoc 210:1753–1756.

Stranden AM, Eckert J, Köhler P. 1990. Electrophoretic characterization of *Giardia* isolated from humans, cattle, sheep, and a dog in Switzerland. J Parasitol 76:660–668.

Svobodova V, Pospisilova D, Svoboda M. 1990. Giardioza psu a kocek - nebezpeci pro cloveka? Veterinarstvi 40:457–458.

Swabby KD, Hibler CP, Wegrzn JG. 1988. Infection of Mongolian gerbils (*Meriones unguiculatus*) with *Giardia* from human and animal sources. In Advances in *Giardia* Research, ed PM Wallis and BR Hammond, pp 75–77. Alberta, Canada: University of Calgary Press.

Swan JM, Thompson RCA. 1986. The prevalence of *Giardia* in dogs and cats in Perth, Western Australia. Aust Vet J 63:110–112.

Thompson RCA, Meloni BP, Lymbery AJ. 1988. Humans and cats have genetically identical forms of *Giardia:* evidence of a zoonotic relationship. Med J Aust 148:207–209.

Tonks MC, Brown TJ, Ionas G. 1991. *Giardia* infection of cats and dogs in New Zealand. N Z Vet J 39:33–34.

Tsuchiya H. 1931. The localization of *Giardia canis* (Hegner, 1922) as affected by diet. J Parasitol 18:232–246.

Vanparijs OFJ, Thienpoint DC. 1973. Canine and feline helminth and protozoan infections in Belgium. J Parasitol 59:327–330.

Warburton ARE, Jones PH, Bruce J. 1994. Zoonotic transmission of giardiasis: a case control study. CDR Rev 4:R32–R36.

Winsland JKD, Nimmo S, Butcher PD, Farthing MJG. 1989. Prevalence of *Giardia* in dogs and cats in the United Kingdom: survey of an Essex veterinary clinic. Trans Roy Soc Trop Med Hyg 83:791-792.

KINETOPLASTIDA

Trypanosomes

The trypanosomes and leishmanial organisms all have a flagellum (or undulipodium of some workers) in some part of their life cycle that is connected to a large mitochondrial body that was called a kinetosome or a kinetoplast by early microscopists. It is the presence of this structure that causes these parasites to be grouped with other organisms within the phylum Kinetoplastida. Some members of the Kinetoplastida are parasites of invertebrates only; others are parasites of invertebrates, as well as plants and animals. One group of these organisms that is parasitic in mammals has a single stage in the vertebrate host, an elongate cell called the trypomastigote. The trypomastigote has a large nucleus and a long flagellum that runs the length of the body from the posterior to the anterior end where there is typically a free portion. Along the body, the flagellum is attached to the cell body of the parasite by a thin layer of cell membranes and cytoplasm; this is what produces the structure called the undulating membrane (so called because as the flagellum beats, the membrane undulates). In cats, the members of the genus *Trypanosoma* that are transmitted by the bites of flies or bugs, *Trypanosoma brucei, Trypanosoma gambiense, Trypanosoma congolense, Trypanosoma evansi,* and *Trypanosoma rangeli,* are members of this first group. A second group is represented by the members of the genus *Leishmania.* In this group, the only stage found in the tissues of the vertebrate host is a round, intracellular form that consists of a nucleus and the large kinetoplast. The members of this genus are transmitted by the bite of a phlebotomine sandfly, where the flagellated form of this parasite is found. The third group of kinetoplastid parasites found in cats is represented by *Trypanosoma cruzi.* This is a diphasic organism that has a stage in tissues of its vertebrate host that is similar to the amastigote stage of the *Leishmania* parasites and a trypomastigote stage that is present in the blood of the vertebrate host during the acute phase of the infection. *Trypanosoma cruzi* is transmitted in the feces of a kissing or triatomid bug.

Trypanosoma Gruby, 1843

The trypanosomes are parasites of all classes of vertebrates. Having been found initially in the blood of fish and frogs, trypanosomes have since been found in reptiles, birds, and mammals. Members of the genus *Trypanosoma* are typically transmitted between hosts by some type of invertebrate vector. One exception is *Trypanosoma equiperdum,* which is transmitted between horses during coitus. Trypanosomes are significant pathogens of humans and animals throughout the tropics. There has, however, been little evidence that they are major pathogens of the domestic cat.

Trypanosoma brucei Plimmer and Bradford, 1899

Trypanosoma brucei is morphologically indistinguishable from *Trypanosoma gambiense* and *Trypanosoma rhodesiense.* Together, these three parasites are considered to form a tsetse-transmitted complex (Hoare, 1967), of which *Trypanosoma gambiense* is almost exclusively human wherein chronic disease is produced, *Trypanosoma rhodesiense* is a zoonosis from African ungulates producing fulminant disease in humans, and *Trypanosoma brucei* occurs mainly in animals and may or may not cause human disease. Hill (1955) summarized the reports of these three species in the cat including several personal communications with workers in the field, but in most cases only very minor notes have been presented by those cited by Hill. Thus, there seems to be little or no literature concerning the infection of cats with *Trypanosoma rhodesiense.* Experimental infections of cats with *Trypanosoma gambiense* have been examined on at least one occasion.

Etymology

The parasite is named after Major David Bruce.

Synonyms

Trypanosoma pecaudi Laveran, 1907; *Trypanosoma togolense* Mesnil and Brimont, 1909; *Trypanosoma ugandae* Stephens and Blacklock, 1913; *Trypanosoma multiforme* Kinghorn et al., 1913; *Trypanosoma anceps* Bruce et al., 1914; *Trypanosoma dukei* Knuth and duToit, 1921.

History

The parasite was found to be the causative agent of nagana in cattle by Sir David Bruce in 1894, who recognized the trypanosome in the blood of cattle and showed that it could be transmitted by inoculation into horses and dogs where it caused acute disease (Hoare, 1967). Bruce also showed that naturally infected tsetse flies were involved in the transmission of the parasite, but it was not until the work of Kleine (1909a, b) that it was shown that a period of development within the tsetse was required for transmission to occur.

Geographic Distribution

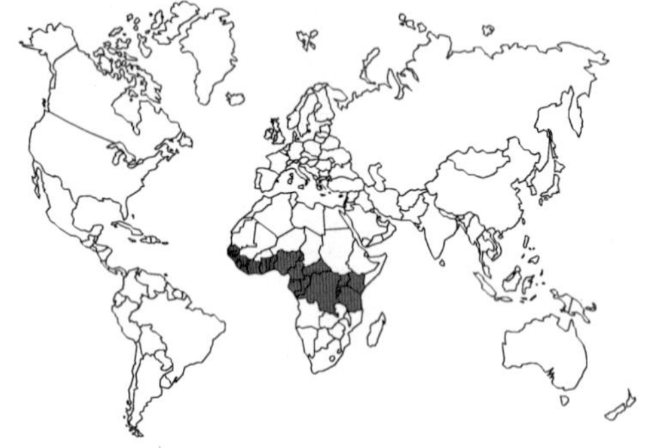

Fig. 1.48.

This parasite is distributed throughout the range of the tsetse fly vector in western Africa. The mammalian reservoirs of infection are considered to be various forms of African antelope.

Location in Host

The parasite is considered to be a parasite of blood and tissue fluids. Although in cats, the parasite has only been observed in the blood.

Parasite Identification

Trypanosoma brucei is the type of trypanosome that has two stages present in the blood, a short and stumpy form with no free flagellum and a long and slender form with a free flagellum. The short form has a length of around 18 μm (range: 12–26 μm), while the long form has a length of 29 μm (range: 23–42 μm).

In Giemsa-stained blood films, the trypanosomes can be examined, and dividing forms can be seen. The slender forms will typically be S shaped with three to five undulations of the undulating membrane throughout the length of the cell body. The free flagellum will be about one-half to one-third of the length of the cell. The nucleus will be near midbody, and the rather small kinetoplast will be near the posterior end of the cell body. In the stumpy forms of the parasite, the cell often takes on more of a C shape or L shape, the nucleus will be near the end of the cell body, and there will be no free flagellum. There will still be around three undulations of the membrane along the cell surface.

Life Cycle

The transmission of *Trypanosoma brucei* typically requires the development within a tsetse fly (genus *Glossina*), wherein development of infective stages occur within the gut and salivary glands (Kleine 1909a, b). The trypanosomes are transmitted to the next host through the bite of the fly. Transmission of the parasite can also be caused by inoculation of blood containing the organisms as might occur with a dirty needle, by the contaminated mouth parts of a horse fly (tabanid), or by transfusion. One study showed that the parasite can also be transmitted by cats feeding on the meat of an infected goat with parasites in circulation; 3 of 17 cats became infected in this manner (Moloo et al., 1973).

In cats inoculated with blood, trypanosomes will appear in the blood stream beginning 5 days after inoculation (Kanthack et al., 1899). When cats were fed goat meat, trypanosomes first appeared in the blood 31 to 38 days after they had been fed the infected meat; these cats were killed soon after the infection was detected in the blood. In cats fed an infected mouse or an infected guinea pig, the prepatent periods were 44 and 25 days, respectively (Laveran and Mesnil, 1912). In general, it is considered that the infected cat seldom lives long enough to play a major role in transmission.

Clinical Presentation and Pathogenesis

Cats that have been experimentally infected die within 22 to 26 days after infection (Kanthack et al., 1899). These cats were noted to develop pyrexia, changes in the eyes including an aqueous flare and conjunctivitis, and edema of the face and eyelids. At necropsy, these cats were found to have pronounced wasting with generalized lymphadenopathy, splenomegaly, hepatomegaly, and pleura and pericardium hemorrhage.

A naturally infected cat was noted to be listless and off its food, with a dry rough haircoat and pale mucous membranes (Hill, 1955). There was edema and erythmea of the head region. In this cat, both eyes were acutely affected with photophobia, lacrimation, conjunctivitis, and keratitis; in the right eye there was pannus, hypopyon, and hypertony. Within 6 days of the initial presentation, the cat became blind and too weak to stand.

Treatment

Treatment of only one infected cat has been reported in the literature (Hill, 1955). This cat was treated with antycide methylsulphate (6 mg/kg body weight) subcutaneously. It began to eat again by the third day after treatment, and the hypopyon began to disappear. Both eyes appeared normal 8 days after treatment. This cat did relapse a few weeks later, again with ophthalmologic signs, and was again treated. Relapse developed again several months later, and following treatment and another relapse, the cat was euthanatized.

Epizootiology

Trypanosoma brucei is considered a parasite of African ungulates that can get into domestic cats by the bite of a tsetse fly.

Hazards to Other Animals

As noted above, cats seldom live long enough after infection to serve as major sources of infection to other animals.

Hazards to Humans

The hazard to humans would be in the veterinary clinic where an accident with a contaminated needle could serve to introduce the parasite into someone supplying veterinary care.

Control/Prevention

There is currently very little known about the control and prevention of the disease in cats. The biology of the parasite would suggest that cats should be protected from tsetse bites and not fed meat of wild game that might be infected.

REFERENCES

Hill DH. 1955. *Trypanosoma brucei* in the cat. Br Vet J 111:77–80.

Hoare, CA. 1967. Evolutionary trends in mammalian trypanosomes. Adv Parasitol 5:47–91.

Kanthack AA, Durham HE, Blandford WFH. 1899. On nagana, or tsetse fly disease. Proc Roy Soc 64:100–118.
Kleine FC. 1909a. Positive Infektiens versuche mit *Trypanosoma brucei* durch *Glossina palpalis.* Dtsch Med Wochenschr 35:469–470.
Kleine FC. 1909b. Weitere Beobachtungen über Tsetsefliegenu nd Trypanosomen. Dtsch Med Wochenschr 35:1956–1958.
Laveran A, Mesnil F. 1912. In Masson's *Trypanosomas et Trypanosomiases.* Paris, France.
Moloo SK, Losos GJ, Kutuza SB. 1973. Transmission of *Trypanosoma brucei* to cats and dogs by feeding on infected goats. Ann Trop Med Parasitol 67:331–334.

Trypanosoma gambiense Dutton, 1902

Etymology

This parasite was named after its location along the Gambia river in West Africa.

Synonyms

Trypanosoma ugandense Castellani, 1903; *Trypanosoma castellanii,* Kruse, 1903; *Trypanosoma hominis* Manson, 1903; *Trypanosoma fordii* Maxwell-Adams, 1903; *Trypanosoma nepveui* Sambon, 1903; *Trypanosoma tullochii* Minichin, 1907; *Trypanosoma rovumense* Beck and Weck, 1913; *Trypanosoma nigeriense* Macfie, 1913; *Castellanella gambiense* (Dutton, 1902) Chalmers, 1918.

History

This is the causative organism of classical "sleeping sickness" in humans. This trypanosome was first discovered in human blood in 1901 by Forde, and Dutton proposed the name *Trypanosoma gambiense* in 1902. Dutton did not suspect that this parasite caused sleeping sickness; Castellani (1903) showed that a trypanosome was present in the cerebrospinal fluid of patients with sleeping sickness in Uganda and suggested that the trypanosome was the causative agent of this disease. Gray and Tulloch (1907) made the ultimate connection between the forms found in acute disease in the blood (as by Forde and Dutton) and the trypomastigotes present in cerebrospinal fluid of sleeping sickness patients. Gray and Tulloch showed that patients with acute disease would go on to develop sleeping sickness. The tsetse fly was shown to be the vector by Bruce and Nabarro (1903) and Kleine (1909).

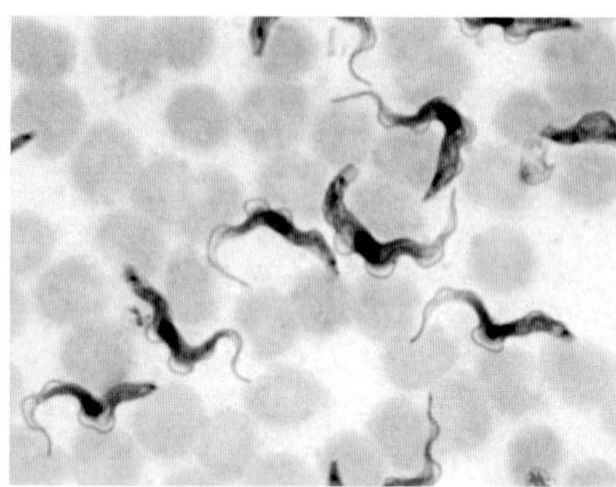

Fig. 1.49. *Trypanosoma gambiense* trypomastigote in the blood of a mouse stained with Giemsa. One of the two trypomastigotes in the center of this photomicrograph is in the process of division as is evidenced by the presence of two kinetoplasts on the posterior end. Dividing forms like this would not be observed in infections with *Trypanosoma cruzi.*

Location in Host

This is a parasite of the blood and tissue fluids (Fig. 1.49); it has not been observed in naturally infected cats.

Parasite Identification

Trypanosoma gambiense is morphologically indistinguishable from *Trypanosoma brucei.*

Clinical Presentation and Pathogenesis

There is only one report describing clinical disease in experimentally infected cats (Bogaert, 1962). Four cats were injected with the parasite. Two died after 4 months of infection, with rapid weight loss, generalized adenopathy, and splenomegaly. After 7 months, a third cat showed a temporary pelvic limb paralysis; histologic examination revealed slight generalized lymphocytic meningitis without trypanosomes in the spinal fluid. At the end of 10 months, the fourth cat showed marked somnolence, myoclonia of the limbs, periodic epileptic seizures, and then a marked ataxia of the cerebellar type. Lymphocytosis, but no parasites, were found in the cerebral spinal fluid. Upon euthanasia and necropsy 11.5 months after infection, this cat showed neurologic changes consistent with cerebral trypanosomiasis: cellular infiltrations in the optic tract, pericapillary infiltrations, and uniform meningitis with the lesions increasingly intense near the ectosyvian convolution and the hippocampus.

Treatment

This has not been attempted in the cat.

Epizootiology

Trypanosoma gambiense is considered a parasite of humans that might get into domestic cats by the bite of a tsetse fly.

Hazards to Other Animals

Unknown.

Hazards to Humans

The hazard to humans would be in the veterinary clinic where an accident with a contaminated needle could serve to introduce the parasite into someone supplying veterinary care.

Control/Prevention

There is currently very little known about the prevalence, control, or prevention of the disease in cats. The biology of the parasite would suggest that cats should be protected from tsetse bites.

REFERENCES

Bogaert L. 1962. Protozoan infections. Chapter IX. In Comparative Neuropathology. New York, NY: Innes JRM and Saunders, Academic Press, pp 473–474.

Bruce D, Nabarro D. 1903. Further information concerning the African sleeping sickness. NY Med J 78:661–662.

Castellani A. 1903. On the discovery of a species of *Trypanosoma* in the cerebro-spinal fluid of cases of sleeping sickness. Proc Roy Soc, Lond 71:501–508.

Dutton JE. 1902. Note on a *Trypanosoma* occurring in the blood of man. Br Med J 2:881–884.

Forde RM. 1902. Some clinical notes on a European patient in whose blood a *Trypanosoma* was observed. J Trop Med Lond 5:261–263.

Gray ACH, Tulloch FMG. 1907. Continuation report on sleeping sickness in Uganda. Rep Sleep Sick Com Roy Soc 8:3–80.

Kleine FC. 1909. Positive Infektiens versuche mit *Trypanosoma brucei* durch *Glossina palpalis*. Dtsch Med Wochenschr 35:469–470.

Trypanosoma evansi (Steel, 1885) Balbiani, 1888

Etymology

This parasite is named after Dr. Griffith Evans, the British veterinarian who discovered the parasite.

Synonyms

Spirochaete evansi Steel, 1885; *Trypanosoma elmassiani* Lignières, 1902; *Trypanosoma soudanense* Laveran, 1907; *Trypanosoma hiipicum* Darling, 1910; *Trypanosoma venezuelense* Mesnil, 1910; *Trypanosoma annamense* Laveran, 1911; *Trypanosoma cameli* Pricolo and Ferror, 1914; *Trypanosoma macracanum* Sergent, Lhéritier and Belleval, 1915; *Trypanosoma ninae kohlyakimov* Yakimoff, 1921.

History

This was the first pathogenic trypanosome to be discovered. Dr. Griffith Evans discovered the organisms in 1880 in the blood of horses and camels in India that were suffering from a disease called surra. Mechanical transmission by biting flies was first shown by Rogers (1901).

Geographic Distribution

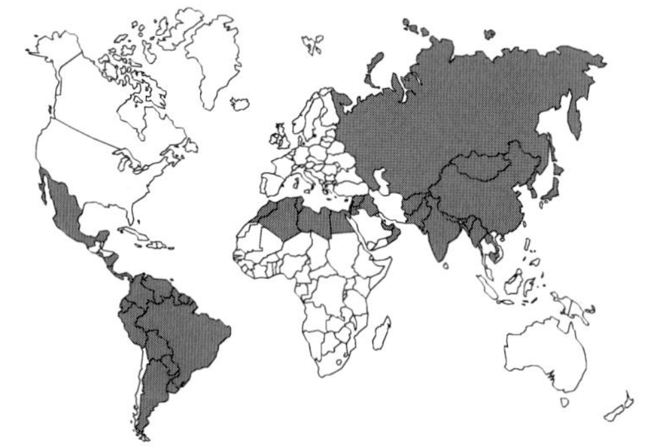

Fig. 1.50.

The organism is found in Africa north of the Sahara, Asia, and Central and South America.

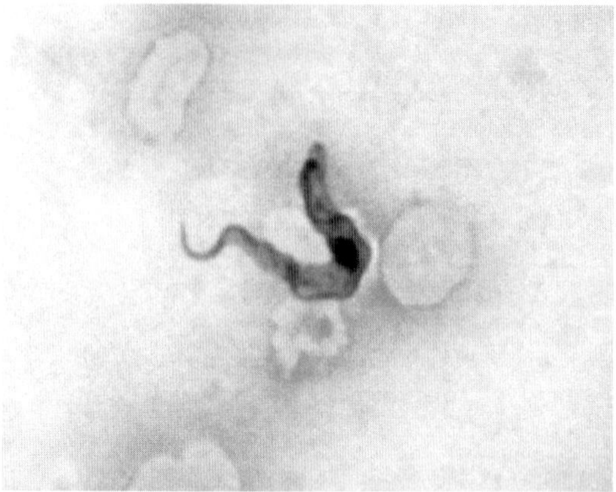

Fig. 1.51. *Trypanosoma evansi* in the blood of a horse. Giemsa stain.

Location in Host

These parasites are parasites of the bloodstream and tissue fluids. In the cat, organisms have only been observed in the blood.

Parasite Identification

The morphology of this parasite (Fig. 1.51) is indistinguishable from that of *Trypanosoma brucei.*

Life Cycle

This parasite is transmitted between hosts by mechanical transmission by biting flies (Rogers, 1901). In South America, transmission has also been shown to be possible through the bite of vampire bats (*Desmodus rotundus*) (Dunn, 1932).

Clinical Presentation and Pathogenesis

Typically, this parasite is thought of as causing disease in horses, camels, elephants, and dogs wherein there is emaciation and edema. There have been few reports in cats.

A naturally infected cat presented with lethargy and inappetence, sunken eyes, and incoordination (Paikne and Dhake, 1974). Poisoning was the expected etiology. The animal died, and a necropsy was performed. Blood smears revealed numerous *Trypanosoma evansi* organisms. There was perivascular cuffing around vessels in the brain.

At least two studies have been performed in which cats have been experimentally infected (Choudhury and Misra, 1972; Scheidle, 1982). In the earlier report, cats were inoculated intraperitoneally. The trypanosomes appeared in the circulation 14 to 15 days after infection. Young cats could succumb during the first peak parasitemia, but if they survived, 4-day-long peaks of parasitemia appeared every 2 weeks. During the peak parasitemias, the cats showed signs of drowsiness, lack of appetite, and facial inflammation. In the later report, three cats were inoculated with 1,500 trypanosomes. Two days after infection, parasites were detectable in the blood; after 2 weeks of infection, there were 70,000 trypanosomes observed per cubic millimeter of blood. The body temperature of the infected cats seldom exceeded 40°C. After 9 days of infection, the cats were severely anemic, which was the major observation at necropsy.

Treatment

Two experimentally infected cats were treated with Berenil, 4-4'-diamidino-diazoamino-benzol-diaceturat (Scheidle, 1982). A second treatment was given 2 days later because the cats still had low parasitemias 1 day after the first treatment. After the second treatment, trypanosomes were not observed for 8 to 20 days, but they then appeared and rose to near the pretreatment levels of 70,000 trypanosomes per milliliter.

Epizootiology

Trypanosoma evansi is considered to use cattle and buffalo as the reservoir hosts. Transmission to horses and dogs is not uncommon, but it is unclear how often cats may be infected.

Hazards to Other Animals

Unknown.

Hazards to Humans

Trypanosoma evansi is not considered to be a human pathogen. However, precautions should be taken to reduce potential hazards to humans in the veterinary clinic where an accident with a contaminated needle could serve to introduce the parasite into someone supplying veterinary care.

Control/Prevention

There is currently very little known about the prevalence, control, or prevention of the disease in cats. The biology of the parasite would suggest that cats should be protected from fly bites.

REFERENCES

Choudhury A, Misra KK. 1972. Experimental infection of *T. evansi* in the cat. Trans Roy Soc Trop Med Hyg 66:672–673.

Dunn LH. 1932. Experiments in the transmission of *Trypanosoma hippicum* Darling with the vampire bat, *Desmodus rotundus murinus* Wagner, as a vector in Panama. J Prevent Med 6:415–424.

Paikne DL, Dhake PR. 1974. Trypanosomiasis in a domestic cat (*Felis catus*). Ind Vet J 51:10.

Rogers L. 1901. The transmission of *Trypanosoma evansi* by horseflies and other experiments pointing to the probable identity of surra and nagana or tsetse-fly disease in Africa. Proc Roy Soc Ser B 68:163–170.

Scheidle G. 1982. Das Infektionsverhalten von *Trypanosoma evansi* (Stamm Manila) in vershiedenen Tierarten. Dissertation, Ludwig-Maximillians-Universität München. 53 pp.

Trypanosoma congolense Broden, 1904

Etymology

This parasite is named after the Congo location in which it was first observed.

Synonyms

Trypanosoma dimorphon Laveran and Mesnil, 1904; *Trypanosoma nanum* Laveran, 1905; *Trypanosoma confusum* Montgomery and Kinghorn, 1909; *Trypanosoma montgomeryi* Laveran, 1909; *Trypanosoma pecorum* Bruce et al., 1910; *Trypanosoma frobeniusi* Weissenborn, 1911; *Trypanosoma Somaliense* Maroglio, 1911; *Trypanosoma cellii* Martogio, 1911; *Trypaonsoms multiforme* Kinghorne et al., 1913; *Trypaonson randae* van Saceghem, 1921; *Trypanosoma urundiense* Chardome and Peel, 1967; *Trypanosoma berghei* Chardome and Peel, 1967; *Trypanosoma mossosense* Chardom and Peel, 1967.

History

This parasite was first observed in the blood of sheep and a donkey in Leopoldville (Kinshasa) of the Congo, and Broden noted that it was small and did not have a free flagellum. This is the major trypanosome of African animals and the most important animal trypanosome in East Africa.

Geographic Distribution

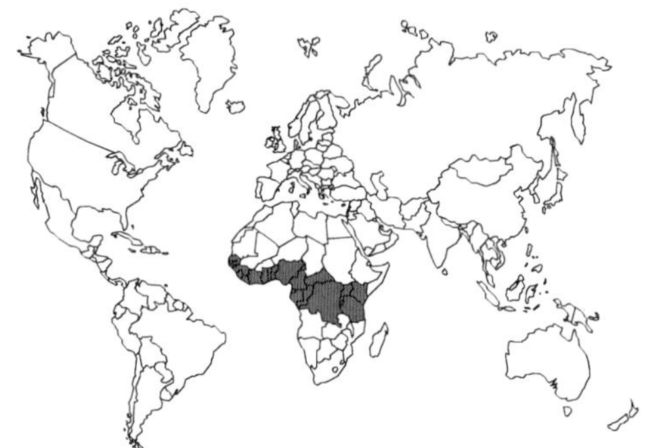

Fig. 1.52.

Tropical Africa south of the Sahara, within the range of the tsetse fly.

Location in Host

Trypanosoma congolense is a parasite mainly of the blood, although it may be found at times in tissue fluids.

Parasite Identification

Trypanosoma congolense is a small trypanosome measuring 9 to 18 μm in length (Fig. 1.53). There is typically no free flagellum observed in Giemsa-stained organisms, and the undulating membrane typically has no more than three to four undulations throughout the length of the cell body. The kinetoplast is relatively small, tends to be marginal, and is just subterminal to the posterior end of the body. In fresh blood, the trypanosome is active but shows no progressive motion through red blood cells, rarely leaving the field of view in the microscope.

Life Cycle

This parasite is transmitted between hosts by the bite of a fly, the tsetse, which serves as a required biological vector of this parasite.

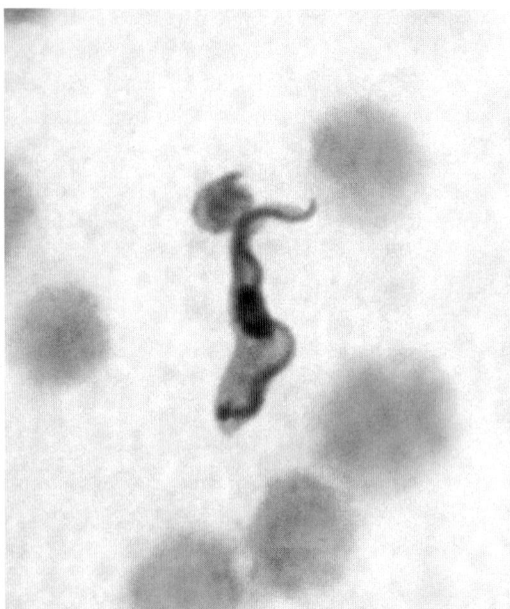

Fig. 1.53. *Trypanosoma congolense* in the blood of a mouse. In this preparation, the flagellum is clearly evident as it undulates along the body of this parasite.

Clinical Presentation and Pathogenesis

This parasite is capable of causing disease in most domestic animals. The disease is typically one of anemia that is considered to be related to an inhibition of hematopoiesis. There have been few reports in cats.

In six cats experimentally infected with *Trypanosoma congolense,* organisms appeared in the blood within 11 to 25 days after infection but were difficult to find throughout the course of the infection (Laveran, 1909). All six cats died within 68 to 85 days after infection. At necropsy, two of the cats were noted to have splenomegally.

Treatment

Treatment has not been tried in cats.

Epizootiology

Trypanosoma congolense is thought to use domestic cattle and wild game as reservoir hosts. It is unclear how often cats may be infected.

Hazards to Other Animals

Unknown.

Hazards to Humans

Trypanosoma congolense is not considered to be a human pathogen. However, precautions should be taken to reduce potential hazards to humans in the veterinary clinic where an accident with a contaminated needle could serve to introduce the parasite into someone supplying veterinary care.

Control/Prevention

There is currently very little known about the prevalence, control, or prevention of the disease in cats. The biology of the parasite would suggest that cats should be protected from fly bites.

REFERENCE

Laveran A. 1909. Au sujet de *Trypanosoma congolense* Broden. Bull Soc Pathol Exot 2:526–528.

Trypanosoma cruzi Chagas, 1909

Etymology

This parasite is named after Dr. Cruz, the director of the institute in which Dr. Chagas worked.

Synonyms

Schizotrypanum cruzi Chagas, 1909; *Trypanosoma triatomae* Kofoid and McCulloch, 1916.

History

This parasite and the life cycle wherein triatomid bugs serve as the vectors were described by Chagas in 1909. Chagas was also the first to observe this trypanosome in the blood of domestic cats.

Geographic Distribution

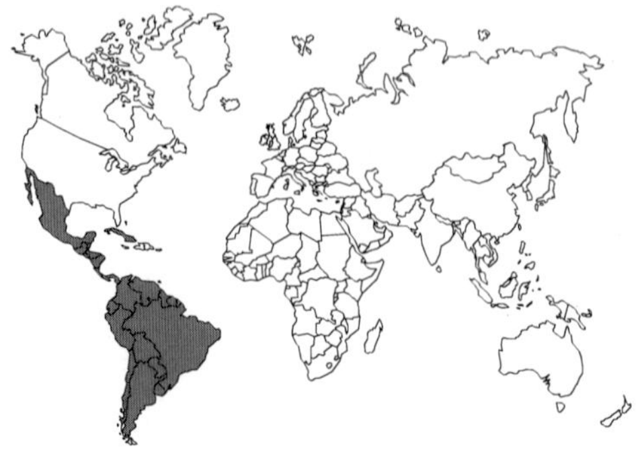

Fig. 1.54.

This organism is found in the southern United States, and throughout Mexico, Central America, and South America down into Argentina.

Location in Host

In the mammalian host, the trypomastigote stage of the parasite is found within the peripheral blood. The amastigote stage is found in reticuloendothelial cells at the site of the initial insect bite and, later, throughout the body. Other cells that may contain the amastigote stage include striated and cardiac muscle cells.

Parasite Identification

The trypomastigote stage of *Trypanosoma cruzi* that is present in peripheral blood is never seen to be dividing, is about 20 μm long, tends to be fixed in a C shape on prepared slides, has one to two undulations of the undulating membrane, and has a relatively large kinetoplast at the posterior end that appears to bulbously expand the cell body (Fig. 1.55). The free flagellum of *Trypanosoma cruzi* that extends from the anterior end is about one-half to two-thirds of the length of the cell body.

The amastigote stage of *Trypanosoma cruzi* is indistinguishable morphologically from that of the *Leishmania* species (see below), although if present in muscle cells, the location is diagnostic (Fig. 1.56) because the leishmanial amastigotes are found only in reticuloendothelial cells. The amastigote stage is round to oval, is 1.5 to 4 μm in diameter, and contains a large nucleus and a smaller kinetoplast. The amastigotes appear slightly larger in impression smears than in histologic sections due to flattening and the different methods of fixation.

Life Cycle

This parasite is transmitted between hosts by triatomid bugs (Chagas, 1909); genera that have been shown to serve as vectors include *Rhodnius, Panstrongylus,* and *Triatoma.* Within bugs that have ingested blood containing trypomastigotes, the parasite undergoes development from the trypomastigote through various stages (Fig. 1.57) to become an infective metacyclic trypomastigote form that is shed in the feces of the bug. Hosts become infected when they rub the feces into the bite wound after the bug has fed on them. Hosts can also become infected by the ingestion of the bugs with the parasites penetrating the mucosa of the mouth. It is also known that the parasite can be transmitted from a mother to her fetus transplacentally. Cats have been experimentally infected by feeding them infected mice (Baretto et al., 1978).

In the vertebrate host, the parasites multiply initially within macrophages and histiocytes at the location of the bite wound. Next there is the development of trypomastigotes within the blood and the development of additional amastigotes in

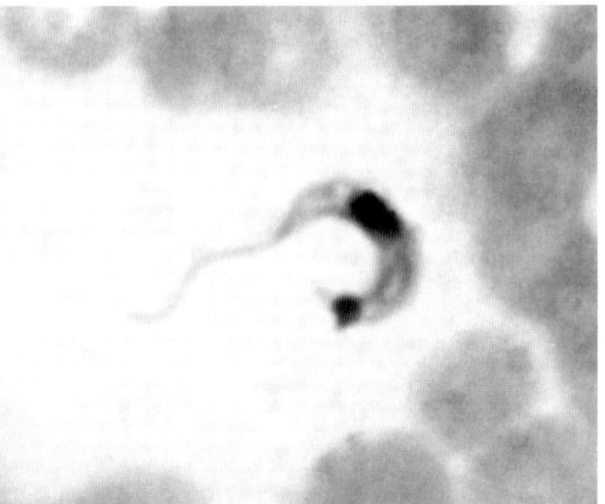

Fig. 1.55. *Trypanosoma cruzi* trypomastigotes in the blood of a mouse, stained with Giemsa. (Preparation courtesy of Dr. L. Leiva, School of Medicine, Louisiana State University.) Note the C shape of the trypomastigote and the very large kinetoplast at the posterior end of the cell.

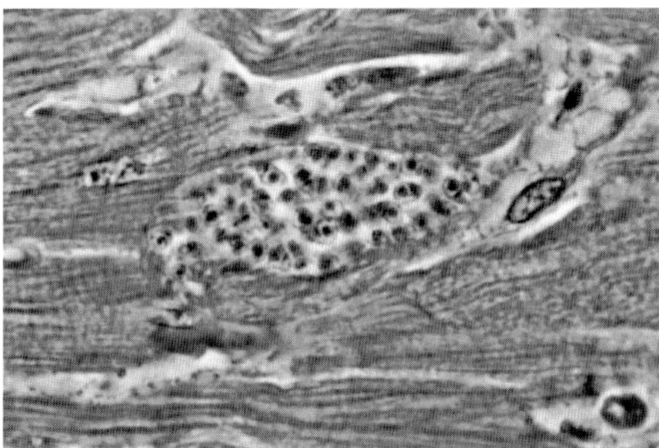

Fig. 1.56. *Trypanosoma cruzi* amastigotes in the heart muscle of an experimentally infected mouse. (Preparation courtesy of Dr. L. Leiva, School of Medicine, Louisiana State University.) Note the small round nucleus and the smaller bar-shaped kinetoplast that can be seen in some of the amastigotes present within this cell.

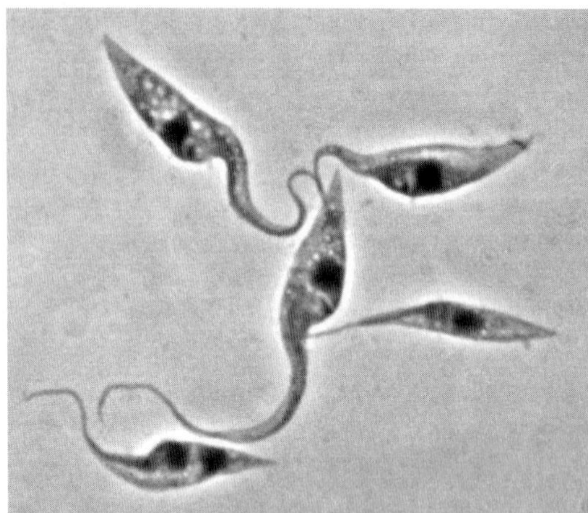

Fig. 1.57. *Trypanosoma cruzi* epimastigote culture forms representative of stages that would be observed in the invertebrate vector. (Preparation courtesy of Dr. L. Leiva, School of Medicine, Louisiana State University.)

other tissues. Ultimately, the blood forms become less common, and the amastigote stages are found within the reticuloendothelial cells of the spleen and liver and within muscle cells, especially the myocardium.

Clinical Presentation and Pathogenesis

Only a single cat has been described as having signs due to *Trypanosoma cruzi* (Talice, 1938). This cat in Montevideo, Uruguay, had signs that included convulsions and transient posterior paralysis.

Diagnosis

Although not well described in the cat, similar methods used in other species are likely to be successful. Blood smears stained with Giemsa may be effective in showing organisms during the first 1 to 2 weeks of infection. After this time the parasitemia becomes subpatent, requiring a concentration technique to identify organisms, or blood culture. Examining the region just above the buffy coat in a microhematocrit tube may show the presence of trypomastigote forms. Serum (1:10 dilution) may be cultured in LIT (liver infusion tryptose broth) at room temperature for 6 weeks, after which the broth may be examined for epimastigote forms. Serum may also be inoculated onto Vero cell cultures and maintained at 37°C for 4 to 6 weeks to identify trypomastigote forms. Inoculation of infected cat blood into weanling laboratory inbred mice (C3H) will usually cause parasitemias to appear 10 to 20 days later. There are currently no immunologic serology tests for cats, although tissue stage organisms could be identified using immunohistochemistry. Polymerase chain reaction tests used for humans or dogs should also work in cats.

Treatment

There are no reports of attempted treatment of infected cats.

Epizootiology

Cats are commonly found to be infected when examined as part of surveys in Latin America (e.g., 3.3 percent of cats in Chile) (Rojas et al., 1973), 2.9 percent of cats in Costa Rica (Zeledon et al., 1975), 28.6 percent of cats in northeastern Brazil (Mott et al., 1978), 26.9 percent of cats in Bolivia (Balderama et al., 1981), 7 to 8.5 percent of cats in Venezuela (Tonn et al., 1983), 63.6 percent of cats in Argentina (Wisnivesky-Colli et al., 1982), and 50 percent of cats in Oaxaca, Mexico (Salazar Schettino et al., 1987). The role of cats in the perpetuation of the parasite would thus appear to be a real one, although studies using immunologic methods that have identified hosts from tratomid bugs' blood meals have shown that in some areas cats are seldom fed on by the bugs (Wisnivesky-Colli, 1982), while other studies have shown that cats are routinely fed on by the vector (Deane, 1964).

Hazards to Other Animals

Trypanosoma cruzi is capable of infecting most vertebrates. Also, if introduced into a poorly maintained facility that might have infestations with the vector, transmission could occur.

Hazards to Humans

Trypanosoma cruzi is a serious human pathogen. Also, prevalence data would suggest that it should often be considered as a potential pathogen in cats that are being treated in Mexico and Central and South America. Precautions must be taken to reduce potential hazards to humans in the veterinary clinic where an accident with a contaminated needle could serve to introduce the parasite into someone supplying veterinary care.

Control/Prevention

Control and prevention of the disease in cats would, in part, be similar to that for humans (i.e., removing the domesticated triatomid vectors from the living quarters). However, the nature of cats to hunt on their own in the wild will continue to place them at great risk of acquiring infections from this parasite either from the bite of the bugs or the ingestion of infected rodents.

REFERENCES

Balderama F, Romero A, Garcia JA, Bermudez H, Serrano R, LaFuente C, Romero F. 1981. Estudio epidemiologico de la enfermedad de Chagas en el Trigal dpto. de Santa Cruz—Bolivia. Bol Inf Cenetrop 3:16–22.

Barreto MP, Ribeiro RS, Neto FMB. 1978. Estudos sobre reservatórios e vectores silvestres do *Trypanosoma cruzi.* LXCVIII: Infecção de mamíferos pela via oral. Rev Brazil Biol 38:455–459.

Chagas C. 1909. Nova tripanozomiaze humana. Estudo sobre a morfologia e o ciclo evolutivo do *Schizotrypanum cruzi,* n. gen. n. sp., agent etiológico de nova entidade morbida do homen. Mem Inst Osw Cruz 1:159–218.

Deane LM. 1964. Animal reservoirs of *Trypanosoma cruzi* in Brazil. Brasil Malario Doenças Trop 16:27–48.

Mott KE, Mota EA, Sherlock I, Hoff R, Muniz TM, Oliveira TS, Draper CC. 1978. *Trypanosoma cruzi* infection in dogs and cats and household seroreactivity to *T. cruzi* in a rural community in northeast Brazil. Am J Trop Med Hyg 27:1123–1127.

Rojas A, Sotelo JM, Villarroel F, Contrerar MC. 1973. La importancia del perro y el gato en la epideiologia de la enfermedad de Chagas. Bol Chile Parasit 28:42–43.

Salazar Schettino PM, Bucio Torres MI, De Haro Arteaga I, Tay Zavalka J, Alonso Guerrero T. 1987. Reservorios y transmisores de *Trypanosoma cruzi* en el estado de Ozxaca. Sal Publ Mex 29:26–32.

Talice RV. 1938. Primeras observaciones en el Uruguay de gatos espontáneamente infectados por el *Trypanosoma cruzi.* Arch Urug med, chir, espesiald 13:61–65.

Tonn RJ, Cedillos RA, Ortegon A, Gonzalez JJ, Carrasquero B. 1983. Reservorios domésticos de *Trypanosoma cruzi* y *Trypanosoma rangeli* en Venezuela. Bol Dir Malariol Saneam Ambient 23:18–26.

Wisnivesky-Colli C, Gürtler RE, Solarz ND, Lauricella MA, Segura EL. 1982. Epidemiological role of humans, dogs, and cats in the transmission of *Trypanosoma cruzi* in a central area of Argentina. Rev Inst Med trop São Paulo 27:346–352.

Zeledon R, Solano G, Burstin L, Schwartzwelder JC. 1975. Epidemiological pattern of Chagas' disease in an endemic area of Costa Rica. Am J Trop Med Hyg 24:214–225.

Trypanosoma rangeli Tejera, 1920

Etymology

This parasite is named after Dr. Rangel.

Synonyms

Trypanosoma escomeli Yorke, 1920; *Trypanosoma guatamalense* De Léon, 1946; *Trypanosoma cebus* Floch and Abonnenc, 1949; *Trypanosoma ariarii* Groot, Renjifo, and Uribe, 1951.

History

This trypanosome, like *Trypanosoma cruzi,* was first discovered in its invertebrate vector (Tejera, 1920). Although nonpathogenic trypanosomes were observed in Latin America after this time, it was some time until the nonpathogenic trypanosomes isolated from the human blood were identified as *Trypanosoma rangeli* (Pifano et al., 1948).

Geographic Distribution

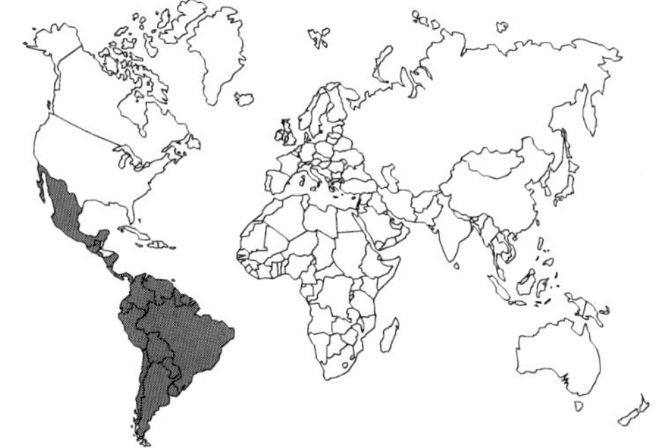

Fig. 1.58.

This organism is found in Central America and South America down into Chile.

Location in Host

In the mammalian host, the trypomastigote stage of the parasite is found within the peripheral blood.

Parasite Identification

The trypomastigote stage of *Trypanosoma rangeli* is the only stage of the parasite found in the vertebrate host. The trypomastigote may be seen to be dividing. The trypomastigote is slender, 26 to 34 μm long; the undulating membrane is well developed and may have four to five undulations throughout its length. The kinetoplast is small and subterminal to the posterior end of the cell. The free flagellum of *Trypanosoma rangeli* that extends from the anterior end is about one-half to two-thirds of the length of the cell body.

Life Cycle

This parasite is transmitted between hosts by the bite of triatomid bugs (Groot, 1952); genera that have been shown to serve as vectors include *Rhodnius* and *Triatoma.* Within bugs that have ingested blood containing trypomastigotes, the parasites develop within the hemolymph and then make their way to the salivary glands. In the vertebrate host, the parasites multiply within the bloodstream.

Clinical Presentation and Pathogenesis

This trypanosome is apparently nonpathogenic in humans, and it would likely be nonpathogenic in cats.

Diagnosis

Trypomastigotes may be identified within a peripheral blood smear, like *Trypanosoma cruzi,* and may be better identified above the buffy coat in a hematocrit tube viewed under 400× magnification. Culture may be attempted in axenic media. *Trypanosoma rangeli* may be distinguished from *Trypanosoma cruzi* morphologically and with mouse infection studies: *Trypanosoma rangeli* does not infect mice.

Treatment

There are no reports of attempted treatment of infected cats.

Epizootiology

Overall, very few cats have been examined for the presence of *Trypanosoma rangeli.* A cat in Venezuela was found to have circulating trypomastigotes of *Trypanosoma rangeli* in its blood (Pifano, 1954). More recently, 8.5 percent of cats in Venezuela were shown to be infected with *Trypanosoma rangeli* (Tonn et al., 1983).

Hazards to Other Animals

Although transmission to other animals could occur, this protozoan is considered to be nonpathogenic.

Hazards to Humans

The role of cats in the epidemiology of this nonpathogenic organism is not known.

Control/Prevention

Control and prevention of the disease in cats would, in part, be similar to that for humans (i.e., removing the domesticated triatomid vectors from the living quarters). However, the nature of cats to hunt on their own in the wild will continue to place them at risk of acquiring infections from this parasite.

REFERENCES

Groot H. 1952. Further observations on *Trypanosoma ariarii* of Colombia, South America. Am J Trop Med Hyg 1:585–592.

Pifano F. 1954. Nueva trypanosomiasis humana de la region neotropica producida por el *Trypanosoma rangeli,* con especial referencia a Venezuela. Arch Venezol Patol Trop Parasitol 2:89–120.

Pifano F, Mayer M, Medina R, Pinto HB. 1948. Primera comprabación de *Trypanosoma rangeli* en el organisms humana por cultiva sangria perifica. Arch Venezol Patol Trop Parasitol 1:1–31.

Tejera E. 1920. Un nouveau flagellé de *Rhodnius prolixus, Trypanosoma* (ou *Crithidia*) *rangeli* n.sp. Bull Soc Path Exot 13:525–530.

Tonn RJ, Cedillos RA, Ortegon A, Gonzalez JJ, Carrasquero B. 1983. Reservorios domésticos de *Trypanosoma cruzi* y *Trypanosoma rangeli* en Venezuela. Bol Dir Malariol Saneam Ambient 23:18–26.

Leishmanial Organisms

The different species of *Leishmania* are continuously in a state of flux due to the lack of easy means of differentiating species. Basically, there are three major groups of organisms: those that cause visceral disease, those that cause cutaneous lesions, and those that cause mucocutaneous lesions. The organisms causing visceral disease are species and various subspecies of *Leishmania donovani.* The organisms causing cutaneous leishmaniasis in the Old World are *Leishmania tropica* (anthroponotic or urban cutaneous leishmaniasis with dry lesions), *Leishmania major* (zoonotic or rural cutaneous leishmaniasis with wet lesions), and *Leishmania aethiopica* (zoonotic cutaneous leishmaniasis of Kenya and Ethiopia with varied lesions). The organisms causing zoonotic cutaneous leishmaniasis in the New World are *Leishmania braziliensis, Leishmania mexicana,* and *Leishmania peruviana.* The organisms causing mucocutaneous leishmaniasis in the New World are typically due to species of *Leishmania braziliensis.*

Leishmania donovani (Laveran and Mesnil, 1903) Ross, 1903

Etymology

This parasite is named after William Leishman, who discovered the organisms in spleen smears, and Charles Donovan, who found the organisms in a splenic puncture biopsy.

Synonyms

Piroplasma donovani Laveran and Mesnil, 1903; *Leishmania chagasi* Chagas et al., 1937.

History

In 1900, William Leishman found organisms in spleen smears of a soldier who died from a fever known as kala-azar (Leishman, 1904), and in 1903 Donovan found the same organisms in a splenic biopsy. Rogers (1904) showed that flagellate forms developed in cultures, and Adler and Ber (1941) showed promastigotes would develop in sandflies and transmit the disease. Nicolle and Comte found *Leishmania donovani* in dogs in Tunisia in 1908.

Geographic Distribution

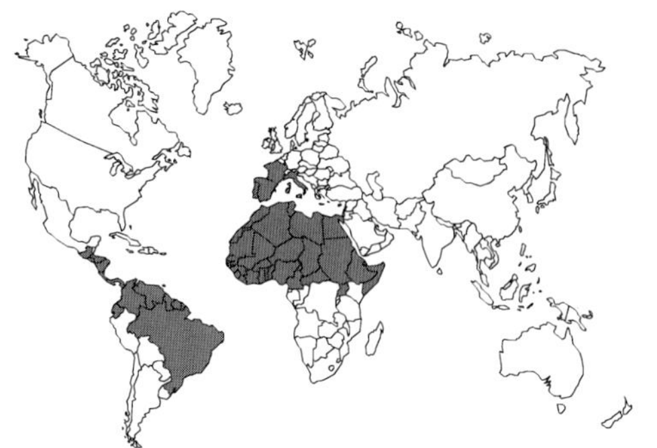

Fig. 1.59.

This organism is found in North Africa, Southern Europe, and the Middle East through India into western China. The disease was brought to the Americas after Columbus and is now endemic in parts of South and Central America. There have been reports of visceral leishmaniasis in cats around Brazil (Mello, 1940) and the Mediterranean—Spain (Gimeno Ondovilla, 1933), Italy (Giordano, 1933), Algeria (Sergent et al., 1912; Bosselut, 1948), Jordan (Morsy et al., 1980), and France (Bergeron, 1927).

Location in Host

In the mammalian host, the only stage that is present is the amastigote that is found within histiocytes, monocytes, and other cells of the reticuloendothelial system. Typically, *Leishmania donovani* is found within the spleen, liver, bone marrow, intestinal mucosa, and mesenteric lymph nodes. Other *Leishmania* species tend to be confined to ulcers on the skin.

Parasite Identification

The amastigote stage of *Leishmania donovani* is indistinguishable morphologically from that of the *Trypanosoma cruzi* and other *Leishmania* species (Fig. 1.60). The amastigote stage is round to oval, is 1.5 to 4 μm in diameter, and contains a large nucleus and a smaller kinetoplast. The amastigotes appear slightly larger in impression smears than in histologic sections due to flattening and the different methods of fixation.

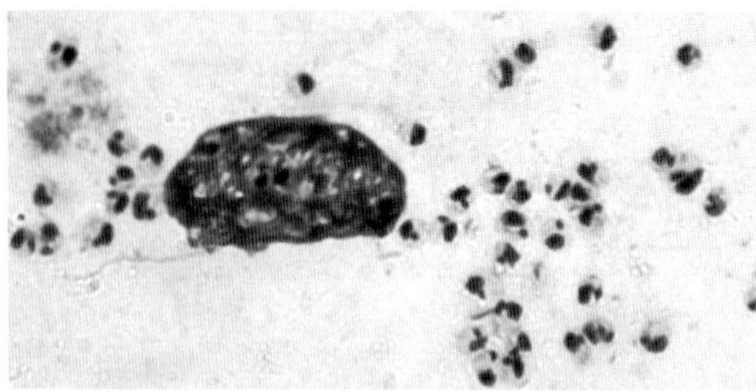

Fig. 1.60. *Leishmania donovani* in impression smear of experimentally infected hamster that was stained with Giemsa stain. (Preparation courtesy of Dr. J. Farrell, College of Veterinary Medicine, University of Pennsylvania.) Note the large host-cell nucleus in the middle that is surrounded by the amastigotes that have a small round nucleus and the bar-shaped kinetoplast.

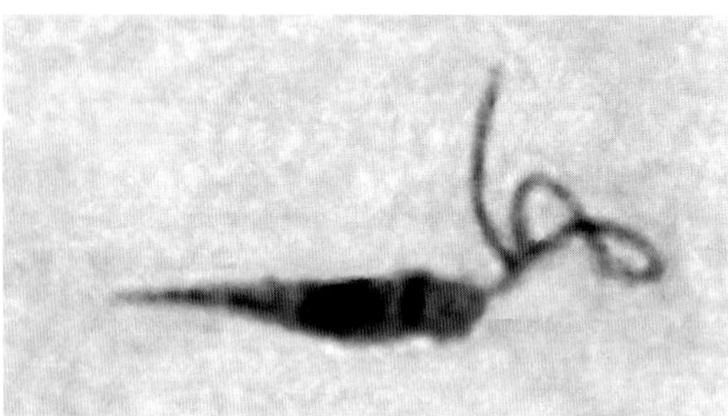

Fig. 1.61. *Leishmania donovani* culture form showing the elongate shape and the presence of the free, anteriorly directed flagellum.

Life Cycle

Within the mammalian host the parasite grows and multiplies within cells of the reticuloendothelial system by simple binary division. *Leishmania donovani* is transmitted between hosts by the bite of infected sandflies (genera: *Phlebotomus* in Europe and Asia, and *Lutzomyia* in the Americas). Within the sandfly are found the flagellated promastigote forms of the parasite that are similar to the stage found in cell-free cultures (Fig. 1.61).

Clinical Presentation and Pathogenesis

Very few of the reports dealing with cats have described clinical signs other than to say that the cats were thin and may have had cutaneous manifestations of the visceral disease. In one case, organisms were found in the spleen (Bergeron, 1927), and in another case amastigotes were seen in bone marrow (Sergent et al., 1912).

The course of infection has been followed in cats with experimentally induced visceral leishmaniasis (Kirkpatrick et al., 1984). Cats inoculated intravenously with amastigotes developed large numbers of organisms in the liver, spleen, and bone marrow. On the other hand, cats inoculated intradermally with promastigotes from culture developed transient (of 3 days duration) palpable nodules at the site of inoculation, but no parasites were recovered from the internal organs of these cats. Of those infected cats that were maintained up to 16 weeks after infection, none developed signs of leishmaniasis or cutaneous lesions. At necropsy, there was no apparent hepatomegaly or splenomegaly. These results describing the failure of the inoculation of promastigotes are not surprising in light of recent work showing the importance that the saliva of the sandfly plays in the development of visceral infection with this parasite.

Diagnosis

Serologic tests exist for the cat but are unreliable as cats are rarely clinically affected even when they are serologically positive. The cutaneous form, the most common, may be diagnosed by identifying organisms within cells on aspirate cytology (Wright's or Giemsa stain) or histopathology of excised lesions. Although not reported in cats, PCR tests on infected tissues should be very sensitive and specific.

Treatment

There are no reports of attempted treatment of infected cats.

Epizootiology

Overall, very few cats have been examined for the presence of *Leishmania donovani.* It has been considered that they do not play a major role as mammalian hosts of this parasite, but at this time, their role is actually not known.

Hazards to Other Animals

Transmission to other animals could occur, but at this time, the significance of the role of the cat in the wild is not known.

Hazards to Humans

Cats could serve as sources of human infection, but they are not considered to be major reservoirs of this parasite. However, personnel need to be protected from possible accidents that could introduce the organisms into their skin.

Control/Prevention

To control and prevent this disease in cats it would be necessary to prevent cats from being bitten by the sandfly vector.

REFERENCES

Adler S, Ber M. 1941. Transmission of *Leishmania tropica* by the bite of *Phlebotomus papatasii.* Ind J Med Test 29:803.

Bergeron PVA. 1927. Un cas de leishmaniose chez le chat. Bull Soc Sci Vet Lyon 30:92–93.

Bosselut H. 1948. Un cas de leishmaniose générale du chat. Arch Inst Pasteur d'Alg 26:14.

Gimeno Ondovilla A. 1933. Contribución a la epidemiología del kala azar. Trabajos Madrid 2:26–27.

Giordano A. 1933. Le chat dans la transmission de la leishmaniose viscérale de la médittéranée. Bull Sez Ital Soc Intern Microbiol 5:330–332.

Kirpatrick CE, Farrell JP, Goldschmidt MH. 1984. *Leishmania chagasi* and *L. donovani:* Experimental infections in domestic cats. Exp Parasitol 58:125–131.

Leishman WB. 1904. Note on the nature of the parasitic bodies found in tropical splenomegaly Br Med J (2249) 1:303.

Mello GB. 1940. Verificão de infecção natural do gato (*Felix domesticus*) por um protozoario do genero *Leishmania.* Bras Med 54:180.

Morsy TA, Michael SA, El Disi AM. 1980. Cats as reservoir hosts of human parasites in Amman, Jordan. J Egypt Soc Parasitol 10:5–18.

Nicolle C, Comte C. 1908. Origine canine du Kala-azar. Compt Rend Acad Sci 146:789–791.

Rogers L. 1904. Preliminary note on the development of *Trypanosoma* in cultures of the Cunningham-Leishman-Donovan bodies of cachexial fever and kala-azar. Lanct (4221) 167:215–216.

Sergent EE, Lombard J, Quilichini M. 1912. La leishmaniose â Alger. Infection simultanée d'un enfant, d'un chien et d'un chat dans la même habitation. Bull Soc Pathol Exot 5:93–98.

Leishmania tropica (Wright, 1903) Lühe, 1906

Etymology

Named for the tropics.

Synonyms

Helicosoma tropica Wright, 1903; *Herpetomonas tropica* Patton, 1912; *Herpetomonas furunculosa* (Wright, 1903) Patton, 1922.

History

The first person to describe the organism was Wright in 1903, who saw them in the cutaneous lesion of an Armenian patient undergoing treatment in Boston. The sandfly was shown to be the vector of this parasite by Sergent et al. (1921).

Geographic Distribution

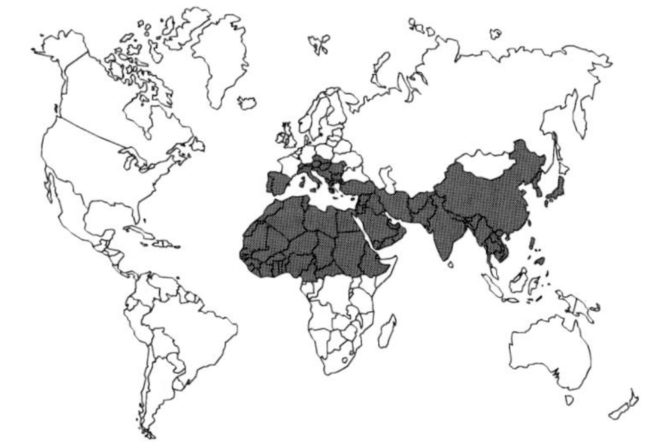

Fig. 1.62.

This organism is found in North Africa, Southern Europe, and the Middle East through India into western China. It is considered that this is mainly a human disease that on occasion also infects animals.

Location in Host

In the mammalian host, the only stage that is present is the amastigote that is found within histiocytes and macrophages in the skin.

Parasite Identification

The amastigote stage of *Leishmania tropica* is indistinguishable morphologically from other *Leishmania* species and that of the *Trypanosoma cruzi.* The amastigote stage is round to oval, is 1.5 to 4 μm in diameter, and contains a large nucleus and a smaller kinetoplast. The amastigotes appear slightly larger in impression smears than in histologic sections due to flattening and the different methods of fixation.

Life Cycle

Within the mammalian host the parasite grows and multiplies within macrophages and histiocytes of the skin at the site of the bite by the sandfly vector. *Leishmania tropica* is transmitted between hosts by the bite of infected sandflies of the genus *Phlebotomus*. Within the sandfly are found the flagellated promastigote forms of the parasite that are similar to the stage found in cell-free cultures.

Clinical Presentation and Pathogenesis

There is a report of two clinical cases of lesions of the *Leishmania tropica* type in cats in Iraq (Machattie et al., 1931). These two cats were found to have ulcers and organisms that were identified as probably being due to *Leishmania tropica*. The cats appeared thin but healthy. One cat had an extensive lesion on the nose, a small ulcerating sore on the left eyelid, and three papules on the left ear. The other cat had a single sore on its nose. Postmortem examination of the cats revealed no organisms within the deeper tissues. A cat from the Marseillaise region was found at autopsy to have numerous skin lesions that contained many organisms that were called *Leishmania infantum* (Dunan et al., 1989). The cat had presented to a local veterinarian with lesions that began as erythematous lesions that later developed pustules. The lesions were on the top of the head and on the neck. After 3 months following anti-inflammatory and antibiotic therapy, the cat was euthanatized at the request of the owner. Only the skin lesions were submitted; thus, it was not possible to ascertain if there were organisms present in other body tissues.

Diagnosis

For cutaneous lesions the diagnosis method of choice is identifying organisms within cells on aspirate cytology (Wright's or Giemsa stain) or histopathology of excised lesions. Although not reported in cats, PCR tests on infected tissues should be very sensitive and specific.

Treatment

There are no reports of attempted treatment of infected cats.

Epizootiology

Overall, very few cats have been examined for the presence of *Leishmania tropica*. It has been considered that they do not play a major role as mammalian hosts of this parasite, and at this time, it is believed that human beings serve as the major reservoir of infection.

Hazards to Other Animals

Transmission to other animals is unlikely. Transmission could occur by direct inoculation of the organisms, but under most circumstances, this would probably not occur.

Hazards to Humans

Cats could serve as sources of human infection, but currently cats are not considered to be major reservoirs of this parasite. However, personnel need to be protected from possible accidents that could introduce the organisms into their skin.

Control/Prevention

Control and prevention of the disease in cats would, in part, be based on reducing the number of cases within the human reservoir of infection.

REFERENCES

Dunan S, Mary C, Garbe L, Breton Y, Olivon B, Ferrey P, Cabassu JP. 1989. A propos d'un cas de leishmaniose chez un chat de la region Marseillaise. Bull Soc Fran Parasitol 7:17–20.

Machattie C, Mills EA, Chadwick CR. 1931. Naturally occurring oriental sore of the domestic cat in Iraq. Trans Roy Soc Trop Med Hyg 25:103–106.

Sergent E, Sergent E, Parrot LM, Dinatien AL, Béguet ME. 1921. Transmission do clou de Biskra par le phlébotome (*Phlebotomus papatasi* Scop.). Compt Rend Acad Sci 173:1030–1032.

Leishmania braziliensis and *Leishmania mexicana*

Etymology

Named for the location in New World tropics.

Synonyms

Leishmania tropica var. *americana* Laveran and Nattan-Larrier, 1912.

History

Spanish explorers soon discovered after conquest that in areas of the Andes there was the possibility of developing lesions of the nares that could prove disfiguring (Weiss, 1943). It is now believed that the lesions of this type are due to several species of leishmaniasis-inducing organisms that are indigenous to the New World.

Geographic Distribution

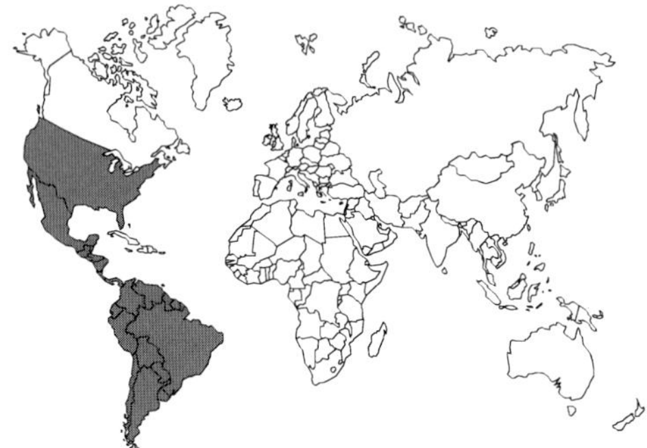

Fig. 1.63.

These organisms are found in the southern United States, Mexico, and Central and South America.

Location in Host

In the mammalian host, the only stage that is present is the amastigote that is found within histiocytes and macrophages in the skin. Some species seem to have a predilection for mucocutaneous areas of the skin.

Parasite Identification

The amastigote stage of these species of *Leishmania* is indistinguishable morphologically from that of other *Leishmania* species and that of the *Trypanosoma cruzi*. The amastigote stage is round to oval, is 1.5 to 4 μm in diameter, and contains a large nucleus and a smaller kinetoplast. The amastigotes appear slightly larger in impression smears than in histologic sections due to flattening and the different methods of fixation.

Life Cycle

Within the mammalian host the parasite grows and multiplies within macrophages and histiocytes of the skin at the site of the bite by the sandfly vector. New World leishmaniasis is transmitted between hosts by the bite of infected sandflies of the genus *Lutzomyia*. Within the sandfly are found the flagellated promastigote forms of the parasite that are similar to the stage found in cell-free cultures.

Clinical Presentation and Pathogenesis

There have been a few reports of cutaneous leishmaniasis in cats in the New World. Craig et al. (1986) reported on lesions in the ear of a 4-year-old long-haired domestic cat in Texas. The cat had no signs of systemic disease and was returned to its owners after a radical pinnectomy. Three other cats (one male and two females) were found to have lesions in Venezuela (Bonfante-Garrido et al., 1991). On the male cat, the lesions occurred on the nose and ears; on the female cats lesions were confined to the nose. In all cases, organisms were observed in impression smears of the lesions.

Diagnosis

For cutaneous lesions the method of diagnosis of choice is identifying organisms within cells on aspirate cytology (Wright's or Giemsa stain) or histopathology of excised lesions. Although not reported in cats, PCR tests on infected tissues should be very sensitive and specific.

Treatment

There are no reports of attempted treatment of infected cats other than surgical excision of the affected tissue.

Epizootiology

Overall, very few cats have been reported to be infected with dermal leishmaniasis. It is believed that small rodents serve as the major reservoirs of infection with this species in the New World.

Hazards to Other Animals

Transmission to other animals could occur through direct inoculation of the organisms, but this would probably be unlikely.

Hazards to Humans

Cats could serve as sources of human infection, but they are not considered to be major reservoirs of this parasite. However, personnel need to be protected from possible accidents that could introduce the organisms into their skin.

Control/Prevention

Control and prevention of the disease in cats would, in part, need to be directed at preventing the cats from coming into contact with infected flies. However, because both the cats and the flies are hunting the same small rodents that serve as reservoirs of this infection, it is likely that it will not be possible to prevent cats that hunt from becoming infected.

REFERENCES

Bonfante-Garrido R, Urdaneta I, Urdaneta R, Alvarado J. 1991. Natural infection of cats with *Leishmania* in Barquisimeto, Venezuela. Trans Roy Soc Trop Med Hyg 85:53.

Craig TM, Barton CL, Mercer SH, Droleskey BE, Jones LP. 1986. Dermal leishmaniasis in a Texas cat. Am J Trop Med Hyg 35:1100–1102.

Weiss P. 1943. Epidemiología y clínica de la leishmaniasis tegumentarias en el Peru. Rev Med Exp Lima 2:209–248.

RHIZOPODA

The sarcodinid parasites of concern are the amebae (spelled by some with an *o,* e.g., "amoebae"). These organisms are characterized by their form of movement, which involves the directional extension of the cell body by processes called pseudopodia; this movement is accomplished without cilia or undulipodia. The feeding stage is called a trophozoite, which ingests particles by surrounding them with cytoplasm of an engulfing pseudopod. Some amebae have a cyst stage that is resistant to environmental extremes. Amebae are found both as free-living forms and as parasitic forms in diverse hosts ranging from cockroaches to humans. Humans are host to several species of ameba, but only one species, *Entamoeba histolytica,* is a serious pathogen of humans, in which it causes large-bowel disease and occasionally hepatic or other deep tissue abscesses. Cats do not appear to be typical hosts of this pathogenic ameba, even though they have been experimentally infected to study the pathogenic effects of this parasite. Cats have, however, on at least one occasion been reported to be infected with this parasite (Kessel, 1928).

Entamoeba histolytica Schaudinn, 1903

Etymology

(*Ent* = internal + *amoeba; histo* = tissue + *lytica* = lysis).

Synonyms

Amoeba coli Lösch, 1878; *Amoeba dysenteriae* Councilman and Lafleur, 1891; *Entamoeba dysenteriae* (Councilman and Lafleur, 1891) Craig, 1905; *Entamoeba tetragena* Hartmann, 1908; *Endamoeba histolytica* (Schaudinn, 1903) Hickson, 1909; *Endamoeba dysenteria* Kofoid, 1920; *Entamoeba dispar* Brumpt, 1925.

History

Disease due to *Entamoeba histolytica* was first observed by Lösch in 1875 in Leningrad. Lösch observed amebae in ulcers of the colon at necropsy and induced disease in a dog by a rectal inoculation with human feces. Work by others, including Councilman and Lafleur, showed that the ameba was the cause of the disease. *Entamoeba histolytica* was distinguished from the nonpathogenic commensal of humans, *Entamoeba coli,* by Schaudinn in 1903.

Geographic Distribution

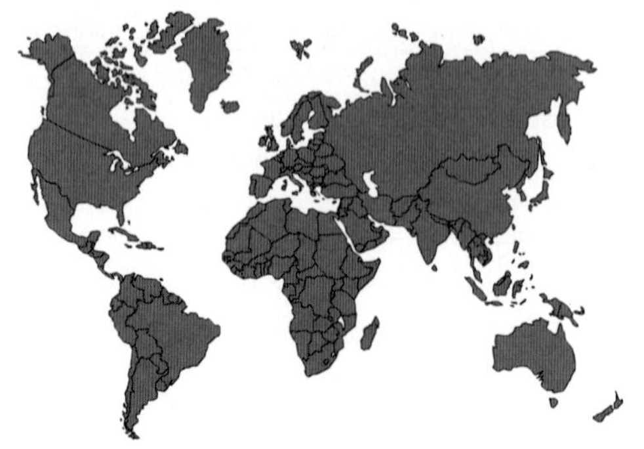

Fig. 1.64.

These organisms are found throughout the world but are more common in the tropics. There is only a single report in which amebae specifically identified as *Entamoeba histolytica* have been found in naturally infected cats.

Location in Host

Entamoeba histolytica is a parasite of the mucosa of the large intestine. Some strains are more pathogenic than others and are capable of causing ulcers within the mucosa and being carried by the bloodstream to other organs, for example, the liver, lung, and brain, where abscesses develop. In experimentally infected cats, abscesses have been observed to develop in the liver.

Parasite Identification

The 8 to 30 µm trophozoite in a fecal smear prepared from fresh feces in physiologic saline will continue to be motile, and finger-shaped, rapidly extended pseudopodia can be observed. The trophozoites of *Entamoeba histolytica* are often seen to contain ingested red blood cells. If the fecal material is stained with a trichrome stain or iron hematoxylin, the characteristic morphology of the nucleus with its small central karyosome and peripheral chromatin granules can be observed.

The spherical cyst, 10 to 20 µm in diameter, is more likely to be observed in formed feces. A fully developed cyst will contain four nuclei, although maturing cysts can contain anywhere from one to four nuclei. The cyst may contain elongate rod-shaped structures, chromatoidal bodies, which will have blunt ends.

Life Cycle

In humans, the typical life cycle includes the feeding, trophozoite stage that is found on or in the mucosa of the large bowel. The trophozoite is the stage that causes disease and is the stage passed in the feces of patients with dysentery. The cyst stage is passed into the environment with the formed feces of individuals that serve as carriers of the infection. The cyst is a relatively resistant form that serves to transport the ameba from host to host in fecal contaminated water.

It is difficult to infect kittens with a *per os* inoculation of cysts of *Entamoeba histolytica,* although it has been done (Dale and Dobell, 1917). More typically, kittens have been experimentally infected by the intrarectal inoculation of cysts or trophozoites obtained from human cases or other experimentally infected cats. In cats that are experimentally infected, amebae can first be detected in dysenteric stools as early as 3 days after infection (Sanders, 1928), with the average prepatent period being about 6 days (Kessel, 1928). As noted above (under Diagnosis), cysts are rarely seen in cats following experimental infection.

Clinical Presentation and Pathogenesis

Diamond and Clark (1993) proposed that there were two morphologically indistinguishable species of *Entamoeba.* One of these species, *Entamoeba histolytica* Schaudinn, 1903 (Walker, 1911), is pathogenic in cats, while a second species, *Entamoeba dispar* Brumpt, 1925, is nonpathogenic in cats. This was a concept originally proposed by Brumpt in 1925 based on pathogenicity of isolates in humans and in experimentally infected kittens. These two isolates of pathogenic and nonpathogenic strains can be differentiated on the basis of electrophoretic enzyme analysis, by using monoclonal antibodies, as well as various DNA probes that hybridize selectively to the DNA of the different ameba isolates. Thus, it would appear that cats that are passing cysts without signs of disease are probably infected with the noninvasive *Entamoeba dispar,* while cats or kittens that develop amebiasis are probably infected with the invasive species *Entamoeba histolytica.*

The experimental inoculation of adult cats with *Entamoeba histolytica* seldom results in infection or disease, although a carrier state has developed in a small number of adult animals (Baetjer and Sellards, 1914); of course, it has not always been clear whether the authors were working with pathogenic or nonpathogenic isolates. Disease occurs mainly in kittens. In the three naturally infected kittens that have been observed to have a pathogenic form of the organism (Kessel, 1928), trophozoites were noted in fecal samples taken soon after the kittens were purchased on the streets of Peking, China. These three kittens developed dysentery and succumbed to the infections within a few days after purchase. Histologic examination of the large bowel revealed lesions similar to those seen in experimentally infected kittens with ulcers containing amebae extending to the level of the muscularis mucosa. Lesions in experimentally infected kittens are typically restricted to the distal fourth of the large bowel, although, in some older animals, lesions have been noted anterior to the ileo-cecal valve. It is difficult to judge whether the observed localization approximates the natural state of disease in the cat because the amebae were often inoculated intrarectally, which may have some effect on where the lesions are produced.

In the experimentally infected kittens, the amebae enter the bottom of the glands in the large intestine and then pass into the connective tissue beneath. This is followed by the degeneration of epithelial cells. As the lesions grow in size and severity, the kitten develops the typical bloody and mucoid stools. A common occurrence in infected cats appears to be a generalized septicemia. Cats typically die within 8 days after infection (Kessel, 1928), but ranges from 4 to 39 days have been reported in cats with dysentery. A few cats have become "carriers" and have been observed apparently healthy 62 days after infection. These carrier cats were without signs of dysentery and without amebae in their stools, but on necropsy they did have lesions (in one an 8 cm bloody patch) containing motile amebae.

Liver abscesses are capable of developing in experimentally infected cats (Wenyon, 1912; Baetjer and Sellards, 1914; Dale and Dobell, 1917). The amebae are first carried to the mesenteric lymph nodes, which become enlarged and in which the amebae multiply. The amebae are then carried to the liver where amebic abscesses typical of those of human amebiasis develop.

In some cats, the observed abscesses have remained less than a centimeter in size and cause superficial bulges of the liver surface. In one case, an extensive internalized abscess developed that occupied about one-quarter of the entire liver (Baetjer and Sellards, 1914). Examination of the abscesses has revealed them to contain numerous amebae. The typical abscess appears to remain free for the most part of contaminating bacteria, although there is extensive necrosis and caseation.

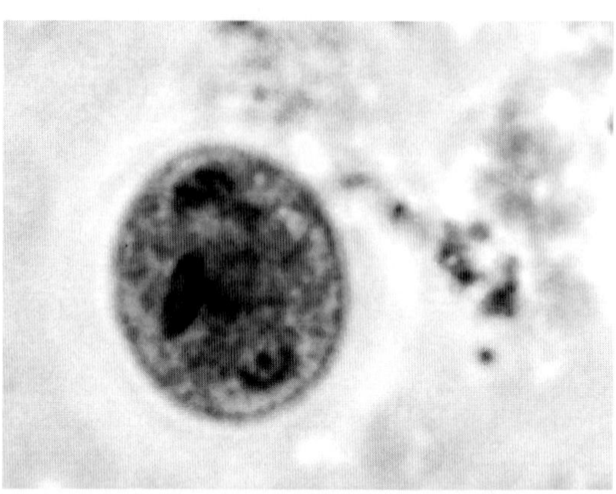

Fig. 1.65. Cyst of *Entamoeba histolytica* in human feces. The cyst was fixed and then stained with iron hematoxylin. Note the characteristic nucleus and kinetoplast and the rounded, dark chromatoidal bodies. In this cyst only one of the four nuclei is visible in the focal plane of the photomicrograph.

Diagnosis

The parasite is diagnosed in formed feces by the identification of the cyst in the feces (Fig. 1.65). In loose or dysenteric stools, a diagnosis requires the identification of the motile trophozoite stage (Fig. 1.66). The only diagnosis made in naturally infected cats has been based on the identification of trophozoites in feces and in histologic sections of the wall of the colon (Kessel, 1928). Typically, cats do not appear to shed cysts, however, Quincke and Roos (1893), who were the first to observe cysts in the feces of humans, observed cysts in the feces of cats that they had infected with cysts from humans. Also, Jungmann et al. (1986) reported 1 of 13 cats in East Berlin to be shedding cysts of an unidentified *Entamoeba* species. It would appear that cats are refractory to infections with the other *Entamoeba* species that infect humans (i.e., *Entamoeba coli* and *Entamoeba hartmanni*) (Wenyon, 1912; Dale and Dobell, 1917); this simplifies the identification of the trophozoite and cyst in cat feces.

Treatment

Kittens were used in a series of trials on the therapeutic effects of a number of ipecacuanha alkaloids (Dale and Dobell, 1917) without any being found to be of significant therapeutic value. There have been no recent reports of attempts to treat infected cats.

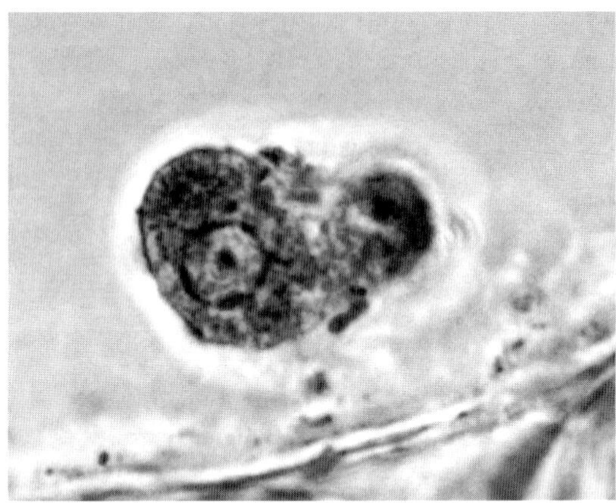

Fig. 1.66. Trophozoite of *Entamoeba histolytica* in human feces. The trophozoite was fixed, then stained with iron hematoxylin, and photographed using phase microscopy. The trophozoite has the characteristic nucleus that is surrounded by chromatin and has a central nucleolus.

Epizootiology

Cats do not appear to be regular hosts of this human pathogen even though cysts have been reported in the feces of cats on several occasions (Baetjer and Sellards, 1914; Jungmann et al., 1986). It would thus appear that kittens are at risk when around water that has been contaminated with human sewage. This parasite has been found in humans throughout the world; it is more common in the warmer climates, but it is present in human populations who live in situations where human feces is not properly disposed of with respect to water and foodstuffs.

Hazards to Other Animals

This is unlikely due to cats seldom shedding the transmission stage, the cyst, in their feces even when infected.

Hazards to Humans

This is a situation where cats are probably mainly at risk of being infected from a human source rather than vice versa.

Control/Prevention

Control and prevention of the disease in cats would be directed at improving the sanitary disposal of human excrement around the world and by providing all people and animals sources with clean drinking water.

REFERENCES

Baetjer WA, Sellards AW. 1914. The behavior of amoebic dysentery in lower animals and its bearing upon the interpretation of the clinical symptoms of the disease in man. Johns Hopkins Hosp Bull 282:237–241.

Brumpt E. 1925. Étude sommaire de l' "*Entamoeba dispar*" n.sp. amibe à kystes quadrinuclés, parasite de l'homme. Bull Acad Méd (Paris) 94:943–952.

Dale HH, Dobell C. 1917. Experiments on the therapeutics of amoebic dysentery. J Pharm Exp Therap 10:399–459.

Diamond LS, Clark CG. 1993. A redescription of *Entamoeba histolytica* Schaudinn, 1903 (Emended Walker, 1911) separating it from *Entamoeba dispar* Brumpt, 1925. J Euk Microbiol 40:340–344.

Jungmann R, Hiepe T, Scheffler C. 1986. Zur parasitären Intestinalfauna bei Hund und Katze mit einem spziellen Beitrag zur *Giardia*-Infektion. Mh Vet Med 41:309–311.

Kessel JH. 1928. Amoebiasis in kittens infected with amoebae from acute and "carrier" human cases and with the tetranucleate amoebae of the monkey and of the pig. Am J Hyg 8:311–355.

Lösch F. 1875. Massenhafte Entwickelung von Amöben im Dickdarm. Arch Path Anat 65:196–211.

Quincke H, Roos E. 1893. Ueber Amöben-Enteritis. Berl Klin Wocheschr 45:1089–1094.

Sanders EP. 1928. Changes in the blood cells of kittens resulting from infections with *Endamoeba histolytica*. Am J Hyg 8:963–989.

Schaudinn F. 1903. Untersuchungen über die Fontpflauzung einigen Rhizopoden (Vorlaufige Mittheilung). Arb K Gsudhtsamte 19:547–576.

Wenyon CM. 1912. Experimental amoebic dysentery and liver-abscess in cats. J Lond Sch Trop Med 2:27–34.

MICROSPORA

Microsporidia are typically parasites of invertebrates (Canning and Lom, 1986). They are characterized by having spores that contain a tubular filament through which the nuclear material is extruded directly into the host cell that is being infected. There have been only four reports of microsporidia infecting domestic cats.

The predominant microsporidian parasite of mammals is *Encephalitozoon cuniculi,* which is considered mainly a parasite of rabbits and small rodents (Fig. 1.68). The spores are passed in the urine, and hosts become infected by the ingestion of the spores. Once ingested, host cells are penetrated, and the organisms are found in the vascular endothelium throughout the body. The major organs affected are the kidney and brain, although organisms can be found in almost any tissue. Carnivores can apparently become infected by the ingestion of infected rodent or lagomorph hosts that contain hundreds to thousands of spores. As noted for dogs and foxes, if hosts become infected while pregnant, there can be transuterine infection with pronounced deleterious effects on the offspring.

Encephalitozoon cuniculi Levaditi, Nicolau, and Schoen, 1923

Etymology

Encephalito (brain) + *zoon* (animal) and *cuniculi* (rabbit).

Schuster (1925) described neuropathology associated with meningoencephalitis in cats infected with *Encephalitozoon* (syn = *Nosema*) *cuniculi* that were apparently normal and healthy. Histopathology performed on a Siamese kitten that had developed spasms, muscle twitching, and depression along with two littermates revealed organisms of *Encephalitozoon* in the brain, kidney, spleen, lymph node, and tunica media of the blood vessels (van Rensburg and du Plessis, 1971). Waller et al. (1983) noted two cats that had low levels of antibody to the spores of *Encephalitozoon cuniculi* out of a population of 22 cats of which 18 had antibody to *Toxoplasma gondii.*

The responses to experimental infection with *Encephalitozoon cuniculi* of 10 3- to 14-day-old kittens and 3 2.5-month-old cats that had also been experimentally infected with FeLV were followed for a period of 3 to 12 weeks (Pang and Shadduck, 1985). Although *Encephalitozoon cuniculi* was observed in tissue sections of the kidneys of all but one cat, most of these cats showed no signs of infection. All the cats developed a subacute or chronic interstitial nephritis of varying severity with the lesions being markedly more severe in the cats that were also infected with FeLV. Meningoencephalitis was observed in 4 of the cats, 1 of which had received FeLV; however, all lesions were mild. Pneumonia was present in 4 of the cats, 3 of which were those also infected with FeLV. Vascular lesions were seen in none of these cats.

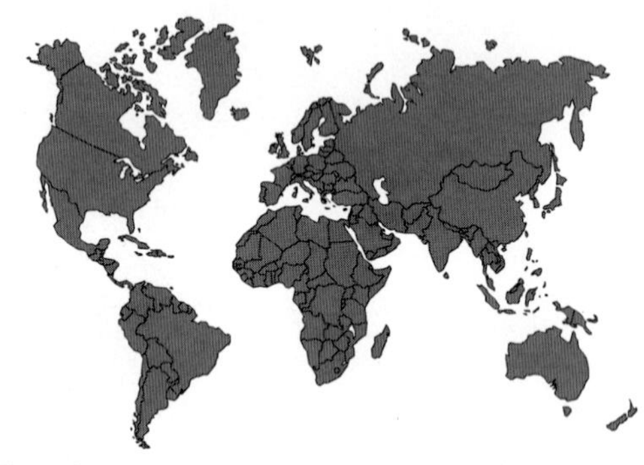

Fig. 1.67.

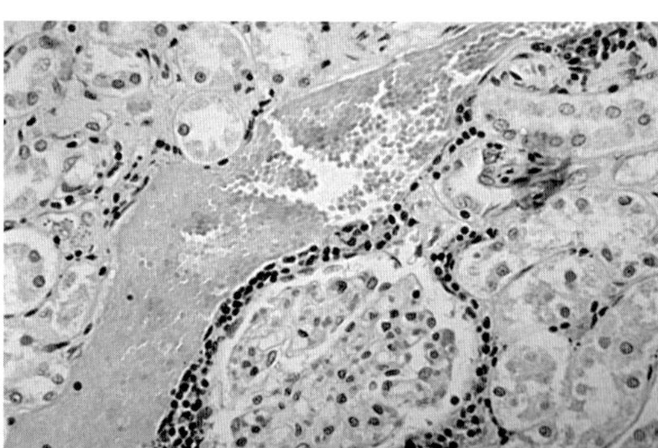

Fig. 1.68. *Encephalitozoon cuniculi* spores in the kidney of an infected rabbit. (Histological section stained with Gram's stain)

REFERENCES

Canning EU, Lom J. 1986. The Microsporidia of Vertebrates. New York, NY: Academic Press. 289 pp.

Levaditi C, Nicolau S, Schoen R. 1923. L'agent étiologique de l'encéphalite épizootique du lapin (*Encephalitozoon cuniculi*). Comptes Rendus Soc Biol 89:1157–1162.

Pang VF, Shadduck JA. 1985. Susceptibility of cats, sheep, and swine to a rabbit isolate of *Encephalitozoon cuniculi.* Am J Vet Res 46:1071–1077.

Schuster J. 1925. Über eine Spontan beim kaninchen auftretende encephalitische Erkrankung. Klinische Wochenschrift 4:550.

van Rensburg IBJ, du Plessis JL. 1971. Nosematosis in a cat: a case report. J S Afr Vet Med Assoc 42:327–331.

Waller T, Uggla A, Bergquist NR. 1983. Encephalitozoonosis and toxoplasmosis diagnosed simultaneously by a novel rapid test; the carbon immunoassay. Proc Third Int Symp Assoc Vet Lab Diagn, pp 171–177.

Microsporidium buyukmihcii Canning and Lom, 1986

Buyukmihci et al. (1977) described an infection of the cornea of the eye of a cat due to a microsporidium that they identified as *Encephalitozoon.* It has since been decided that this parasite is not the same species as *Encephalitozoon cuniculi* based on the number of coils of the tube within the spore as discerned from their published photograph. This parasite has been assigned the name *Microsporidium buyukmihcii.* In the cat, the right central cornea developed numerous opacities arranged in a stellate pattern. A superficial keratectomy was performed. Histopathology and electron microscopy of the specimen revealed microsporidian organisms measuring 1.5 to 4 µm with 15 to 16 coils of the polar tube. A year after the procedure the cat was known to be in good health without a recurrence of the eye lesion. The typical host of this species and how this cat became infected are not known.

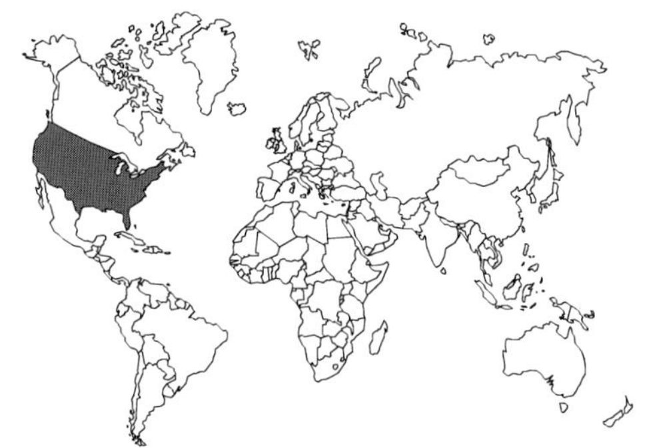

Fig. 1.69.

REFERENCES

Buyukmihci N, Bellhorn RW, Hunziker J, Clinton J. 1977. *Encephalitozoon* (*Nosema*) infection of the cornea in a cat. J Am Vet Med Assoc 171:355–357.

2 THE TREMATODES

The trematodes are a group of organisms that are related to the planarian studied in biology class. The planarian belongs to the free-living form of platyhelminth called the turbellarian. The trematodes differ from their free-living turbellarian relatives in that trematodes are all parasitic and lack the cilia that cover the body surface of the adult turbellarian.

There are two kinds of trematodes: monogenetic and digenetic. This terminology refers to whether or not there is development through morphologically dissimilar stages in some type of intermediate host (i.e., whether or not there is an "alternation of generations"). The digenetic trematodes undergo a form of development wherein a larval stage develops in a mollusk and the adult develops in a different host. This dissimilar nature of the larval and adult forms caused the larvae and adults to be considered separate entities until the work of Steenstrup in 1842 showed them to be the same animals. This problem of stage identification did not exist for the monogenetic trematodes that look like adults when they hatch from eggs. The monogenetic trematodes are parasites of fish, amphibians, and other hosts and are only important if their eggs are found in the feces of a cat that has eaten an infected host. A wide variety of digenetic trematodes, on the other hand, commonly infect cats.

The digenetic trematodes undergo their first larval development in a mollusk, typically a snail. The snail is infected with a ciliated stage, the miracidium, that hatches from the egg produced by the adult trematode. In most cases, after the larva develops through one to several stages within the snail, a proliferative stage is reached that produces the cercaria, the stage that ultimately leaves the snail. After leaving the snail, the cercaria may take one of several routes, it may encyst on vegetation, it may encyst in the tissues of a second intermediate host that will ultimately be eaten by the final host, or it may (in the case of schistosomes only) penetrate directly into the final host. Cats typically become infected by either eating an infected host or via the penetration of the skin. Feline feeding habits are such that cats seldom fall prey to the trematodes that utilize vegetation.

Digenetic trematodes can be classified in several ways. The "natural" classification used by taxonomists takes into account many characteristics of biology and morphology to place similar organisms into similar groups. Due to the very large numbers of trematodes, this system unfortunately is often considered cumbersome by practitioners. Another means of classification is the mode of infection for the final host. Thus, the adult trematodes could be listed as those, for example, from fish, crabs, lizards, or direct penetration. Again, although useful for epizootiology and prevention, this is not of great use to the practitioner. Thus, the trematodes presented in Table 2.1 are given as to where they are typically found within the body of the final host. At the end of the chapter, Table 2.2 lists how cats become infected and the geographical distribution of the species discussed in this chapter.

TREMATODES OF THE BUCCAL CAVITY

CLINOSTOMATIDAE

Trematodes of the buccal cavity are not uncommon in fish-eating reptiles and birds. They are, however, rare in mammals, and only three species of a single genus, *Clinostomum,* have been reported from cats.

The genus *Clinostomum* (Figs. 2.2 and 2.3) and other clinostomatids are characterized by the possession of a retractile oral sucker that appears to be surrounded by a collar-like fold of tegument.

Table 2.1. Where trematodes are typically found within the body of the final host

Trematodes of the buccal cavity
- CLINOSTOMATIDAE
  - *Clinostomum falsatum* Ortlepp, 1963
  - *Clinostomum kalappahi* Bhalerao, 1947
  - *Clinostomum abdoni* Tubangui and Garcia, 1939

Trematodes of the intestine
- CYATHOCOTYLIDAE
  - *Mesostephanus milvi* Yamaguti, 1939
  - *Prohemistomum vivax* (Sonsino, 1893) Azim, 1933
- DIPLOSTOMATIDAE
  - *Alaria marcianae* (LaRue, 1917) Walton, 1949
  - *Cynodiplostomum azimi* (Gohar, 1933) Dubois, 1936
  - *Fibricola minor* Dubois, 1936
  - *Pharyngostomum cordatum* (Diesing, 1850) Ciurea, 1922
- ECHINOSTOMATIDAE
  - Echinochasminae
    - *Echinochasmus perfoliatus* (Ratz, 1908) Dietz, 1909
    - *Echinochasmus breviviteilus* Fahmy, Khalifa, Sakla, 1981
    - *Echinochasmus liliputanus* (looss, 1896) Odhner, 1911
    - *Echinochasmus caninum* (Verma, 1935) Chatterji, 1954
    - *Stephanoprora denticulatoides* Isaichikoff, 1925
  - Echinostominae
    - *Artyfechinostomum surfrartyfex* (Schrank, 1788) Lühe, 1909
    - *Isthmiophora melis* (Schrank, 1788) Lühe, 1909
    - *Echinoparyphium* Dietz, 1909
- HETEROPHYIDAE
  - Apaphallinae
    - *Apophallus donicus* (Skrjabin and Lindtrop, 1919) Cameron, 1936
    - *Apophallus venustus* (Ransom, 1920) Cameron, 1936
    - *Apophallus muehlingi* (Jägerskiöld, 1899) Lühe, 1909
  - Ascocotylinae
    - *Ascocotyle ascolonga* (Witenberg, 1929) Travassos, 1930
    - *Ascocotyle longicollis* (Kuntz and Chandler, 1956) Sogandares-Bernal and Lumsden, 1963
    - *Ascocotyle minuta* Looss, 1899
    - *Ascocotyle angrense* Travassos, 1916
    - *Ascocotyle longa* Ransom, 1921
    - *Ascocotyle pachycystis* Schroeder and Leigh, 1965
    - *Ascocotyle arnoldoi* (Travassos, 1928) Soganderes-Bernal and Lumsden, 1963
  - Centrocestinae
    - *Centrocestus caninus* Leiper, 1913
    - *Pygidiopsis genata* Looss, 1907
    - *Pygidiopsis summa* Onji and Nishio, 1916
    - *Pygidiopsis spindalis* Martin, 1951
  - Cryptocotylinae
    - *Cryptocotyle lingua* (Creplin, 1825) Fischoeder, 1903
    - *Cryptocotyle concavum* (Creplin, 1825) Lühe, 1899
    - *Cryptocotyle quinqueangularis* (Skrjabin, 1923)
  - Euryhelminthinae
    - *Euryhelmis squamula* (Rudolphi, 1819) Poche, 1926
    - *Euryhelmis monorchis* Ameel, 1938
    - *Euryhelmis pacifica* Senger and Macy, 1952
  - Galactosominae
    - *Galactosomum fregatae* Prudhoe, 1949
  - Haplorchiinae
    - *Haplorchis pumilio* (Looss, 1896) Looss, 1899
    - *Haplorchis yokogawai* (Katsuta, 1932) Chen, 1936
    - *Haplorchis taichui* (Nishigori, 1924) Witenberg, 1930
    - *Haplorchis sprenti* Pearson, 1964
    - *Haplorchis parataichui* Pearson, 1964
    - *Procerovum varium* Onji and Nishio, 1916
    - *Procerovum calderoni* (Africa and Garcia, 1935) Price, 1940
    - *Stellantchasmus falcatus* Onji and Nishio, 1916
  - Heterophyinae
    - *Heterophyes heterophyes* (von Siebold, 1852) Stiles and Hassall, 1900

Table 2.1. (Continued)

Heterophyes aequalis Looss, 1902
Heterophyopsis continua (Onji and Nishi, 1916) Tubangui and Africa, 1938
Metagoniminae
Metagonimus yokogawai (Katsurada, 1912) Katsurada, 1912
Metagonimus takahashii Suzuki, 1930
Dexiogonimus ciureanus Witenberg, 1929
Stictodoriinae
Stictodora sawakinensis Looss, 1899
Stictodora thapari Witenberg, 1953
MICROPHALLIDAE
Microphalloides vajrasthirae Waikagul, 1983
PLAGIORCHIDAE
Plagiorchis massino Petrov and Tikhonov, 1927
NANOPHYETIDAE
Nanophyetus salmincola Chapin, 1928

Trematodes of the pancreatic duct
DICROCOELIDAE
Eurytrema procyonis Denton, 1942

Trematodes of the gallbladder and bile ducts
DICROCOELIDAE
Euparadistomum pearsoni Talbot, 1970
Euparadistomum buckleyi Singh, 1958
Euparadistomum heiwschi Buckley and Yeh, 1958
Platynosomum concinnum (Braun, 1901) Purvis, 1933
OPISTHORCHIDAE
Amphimerius pseudofelineus (Ward, 1901) Barker, 1911
Clonorchis sinensis (Cobbold, 1875) Looss, 1907
Opisthorchis felineus (Rivolta, 1884) Blanchard, 1895
Opisthorchis viverrini (Poirier, 1886) Stiles and Hassall, 1896
Paropisthorchis caninus Stephens, 1912
Metorchis conjunctus (Cobbold, 1860) Looss, 1899
Metorchis albidus (Braun, 1893) Looss, 1899
Metorchis orientalis Tanabae, 1919
Parametorchis complexum (Stiles and Hassall, 1894) Skrjabin, 1913
P*seudamphistomum truncatum* (Rudolphi, 1819) Lühe, 1909

Trematodes of the nasal fossae
ORCHIPEDIDAE
Orchipedum isostoma (Rudolphi, 1819)
TROGLOTREMATIDAE
Troglotrema mustelae Wallace, 1932

Trematodes of the lungs
TROGLOTREMATIDAE
Paragonimus westermani (Kerbert, 1878) Braun, 1899
Paragonimus pulmonalis (Baelz, 1880) Miyazaki, 1978
Paragonimus miyazakii Kamo, Nishida Hatsushika, and Tomimura, 1961
Paragonimus heterotremus Chen and Hsia, 1964
Paragonimus siamensis Miyazaki and Wykoff, 1965
Paragonimus skrjabini Chen, 1960
Paragonimus ohirai Miyazaki, 1939
Paragonimus kellicotti Ward, 1908
Paragonimus mexicanus Miyazaki and Ishii, 1968
Paragonimus inca Miyazaki, Mazabel, Grados, and Uyema, 1975
Paragonimus peruvianus Miyazaki, Ibáñez, and Miranda, 1969
Paragonimus caliensis Little, 1968
Paragonimus amazonicus Miyazaki, Grados, and Uyema, 1973
Paragonimus africanus Voelker and Vogel, 1965
Paragonimus uterobilateralis Voelker and Vogel, 1965

Trematodes of the blood vessels
SCHISTOSOMATIDAE
Heterobilharzia americana Price, 1929
Ornithobilharzia turkestanica (Skrjabin, 1913)
Schistosoma japonicum (Katsurada, 1904) Stiles, 1905

Trematodes of the buccal cavity
CLINOSTOMATIDAE
Clinostomum falsatum Ortlepp, 1963
Clinostomum kalappahi Bhalerao, 1947
Clinostomum abodoni Tubangui and Garcia, 1939

Fig. 2.1. Trematodes of the buccal cavity.

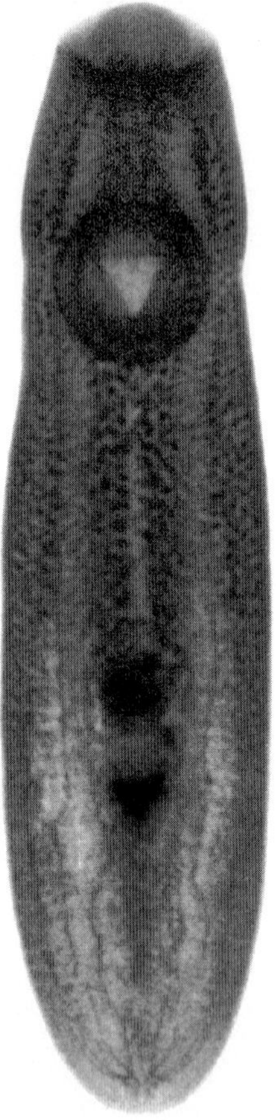

Fig. 2.2. *Clinostomum marginatum.* Sample clinostomatid removed from the mouth of a heron.

The ventral sucker is relatively large and anterior to midbody. The testes and ovary are in the posterior of the body. The adults are found in the mouths of reptiles and birds.

Clinostomum falsatum Ortlepp, 1963

Etymology

Clino (bent) + *stoma* (mouth) and *falsatum* for bill-hooked.

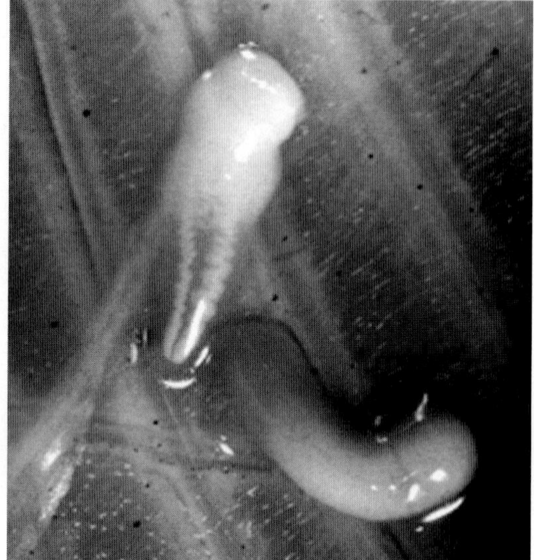

Fig. 2.3. Metacercariae of *Clinostomum* sp. teased from the tissues of a rainbow trout *(Salmo gairdneri).* The metacercariae have also been removed from the metacercarial cyst wall to reveal the contained trematode. (Photo kindly provided by Dr. Gary Conbay, Atlantic Veterinary College, PEI, Canada).

Synonyms

None.

History

This parasite was described from the oral mucosa of a cat in Durban, South Africa. A second collection of similar specimens was made from the mouth of a cat in Lydenburg.

Geographic Distribution

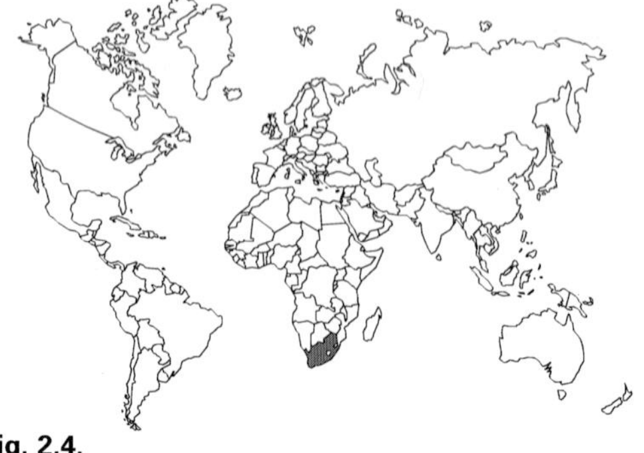

Fig. 2.4.

South Africa.

Location in Host

Mouth.

Parasite Identification

These are small trematodes that are less than 5 mm long. The oral sucker, which is retractable as evidenced by a collar-like fold in the tegument of the fluke at the base of the oral sucker, is about one-third the diameter of the ventral sucker that is located slightly anterior to midbody. The genital opening is posterior to the ventral sucker, and the ovary is in the posterior of the body between the testes.

The oval eggs are large, 95–116 μm long by 65–74 μm wide, operculate, and not embryonated when they leave the fluke.

Life Cycle

The life cycle of *Clinostomum falsatum* has not been elucidated. Other clinostomatids are typically found as adults in the mouth or esophagus of aquatic reptiles and birds. Miracidia develop in eggs that leave the bird, and in the water the miracidia hatch and penetrate a snail host. After sporocyst and redial generations, brevifurcate, pharyngeate cercariae with pigmented eyespots are produced. These cercariae seek out freshwater fish, which they penetrate and then encyst as metacercariae in muscle and connective tissues. The metacercaria contains some reproductive structures and takes only a few days to develop to the adult stage after a fish is eaten by a final host.

Clinical Presentation and Pathogenesis

The clinical presentation has been described by Dr. Coetzee (in Ortlepp, 1963) as follows: "An Indian resident at Badfontein brought in a male domestic cat in fairly good condition with the information that it had worms in its mouth." Subsequent examination revealed a granulomatous growth in the soft tissues (frenulum) under the tongue. The parasites were firmly attached within the growth and required removal with forceps.

Treatment

Physical removal.

Epizootiology

Cats become infected by eating fish containing the metacercariae. The flukes are capable of developing to the adult stage in a few days.

Hazards to Other Animals

None.

Hazards to Humans

None.

Control/Prevention

Prevent cats from eating raw fish.

REFERENCES

Ortlepp RJ. 1963. Clinostomid trematodes as aberrant parasites in the mouth of the domestic cat *(Felis catus domesticus)*. Onderstepoort J Vet Res. 30:137–144.

Clinostomum kalappahi Bhalerao, 1947

Etymology

Clino (bent) + *stoma* (mouth) and *Kalappah* for Dr. Kalappah.

Synonyms

None.

History

First described by Dr. Bhalerao (1947), these flukes were originally collected from the mouth of a cat in India by Dr. Belliappa. This cat had been treated a year previously for the same condition by another veterinarian. A second cat treated by Dr. Belliappa was found to have about 40 trematodes under its tongue and on the sides of its mouth and was noticed to be holding its mouth open.

Geographic Distribution

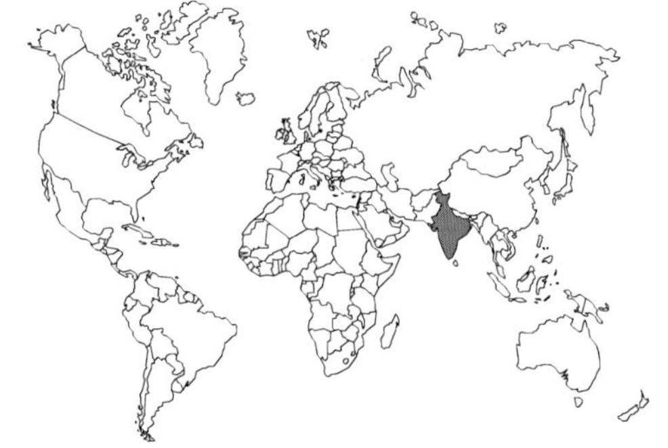

Fig. 2.5.

India.

Location in Host

Mouth.

Parasite Identification

The description of this trematode by Bhalerao is insufficient for discrimination between this and *Clinostomum falsatum.* Based on the original description of Belliappa, it would appear that these flukes are larger than those recovered from cats in South Africa.

Life Cycle

The life cycle of *Clinostomum kalappahi* has not been elucidated. See *Clinostomum falsatum* for a general description.

Clinical Presentation and Pathogenesis

The clinical presentation has been described by Belliappa (1944). Historically, cats may present with anorexia and depression. The temperature is usually normal. Microscopic examination of the feces is usually negative. Cats will champ their jaws often, suggestive of some foreign body stuck up inside the mouth, and they may hypersalivate. On oral examination, a large number of papillomatous outgrowths may be present under the tongue on either side of the frenulum. The growths may reach an inch in length. Slight movements may be seen at the free end of the growths, and parasites (up to 20) may be removed with forceps.

Treatment

Physical removal.

Epizootiology

Cats become infected by eating fish containing the metacercariae. The flukes are capable of developing to the adult stage in a few days.

Hazards to Other Animals

None.

Hazards to Humans

None.

Control/Prevention

Prevent cats from eating raw fish.

REFERENCES

Belliappa AB. 1944. On a species of *Clinostomum* in a cat. Indian Vet J 21:101–102.

Bhalerao AB. 1947. *Clinostomum kalappahi* n. sp. (Trematoda) from the mouth of cats in the Coorg. Helm Abst 16:No 576c.

Clinostomum abdoni Tubangui and Garcia, 1939

Etymology

Clino (bent) + *stoma* (mouth) and *abdoni* for Dr. Abdon who originally found the fluke in the mouth of a cat.

Synonyms

None.

History

This parasite was described from a single specimen obtained from a pocket under the tongue of the mouth of a cat in the Philippines.

Geographic Distribution

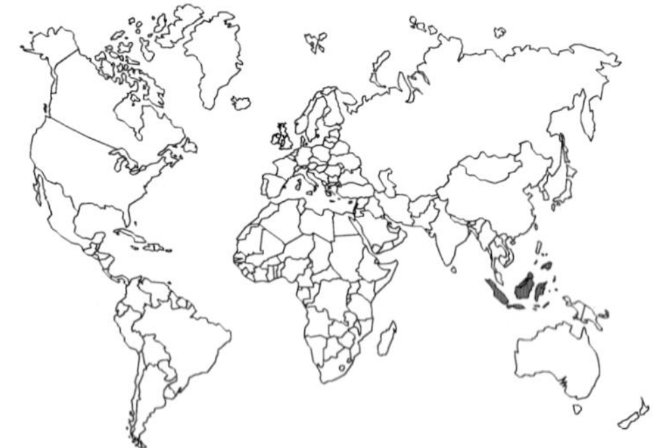

Fig. 2.6.

Surigao, Mindanao, Philippines.

Location in Host

Mouth, pocket under the tongue.

Parasite Identification

This trematode is 6.8 mm long and 1.65 mm wide with no markedly noticeable cuticular spines. The acetabulum is much larger than the oral sucker. The testes are tandem. The oral sucker, which is retractable as evidenced by a collar-like fold in the tegument of the fluke at the base of the oral sucker, is about one-third the diameter of the ventral sucker that is located slightly anterior to midbody. The genital opening is in the posterior third of the body, and the uterus fills the body between the acetabulum and the genital pore.

The oval eggs are large, 100 to 109 μm long by 60 to 64 μm wide, operculate, and not embryonated when they leave the fluke.

Life Cycle

The life cycle of *Clinostomum abdoni* has not been elucidated, but the authors of the original description felt that it was highly likely that the normal host was a piscivorous bird. For a general presentation see *Clinostomum falsatum.*

Clinical Presentation and Pathogenesis

The only clinical sign was the presence of the pocket under the tongue that housed the fluke at the time of its collection.

Treatment

Physical removal.

Epizootiology

Cats become infected by eating fish containing the metacercariae. The flukes are capable of developing to the adult stage in a few days.

Hazards to Other Animals

None.

Hazards to Humans

None.

Control/Prevention

Prevent cats from eating raw fish.

REFERENCES

Tubangui MA, Garcia EJ. 1939. *Clinostomum abdoni* sp. nov. a trematode parasite of the cat in the Philippines. Philipp J Sci 70:397–401.

TREMATODES OF THE SMALL INTESTINE

This is by far the largest group of trematodes found in the cat (Fig. 2.7). Trematodes differ from other helminths in that they are often less discriminating in their requirements for a final host. For this reason, cats can harbor a large number of trematodes that they share with other animals that might eat the same intermediate hosts containing the arrested metacercarial stage. For example, if a trematode uses a fish as a second intermediate host, it might grow to adulthood in a cat, a dog, a piscivorous bird, an otter, or a raccoon. Thus, it is sometimes difficult to be certain whether the "true" final host is the cat or some other animal. Also, there are reports of worms being recovered on single or only a few occasions because cats are becoming infected when they accidentally ingest a metacercarial-containing meal meant for another host.

CYATHOCOTYLIDAE

One group of trematodes found in the intestine of cats is the cyathocotylids, represented by the genera *Mesostephanus* and *Prohemistomum.* The adults of these trematodes parasitize the intestine of piscivorous reptiles, birds, and mammals. These flukes are characterized by the presence of a glandular tribocytic organ that is present in addition to the ventral sucker (The ventral sucker is absent in some genera.). The body may be weakly divided into forebody and hindbody regions, and a cirrus sac is present at the posterior end of the body.

Besides natural infections with *Mesostephanus milvi* and *Prohemistomum vivax* (discussed below), cats have been reported to have been experimentally infected with *Mesostephanus appendiculatus* in Romania and with *Prohemistomum vivax* in Egypt by feeding them infected fish (Chandler, 1950).

REFERENCES

Chandler AC. 1950. *Mesostephanus longisaccus* a new cyathocotylid trematode from a dog. J Parasitol 46:90.

CYATHOCOTYLIDAE
Mesostephanus milvi Yamaguti, 1939
Prohemistomum vivax (Sonsino, 1893) Azim, 1933
DIPLOSTOMATIDAE
Alaria marcianae (LaRue, 1917) Walton, 1949
Cynodiplostomum azimi (Gohar, 1933) Dubois, 1936
Fibricola minor Dubois, 1936
Pharyngostomum cordatum (Diesing, 1850) Ciurea, 1922
ECHINOSTOMATIDAE
Echinochasminae
Echinochasmus perfoliatus (Ratz, 1908) Dietz, 1909
Echinochasmus breviviteilus Fahmy, Khalifa, Sakla, 1981
Echinochasmus liliputanus (Looss, 1896) Odhner, 1911
Episthmium caninum (Verma, 1935) Chatterji, 1954
Stephanoprora denticulatoides Isaichikoff, 1925
Echinostominae
Artyfechinostomum sufrartyfex (Schrank, 1788) Lühe, 1909
Isthmiophora melis (Schrank, 1788) Lühe, 1909
Echinoparyphium Dietz, 1909
HETEROPHYIDAE
Apophallinae
Apophallus donicus (Skrjabin and Lindtrop, 1919) Cameron, 1936
Apophallus venustus (Ransom, 1920) Cameron, 1936
Apophallus muehlingi (Jägerskiöld, 1899) Lühe, 1909
Ascocotylinae
Ascocotyle ascolonga (Witenberg, 1929) Travassos, 1930
Ascocotyle longicollis (Kuntz and Chandler, 1956) Soganderes-Bernal and Lumsden, 1963
Ascocotyle minuta Looss, 1899
Ascocotyle angrense Travassos, 1916
Ascocotyle longa Ransom, 1921
Ascocotyle pachycystis Schroeder and Leigh, 1965
Ascocotyle arnoldoi (Travassos, 1928) Soganderes-Bernal and Lumsden, 1963
Centrocestinae
Centrocestus caninus Leiper, 1913
Pygidiopsis genata Looss, 1907
Pygidiopsis summa Onji and Nishio, 1916
Pygidiopsoides spindalis Martin, 1951
Cryptocotylinae
Cryptocotyle lingua (Creplin, 1825) Fischoeder, 1903
Cryptocotyle concavum (Creplin, 1825) Lühe, 1899
Cryptocotyle quinqueangularis (Skrjabin, 1923)
Euryheminthinae
Euryhelmis squamula (Rudolphi, 1819) Poche, 1926
Euryhelmis monorchis Ameel, 1938
Euryhelmis pacifica Senger and Macy, 1952
Galactosominae
Galactosomum fregatae Prudhoe, 1949
Haplorchiinae
Haplorchis pumilio (Looss, 1896) Looss, 1899
Haplorchis yokogawai (Katsuta, 1932) Chen, 1936
Haplorchis taichui (Nishigori, 1924) Witenberg, 1930
Haplorchis sprenti Pearson, 1964
Haplorchis parataichui Pearson, 1964
Procerovum varium Onji and Nishio, 1916
Procerovum calderoni (Africa and Garcia, 1935) Price, 1940
Stellantchasmus falcatus Onji and Nishio, 1916
Heterophyinae
Heterophyes heterophyes (von Siebold, 1852) Stiles and Hassall, 1900
Heterophyes aequalis Looss, 1902
Heterophyopsis continua (Onji and Nishi, 1916) Tubangui and Africa, 1938
Metagoniminae
Metagonimus yokogawai (Katsurada, 1912) Katsurada, 1912
Metagonimus takahashii Suzuki, 1930
Dexiogonimus ciureanus Witenberg, 1929
Stictodoriinae
Stictodora sawakinensis Looss, 1899
Stictodora thapari Witenberg, 1953
MICROPHALLIDAE
Microphalloides vajrasthirae Waikagul, 1983
PLAGIORCHIDAE
Plagiorchis massino Petrov and Tikhonov, 1927
NANOPHYETIDAE
Nanophyetus salmincola Chapin, 1928

Fig. 2.7. Trematodes of the intestine.

Mesostephanus milvi Yamaguti, 1939

Etymology

Meso (middle) + *stephanus* (crown) (referring to the organization of the vitellaria in the middle of the body) and *milvi* for the generic name of the kite, *Milvus migrans,* host from which it was originally described.

Synonyms

Prohemistomum milvi (Yamaguti, 1939) Dubois, 1951; *Mesostephanus indicus* Vidyarthi, 1948; *Gelanocotyle milvi* (Yamaguti, 1939) Sudarikov, 1961.

History

This species was first described from worms collected from a kite, *Milvus migrans lineatus,* in

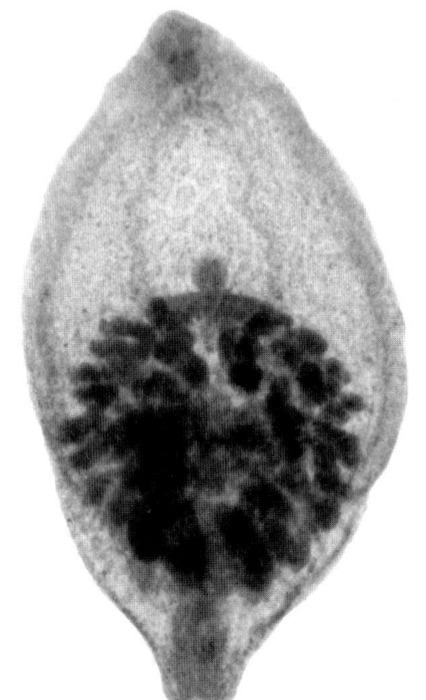

Fig. 2.8. *Mesostephanus milvi* recovered from a cat in Egypt.

Japan. Specimens were recovered from two cats from the Daqahliya province of Egypt (Dubois and Pearson, 1963) and again in four cats of the Assiut province by Fahmy et al. (1984).

Geographic Distribution

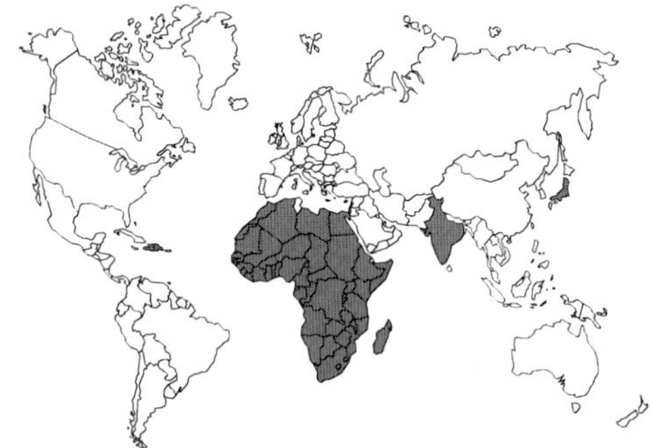

Fig. 2.9.

Japan, India, Africa—although it has only been reported from cats in Egypt.

Location in Host

Small intestine.

Parasite Identification

These are very small trematodes that are 1.5 to 2 mm long and about twice as long as they are wide. The small oral sucker, about 100 µm in diameter, is similar in size to the ventral sucker. The ventral sucker is located at midbody, and just behind the ventral sucker is the circular tribocytic organ that is about one-third of the body's width. The sexual organs are located posterior to the ventral sucker, and there is a small elongation of the posterior end of the body.

The oval eggs are large, yellowish-brown, operculate, 100 µm long by 60 to 70 µm wide, and not embryonated when they leave the fluke. (The eggs are embryonated according to Fahmy et al., 1984.)

Life Cycle

The life cycle of *Mesostephanus milvi* has not been elucidated. The life cycle of another cyathocotylid, *Prohemistomum vivax,* has been investigated (see below).

Clinical Presentation and Pathogenesis

Asymptomatic.

Treatment

Probably praziquantel, but not reported.

Epizootiology

Cats become infected by eating fish containing the metacercariae. The flukes are capable of developing to the adult stage in a few days.

Hazards to Other Animals

None.

Hazards to Humans

None.

Control/Prevention

Prevent cats from eating raw fish.

REFERENCES

Dubois G, Pearson JC. 1963. Les Strigeida (Trematoda) d'Egypte (Collection William H. Walls). Ann Parasitol 38:77–91.

Fahmy MA, Arafa MS, Khalifa R, Abdel-Rahman AM, Mounib ME. 1984. Studies on helminth parasites in some small mammals in Assiut Governorate. 1. Trematode parasites. Assiut Vet Med J 11:43–52.

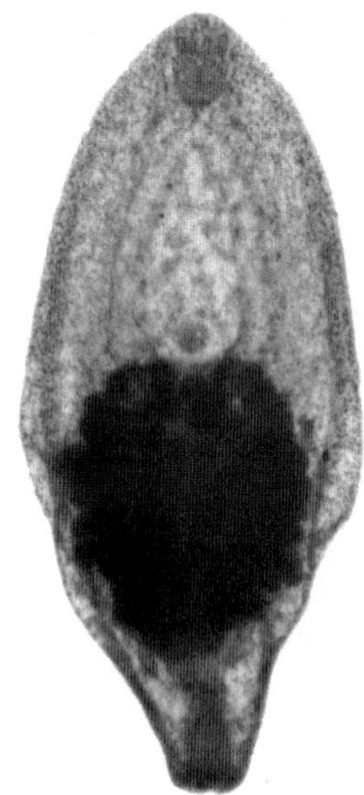

Fig. 2.10. *Prohemistomum vivax* recovered from a cat in Egypt.

Prohemistomum vivax (Sonsino, 1893) Azim, 1933

Etymology

Pro (anterior) + *hemi* (half) + *stomum* (mouth) and *vivax* (lively).

Synonyms

Prohemistomum spinulosum Odhner, 1913.

History

This species was first described from worms collected from a kite, *Milvus migrans aegypticus.*

Geographic Distribution

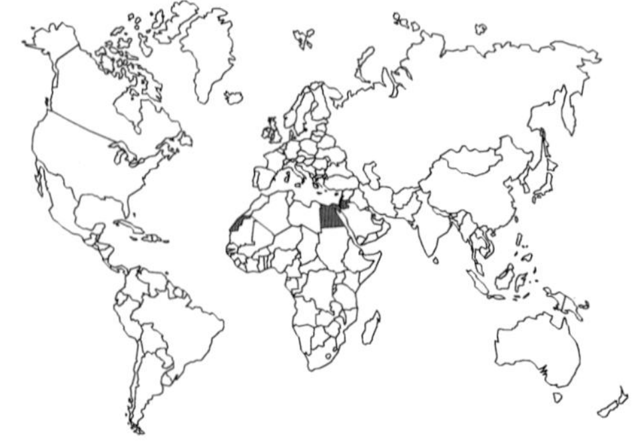

Fig. 2.11.

Egypt (Abo-Shady et al., 1983, and Fahmy et al., 1984, found this parasite in 19 of 29 stray cats) and Israel (Witenberg, 1934).

Location in Host

Small intestine.

Parasite Identification

These are very small trematodes that are about 1 mm in length. They differ from *Mesostephanus* in that the overall body shape is oval rather than elongate.

Life Cycle

The life cycle of *Prohemistomum vivax* was initially elucidated by Azim (1933) under the synonym *Prohemistomum spinulosum.* Azim found that brackish and freshwater fish (*Gambusia affinis* and *Tilapia nilotica*) could serve as the second intermediate host. More recently, El-Naffar et al. (1985) showed that the metacercaria of this fluke is found in the muscles of several fish genera, including *Tilapia, Hydrocyon, Alestes, Schibe,* and *Eutropius.* The adult parasites were recovered from the duodenum, jejunum, and ileum of kittens about 6 days after they were fed the metacercariae harvested from fish in Lake Nasser, Egypt. Work with the related species *Prohemistomum chandleri* has disclosed that the metacercaria contains some reproductive structures and appears to require only a few days to develop to the adult stage after a fish is eaten by a final host (Vernberg, 1952).

Clinical Presentation and Pathogenesis

Asymptomatic.

Treatment

Probably praziquantel, but not reported.

Epizootiology

Cats become infected by eating fish containing the metacercariae. The flukes are capable of developing to the adult stage in a few days.

Hazards to Other Animals

None.

Hazards to Humans

None.

Control/Prevention

Prevent cats from eating raw fish.

REFERENCES

Abo-Shady AF, Ali MM, Abdel-Magied S. 1983. Helminth parasites of cats in Dakahlia, Egypt. J Egypt Soc Parasitol 13:129–133.

Azim MA. 1933. On *Prohemistomum vivax* (Sonsino, 1892) and its development from cercaria vivax Sonsino, 1892. Ztschr Parasitenk 5:432–436.

El-Naffar MK, Saoud MF, Hassan IM. 1985. Role played by fish in transmitting some trematodes of dogs and cats at Asswan Province, A.R. Egypt. Assiut Vet Med J 14:57–67.

Fahmy MA, Arafa MS, Khalifa R, Abdel-Rahman AM, Mounib ME. 1984. Studies on helminth parasites in some small mammals in Assiut Governorate. 1. Trematode parasites. Assiut Vet Med J 11:43–52.

Vernberg WG. 1952. Studies on the trematode family Cyathocotylidae Poche, 1926, with the description of a new species of *Holostephanus* from fish and the life history of *Prohemistomum chandleri* sp. nov. J Parasitol 38:327–340.

Witenberg G. 1934. Parasitic worms of dogs and cats in Palestine. Vet Rec 14:232–239.

DIPLOSTOMATIDAE

Another group of trematodes found in the small intestine of cats is the diplostomatids; adult diplostomatids occur in the intestine of birds and mammals. These trematodes are similar to the cyathocotylids in that they possess a tribocytic organ. However, they are typically divided into a marked forebody and hindbody. Cyathocotylids also possess an organ called the cirrus sac that is absent in the diplostomatids.

Four species of diplostomatid have been reported in cats. One of these species, *Alaria marcianae,* has been shown capable of infecting young cats through the milk of queens that contain larval stages in their tissues.

Alaria marcianae (La Rue, 1917) Walton, 1949

Etymology

Alaria (winged—referring to the alate nature of the forebody) and *marcianae* for the specific name of the garter snake, *Thamnophis marcianus,* from which the mesocercarial stage was first recovered by La Rue (1917).

Synonyms

Cercaria marcianae La Rue, 1917; *Agamodistomum marcianae* (La Rue, 1917) Cort, 1918.

History

This species was first collected as a larval form, the mesocercaria, from the tissues of the garter snake and described as *Cercaria marcianae.* It was later demonstrated that the larval stage was present in frogs and that snakes may serve as paratenic hosts (Cort, 1918). The sporocyst and cercarial stages were described from naturally infected snails, and the cercariae shown to be capable of developing in tadpoles by Cort and Brooks (1928). Cuckler (1941) recovered adult worms from cats fed mesocercariae from naturally infected frogs. Burrows and Lillis (1965) described the adult form for the first time from naturally infected cats.

Geographic Distribution

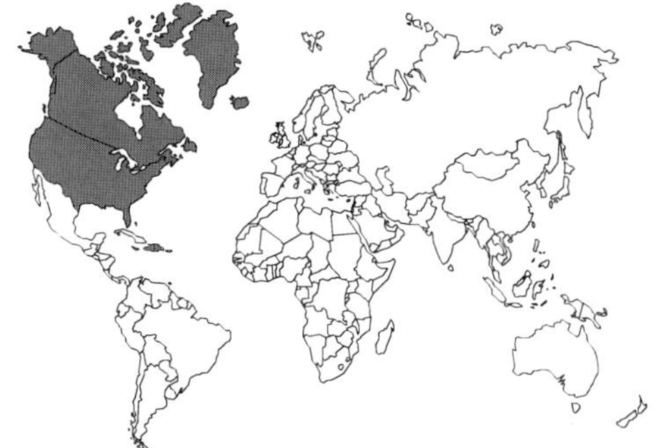

Fig. 2.12.

North America.

Location in Host

Small intestine.

Parasite Identification

These are very small trematodes that are 1.2 to 1.6 mm long with a distinct forebody and hindbody (Figs. 2.13 and 2.14). On each side of the small oral sucker are two anteriorly directed tentacles associated with pseudosuckers that are about 100 µm long. The oral sucker is about 100 µm wide. The forebody is concave ventrally, and the lateral margins fold in and partially overlap

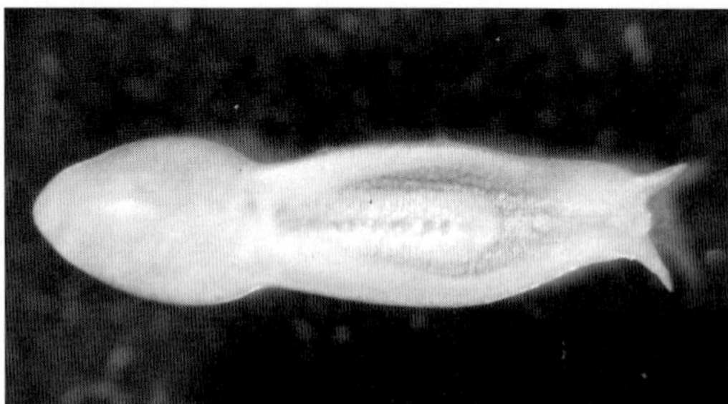

Fig. 2.13. *Alaria marcianae* adult showing the alate tentacles associated with the pseudosucker on either side of the head and the division of the body into distinct forebody and hindbody sections.

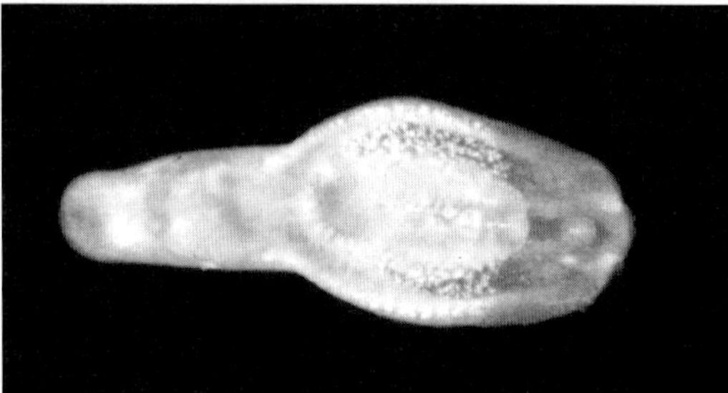

Fig. 2.14. *Alaria marcianae* adult showing how the alae are not always obvious on the anterior end. In the center of the body between the junctions of the fore- and hindbody can be observed the tribocytic organ.

the ventral surface of the body. The ventral sucker is about the same diameter as the oral sucker and is located in the middle of the forebody. The tribocytic organ is just posterior to the ventral sucker and is approximately 150 to 200 μm wide and slightly more than twice as long as it is wide. The vitellaria are almost exclusively in the forebody. The sexual organs are located mainly in the hindbody. The posterior testis is bilobed with one lobe on each side of the body. The anterior testis appears only on one side of the body and is slightly smaller than a lobe of the posterior testis. The ovary is just anterior to the anterior testis.

The oval eggs are large, 110 to 127 μm long by 65 to 72 μm wide, operculate, and not embryonated when they leave the fluke (Fig. 2.15). When the eggs become embryonated after several weeks in fresh water, the miracidium has two dark eyespots (Fig. 2.16).

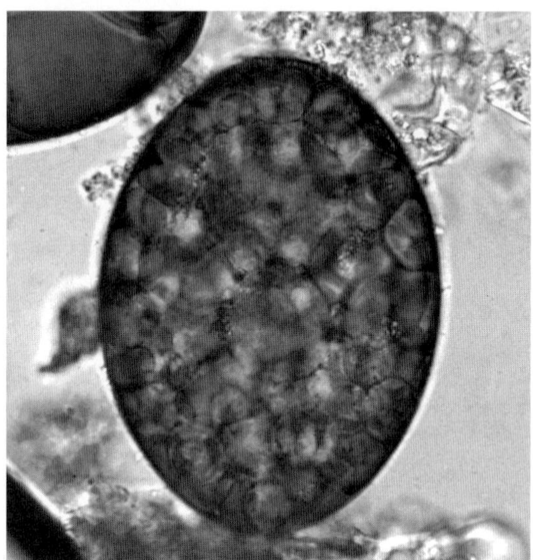

Fig. 2.15. *Alaria marcianae* egg as it appears when passed in the feces.

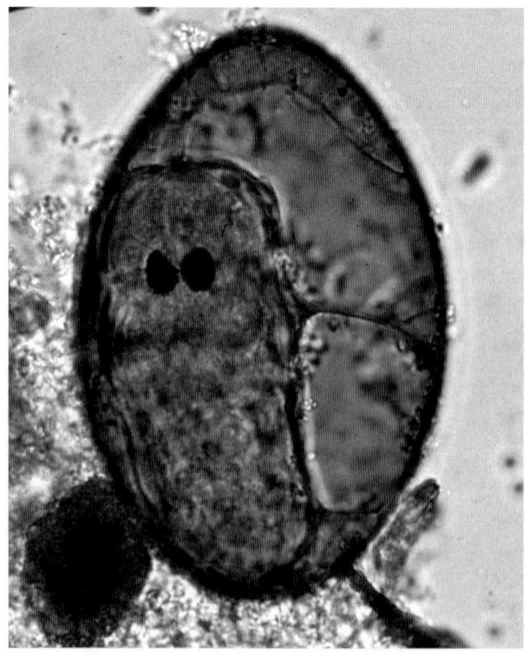

Fig. 2.16. *Alaria marcianae* egg containing a developed miracidium with dark pigmented eyespots.

Life Cycle

The life cycle of *Alaria marcianae* was initially elucidated by Johnson (1968) and then expanded by Shoop and Corkum (1982 and 1983). The eggs are passed in the feces of the final host in an undeveloped state. After development, the eggs contain miracidia that possess two pigmented eyespots. The miracidia then seek out a snail host of the genus *Helisoma* in which they develop into sporocysts. From the sporocysts longifurcous cercariae are released that possess both oral and ventral suckers, a pharynx, unpigmented eyespots, and well-developed penetration glands. The cercariae penetrate and develop in tadpoles. The stage in the tadpole is termed a mesocercaria due to its resemblance to an enlarged cercarial body without the tail. Mesocercariae are capable of being passed between carnivorous paratenic hosts. When the mesocercariae are ingested by the final host, the mesocercariae typically migrate through the lungs where they develop through the metacercarial stage before returning to the intestine where they develop to adults. Eggs are produced in the feces of cats 19 days after infection. The work of Shoop and Corkum showed that it is possible for mesocercariae to be transmitted between mammalian paratenic hosts by transmammary transmission. Also, if queens become infected with mesocercariae while nursing they can pass the infection onto their offspring through the milk.

Clinical Presentation and Pathogenesis

There are no reports of *Alaria marcianae* causing clinical disease in cats. However, the migration through the lung could cause migrating tracts through the lung parenchyma.

Treatment

Probably praziquantel, but not reported.

Epizootiology

Cats become infected by eating frogs, reptiles, or small mammals and birds that contain mesocercariae in their tissues. It is also possible for kittens to become infected through the milk of the queen. Other hosts of *Alaria marcianae* include the opossum, *Didelphis virginiana,* raccoon, *Procyon lotor,* striped skunk, *Mephitis mephitis,* spotted skunk, *Spiglogale putrorius,* red fox, *Vulpes fulva,* gray fox, *Urocyon cinereoargeteus,* and the dog.

Hazards to Other Animals

None. Although other hosts are infected, the major means of infection is through the ingestion of the intermediate host, which requires that the appropriate snail also be available.

Hazards to Humans

There have been reports of *Alaria* causing disease in humans. The first report was a single worm in the eye of a woman from Ontario, Canada (Shea et al., 1973); it was believed that the woman may have been infected by rubbing her eyes while cleaning frog legs for cooking. A second case was fatal (Fernandes et al., 1976; Freeman et al., 1976) and also occurred in Ontario. In this case, numerous mesocercariae were recovered from a patient who was suffering from severe respiratory distress who ultimately died. The mesocercariae in this case were identified as those of *Alaria americana* (= *Alaria canis*). It was never determined how the man became infected although it is suspected that he may have eaten raw or undercooked frog legs. A third case involved two intradermal swellings in the thigh and iliac crest of a man in Louisiana (Beaver et al., 1977). In this case, the mesocercaria has been stated to be similar if not identical to that of *Alaria marcianae* (Shoop and Corkum, 1981). It is believed that this man may have become infected by the ingestion of undercooked game, perhaps a raccoon. There have been other cases of ocular infection (McDonald et al., 1994), and a case of a pulmonary nodule in the lung of a man who ate undercooked goose meat (Kramer et al., 1996).

Control/Prevention

With cats that hunt, it will be very difficult to prevent infection with this parasite.

REFERENCES

Beaver PC, Little MD, Tucker CF, Reed RJ. 1977. Mesocercaria in the skin of man in Louisiana. Am J Trop Med Hyg 26:422–426.

Burrows, RB, Lillis, WG. 1965. Trematodes of New Jersey dogs and cats. J Parasitol 51:570–574.

Cort WW. 1918. The excretory system of *Agamodistomum marcianae* (La Rue), the agamodistome stage of a fork-tailed cercaria. J Parasitol 4:130–134.

Cort WW, Brooks ST. 1928. Studies on the holostome cercariae form Douglas Lake Michigan. Trans Am Microsc Soc 47:179–221.

Cuckler AC. 1941. Morphological and biological studies on certain strigeid trematodes of mammals.

PhD thesis, University of Minnesota, Minneapolis, Minn. 102 pp.

Fernandes BJ, Cooper JD, Cullen JB, Freeman RS, Ritchie AC, Scott AA, Stuart PF. 1976. System infection with *Alaria americana* (Trematoda). CMA J 115:1111–1114.

Freeman RS, Stuyart PF, Cullen JB, Ritchie AS, Mildon A, Fernandes BJ, Bonin R. 1976. Fatal human infection with mesocercariae of the trematode *Alaria americana.* Am J Trop Med Hyg 25:803–807.

Johnson AD. 1968. Life history of *Alaria marcianae* (La Rue, 1917) Walton, 1949 (Trematode. Diplostomatidae). J Parasitol 54:324–332.

Kramer MH, Eberhard ML, Blankenberg TA. 1996. Respiratory symptoms and subcutaneous granuloma caused by mesocercariae: a case report. Am J Trop Med Hyg 55:447–448.

La Rue GR. 1917. Two new larval trematodes from *Thamnophis marciana* and *Thamnophis eques.* Occas Papers Mus Zool Univ Mich 35:1–12.

McDonald HR, Kazacos KR, Schatz H, Johnson RN. 1994. Two cases of intraocular infection with *Alaria mesocercaria* (Trematoda). Am J Ophthalmol 117:447–455.

Shea M, Maberley AL, Walters J, Freeman RS, Fallis AM. 1973. Intraretinal larval trematode. Trans Am Acad Ophthalmol Otol 77:784–791.

Shoop WL, Corkum KC. 1981. Epidemiology of *Alaria marcianae* mesocercariae in Louisiana. J Parasitol 67:928–931.

Shoop WL, Corkum KC. 1982. Transmammary infection of newborn by larval trematodes. Science 223:1082–1083.

Shoop WL, Corkum KC. 1983. Transmammary infection of paratenic and definitive hosts with *Alaria marcianae* (Trematodea) mesocercariae. J Parasitol 69:731–735.

Cynodiplostomum azimi (Gohar, 1933) Dubois, 1936

Etymology

Cyno (dog) + *diplo* (two) + *stomum* (mouth) and *azimi* for Dr. Azim.

Synonyms

Diplostomum azimi Gohar, 1933; *Cynodiplostomum namrui* Kuntz and Chandler, 1956.

History

This trematode was originally described from a dog in Cairo, Egypt, by Gohar (1933). It was later placed in the newly created genus *Cynodiplostomum* by Dubois in 1936.

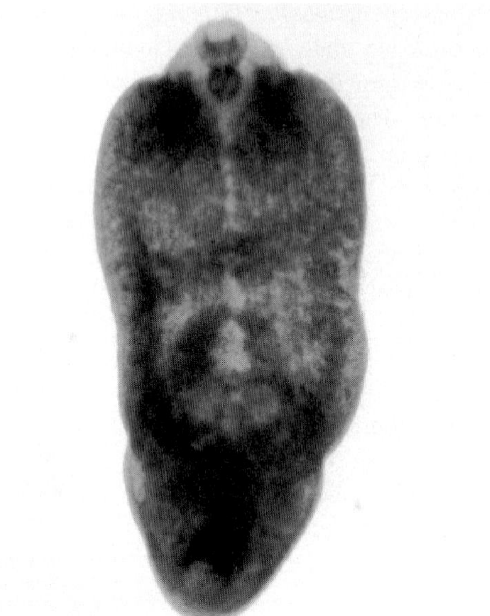

Fig. 2.17. *Cynodiplostomum azimi* collected from a domestic cat in Egypt.

Geographic Distribution

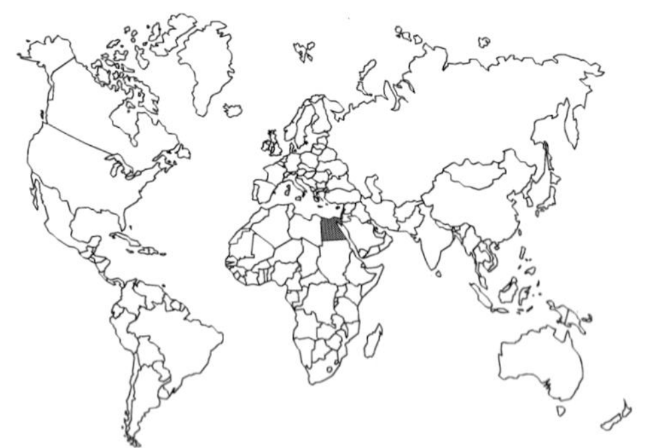

Fig. 2.18.

Egypt.

Location in Host

Small intestine.

Parasite Identification

These are small trematodes that are 0.75 to 1.2 mm long and about twice as long as they are wide. They differ from *Alaria* (described above) in that the tribocytic organ is more circular, the vitellaria are in the forebody and hindbody, and the ovary is opposite to the anterior testis rather than anterior to this testis. Eggs measure 100 to 110 μm by 60 to 67 μm.

Life Cycle

The life cycle of this genus is not known. It is believed to be similar to *Alaria* and other related forms.

Clinical Presentation and Pathogenesis

There are no reports of clinical disease in cats. The only report is from the necropsy of stray cats in Egypt without any mention of clinical presentation.

Treatment

Probably praziquantel, but not reported.

Epizootiology

This parasite was found in 7 of 48 Egyptian cats; in the same study, it was found in two of three dogs (Kuntz and Chandler, 1956). A very similar parasite, *Diplostomum tregenna,* was reported from 5 percent of dogs in Cairo (Azim, 1938), and this may be the same parasite.

Hazards to Other Animals

None. Although other hosts are infected, the major means of infection is through the ingestion of the intermediate host, which requires that the appropriate snail also be available.

Hazards to Humans

None.

Control/Prevention

It is not known what intermediate host harbors the larval stage, although fish are the suspected host.

REFERENCES

Azim MA. 1938. On the intestinal helminths of dogs in Egypt. J Egypt Med Assoc 21:118–122.

Dubois G. 1936. Noveaux principes de classification des Trématodes du groupe des Strigeida. Note préliminaire. Rev Suiss Zool 43:507–515.

Gohar M. 1933. *Diplostomum azimi* sp. n., a new trematode parasite of the dog. Ann Mag Nat Hist 11:302–306.

Kuntz RE, Chandler AC. 1956. Studies on Egyptian trematodes with special reference to the Heterophyids of mammals. I. Adult flukes, with descriptions of *Phagicola longicollis* n. sp., *Cynodiplostomum namrui* n. sp., and a *Stephanoprora* from cats. J Parasitol 42:445–459.

Fibricola minor Dubois, 1936

Etymology

Fibri = fiber + *cola* = colon and *minor* for the small size.

Synonyms

None.

History

This worm was originally described from Australian rodents, *Hydromys chrysogaster,* by Dubois (1936).

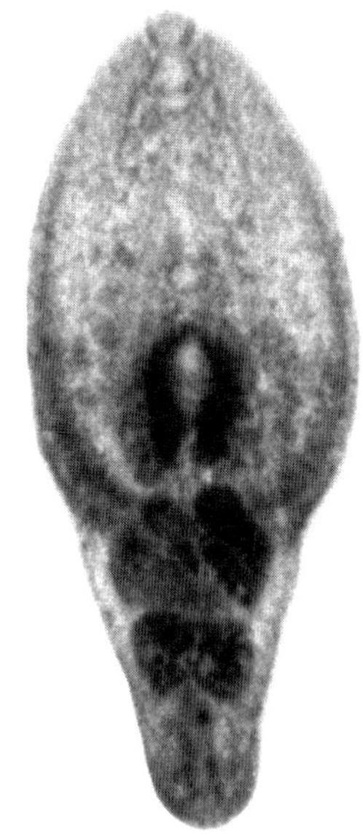

Fig. 2.19. *Fibricola texensis* collected from the small intestine of a raccoon in Texas.

Geographic Distribution

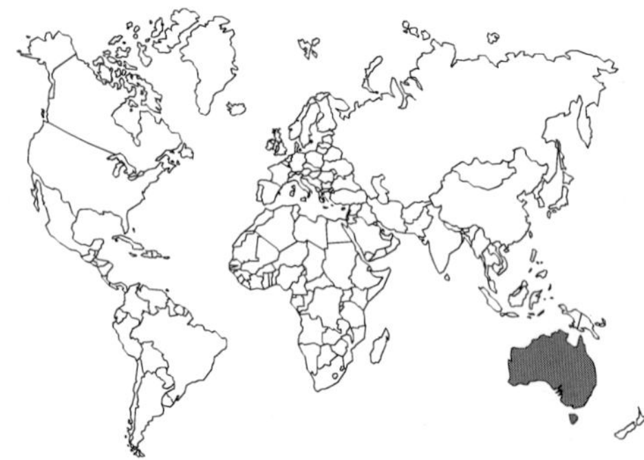

Fig. 2.20.

Seven specimens of this species were collected from a cat in Ross, Tasmania, Australia (Dubois, 1978). Four of 59 cats (6.8 percent) collected from the Tasmanian midlands were found to be infected with this parasite (Gregory and Munday, 1976).

Location in Host

Small intestine.

Parasite Identification

These are small trematodes about 0.5 to 0.75 mm long. *Fibricola* differs from *Alaria* and *Cynodiplostomum* in that it has no pseudosuckers on either side of the oral sucker and the testes are tandem.

Life Cycle

The life cycle of this species is not known. It has been described for the related American species *Fibricola texensis* (Chandler 1942; Leigh, 1954). Eggs passed into the environment in the feces of the natural host, the raccoon, require about 2 weeks of development before they hatch. The miracidium penetrates a snail of the genus *Physa* wherein it produces sporocysts. The cercaria that is produced is pharyngeate and longifurcate with colorless eyespots; the body is covered with small spines. The cercaria penetrates tadpoles and develops to the metacercarial stage. The metacercariae have been experimentally passed to chameleons and frogs by feeding of metacercariae from tadpoles. In the raccoon, the adults developed in 10 days after being fed metacercariae. Feeding metacercariae of *Fibricola texensis* to kittens did not result in patent infections. In Korea, metacercariae of *Fibricola seoulensis* harvested from the viscera of a snake, *Natrix tigrina lateralis,* have been shown to be capable of developing to the adult stage in cats (Hong et al., 1983).

Clinical Presentation and Pathogenesis

There are no reports of clinical disease in cats. The only report is from the necropsy of stray cats in Tasmania without any mention of clinical presentation.

Treatment

Probably praziquantel, but not reported.

Epizootiology

The rodents serve as the major host of this parasite, and cats are probably only incidentally infected.

Hazards to Other Animals

None. Although other hosts are infected, the major means of infection is through the ingestion of the intermediate host, which requires that the appropriate snail also be available.

Hazards to Humans

None.

Control/Prevention

It is not known what intermediate host harbors the larval stage, although frogs and other paratenic hosts are possibilities.

REFERENCES

Chandler AC. 1942. The morphology and life cycle of a new strigeid, *Fibricola texensis,* parasitic in raccoons. Trans Am Microsc Soc 61:156–167.

Dubois G. 1978. Notes helminthologiques IV. Strigeidae Railliet, Diplostomidae Poirier, Proterdiplostomidae Dubois et Cyathocotylidae Poche (Trematoda). Rev Suiss Zool 85:607–615.

Gregory GG, Munday BL. 1976. Intestinal parasites of feral cats from the Tasmanian Midlands and King Island. Aust Vet J 52:317–320.

Hong SJ, Lee SH, Seo BS, Hong ST, Chai JY. 1983. Studies on intestinal trematodes in Korea. IX.

Recovery rate and development of *Fibricola seoulensis* in experimental animals. Korean J Parasitol 21:224–233.
Leigh WH. 1954. Notes on the life history of *Fibricola texensis* (Chandler, 1942) in Florida. J Parasitol 40:45.

Pharyngostomum cordatum (Diesing, 1850) Ciurea, 1922

Etymology

Pharyngo (pharynx) + *stomum* (mouth) and *cordatum* for heart shaped.

Synonyms

Hemistomum cordatum Diesing, 1850; *Alaria cordata* (Diesing, 1850) Railliet, 1919; *Pharyngostomum congolense* Van den Berghe, 1939; *Pharyngostomum fausti* (Skrjabin and Popov, 1930).

History

This worm was first described from *Felis sylvestris* by Diesing (1850). It was considered solely a parasite of cats until it was discovered in cheetahs and genets in Africa.

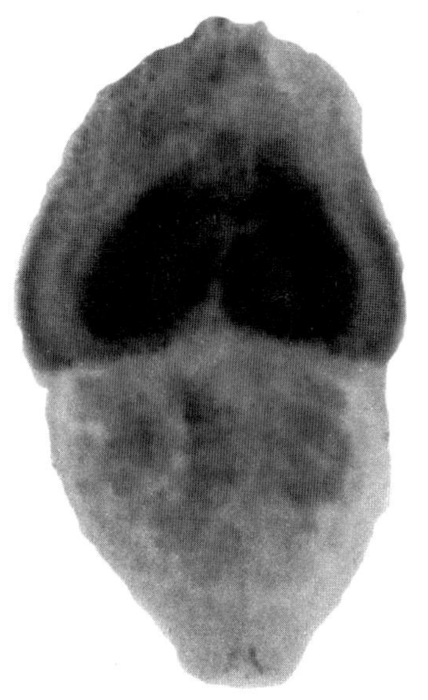

Fig. 2.21. *Pharyngostomum cordatum* collected from domestic cat in Taiwan.

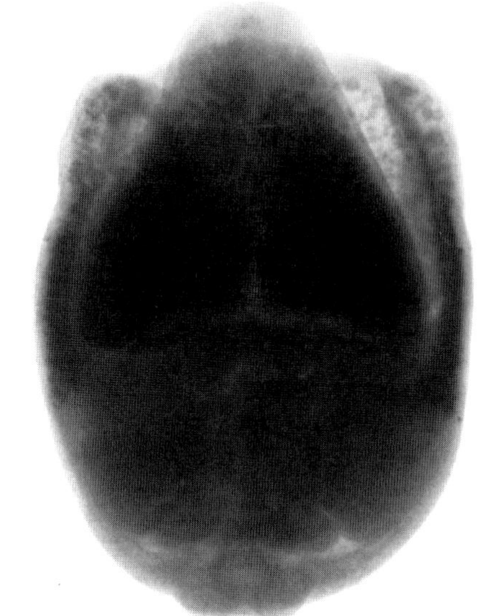

Fig. 2.22. *Pharyngostomum cordatum* collected from domestic cat in Taiwan. Note the division into fore- and hindbodies and the ability of the two body portions to telescope into each other to give the compressed appearance seen in Fig. 2.22 when it is compared with Fig. 2.21.

Geographic Distribution

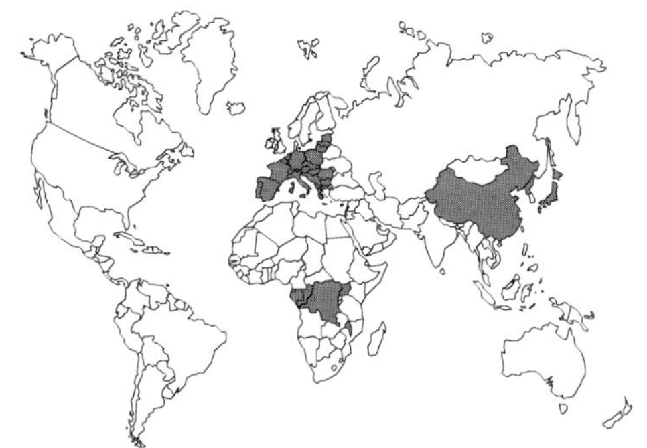

Fig. 2.23.

Besides cats of Europe this trematode has been reported from domestic cats in China (Faust, 1927; Chen, 1934). It has also been reported from Japan (Kifune et al., 1967; Kurimoto, 1976) and Korea (Cho and Lee, 1981). It has been found in the lower Volga of Russia and in cats from Astrakhan. Skrjabin and Popov (1930) described a species *Pharyngostomum fausti* from the delta of the Volga; this is considered a synonym according to Baer and Dubois (1951). *Pharyngostomum cordatum* has been reported from a cheetah in Tanganika (Baer and Dubois, 1951) and from a genet in the Congo (Vanden Berghe, 1939).

Location in Host

Upper small intestine.

Parasite Identification

These trematodes are about 2 to 3 mm long. *Pharyngostomum* differs from *Alaria, Cynodiplostomum,* and *Fibricola* in that it has a very large tribocytic organ that fills the hollow on the ventral surface of the forebody. The egg is 100 μm long and 70 μm wide.

The average number of eggs produced by each worm is about 1,000 per day (To et al., 1988); thus, a gram of feces from an infected cat harboring a single fluke would be between 13 to 70 eggs.

Life Cycle

The life cycle of this species was examined by Wallace (1939). Eggs passed into the environment in the feces of the cat require about 3 to 4 weeks of development before miracidia bearing pigmented eyespots hatch. The miracidium penetrates a snail of the genus *Segmentina* wherein it produces sporocysts. The cercaria that is produced is pharyngeate and longifurcate with colorless eyespots; the body is covered with small spines. The cercaria penetrates tadpoles or adult frogs and develops to the metacercarial stage. Metacercariae can exist in various paratenic hosts including toads, snakes, turtles, and shrews. In experimentally infected cats, developing trematodes were present in the intestine 2 days after treatment. Eggs first appeared in the feces 31 days after infection; another report found the prepatent period to be 28 to 34 days (Kurimoto, 1976). Metacercariae recovered from the European grass snake, *Rhabdophis tigrina,* in Korea were shown to be capable of developing to adults in cats but not in other experimental hosts including mice, rats, hamsters, ducklings, and a dog; in the cats that were infected, adult flukes were recovered 5 weeks after being fed the metacercariae (Chai et al., 1990).

Clinical Presentation and Pathogenesis

The main clinical sign of pharnygostomiasis is chronic diarrhea (Sugano, 1985), probably as a result of a loss of the epithelium at the attachment sites of the trematodes (Uchida and Itagaki, 1980; Okada et al., 1984). The trematode imbeds itself amongst the villi and pulls bits of mucosa into the anterior spoon-shaped region of the body.

Treatment

Thirty-five cats were treated successfully with praziquantel (30 mg/kg subcutaneously). The treatment completely eliminated eggs from the feces and removed the signs of diarrhea (Fukase et al., 1987).

Epizootiology

The cat appears to serve as the major host of this parasite. The metacercaria has been recovered from the thigh muscles of frogs in Japan (Kajiyama et al., 1980).

Hazards to Other Animals

None. Although other hosts are infected, the major means of infection is through the ingestion of the intermediate host, which requires that the appropriate snail also be available.

Hazards to Humans

None.

Control/Prevention

This will be exceedingly difficult in cats that hunt.

REFERENCES

Baer JG, Dubois G. 1951. Note sur le genre *Pharyngostomum* Ciurea, 1922 (Trematoda: Strigeida). Bull Soc Neuchâtel Sci Nat 74:77–82.

Chai JY, Sohn WM, Chung HL, Hong ST, Lee SH. 1990. Metacercariae of *Pharyngostomum cordatum* found from the European grass snake, *Rhabdophis tigrina,* and its experimental infection to cats. Korean J Parasitol 28:175–181.

Chen HT. 1934. Helminths of cats in Fukien and Kwangtung provinces with a list of those recorded from China. Lingnan Sci J 13:261–273.

Cho SY, Lee JB. 1981. *Pharyngostomum cordatum* (Trematoda: Alariidae) collected from a cat in Korea. Korean J Parasitol 19:173–174.

Diesing CM. 1850. Systema Helminthus, Band I, Vienna, Austria.

Faust EC. 1927. Studies on Asiatic holostomes (Class Trematoda). Rec Ind Mus 29:215–227.

Fukase T, Sugano H, Chinone S, Itagaki H. 1987. Anthelmintic effect of praziquantel on *Pharyngos-*

tomum cordatum in naturally infected domestic cats. J Jap Vet Med Assoc 40:640–643.
Kajiyama M, Nakamoto M, Suzuki N. 1980. Studies on *Pharyngostomum cordatum* (Diesing, 1850). 3. An epidemiological survey in the vicinity of Yamaguchi City, Japan. Yamaguchi J Vet Med 7:1–6.
Kifune T, Shiraishi S, Takao Y. 1967. Discovery of *Pharnygostomum cordatum* (Diesing, 1850) in cats from Kyushu, Japan (Trematoda; Strigeoidea; Diplostomatidae) Jap J Parasitol 16:403–409.
Kurimoto H. 1976. Study on the life history of *Pharyngostomum cordatum* (Diesing, 1850) I. The second intermediate host in Japan and experimental infection to the final host. Jap J Parasitol 25:241–246.
Okada R, Imai S, Ishii T. 1984. Scanning electron microscopic observations on the parasitism of *Pharyngostomum cordatum* (Diesing, 1850). Jap J Parasitol 33:333–339.
Skrjabin KI, Popov NP. 1930. *Pharyngostomum fausti* n. sp. Tierärztl Rundschau 35:709–710.
Sugano H. 1985. Chemotherapy of *Pharyngostomum* infection in dogs and domestic cats. J Jap Vet Med Assoc 38:297–301.
To M, Okuma H, Ishida Y, Imai S, Ishii T. 1988. Fecundity of *Pharyngostomum cordatum* parasitic in domestic cats. Jap J Vet Sci 50:908–912.
Uchida A, Itagaki H. 1980. Distribution of metacercariae of *Pharyngostomum cordatum* in Aichi prefecture and pathological findings on cats infected. J Jap Vet Med Assoc 33:594–597.
Vanden Berghe L. 1939. Un strigéidé nouveau du Congo Belge, *Pharyngostomum congolense.* Rev Zool et Botan Africaines 32:654–660.
Wallace FG. 1939. The life cycle of *Pharyngostomum cordatum* (Diesing) Ciurea (Trematoda: Alariidae). Trans Am Microsc Soc 58:49–61.

ECHINOSTOMATIDAE

Another group of trematodes parasitic in the small intestine of cats are the echinostomatids. Echinostomes are characterized by the possession of a group of large spines around the oral sucker. Several genera have been reported from cats. Typically, animals become infected with echinostomes by the ingestion of fish containing metacercariae.

A number of genera have been reported from cats: *Echinochasmus, Episthmium, Stephanoprora, Artyfechinostomum, Isthmiophora,* and *Echinoparyphium. Echinochasmus, Episthmium,* and *Stephanoprora* are similar in that the collar spines, a single row, tend to be interrupted dorsally behind the mouth. *Artyfechinostomum, Isthmiophora,* and *Echinoparyphium* have a double row of spines around the mouth that is not interrupted dorsally. The first three genera tend to utilize fish as intermediate hosts, while the latter three species utilize snails and frogs. The only species that is a parasite commonly isolated from cats is *Echinochasmus perfoliatus,* which is found in cats in Eurasia and North Africa.

Echinochasmus perfoliatus (Ratz, 1908) Dietz, 1909

Etymology

Echino (spined) + *chasmus* (hiatus) (for the discontinuous spination) and *per* (= extremely) + *foliatus* (= leaf-like).

Synonyms

Echinostomum perfoliatum Ratz, 1908; *Echinochasmus perfoliatus* var. *shieldsi* Tubangui, 1922; *Echinochasmus perfoliatus* var. *japonicus* Tanabe, 1922; *Echinochasmus perfoliatus* var. *aegyptius* Fahmy et al., 1981.

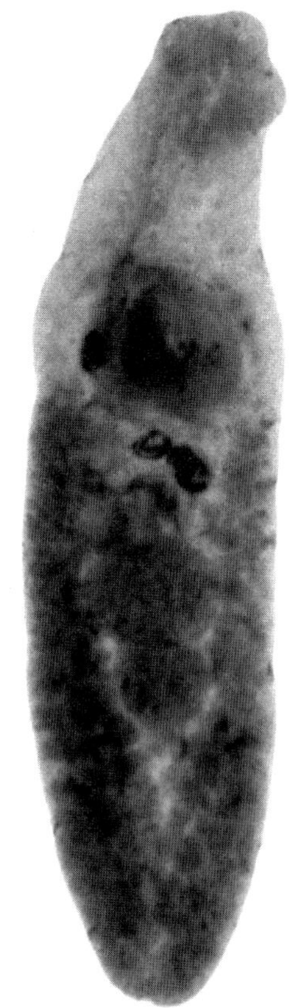

Fig. 2.24. *Echinochasmus perfoliatus* collected from a cat in Egypt.

History

This worm was originally described from dogs and cats in Hungary (Ratz, 1908). Further work has shown it to be present in cats in Russia and Asia.

Geographic Distribution

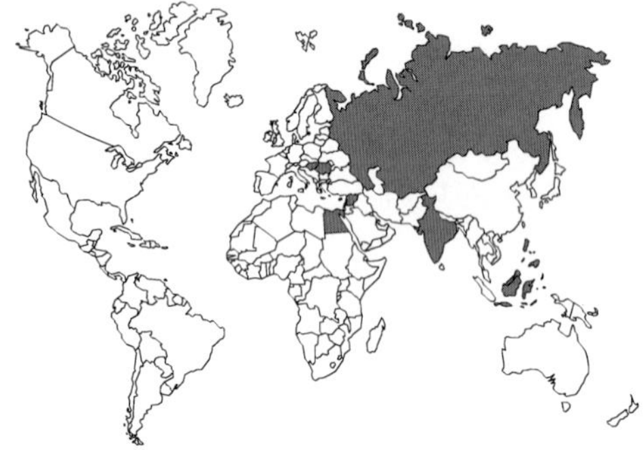

Fig. 2.25.

This trematode is a common parasite of cats in Italy, Hungary, Romania, Russia, Egypt, Israel, and the Far East (Wu, 1938; Fahmy et al., 1981; Fahmy et al., 1984; Abo-Shady et al., 1983).

Location in Host

Small intestine.

Parasite Identification

This worm is elongate, measuring 1 to 12 mm in length. The genus *Echinochasmus* is characterized by the possession of a single row of typical echinostomatid hooks on the anterior collar. *Echinochasmus* differs from other genera of echinostomes in that this circle of hooks is discontinuous in both the ventral and dorsal aspects of the body. The testes are large, globose structures that occur in tandem just posterior to the midline of the body. The ventral sucker is located at the beginning of the second third of the body.

The eggs are rather large, being 90 to 135 μm long by 55 to 95 μm in width.

Life Cycle

Cats have been experimentally infected by feeding them fish containing metacercariae (Ciurea, 1922). The snail intermediate hosts are species of the freshwater genus *Parafossarulus*. The cercariae are of the echinostome type (i.e., they have a tail that is not forked, oral and ventral suckers, and small hooks similar to those of the adult arranged in a row on the head collar). The cercariae enter fish by being swept into the pharynx, and the metacercariae are found encysted in the gills of numerous different freshwater fish. The adult forms develop within 7 to 10 days after the fish is eaten.

Clinical Presentation and Pathogenesis

Thought to be asymptomatic.

Treatment

Probably praziquantel, but not reported.

Epizootiology

Cats become infected by eating raw fish.

Hazards to Other Animals

None. Although other hosts are infected, the major means of infection is through the ingestion of the fish intermediate host, which requires that the appropriate snail also be available. Thus, infection of these other hosts will typically only occur in the wild.

Hazards to Humans

Humans have been infected with this trematode. Due to the large number of infected fish it is believed the infection is less common in people than might otherwise be the case because of the location of the metacercariae in the gill tissue of the fish host, which is often discarded when the fish is eaten.

Control/Prevention

Prevention of the ingestion of raw fish heads.

REFERENCES

Abo-Shady AF, Ali MM, Abdel-Magied S. 1983. Helminth parasites of cats in Dakahlia, Egypt. J Egypt Soc Parasitol 13:129–133.

Ciurea I. 1922. Sur quelques trématodes de renard et du chat sauvage. Comptes Rendus Soc Biol 87:268–299.

Fahmy MA, Khalifa R, Sakla AA. 1981. Study of two echinochasmid parasites (Trematoda. Echinochasmidae) from Upper Egyptian cats. Assiut Vet Med J 8:73–75.
Fahmy MA, Arafa MS, Khalifa R, Abdel-Rahman AM, Mounib ME. 1984. Studies on helminth parasites in some small mammals in Assiut Governorate. 1. Trematode Parasites. Assiut Vet Med J 11:43–52.
Ratz I. 1908. Húserökben élö trematodák. Allat Közlem 7:15–20.
Wu K. 1938. Helminthic fauna in vertebrates of the Hangchow area. Peking Nat Hist Bull 12:1–8.

Echinochasmus breviviteilus Fahmy, Khalifa, Sakla, 1981

This trematode was discovered and described on the basis of five specimens collected from the upper part of the small intestine of one naturally infected stray cat from Assiut, Egypt.

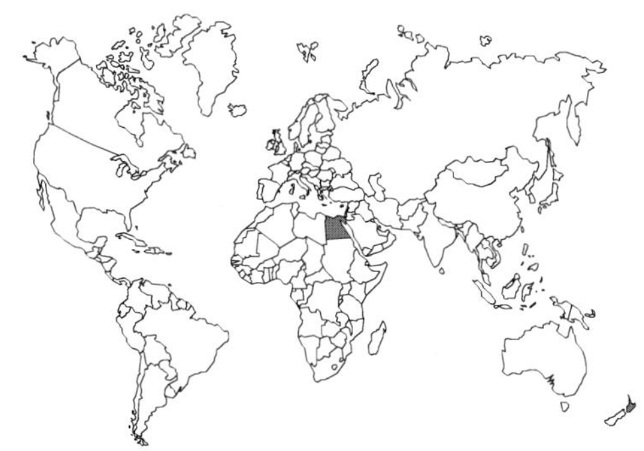

Fig. 2.26.

REFERENCES

Fahmy MA, Khalifa R, Sakla AA. 1981. Study on two echinochasmid parasites (Trematoda. Echinochasmidae) from Upper Egyptian cats. Assiut Vet Med J 8:73–75.

Echinochasmus liliputanus (Looss, 1896) Odhner, 1911

This small trematode (hence the name "liliputanus") was originally described from a hawk (*Pernis apivorus*) and from a kite (*Milvus migrans*). It was redescribed from 4 of 27 cats in Palestine where it was also found in a heron (*Ardea cicerea*) (Witenberg, 1932). Most recently, it was found in 11 of 48 Egyptian cats (Kuntz and Chandler, 1956).

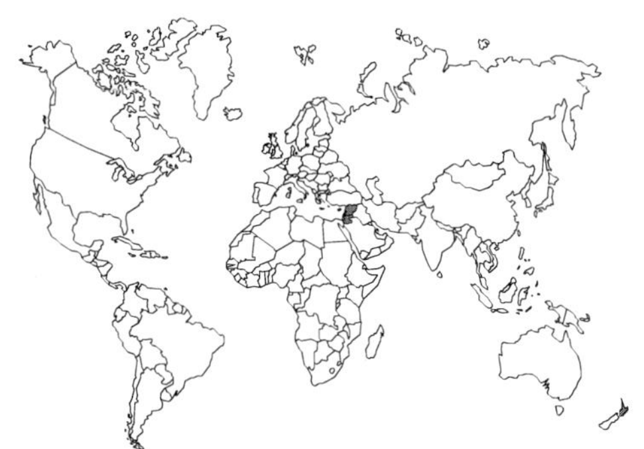

Fig. 2.27.

REFERENCES

Kuntz RE, Chandler AC. 1956. Studies on Egyptian trematodes with special reference to the heterophyids of mammals. I. Adult flukes, with descriptions of *Phagicola longicollis* n. sp., *Cynodiplostomum namrui* n.sp., and a *Stephanoprora* from cats. J Parasitol 42:445–459.
Witenberg G. 1932. Über zwei in Palästina in Hunden und Katzen parasitierende *Echinochasmus*-Arten (Trematoda). Z Parasitenk 5:213–216.

Episthmium caninum (Verma, 1935) Chatterji, 1954

Etymology

Epi (dorsal) + *isthmium* (constriction) (for the break in the spines around the mouth) and *caninum* for the canine host.

Synonyms

Episthochasmus caninum Verma, 1935; *Echinochasmus corvus* (Bhalerao, 1926) Gupte and Pande, 1963. Some consider *Episthmium* a subgenus of *Echinochasmus;* Gupta and Pande (1963) thought this parasite to be synonymous with the species occurring in the crow.

History

This worm was originally described from dogs in Calcutta (Verma, 1935). This fluke has also been rarely reported from the cat (Pande, 1973).

Geographic Distribution

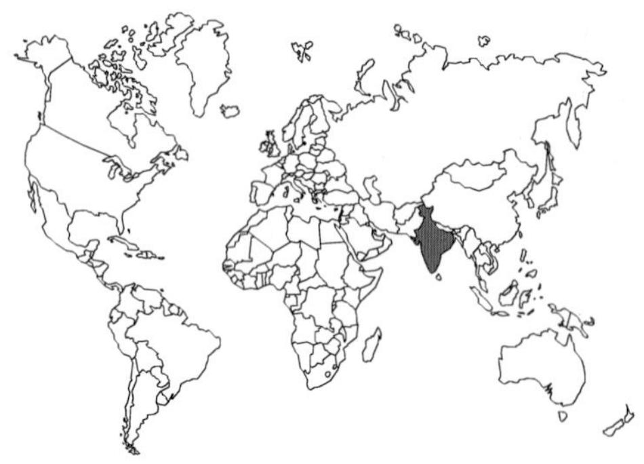

Fig. 2.28.

A rare parasite of cats reported from Lucknow, India (Pande, 1973).

Location in Host

Small intestine.

Parasite Identification

This worm is elongate, measuring 1 to 2 mm in length. The genus *Episthmium* differs from *Echinochasmus* in that the vitelline follicles extend anterior to the ventral sucker.

The eggs are 80 to 85 μm long by 63 to 66 μm wide.

Life Cycle

Not definitely known, probably utilizes fish much in the same manner as *Echinochasmus perfoliatus.*

Clinical Presentation and Pathogenesis

Thought to be asymptomatic.

Treatment

Probably praziquantel, but not reported.

Epizootiology

Cats probably become infected by eating raw fish; it may be that the normal host is a bird such as the crow (Gupta and Pande, 1963).

Hazards to Other Animals

None. Although other hosts are infected, the major means of infection is through the ingestion of the fish intermediate host, which requires that the appropriate snail also be available. Thus, infection of these other hosts will typically only occur in the wild.

Hazards to Humans

None known.

Control/Prevention

Probably prevention of the ingestion of raw fish.

REFERENCES

Gupta VP, Pande BP. 1963. On a trematode of the genus *Echinochasmus* Dietz, 1909, with remarks on the species occurring in Indian carnivores. Parasitology 53:169–175.

Pande KC. 1973. Studies on some known and unknown trematode parasites. Ind J Zootomy 14:197–219.

Verma SC. 1935. Studies on the Indian species of the genus *Echinochasmus.* Part I. and on an allied new genus *Episthochasmus.* Proc Ind Acad Sci 1:837–856.

Stephanoprora denticulatoides Isaichikoff, 1925

Etymology

Stephano (crown) + *prora* (forward) and *denticulatoides* (like *denticulate,* another species of *Stephanoprora* described from European birds).

Synonyms

Beaver (1937) considered *Stephanoprora denticulatoides* a synonym of *Stephanoprora polycesta.* Kuntz and Chandler (1956) redescribed the parasite based on worms recovered from cats in Egypt.

History

This worm was originally described from dogs in the Crimea (Isaichikoff, 1925). The only report from cats is that of Kuntz and Chandler (1956).

Geographic Distribution

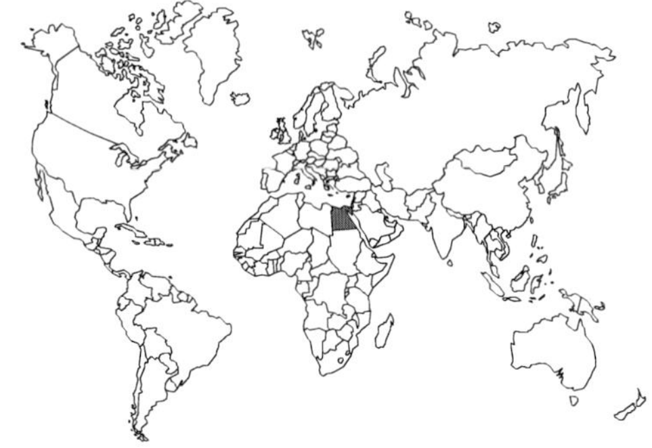

Fig. 2.29.

Crimea and the Mediterranean coast of Egypt.

Location in Host

Small intestine.

Parasite Identification

This worm is elongate in shape, measuring 0.75 to 1.2 mm in length and being about 10 times longer than it is wide. The genus *Stephanoprora* is very similar to *Echinochasmus* (see above) and is considered by some to be a subgenus within *Echinochasmus* (Chatterji, 1954). This parasite differs from *Echinochasmus* in that the vitellaria of *Stephanoprora* are restricted to the posterior part of the body. Thus, species of *Episthmium* have anteriorly extending vitellaria, species of *Echinochasmus* have vitellaria that extend to the level of the ventral sucker, and species of *Stephanoprora* have vitellaria restricted to the posterior of the body.

The eggs are 100 to 110 μm long by 60 to 67 μm in width.

Life Cycle

The life cycle, although not known, is probably similar to that of *Echinochasmus.*

Clinical Presentation and Pathogenesis

Thought to be asymptomatic.

Treatment

Probably praziquantel, but not reported.

Epizootiology

Cats become infected by eating raw fish.

Hazards to Other Animals

None. Although other hosts are infected, the major means of infection is through the ingestion of the fish intermediate host, which requires that the appropriate snail also be available. Thus, infection of these other hosts will typically only occur in the wild.

Hazards to Humans

None.

Control/Prevention

Prevention of the ingestion of raw fish.

REFERENCES

Beaver PC. 1937. Notes on *Stephanoprora polycestus* (Dietz) from the American crow. Trans Ill State Acad Sci 29:247–250.

Chatterji PN. 1954. On a new species of *Echinochasmus* from the intestine of a dog. Ind J Helminthol 6: 1–6.

Isaichikoff IM. 1925. Parasitic worms of domestic carnivores in Crimea. Uchen Trudy Sibirsk Vet 6:47–104.

Kuntz RE, Chandler AC. 1956. Studies on Egyptian trematodes with special reference to the heterophyids of mammals. I. Adult flukes, with descriptions of *Phagicola longicollis* n. sp., *Cynodiplostomum namrui* n. sp., and a *Stephanoprora* from cats. J Parasitol 42:445–459.

Artyfechinostomum sufrartyfex Lane, 1915

Etymology

According to Lane (1915) the worm *Artyfechinostomum sufrartyfex* was named for Dr. E. Smythe of Suffry in Assam, India: "By the kind courtesy of Dr. E. Smythe of Suffry in Assam, India, of whose kindness the name given to the parasite is intended as a slight acknowledgment I have received, on two occasions, consignments of flukes." In 1917, Lane wrote that "In mentioning *Artyfechinostomum sufrartyfex* Leiper refers to the name as 'New and distinctive'; while Odhner is impelled to call it 'terrible.' It would appear

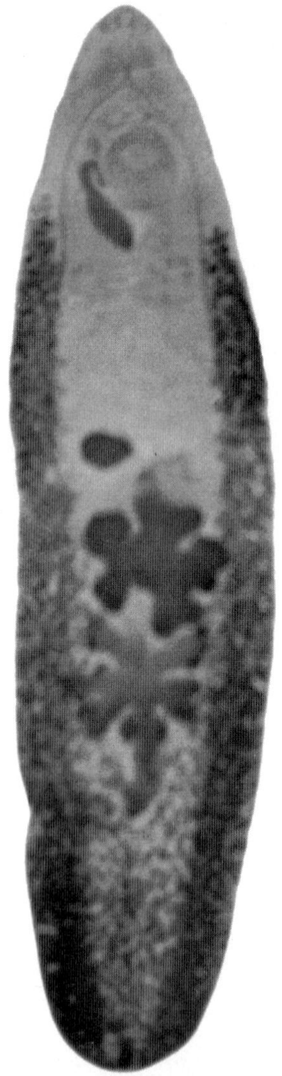

Fig. 2.30. *Artyfechinostomum surfrartyfex* collected from a pig.

therefore to be wise for the future to avoid the attempt to obtain both the alliteration so useful in indicating a type species and the complimentary inclusion of the name of a donor, unless the result can be reached by a less cacophonous combination of syllables than was the case in this effort."

Synonyms

Leiper (1911) is not certain whether or not this worm is the same as *Echinostoma malayanum.* According to Lie Kian Joe (1963a) the two worms are the same, and he presents a long list of potential generic and specific synonomies.

History

The first member of this genus was recovered from a girl in Assam, India, and named *Artyfechinostomum sufrartyfex* Lane, 1915. Other specimens described as *Echinostoma malayanum* have been recovered from humans in Malaysia, Thailand, North Sumatra, and the Sino-Tibetan border.

Geographic Distribution

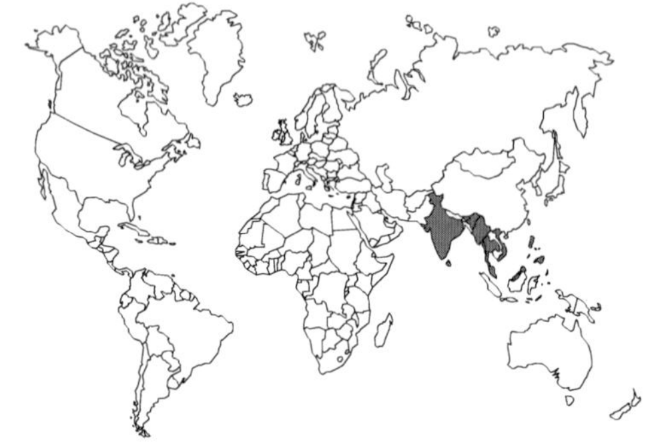

Fig. 2.31.

India; this parasite was reported from 1 cat out of 110 cats that were surveyed (Rajavelu and Raja, 1989). If the parasite is the same as *Echinostoma malayanum,* the range extends into southeast Asia.

Location in Host

Small intestine.

Parasite Identification

The flukes are 8 to 11 mm in length. The genus is characterized by the body being enlarged posteriorly. The ventral sucker is large. The testes are in the posterior part of the body, tandem, and deeply lobed. The eggs are about 120 to 130 μm long and about 80 to 90 μm in diameter.

Life Cycle

Unknown. However, based on the life cycle of *Echinostoma malayanum,* it would appear that the typical host is the pig. *Artyfechinostomum surfrartyfex* has been recovered from pigs in India (Bhalerao, 1931). It seems that this host utilizes two different snails as the intermediate hosts and that pigs become infected by ingesting the second snail host that contains metacercariae. When there are no pigs present, the cycle can be maintained in the wild rat population. Metacercariae can also be found in tadpoles and frogs, and it has been postulated that this is how dogs become infected (Lie Kian Joe, 1963b). It would seem that this is how cats also might obtain an infection with this parasite.

Clinical Presentation and Pathogenesis

In humans, infection has been associated with vomiting (Lane, 1915), but in a light infection in a 5-year-old child, there were no special signs of infection (Lie Kian Joe and Virik, 1963). It is thought to be asymptomatic in cats.

Treatment

Probably praziquantel, but not reported.

Epizootiology

Normal host not known.

Hazards to Other Animals

None. Although other hosts are infected, the major means of infection is through the ingestion of the second snail or amphibian paratenic intermediate host, which requires that the two appropriate snails be available. Thus, infection of these other hosts will typically only occur in the wild.

Hazards to Humans

This trematode has been reported on one occasion from an 8-year-old girl. She vomited one worm and passed 62 after treatment.

Control/Prevention

Cats are probably being infected by eating infected frogs, tadpoles, or snails. This is an infection that would be very difficult to control in cats that enjoy hunting.

REFERENCES

Bhalerao GC. 1931. Trematode parasites of pigs in Bengal. Rec Ind Mus 31:475–482.

Lane C. 1915. *Artyfechinostomum sufrartyfex.* A new parasite echinostome of man. Ind J Med Res 2:977–983.

Lane C. 1917. Are *Echinostomum malayanum* and *Artyfechinostomum sufrartyfex* identical? Ind J Med Res 4:440–441.

Lie Kian Joe. 1963a. Studies on Echinostomatida in Malaya. III. The adult *Echinostoma malayanum* Leiper, 1911 (Trematoda: Echinostomatidae) and the probable synonymy of *Artyfechinostomum sufrartyfex* Lane, 1915. Z Parasitenk 23:124–135.

Lie Kian Joe. 1963b. Studies on Echinostomatida in Malaya. IV. The animal hosts of *Echinostoma malayanum* Leiper, 1911 (Trematoda). Z parasitenk 23:136–140.

Lie Kian Joe, Virik HK. 1963. Human infection with *Echinostoma malyanum* Leiper, 1911 (Trematoda: Echinostomatidae). J Trop Med Hyg 66:77–82.

Rajavelu G, Raja EE. 1989. A note on *Artyfechinostomum malayanum* in cats with special reference to taxonomic position. Cheiron 18:46–48.

Isthmiophora melis (Schrank, 1788) Lühe, 1909

This trematode, along with *Euparyphium beaveri* and *Echinostoma melis,* make up a group that is mainly a parasite of otters and badgers that on rare occasions find their way into dogs. It seems that it is also possible that this trematode could be found in cats. The life cycle, like that of *Artyfechinostomum,* appears to involve infection via the ingestion of frogs, which is how cats are likely to be infected.

Echinoparyphium Dietz, 1909

Specimens identified as belonging to the genus *Echinoparyphium* were recovered from 16 of 59 cats in the midlands of Tasmania (Gregory and Munday, 1976). The species of fluke was not identified, and no pathology or signs due to the parasites were described. The life cycle of these parasites also involves tadpoles and frogs as intermediate hosts.

REFERENCES

Gregory GG, Munday BL. 1976. Intestinal parasites of feral cats from the Tasmanian Midlands and King Island. Aust Vet J 52:317–320.

HETEROPHYIDAE

Another major group of trematodes that is found in the small intestine of cats is the heterophyids. This family of trematodes is characterized by a very small body in the adult fluke and a fusion of the male and female reproductive tracts just prior to exit from the body to form a hermaphroditic duct. There are many genera within this family, and numerous species have been reported from the cat. Cats become infected by the ingestion of fish or sometimes amphibia that contain the metacercariae. The fish are infected by a swimming cercarial stage that typically has eyespots and a long tail and that penetrates the skin of the fish host. The adults of this trematode family seem to be able to develop in a number of different hosts, both birds and mammals, and thus the same species is often found in several different host species as an adult.

There are 10 subfamilies of heterophyids represented in cats. The differences are mainly morphologic. The first, the Apophallinae, are characterized by having their vitellaria distributed throughout the posterior part of the body and no spines on the oral sucker. The second subfamily, the Ascocotylinae, has an oral sucker that has a cone-shaped extension into the esophagus of the adult fluke and the presence of a circumoral crown of spines. This subfamily, according to Soganderes-Bernal and Lumsden (1963), is represented by a single genus *Ascocotyle;* this single genus incorporates many of the parasites of the cats that were originally reported under the generic names *Parascocotyle* and *Phagicola.* The third subfamily, the Centrocestinae, is characterized by a small circle of spines around the oral sucker that has no esophageal extension. The Cryptocotylinae are much like the Centrocestinae, but there are no spines around the mouth. The Euryhelminthinae are characterized by the possession of bodies that are wider than they are long. The Galactosominae are characterized by having an elongate body, by the uterus extending all the way to the posterior of the body, and by relatively large oral suckers. The Haplorchiinae are identified by their possession of a single testis. The Heterophyinae are characterized by their possession of an extra ventral sucker that is next to the ventral sucker and that is used in copulation. The Metagoniminae are characterized by their having an oral sucker that is rather small and subterminal and with the genital opening and ventral sucker often being off the midline of the body. The tenth group, the Stictodoriinae, is characterized by having a subterminal oral sucker and a ventral sucker that is a nonsuctorial organ with numerous spines that project into the genital opening.

REFERENCES

Leiper RT. 1911. A new echinostome parasite in man. J London Schl Trop Med 1:27–28.

Soganderes-Bernal F, Lumsden RD. 1963. The generic status of the heterophyid trematodes of the *Ascocotyle* complex, including notes on the systematics and biology of *Ascocotyle angrense* Travassos, 1916. J Parasitol 49:264–274.

Apophallinae

There are three representatives of this subfamily that have been reported from cats. Some might consider the two species *Apophallus donicus* and *Apophallus venustus* the same species. These two species are not uncommon in cats that eat fish. The other species, *Apophallus muehlingi,* is probably a parasite of gulls that is capable of developing in the cat under appropriate conditions.

Apophallus donicus (Skrjabin and Lindtrop, 1919) Cameron, 1936

Etymology

Apo (away from) + *phallus* (phallus) (the opening of the genital sinus is anterior to the ventral sucker) and *donicus* for the Don River.

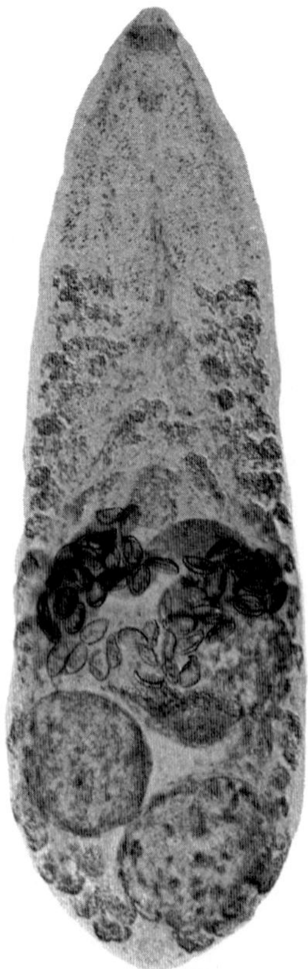

Fig. 2.32. *Apophallus donicus* from a cat in Europe.

Synonyms

Rossicotrema donicum Skrjabin and Lindtrop, 1919; *Tocotrema donicum* (Skrjabin and Lindtrop, 1919) Witenberg, 1929; *Apophallus donicus* (Skrjabin and Lindtrop, 1919) Price, 1931.

History

This trematode was described by Skrjabin and Lintrop (1919) from specimens collected from cats and dogs in Russia under the name *Rossicotrema donicum.* There has been considerable debate over the validity of the genus and even the species. However, using the classification of Cameron (1936) (see the history of *Apophallus venustus,* below), it would appear that there are two distinct species that conveniently fit within the genus *Apophallus* that was originally created by Lühe (1909).

Geographic Distribution

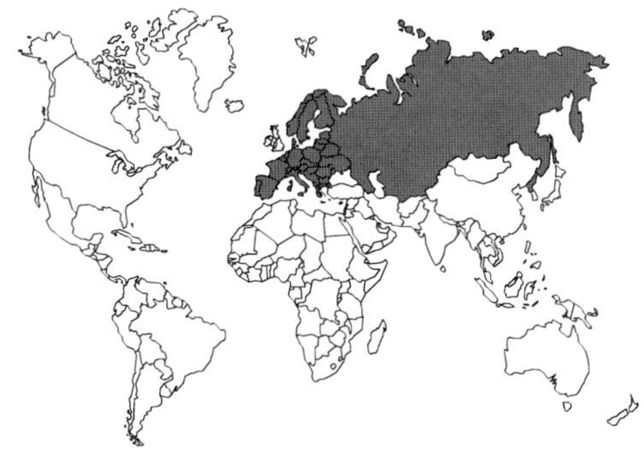

Fig. 2.33.

Russia and other parts of Europe. It was reported in 1966 from a cat in the Netherlands (Jansen, 1966).

Location in Host

Small intestine.

Parasite Identification

This worm is less than 1.14 mm in length. The ventral sucker is small, the large, globular testes are located obliquely in the posterior of the body, and the vitellaria extend only to the ventral sucker. The eggs are 35 to 40 μm long by 26 to 32 μm in width. Supposedly, this species differs from *Apophallus venustus* in that the vitellaria in *Apophallus donicus* remain lateral, while those in *Apophallus venustus* are continuous across the body.

Life Cycle

The life cycle was examined by Ciurea (1933). When cats were fed freshwater fish containing the metacercarial stage, eggs were present in the uteri of the developed adult worms within 2.5 days after infection.

Clinical Presentation and Pathogenesis

Thought to be asymptomatic although it is expected that the small trematodes deeply embedded within the small intestinal mucosa may cause some pathology.

Treatment

Probably praziquantel, but not reported.

Epizootiology

Cats become infected by eating raw fish. Animals other than the cat that have been shown to serve as hosts of the adult fluke include the dog, fox (*Vulpes lagopus*), and weasel (*Mustela sarmatica.*) It has also been found in numerous piscivorous birds: *Mergus merganser, Nycticorax nycticorax, Buteo buteo,* and *Ciconia ciconia.*

Hazards to Other Animals

None. Although other hosts are infected, the major means of infection is through the ingestion of the fish intermediate host, which requires that the appropriate snail also be available. Thus, infection of these other hosts will typically only occur in the wild.

Hazards to Humans

None. Humans theoretically could become infected if they ingested an infected piscine host.

Control/Prevention

Prevention of the ingestion of raw fish.

REFERENCES

Cameron TWM. 1936. Studies on the heterophyid trematode, *Apophallus venustus* (Ransom, 1920) in Canada. Part I. Morphology and taxonomy. Can J Res 14:59–69.

Ciurea I. 1933. Les vers parasites de l'homme, des mammifères et des oiseaux provenant des poissons du Danube et de la Mer Noire. Premier Mémoire. Trématodes, famille Heterophyidae Odhner, avec

un essai de classification des Trématodes de la superfamille Heterophyoidea Faust. Arch Roum Pathol Exp et de Microbiol 6:5–134.
Jansen J. 1966. *Apophallus donicus* (Skrjabin et Lindtrop, 1919) bij een kat. Tijdschr Diergeneesk 91:614–615.
Lühe M. 1909. Parasitische Plattwürmer. I. Trematoden. Süsswasserfauna Deutschlands Heft. 17. Jena.
Skrjabin KI, Lindtrop GT. 1919. Trematodes intestinales des chiens du Don. don Izvest Donsk Vet Inst 1:30–43.

Apophallus venustus (Ransom, 1920) Cameron, 1936

Etymology

Apo (away from) + *phallus* (phallus) (the genital opening is anterior to the ventral sucker) and *venustus* (= handsome, comely in appearance).

Synonyms

Cotylophallus venustus Ransom, 1920; *Tocotrema donicum* (Skrjabin and Lindtrop, 1919) Witenberg, 1929; *Apophallus donicus* (Skrjabin and Lindtrop, 1919) Price, 1931; *Rossicotrema venustus* (Ransom, 1921) Ciurea, 1933.

History

Cameron (1936) considered *Apophallus venustus* a species distinct from its European counterpart *Apophallus donicus.* The morphological distinctions that he noted were in the anterior extent of the vitellaria (to the esophageal bifurcation in *Apophallus venustus,* to the ventral sucker in *Apophallus donicus*), *Apophallus venustus* having a body that is slightly longer and having eggs that are slightly larger.

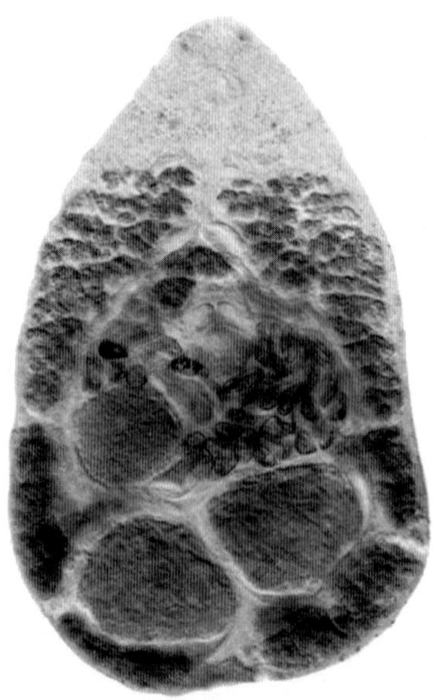

Fig. 2.34. *Apophallus venustus* from a cat in Washington, D.C.

Geographic Distribution

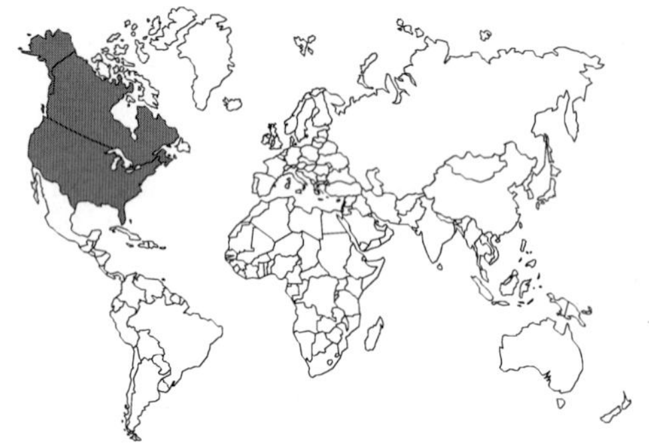

Fig. 2.35.

North America, mainly eastern North America. The Alaskan fox from which it was originally described was from the National Park Zoo in Washington, D.C. The original description also included specimens collected from a cat in the Washington, D.C., area (Ransom, 1920).

Location in Host

Small intestine.

Parasite Identification

This worm is small, less than 1.44 mm in length, but typically slightly larger than *Apophallus donicus.* The ventral sucker is small, the large, globular testes are located obliquely in the posterior of the body, and the vitellaria extend anterior to the ventral sucker, often to the level of the esophageal bifurcation.

The eggs are 26 to 32 μm long by 18 to 22 μm in width.

Life Cycle

The life cycle was examined by Cameron (1937). The snail *Goniobasis livescens* becomes infected by ingesting the embryonated egg from which the miracidium then hatches. From the stages in the snail, cercariae are produced that have long, unbranched tails, with flanges, and pigmented eyespots. These cercariae penetrate the skin of fish and then produce metacercariae in the musculature. Cats become infected by ingesting the infected freshwater fish (e.g., catfish and sunfish). The prepatent period appears to be 1 to 3 weeks, and the adult flukes appear to live only a few months.

Clinical Presentation and Pathogenesis

Thought to be asymptomatic even though the parasite becomes embedded in the mucosa of the ilium.

Treatment

Probably praziquantel, but not reported.

Epizootiology

Cats become infected by eating raw fish. Animals other than the cat that have been shown to serve as hosts of the adult fluke include the dog, raccoon (*Procyon lotor*), Alaskan fox (*Vulpes lagopus*), harbor seal (*Phoca vitulin*), and the great blue heron (*Ardea herodias*).

Hazards to Other Animals

None. Although other hosts are infected, the major means of infection is through the ingestion of the fish intermediate host, which requires that the appropriate snail also be available. Thus, infection of these other hosts will typically only occur in the wild.

Hazards to Humans

None. Humans theoretically could become infected if they ingested an infected piscine host.

Control/Prevention

Prevention of the ingestion of raw fish.

REFERENCES

Cameron TWM. 1936. Studies on the heterophyid trematode, *Apophallus venustus* (Ransom, 1920) in Canada. Part I. Morphology and taxonomy. Can J Res 14:59–69.

Cameron TWM. 1937. Studies on the heterophyid trematode *Apophallus venustus* (Ransom, 1920) in Canada. Part II. Life history and bionomics. Can J Res 15:38–51.

Ransom BH. 1920. Synopsis of the trematode family Heterophyidae with descriptions of a new genus and five new species. Proc U.S. Nat Mus 57:527–573.

Apophallus muehlingi (Jägerskiöld, 1899) Lühe, 1909

This trematode (called *Tocotrema muehlingi* by Looss, 1899) is usually reported from gulls. It has also been reported once from an infected cat in Europe (Witenberg, 1929).

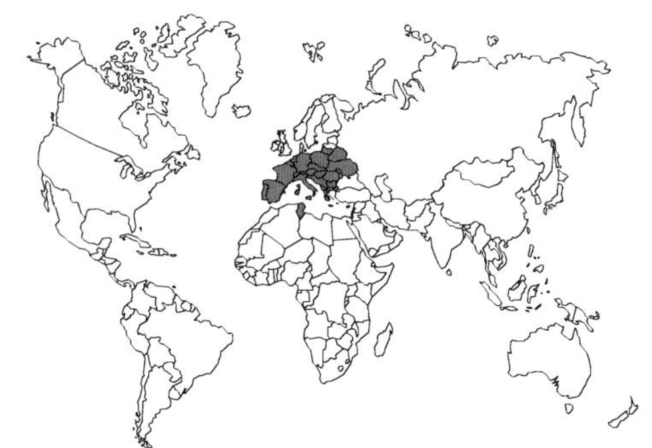

Fig. 2.36.

REFERENCES

Witenberg G. 1929. Studies on the trematode family Heterophyidae. Ann Trop Med Parasitol 23:131–239.

Ascocotylinae

The Ascocotylinae is a group of trematodes that is characterized by an elongation of the oral sucker (Fig. 2.38). The genus *Ascocotyle* now contains worms that were previously included in

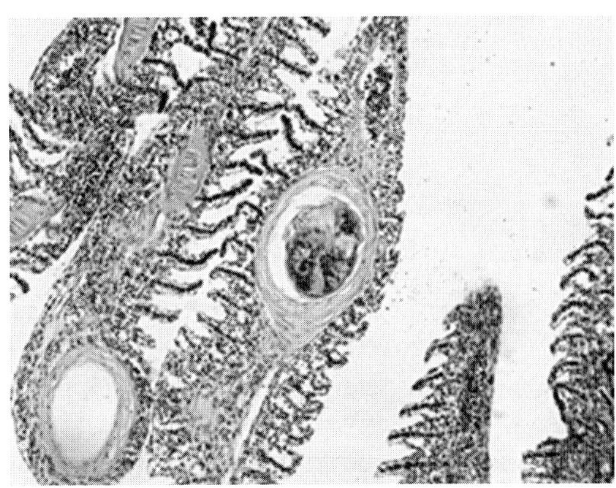

Fig. 2.37. Metacercariae of an *Ascocotyle* sp. viewed in a histological section of a gill of a killifish (*Fundulus* sp.).

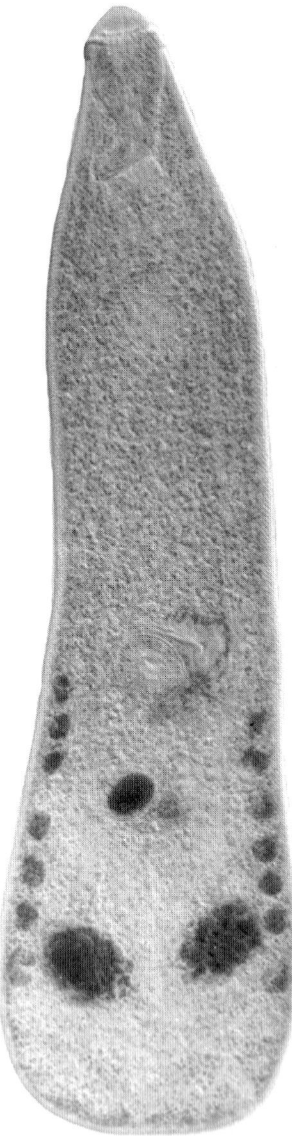

Fig. 2.38. *Ascocotyle chandleri* from a roseatte spoonbill (*Ajaia ajaja*). Note the elongated oral sucker.

the genera *Phagicola, Leighia,* and *Parascocotyle*. There are seven different species of *Ascocotyle* that have been reported from cats. All these trematodes gain access to cats through the cats' ingestion of fish containing the metacercarial stage. It appears that many of these trematodes are parasites of other animals but that they are capable of developing in the cat if it happens to ingest the infected fish.

Ascocotyle ascolonga (Witenberg, 1929) Travassos, 1930

Etymology

Asco (tube) + *cotyle* (disk) (referring to the shape of the anterior sucker being elongated within the body) and *asco* (tube) + longus (long).

Synonyms

Parascocotyle ascolonga Witenberg, 1929; *Phagicola ascolonga* (Witenberg, 1929) Price, 1932.

History

This parasite was originally described from specimens collected in small numbers from dogs and cats in Palestine (Witenberg, 1929).

Geographic Distribution

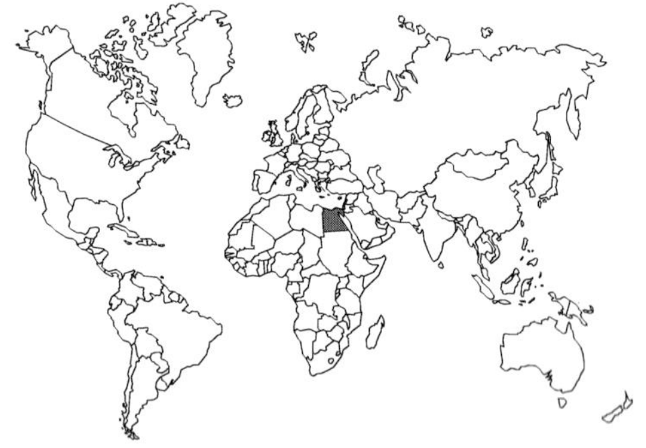

Fig. 2.39.

Palestine. This fluke has been reported from Egypt (Azim, 1938) where it was also collected from 17 of 48 cats under the name *Phagicola ascolonga* (Witenberg, 1929) Price, 1932 (Kuntz and Chandler, 1956).

Location in Host

Small intestine.

Parasite Identification

This small fluke is 0.5 to 0.7 mm in length with a width of 0.1 to 0.3 mm. The body is covered with small, scale-like spines. The oral aperture is surrounded by a single row of 16 large spines. There is a funnel-like appendix on the oral sucker that has been the basis for the various other generic placements of this species. The testes lie side by side in the hind extremity of the body.

The eggs are 18 μm long by 9 μm in width, have thin shells, are somewhat narrowed anteriorly, and have distinctly visible opercula.

Life Cycle

Dogs were experimentally infected by feeding them brackish-water fish (*Tilapia simonis* and *Tilapia galilea*) that contained metacercariae (Witenberg, 1929).

Clinical Presentation and Pathogenesis

Thought to be asymptomatic.

Treatment

Probably praziquantel, but not reported.

Epizootiology

Cats probably are infected by eating raw fish.

Hazards to Other Animals

None. Although other hosts are infected, the major means of infection is through the ingestion of the fish intermediate host, which requires that the appropriate snail also be available. Thus, infection of these other hosts will typically only occur in the wild.

Hazards to Humans

None. Humans theoretically could become infected if they ingested an infected piscine host.

Control/Prevention

Prevention of the ingestion of raw fish.

REFERENCES

Azim MA. 1938. On the intestinal helminths of dogs in Egypt. J Egypt Med Assoc 21:118–122.

Kuntz RE, Chandler AC. 1956. Studies on Egyptian trematodes with special reference to the heterophyids of mammals. I. Adult flukes, with descriptions of *Phagicola longicollis* n. sp., *Cynodiplostomum namrui* n. sp., and a *Stephanoprora* from cats. J Parasitol 42:445–459.

Witenberg G. 1929. Studies on the trematode family Heterophyidae. Ann Trop Med Parasitol 23:131–239.

Ascocotyle longicollis (Kuntz and Chandler, 1956) Soganderes-Bernal and Lumsden, 1963

Etymology

The *longicollis* refers to the length of the elongation of the oral sucker.

Synonyms

Phagicola longicollis Kuntz and Chandler, 1956.

History

This parasite was originally described from specimens collected from 22 of 48 cats in Egypt.

Geographic Distribution

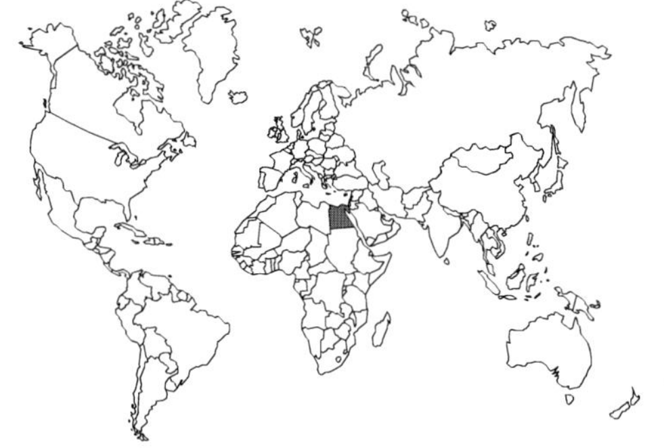

Fig. 2.40.

Egypt.

Location in Host

Small intestine.

Parasite Identification

This fluke is 0.6 to 1 mm in length. The oral sucker bears approximately 20 hooklets and leads into the conical prepharynx that is characteristic of this genus. The genital opening is just anterior to the ventral sucker, which is at the beginning of the posterior third of the body. Most of the reproductive organs are posterior to the ventral sucker. The paired testes are symmetrical and located at the posterior end of the body.

The eggs are 18 to 20 μm long by 10 μm in width.

Life Cycle

Cats were found to be naturally infected with this parasite. Adult worms were recovered from dogs fed brackish-water fish (*Mugil* and *Telapia* species) containing metacercariae (Fahmy and Selim, 1959).

Clinical Presentation and Pathogenesis

Thought to be asymptomatic.

Treatment

Probably praziquantel, but not reported.

Epizootiology

Cats probably become infected by eating raw fish with the parasite. Dogs also seem to serve as final hosts.

Hazards to Other Animals

None. Although dogs are also infected, the major means of infection is through the ingestion of the fish intermediate host, which requires that the appropriate snail also be available. Thus, infection of these other hosts will typically only occur in the wild.

Hazards to Humans

None. Humans theoretically could become infected if they ingested an infected piscine host.

Control/Prevention

Prevention of the ingestion of raw fish.

REFERENCES

Fahmy MAM, Selim MK. 1959. Studies on some trematode parasites of dogs in Egypt with special reference to the role played by fish in their transmission. Z Parasitenk 19:3–13.

Ascocotyle minuta Looss, 1899

Etymology

Asco (tube) + *cotyle* (disk) (referring to the shape of the anterior sucker being elongated within the body) and *minuta* (small) (referring to the small size).

Synonyms

Phagicola minuta (Looss, 1899) Faust, 1920; *Parascocotyle minuta* (Looss, 1899) Stunkard and Haviland 1924.

History

This parasite was originally described from dogs and cats in Egypt; it was also found at this time in a heron, *Ardea cinerea*.

Geographic Distribution

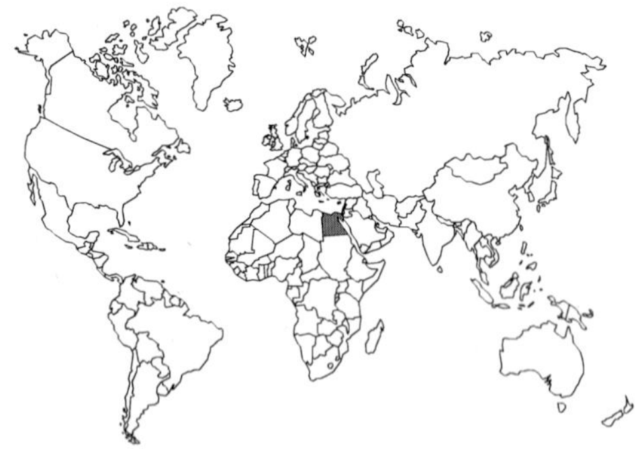

Fig. 2.41.

Egypt.

Location in Host

Small intestine.

Parasite Identification

This small fluke is less than 0.5 mm in length. The oral sucker bears approximately 18 to 20 hooklets and leads into the conical prepharynx that is characteristic of this genus. The genital opening is just anterior to the ventral sucker. Most of the reproductive organs are posterior to the ventral sucker. The paired testes are symmetrical and located at the posterior end of the body.

The eggs have a golden brown shell and are 23 to 24 µm long by 14 µm in width.

Life Cycle

Assumed to use a piscine intermediate host.

Clinical Presentation and Pathogenesis

Thought to be asymptomatic.

Treatment

Probably praziquantel, but not reported.

Epizootiology

Cats probably become infected by eating raw fish.

Hazards to Other Animals

None. Although other hosts are infected, the major means of infection is through the ingestion of the fish intermediate host, which requires that the appropriate snail also be available. Thus, infection of these other hosts will typically only occur in the wild.

Hazards to Humans

None. Humans theoretically could become infected if they ingested an infected piscine host.

Control/Prevention

Prevention of the ingestion of raw fish.

REFERENCES

Looss A. 1899. Weitere Beiträge sur Kenntnis der Trematodenfauna Aegyptens, zugleich Versuch einer natürlichen Gliederung des Genus *Distomum* Retzius. Zool Jahrb Syst 12:521–784.

Ascocotyle angrense Travassos, 1916

This parasite was originally described from a heron, *Butorides striata,* in Brazil. The only report of this parasite from the small intestine of a cat is from an experimental infection (Sogandares-Bernal and Lumsden, 1963). The parasite is distributed along the east coast of North America, Yucatan, and Rio de Janeiro, Brazil. This small fluke is 0.46 to 0.79 mm in length with an oral sucker bearing approximately 20 hooklets. The eggs are 16 to 24 µm long by 16 to 20 µm in width. Cats were experimentally infected with this trematode when fed fish (poeciliid and cyprinodont) gills that contained metacercariae in their filaments. The prepatent period in cats is not stated, but rats passed eggs within 48 hours after exposure. Clinical signs in the experimental animals were not monitored. Natural hosts include a long list of fish intermediate hosts (e.g., *Fundulus, Lucania,* and *Mollienesia*), and as final hosts, a long list of birds and mammals (e.g., wood duck, *Aix sponsa,* egret, *Casmerodius albus,* muskrat, *Ondatra zibethicus,* raccoon, and rat, *Rattus norvegicus*).

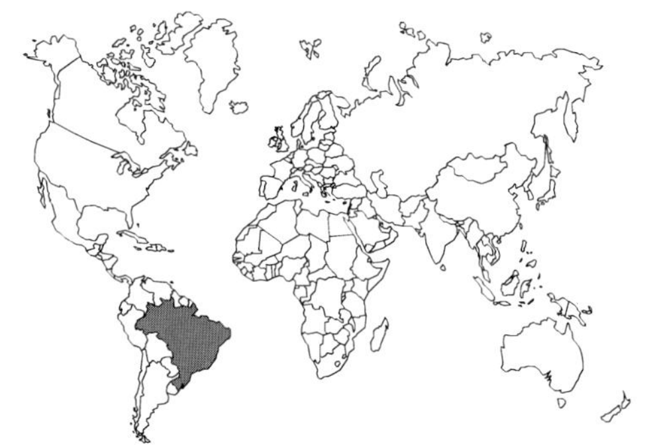

Fig. 2.42.

REFERENCES

Sogandares-Bernal F, Lumsden RD. 1963. The generic status of the heterophyid trematodes of the *Ascocotyle* complex, including notes on the systematics and biology of *Ascocotyle angrense* Travassos, 1916. J Parasitol 49:264–274.

Ascocotyle longa Ransom, 1921

This parasite was originally described from an Alaskan fox (*Vulpes lagopus*) that died in the National Zoo in Washington, D.C. It has been reported from dogs in Cairo and Alexandria (Azim, 1938). However, others have felt that this was a misidentification of a species that they described as *Phagicola longicollis* (see above) (Kuntz and Chandler, 1956). Cats were experimentally infected with Venezuelan mullet meat containing parasites identified as *Phagicola longa* (Conroy, 1986).

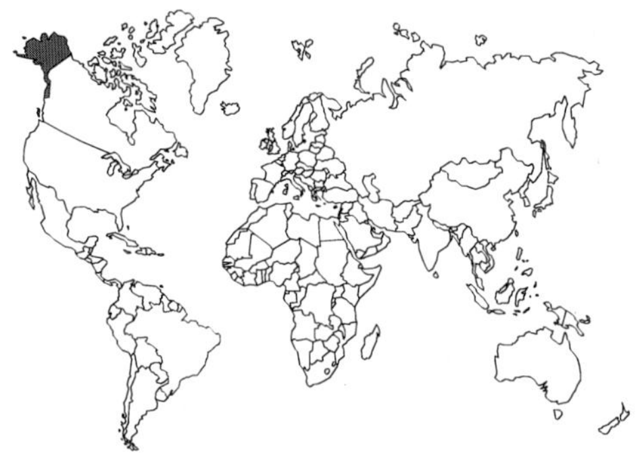

Fig. 2.43.

REFERENCES

Azim MA. 1938. On the intestinal helminths of dogs in Egypt. J Egypt Med Assoc 21:118–122.

Conroy GA de. 1986. Investigaciones sobre la fagicolosis en lisas (Mugilidae) de aguas americanas. I. Estudios taxonómicos de *Phagicola* sp. (Trematoda: Heterophyidae) en mugílidos sudamericanos. Rev Iber Parasitol 46:39–46.

Kuntz RE, Chandler AC. 1956. Studies on Egyptian trematodes with special reference to the Heterophyids of mammals. I. Adult flukes, with descriptions of *Phagicola longicollis* n. sp., *Cynodiplostomum namrui* n. sp., and a *Stephanoprora* from cats. J Parasitol 42:445–459.

Ascocotyle pachycystis Schroeder and Leigh, 1965

As part of the study of the life cycle of this parasite that typically infects raccoons, kittens were experimentally infected (Schroeder and Leigh, 1965). *Littotadinops tenuipes* is the snail in which development occurs. The cercariae that are produced have pigmented eyespots and short unbranched tails with lateral fins. These cercariae penetrate the fins of brackish-water fish (*Cyprinodon variegatus*) and then migrate to the bulbus arteriosus of the heart where very large numbers might occur. When kittens were fed fish containing metacercariae, some developed infections while others appeared refractory.

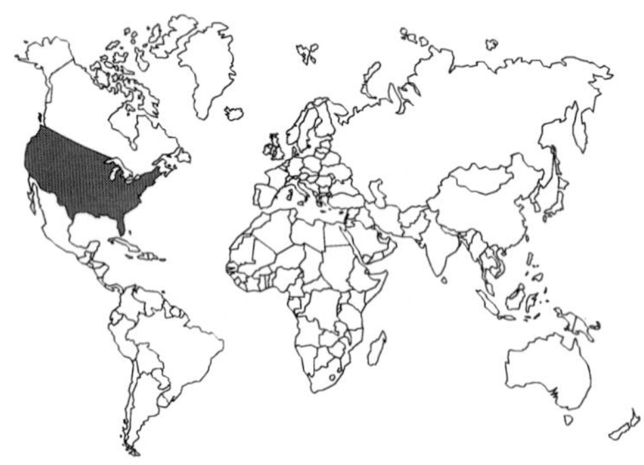

Fig. 2.44.

REFERENCES

Schroeder RE, Leigh WH. 1965. The life history of *Ascocotyle pachycystis* sp. n., a trematode (Digenea: Heterophyidae) from the raccoon in south Florida. J Parasitol 51:594–599.

Ascocotyle arnoldoi (Travassos, 1928) Soganderes-Bernal and Lumsden, 1963

This worm was originally described from mice, dogs, and an albatross. However, this trematode has been reported from 3 percent of cats in São Paulo, Brazil and in 6 percent of cats in Chile. Clinical signs due to this worm have not been described.

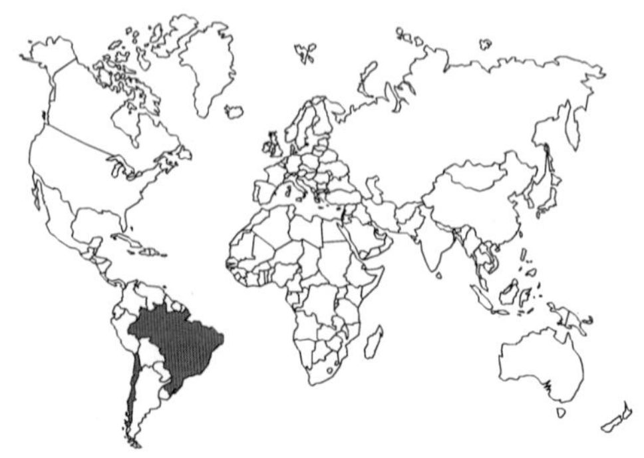

Fig. 2.45.

Centrocestinae

The Centrocestinae is characterized by a fairly large oral sucker that has a double crown of spines. The body is small, and oval to pear shaped. These parasites are transmitted to cats through the ingestion of freshwater fish. Included here with *Centrocestus,* the type genus of this subfamily, are also two genera of heterophyid trematodes that others are likely to place in other subfamilies. These two genera, *Pygidiopsoides* and *Pygidiopsis,* have characters that are somewhat *Centrocestus*-like, and for the sake of simplicity, it seemed warranted to use the more general treatment of lumping the three genera together. These latter two genera appear to be transmitted by brackish-water fish.

Centrocestus caninus Leiper, 1913

Etymology

Centro (spined) + *cestus* (girdle) (for a ring of small spines around the oral opening) and *caninus* for the canine host.

Synonyms

Centrocestus cuspidatus Leiper, 1913; *Stephanopirumus longus* Onji and Nishio, 1916; *Stamnosoma formosanum* Nishigori, 1924; *Centrocestus yokogawai* Kobayasi, 1942.

History

This parasite was first described by Leiper from a dog in Taiwan (Leiper, 1913).

Geographic Distribution

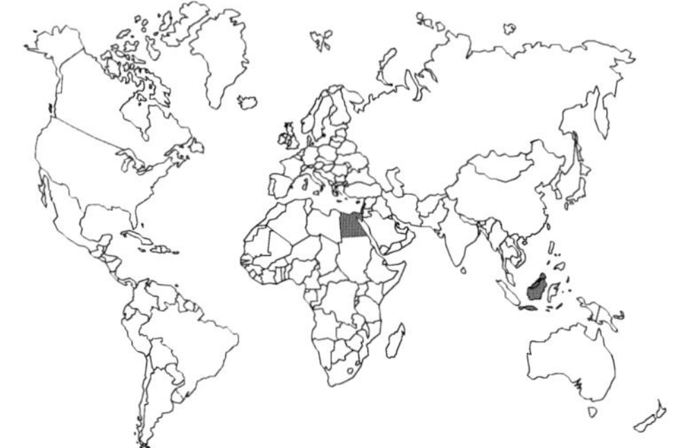

Fig. 2.46.

This parasite has been reported from Egypt, the islands of Taiwan and Hainan, and from Malaysia (Chen, 1941; Rohde, 1962).

Location in Host

Small intestine.

Parasite Identification

This small worm has two rows of spines (a total of 30 to 36 spines) on the oral sucker. The testes are terminal and the vitellaria do not extend into the middle of the body.

The eggs are 33 μm long by 16 to 17 μm in width; the eggs are relatively thin shelled and bear minute spines.

Life Cycle

The life cycle has been examined by Nishigori (1924) and Chen (1941). The miracidia develop in snails of the genus *Semisulcospira,* and the simple-tailed cercariae with eyespots encyst in the gills of various freshwater fish, including *Macropodus opervularis, Puntius semifasciolatus, Carassius auratus,* and *Misgurnus anguillicaudatus,* and in the stomach wall and muscle of frogs, *Rana limnocharis,* and toads, *Bufo melanostictus.* When cats were experimentally infected, eggs were present 11 to 17 days after the cats were fed metacercariae.

Clinical Presentation and Pathogenesis

Thought to be asymptomatic.

Treatment

Probably praziquantel, but not reported.

Epizootiology

Cats become infected by eating raw fish or frogs. Animals other than the cat that have been shown to serve as hosts of the adult fluke include the various herons and egrets. Humans and dogs have been experimentally infected through the feeding of infected fish.

Hazards to Other Animals

None. Although other hosts are infected, the major means of infection is through the ingestion of the fish intermediate host, which requires that the appropriate snail also be available. Thus, infection of these other hosts will typically only occur in the wild.

Hazards to Humans

Humans have been experimentally infected by feeding them fish containing the metacercarial stage of this parasite.

Control/Prevention

Prevention of the ingestion of raw fish.

REFERENCES

Chen HT. 1941. The metacercaria and adult of *Centrocestus formosanus* (Nishigori, 1924), with notes on the natural infection of rats and cats with *C. armatus* (Tanabe, 1922). J Parasitol 28:285–298.

Leiper RT. 1913. Seven helminthological notes. J Lond School Trop Med 2:175–178.

Nishigori M. 1924. On a new species of fluke, *Stamnosoma formosanum,* and its life history. Taiwan Igakkai Zasshi 234:181–238.

Rohde K. 1962. Helminthen aus Katzen und Hunden in Malaya; Bemerkungen zu ihrer epidemiologischen Bedeutung für den Menschen. Z Parasitenk 22:237–244.

Pygidiopsis genata Looss, 1907

Etymology

Pygidiopsis (*pygid* = posterior; *opsi* = late) along with *genata* (referring to the genital opening).

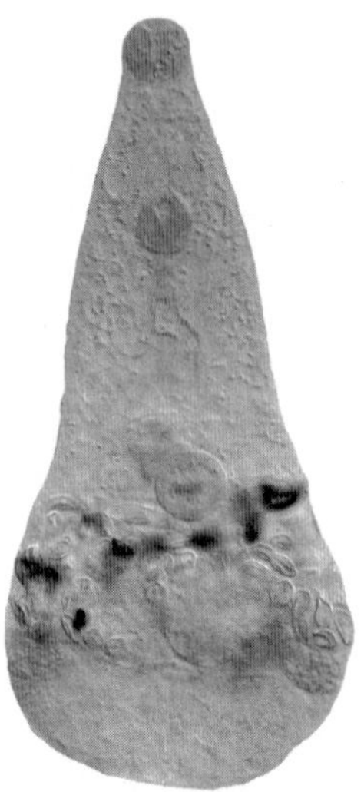

Fig. 2.47. *Pygidiopsis genata* from the small intestine of a domestic cat in Cairo, Egypt.

Synonyms

None.

History

This parasite was described by Looss (1907) from specimens recovered from a pelican, *Pelecanus onocrotalus.*

Geographic Distribution

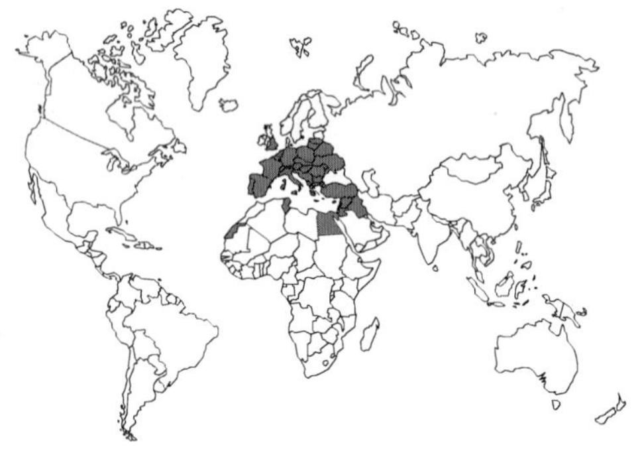

Fig. 2.48.

Naturally infected cats have been found in Europe, Egypt (29.2 percent of stray cats in Dakahlia) (Abo-Shady et al., 1983), and Asia.

Location in Host

Small intestine.

Parasite Identification

The posterior end of the body is wider than the anterior. The entire body is covered with small spines. *Pygidiopsis* has two symmetrical testes and a single gonotyl. The worm is 0.4 to 0.7 mm long and 0.2 to 0.4 mm wide. The body is covered with small spines, and 16 larger spines surround the mouth. The eggs are 18 to 22 μm long by 9 to 12 μm wide.

Life Cycle

The snail intermediate host is *Melania tuberculata.* The cercariae have a dorsal fin and eyespots. The cercariae encyst in brackish-water fish of the genus *Tilapia* (Boulos et al., 1981). Cats have been experimentally infected by the feeding of infected fish.

Clinical Presentation and Pathogenesis

Thought to be asymptomatic.

Treatment

Probably praziquantel, but not reported.

Epizootiology

Cats become infected by eating raw fish. Chicks have also been shown to serve as experimental hosts of this trematode, and it is likely that the natural host is a marine bird.

Hazards to Other Animals

None. Although other hosts are infected, the major means of infection is through the ingestion of the fish intermediate host, which requires that the appropriate snail also be available. Thus, infection of these other hosts will typically only occur in the wild.

Hazards to Humans

Humans have been reported to be infected with this parasite in Egypt (Boulos et al., 1981). Infections were probably acquired by the ingestion of raw fish.

Control/Prevention

Prevention of the ingestion of raw fish.

REFERENCES

Abo-Shady AF, Ali MM, Abdel-Magied S. 1983. Helminth parasites of cats in Dakahlia, Egypt. J Egypt Soc Parasitol 13:129–133.

Boulos LM, Abdou LA, Girgis RS. 1981. Histopathological and histochemical studies on experimentally infected hamsters with *Pygidiopsis genata.* J Egypt Soc Parasitol 11:67–76.

Looss A. 1907. Notizen sur Helminthologie Aegyptiens. VII. Ueber einige neue Trematoden der ägyptischen Fauna. Centralbl Bakt Parasitenk Infekt 43:478–490.

Pygidiopsis summa Onji and Nishio, 1916

This small trematode (0.3 to 0.5 mm long by about 0.2 mm wide) has been found in the small intestine of cats in Japan and Korea (Eom et al., 1984). It has also been reported from avian hosts. In Korea, human infections have been reported in a patient with a history of eating the flesh of raw, brackish-water fish (Seo et al., 1981). After they were treated, patients passed up to 4,000 of these. The eggs are 18–20 μm by 9–11 μm.

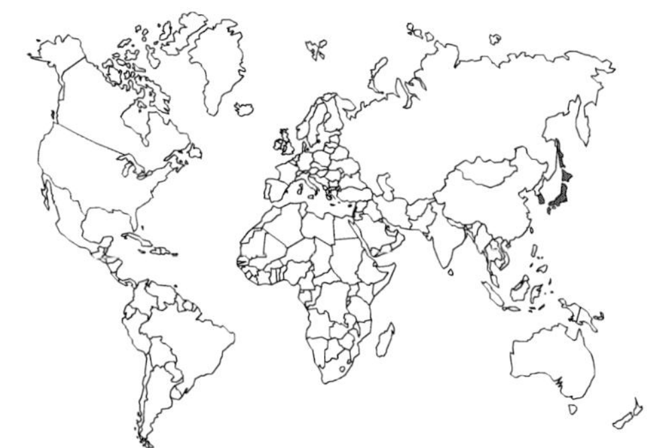

Fig. 2.49.

REFERENCES

Eom KS, Son SY, Lee JS, Rim HJ. 1984. Heterophyid trematodes (*Heterophyopsis continua, Pygidiopsis summa* and *Heterophyes heterophyes nocens*) from domestic cats in Korea. Korean J Parasitol 23:197–202.

Seo BS, Hong ST, Chai JY. 1981. Studies on intestinal trematodes in Korea. III. Natural human infections of *Pygidiopsis summa* and *Heterophyes heterophyes nocens.* Seoul J Med 22:228–235.

Pygidiopsoides spindalis Martin, 1951

This parasite, *Pygidiopsoides* (*Pygidiopsis*-like) along with *spindalis* (referring to the spindle-shaped body), was described from adults recovered from the small intestines of cats and chicks fed metacercariae from fish in southern California. Because this parasite has only one testis, it has been placed by some in the subfamily Haplorchiinae; however, based on larval morphology, it appears more related to members of the Centrocestinae (Martin, 1964). This worm is distinguished from the other members of the Centrocestinae by the presence of a common muscular genital ejector. Unlike specimens of *Pygidiopsis,* this trematode has a single testis and two gonotyls.

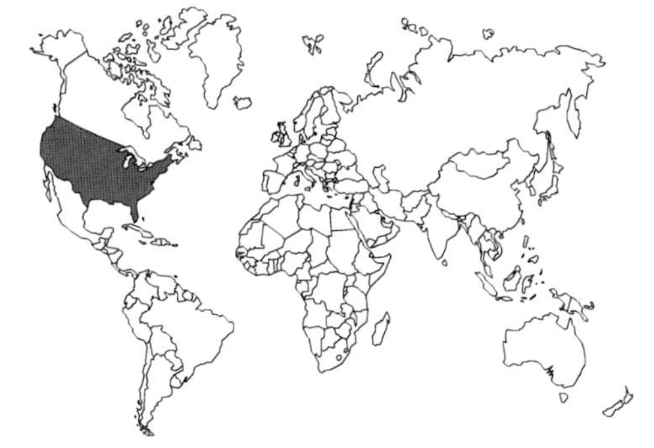

Fig. 2.50.

Pygidiopsoides spindalis adults are 0.22 to 0.43 mm long and 0.06 to 0.10 mm wide. The body is covered with small spines, and 14 spines surround the mouth. The eggs are 26 to 28 μm long by 13 to 15 μm wide.

Life Cycle

The life cycle has been examined by Martin (1951, 1964). The miracidia develop in snails, *Certhidea californica,* that live in intertidal areas. The cercariae have simple tails without fins and two large eyespots. The cercariae penetrate the gills of brackish-water fish, *Fundulus parvipinnis,* and they work their way to the body process of the gill where they encyst. The adult trematodes were recovered from cats 4 to 6 days after being fed infected fish.

REFERENCES

Martin WE. 1951. *Pygidiopsoides spindalis* n. gen., n. sp., (Heterophyidae; Trematoda), and its second intermediate host. J Parasitol 37:297–300.

Martin WE. 1964. Life cycle of *Pygidiopsoides spindalis* Martin, 1951 (Heterophyidae: Trematoda) Trans Am Microsc Soc 83:270–272.

Cryptocotylinae

This subfamily of heterophyids is characterized by the possession of a large genital atrium that incorporates the ventral sucker. There are three species of this parasite that have been recovered from the cat.

Cryptocotyle lingua (Creplin, 1825) Fischoeder, 1903

Etymology

Crypto (hidden) + *cotyle* (disk) (for the small ventral sucker being incorporated, hidden within, the muscular ring of small spines around the oral opening) and *lingua* for the tongue-like shape of the body.

Synonyms

Hallum caninum Wigdor, 1918.

History

This parasite was first described by Creplin in 1825 and placed by Fischoeder in the genus *Cryptocotyle* in 1903.

Geographic Distribution

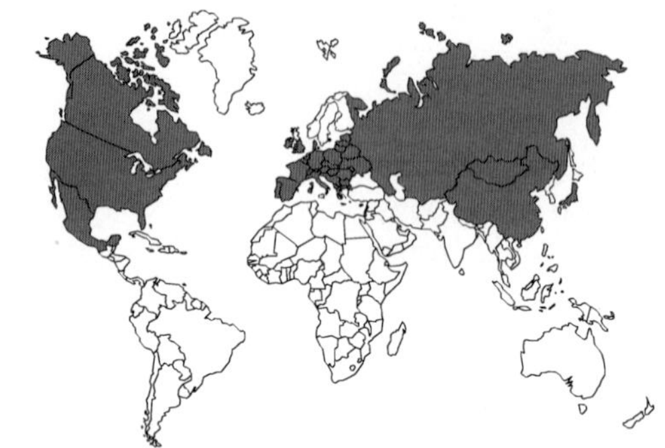

Fig. 2.51.

This parasite has been reported from North America (Burrows and Lillis, 1965), Europe, and Asia.

Location in Host

Small intestine.

Parasite Identification

This small worm (1.29 to 1.46 mm long by 0.59 to 0.77 wide) differs from *Cryptocotyle concavum* in that the body is more tongue-shaped.

The eggs are 34 to 38 μm long by 16 to 20 μm in width.

Life Cycle

The typical final hosts are gulls and terns. The life cycle was examined by Stunkard (1930) and by Stunkard and Willey (1929), who experimentally infected cats. The snail hosts are the brackish-water and seawater snails *Littorina littorea* and *Littorina rudis.* The cercariae that are released encyst in cunner and other saltwater fish. Cats become infected by eating the brackish-water fish. The worms rapidly grow to adults, producing patent infections in a week to 20 days.

Clinical Presentation and Pathogenesis

Although experimental infections in cats produced worm development between the intestinal villi, no clinical signs developed.

Treatment

Probably praziquantel, but not reported.

Epizootiology

Cats, like the typical bird hosts, become infected by eating raw fish. Animals other than the cat that have been shown to serve as hosts of the adult fluke include the dog.

Hazards to Other Animals

None. Although other hosts are infected, the major means of infection is through the ingestion of the fish intermediate host, which requires that the appropriate snail also be available. Thus, infection of these other hosts will typically only occur in the wild.

Hazards to Humans

Humans could possibly be infected if they ingested the fish intermediate host.

Control/Prevention

Prevention of the ingestion of raw fish.

REFERENCES

Burrows RB, Lillis WG. 1965. Trematodes of New Jersey dogs and cats. J Parasitol 51:570–574.

Stunkard HW. 1930. Life history of *Cryptocotyle lingua* (Crepl.) from the gull and tern. J Morph Physiol 50:143–191.

Stunkard HW, Willey CH. 1929. The development of *Cryptocotyle* (Heterophyideae) in its final host. Am J Trop Med 9:117–128.

Cryptocotyle quinqueangularis (Skrjabin, 1923)

Etymology

Crypto (hidden) + *cotyle* (disk) (for the small ventral sucker being incorporated, hidden within, the muscular ring of small spines around the oral opening) and *quinqueangularis* for the five-sided nature of this worm.

Synonyms

Ciureana quinqueangularis (Skrjabin, 1923).

History

This parasite was first described by Skrjabin from specimens recovered from domestic cats in the former USSR.

Geographic Distribution

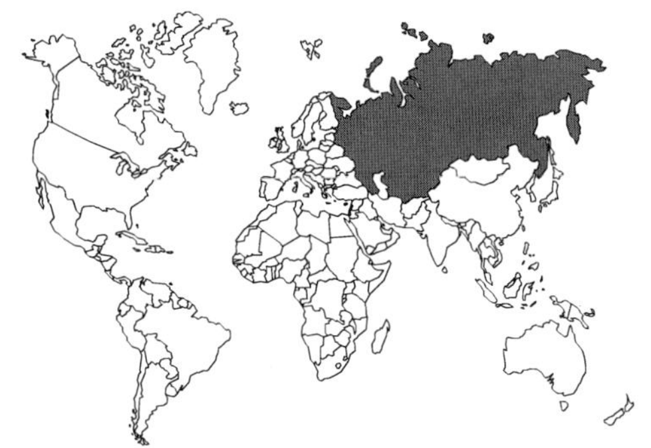

Fig. 2.52.

This parasite has been reported from the former USSR.

Location in Host

Small intestine.

Parasite Identification

This small worm differs from the other species of *Cryptocotyle* in that the body is five sided and has vitellaria extending anteriorly to the level of the intestinal bifurcation.

The eggs tend to be lopsided (i.e., the ovals are longer on one side than the other). The dimensions are 38 μm long by 15 μm in width.

Life Cycle

The typical final hosts are probably gulls and terns; however, the only specimens recovered have been from the cat.

Clinical Presentation and Pathogenesis

Thought to be asymptomatic.

Treatment

Probably praziquantel, but not reported.

Epizootiology

Cats probably become infected by eating raw fish.

Hazards to Other Animals

None known.

Hazards to Humans

Humans could possibly be infected if they ingested the presumed fish intermediate host.

Control/Prevention

Probably the prevention of the ingestion of raw fish.

REFERENCES

Skrjabin KI. 1923. Studies on the parasitic worms of carnivores II–IV. Trudy Gos Inst Exsp Vet 1:67–71.

Cryptocotyle concavum (Creplin, 1825) Lühe, 1899

This species of *Cryptocotyle* was named *concavum* for its concave body shape. *Cryptocotyle echinata* (Linstow, 1878) is a synonym for this first species of *Cryptocotyle* to be described. Specimens have been collected from birds in Europe, North Africa, and North America. The flukes are found in the small intestine and are about 1 mm long with an oval body containing vitellaria that extend anteriorly to a midpoint between the ventral sucker and the bifurcation of the intestine. The eggs are 34 to 38 μm long by 16 to 20 μm in width. It has been shown that cats can be infected if they are fed infected fish.

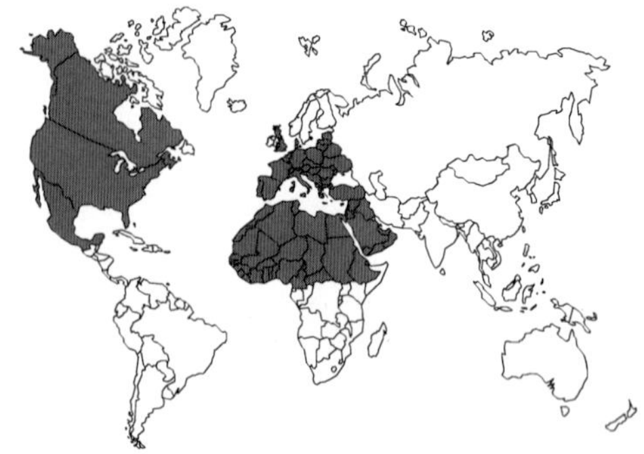

Fig. 2.53.

REFERENCES

Issaitschikoff IM, Weinberg M. 1926. Sur le dévelopment du trematode *Cryptocotyle concavum* (Crepl.). Comptes Rendu Soc Biol 94:305–308.

Euryhelminthinae

This subfamily of the Heterophyidae is composed of wide-bodied trematodes that are typically found in mustelid hosts. These trematodes appear to use amphibians as the host that contains the metacercarial stage.

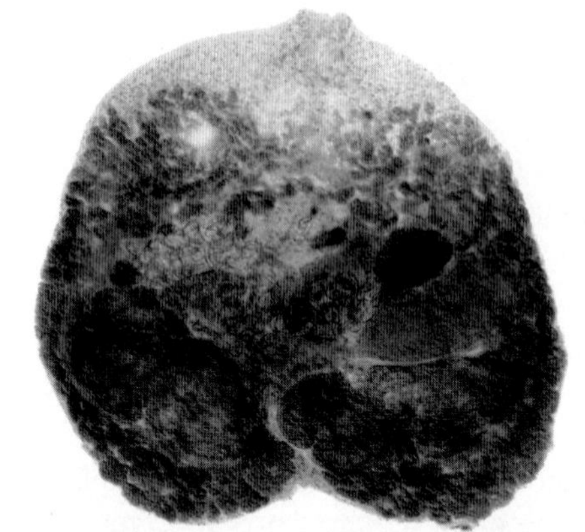

Fig. 2.54. *Euryhelmis squamula* from a raccoon in Georgia, USA. Note the wide body of this genus of organisms.

Euryhelmis squamula (Rudolphi, 1819) Poche, 1926

Etymology

Eury = wide and *helmis* = worm; *squamula* refers to the scale-like shape of the body.

Synonyms

Eurysoma of Dujardin, 1845; the name was already used for other organisms.

History

This fluke is known from mustelids and foxes in Europe and from mustelids and raccoons in North America. The metacercariae were first found encysted under the skin of a frog (Zeller, 1867).

Geographic Distribution

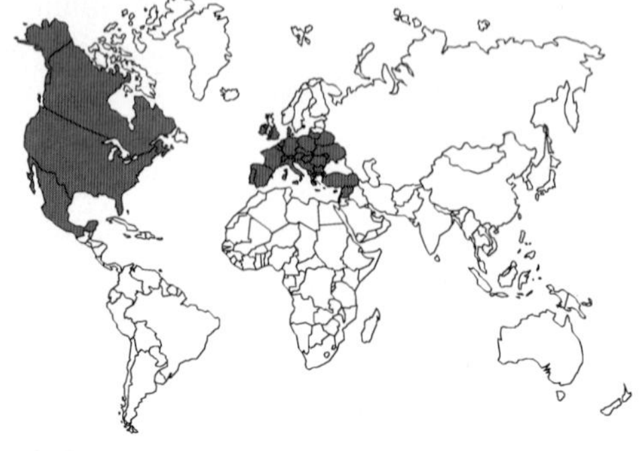

Fig. 2.55.

This trematode appears to have a holarctic distribution having been found in Europe and North America.

Location in Host

Small intestine.

Parasite Identification

The genus *Euryhelmis* is characterized by being a very wide trematode. This trematode differs from *Euryhelmis monorchis* in that it possesses two testes. The trematodes are about 1 mm long by 1 mm in width.

Life Cycle

The life cycle was elucidated by Anderson and Pratt (1965). The snail used by the parasite in Oregon was *Bythinella hemphilli.* The cercariae produced were found to have a tail that was one-third longer than the body with a dorsal fin fold. The cercariae penetrated and encysted under the skin of frogs (*Ascaphus truei* and *Rana aurora*). Metacercariae have also been recovered from the newt (*Triturus cristatus*) and toads. Cats have been experimentally infected by being fed metacercariae (McIntosh, 1936).

Clinical Presentation and Pathogenesis

Thought to be asymptomatic.

Treatment

Probably praziquantel, but not reported.

Epizootiology

Cats would become infected by eating raw frogs, toads, or newts.

Hazards to Other Animals

None known; however, due to the requirements for two intermediate hosts, it is unlikely that an infected cat would pose a direct threat to other animals.

Hazards to Humans

Humans might be infected if they were to eat uncooked or improperly cooked frog legs.

Control/Prevention

The prevention of the ingestion of amphibia.

REFERENCES

Anderson GA, Pratt I. 1965. Cercaria and first intermediate host of *Euryhelmis squamula.* J Parasitol 51:13–15.

McIntosh A. 1936. The occurrence of *Euryhelmis squamula* (Rud., 1819) in the United States. J Parasitol 22:536.

Zeller E. 1867. Ueber das enkystierte Vorkommen von *Distomum squamula* Rud. in braunen Grasfrosh. Z Wissensch Zool 17:215–220.

Euryhelmis monorchis Ameel, 1938

This trematode parasite (*Eury* = wide and *helmis* = worm along with *monorchis* = single testis) is a parasite of mink in North America (Fig. 2.56). The worm tends to be wider (0.6 mm) than long (0.4 mm). It resembles the parasite, *Euryhelmis squamula* of the European polecat, *Putorius putorius.* The life cycle involves a freshwater snail, *Pomatiopsis lapidaria,* along with frogs, *Rana clamatans, Rana pipiens,* and *Rana palustris* as the second host (Ameel, 1938). A cat was experimentally infected with this parasite by feeding it metacercariae, and cats could perhaps become naturally infected. The eggs are operculate, are undeveloped when laid, and measure 29 μm by 14 μm.

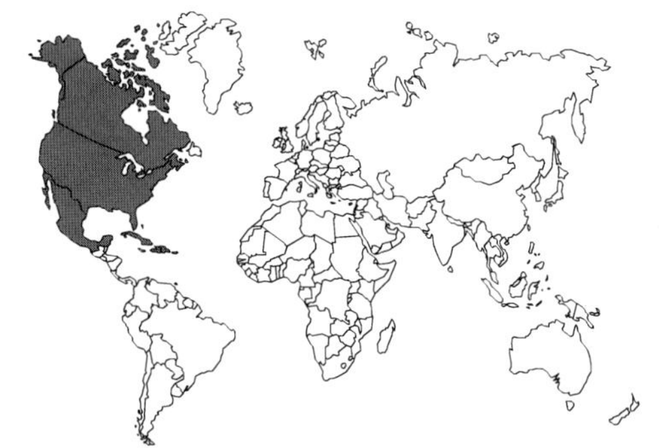

Fig. 2.56.

REFERENCES

Ameel DJ. 1938. The morphology and life cycle of *Euryhelmis monorchis* n. sp. (Trematoda) from the mink. J Parasitol 24:219–224.

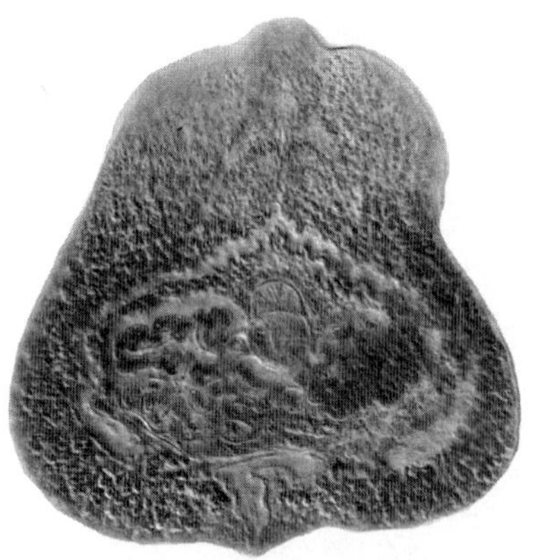

Fig. 2.57. *Euryhelmis monorchis* from an experimentally infected white rat. The large single dark testis can be observed on the right side of this specimen.

Euryhelmis pacifica Senger and Macy, 1952

This trematode parasite was found in mink and muskrats in Oregon (Senger and Macy, 1952). The specimens were described as a new species due to their being pyriform rather than flat in shape. The difference is such that the species can easily be distinguished in mixed infections (Schell, 1964). The metacercariae are found in the Pacific giant salamander, *Dicamptodon ensatus,* and in the tailed frog, *Ascaphus truei.* When metacercariae from the frogs were fed to cats, the cats were found to harbor adult specimens of this fluke 30 days after infection.

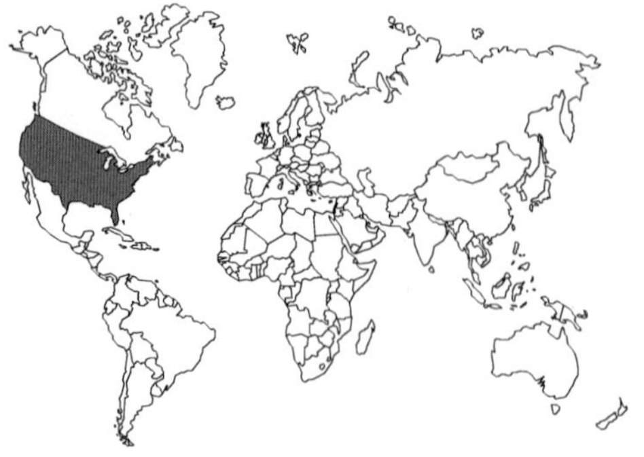

Fig. 2.58.

REFERENCES

Schell SC. 1964. *Bunoderella metteri* gen and sp. n. (Trematoda: Allocreadiidae) and other trematode parasites of *Ascaphus truei* Stejneger. J Parasitol 50:652–655.

Senger CM, Macy RW. 1952. Helminths of northwest mammals. Part III. The description of *Euryhelmis pacificus* n. sp., and notes on its life cycle. J Parasitol 38:481–486.

Galactosominae

This subfamily of the Heterophyidae is characterized by its possession of an elongate body with a well-developed oral sucker. The testes are tandem in the posterior of the body posterior to the ovary.

Galactosomum fregatae Prudhoe, 1949

This trematode parasite (*Galacto* = milk and *somum* = body) (Fig. 2.60) was originally collected from a magnificent frigate bird (*Fregata magnificens*) in the West Indies. This parasite was also described from 3 of 110 stray cats examined in Madras, India (Rajavelu and Raja, 1988). Other species of this genus are found in gulls. Related species develop in marine snails, and the monostomate, very long-tailed cercariae enter and encyst in the brain of mullet, *Mugil auratus.* Birds, and probably the cat, become infected by the ingestion of infected brackish-water fish.

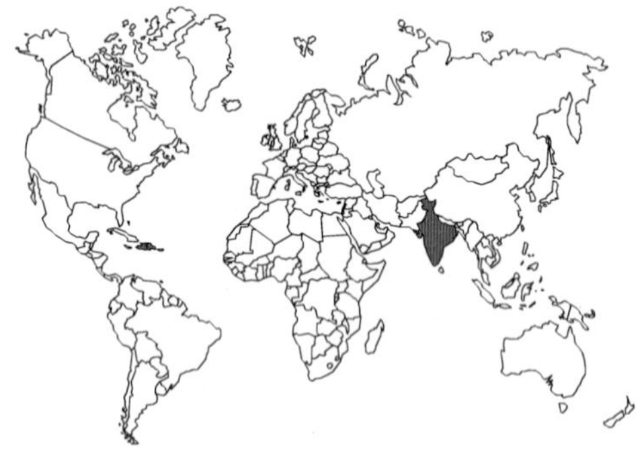

Fig. 2.59.

REFERENCES

Rajavelu G, Raja EE. 1988. On helminth parasites in domestic cat in Madras. Cheiron 17:11–14.

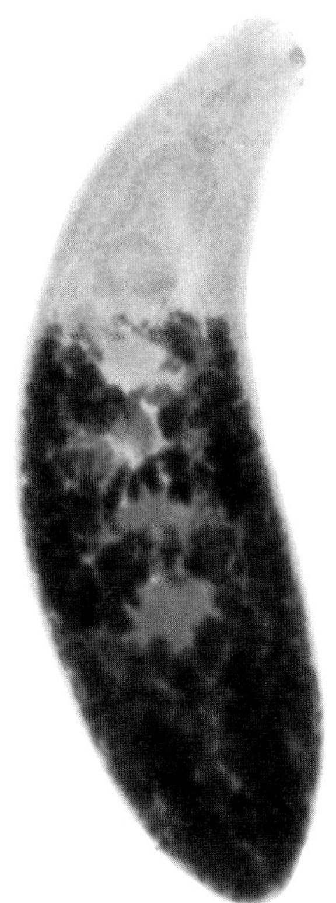

Fig. 2.60. *Galactosomum fregatae* from the intestine of a pelican in Panama.

Haplorchiinae

This subfamily of heterophyids is characterized by the possession of a single testis, although one of the genera in this family, *Stellantchasmus,* actually has two testes. There are three genera within this subfamily, *Haplorchis, Procerovum,* and *Stellantchasmus. Procerovum* specimens differ from those of *Haplorchis* in that they possess a highly muscular ejaculatory duct called an expulsor. *Stellantchasmus* specimens differ from those of *Haplorchis* and *Procerovum* in that they possess two testes while possessing an expulsor as in *Procerovum.*

Haplorchis pumilio (Looss, 1896) Looss, 1899

Etymology

Haplorchis = single testis and *pumilio* = a dwarf.

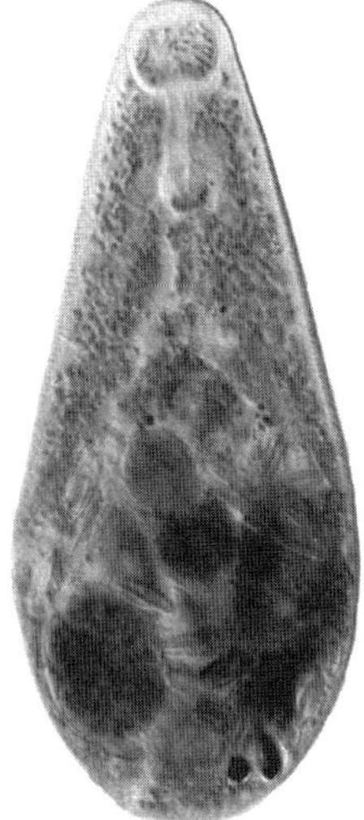

Fig. 2.61. *Haplorchis pumilio* from the small intestine of a domestic cat in Cairo, Egypt. Note the large single testis in the posterior of the body.

Synonyms

Monostomum pumilio Looss, 1896; *Monorchotrema taihokui* Nishigori, 1924; *Haplorchis taihokui* Yamaguti, 1958; *H. milvi* Gohar, 1934; and *Kasr aini* Khalil, 1932.

History

This fluke was originally described from a pelican, *Pelecanus onocrotalus,* and a kite, *Milvus migrans,* in Cairo, Egypt. *Haplorchis pumilio* has been described from numerous hosts as a new species; it has also been confused with other species (i.e., *Haplorchis taichui*) and with parasites in other genera (i.e., *Stellantochasmus falcatus*) (Pearson, 1964).

Geographic Distribution

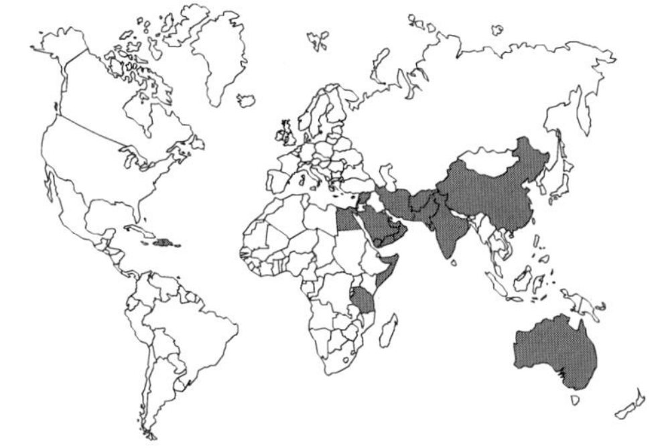

Fig. 2.62.

This trematode has a wide distribution. It has been reported from Egypt, Israel, Tunisia, China, Taiwan, India, and Australia.

Location in Host

Small intestine.

Parasite Identification

The genus *Haplorchis* (as is the related *Procerovum*) is characterized by possession of a single testis. The ventral sucker is posterior to the bifurcation of the intestine and contains the typical sucker/genital complex. *Haplorchis* can be differentiated from *Procerovum* by the possession in the latter of a very muscular wall on the seminal vesicle, called an expulsor, that runs along the intestinal cecum on the left side.

The species *Haplorchis pumilio* is a small fluke, 0.25 to 7.2 mm long by 0.1 to 0.19 mm wide. It differs from other species of *Haplorchis* in that the anterior edge of the ventral sucker is not lined with spines but with what has been called bars that number from 32 to 40. The eggs measure 29 to 32 μm by 15.5 to 17.5 μm.

Life Cycle

The life cycle has been elucidated by feeding kittens freshwater fish, *Gambusia,* infected with cercariae that had developed in the snail *Pirenella conica* (Kuntz and Chandler, 1956).

Clinical Presentation and Pathogenesis

Not reported, so thought to be asymptomatic.

Treatment

Probably praziquantel, but not reported.

Epizootiology

Cats probably become infected by eating raw fish. Other animals that have been found naturally infected include, among others, pelicans, kites, dogs, foxes (*Vulpes vulpes*), shrews (*Crocidura olivieri*), gulls, and human beings.

Hazards to Other Animals

None known; however, due to the requirements for two intermediate hosts, it is unlikely that an infected cat would pose a direct threat to other animals.

Hazards to Humans

Humans have been infected, probably by the ingestion of the infected fish intermediate hosts.

Control/Prevention

The prevention of the ingestion of raw fish.

REFERENCES

Kuntz RE, Chandler AC. 1956. Studies on Egyptian trematodes with special reference to the Heterophyids of mammals. I. Adult flukes, with descriptions of *Phagicola longicollis* n. sp., *Cynodiplostomum namrui* n. sp., and a *Stephanoprora* from cats. J Parasitol 42:445–459.

Pearson JC. 1964. A revision of the subfamily Haplorchiinae Looss, 1899 (Trematoda: Heterophyidae). Parasitology 54:601–676.

Haplorchis yokogawai (Katsuta, 1932) Chen, 1936

Etymology

Haplorchis = single testis and *yokogawai* = for Dr. Yokogawa.

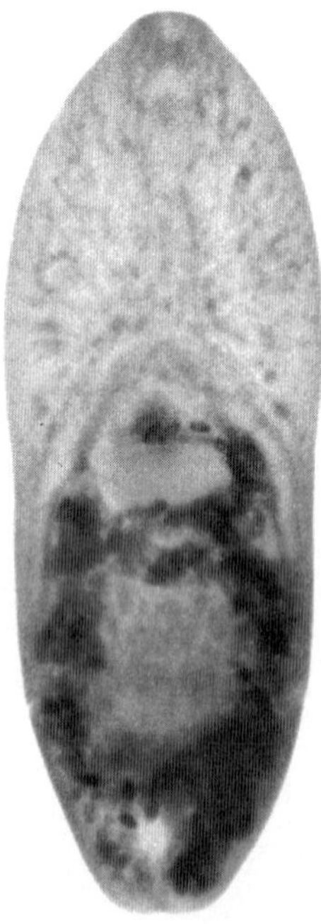

Fig. 2.63. *Haplorchis yokogawai* recovered from the intestine of a cat in Cairo, Egypt.

Synonyms

Monorchotrema yokogawai Katsuta, 1932; *Monorchotrema taihokui* Nishigori, 1924; *Monorchotrema taihokui* Africa and Garcia, 1935; *Haplorchis vagabundi* Baugh, 1963.

History

This fluke was originally described from specimens collected from dogs, cats, and human beings that were experimentally infected (Katsuta, 1931).

Geographic Distribution

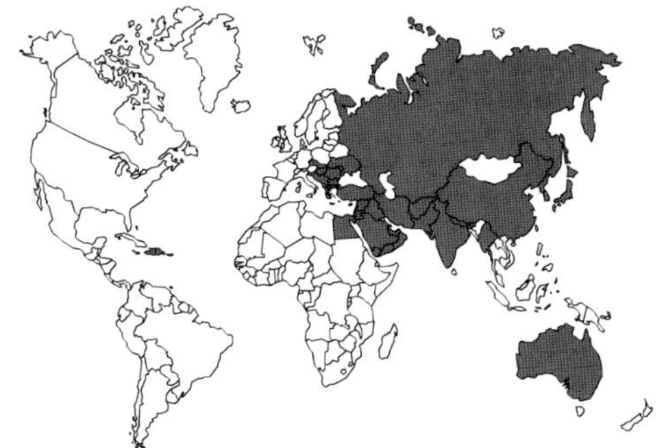

Fig. 2.64.

This trematode has a wide distribution throughout Asia and the Mediterranean. It has been reported from cats in Taiwan, China, Java, Egypt, and Hawaii, from avian hosts in India, and from the cat, a water rat (*Hydromys chorogaster*), and a whistling eagle (*Haliastur sphenurus*) in Australia (Pearson, 1964).

Location in Host

Small intestine, within the first half.

Parasite Identification

Haplorchis yokogawai differs from the other species of *Haplorchis* found in the cat in that the ventral sucker is covered with a small number of very small spines rather than with hooks as in *Haplorchis pumilio* or a few large spines as in *Haplorchis taihokui.*

The species *Haplorchis yokogawai* is a small fluke that is rather wide, 0.23 to 0.34 mm long by 0.2 to 0.28 mm wide. The eggs measure 29 to 30 μm by 13 to 17 μm.

Life Cycle

The life cycle has been elucidated by the feeding of infected brackish-water mullet to human beings (Katsuta, 1931). The metacercariae are encysted in the scales, gills, and fins of mullet, but not in the muscles. The snail host in Hawaii is *Stenomelania newcombi,* where two generations of rediae develop in the digestive gland of the snail (Martin, 1958). The cercariae have a very long flagellum and lateral fins near the body. When experimentally infected fish were fed to cats, the adult worms were found to contain eggs within 10 days after infection (Martin, 1958).

Clinical Presentation and Pathogenesis

Not reported. The fact that the eggs are carried to ectopic locations in humans (see "Hazards to Humans") would suggest that similar events could occur in other hosts including the cat.

Treatment

Probably praziquantel, but not reported.

Epizootiology

Cats become infected by eating raw fish. Other hosts that ingest infected raw fish are also likely to become infected. The normal natural hosts are probably piscivorous birds.

Hazards to Other Animals

None known; however, due to the requirements for two intermediate hosts, it is unlikely that an infected cat would pose a direct threat to other animals.

Hazards to Humans

Humans have been infected by the ingestion of the infected fish intermediate hosts. Eggs of *Haplorchis yokogawai* have been found in cardiac lesions of persons with cardiac failure and in the epicardiac layer of the heart (Africa et al., 1937).

Control/Prevention

The prevention of the ingestion of raw fish.

REFERENCES

Africa JE, de Leon W, Garcia EY. 1937. Heterophyidiasis. VI. Two more cases of heart failure associated with the presence of eggs in sclerosed veins. J Philipp Isl Med Assoc 17:605–609.

Katsuta I. 1931. Studies on trematodes whose second intermediate hosts are fishes from the brackish waters of Formosa. III. On a new trematode *Monorchotrema yokogawai* of which the mullet is the second intermediate host. J Med Assoc Formosa 31:25–26.

Martin WE. 1958. The life histories of some Hawaiian Heterophyid trematodes. J Parasitol 44:305–323.

Pearson JC. 1964. A revision of the subfamily Haplorchiinae Looss, 1899 (Trematoda. Heterophyidae). Parasitology 54:601–676.

Haplorchis taichui (Nishigori, 1924) Witenberg, 1930

Etymology

Haplorchis = single testis and *taichui* = for Dr. Taichu.

Synonyms

Monorchotrema yokogawai Katsuta, 1932; *Monorchotrema taihokui* Nishigori, 1924; *Monorchotrema taihokui* Africa and Garcia, 1935; *Haplorchis rayi* Saxena, 1955.

History

This fluke was originally described from specimens collected from a night heron, *Nycticorax nycticorax* in Taiwan. Experimental infections have been produced in human beings, dogs, cats, and mice (Faust and Nishigori, 1926).

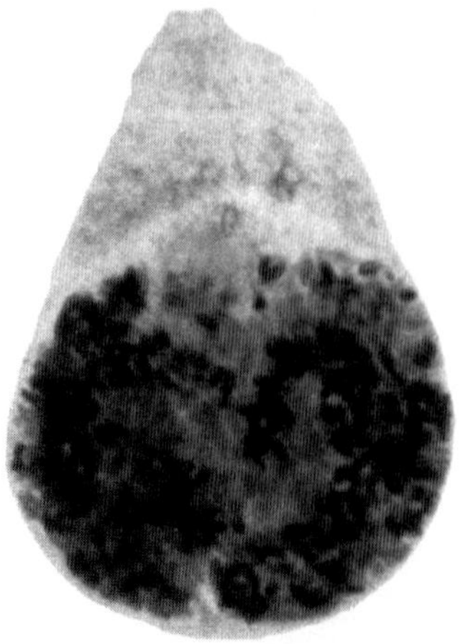

Fig. 2.65. *Haplorchis taichui* from a kite, *Milvus migrans,* in Egypt.

Geographic Distribution

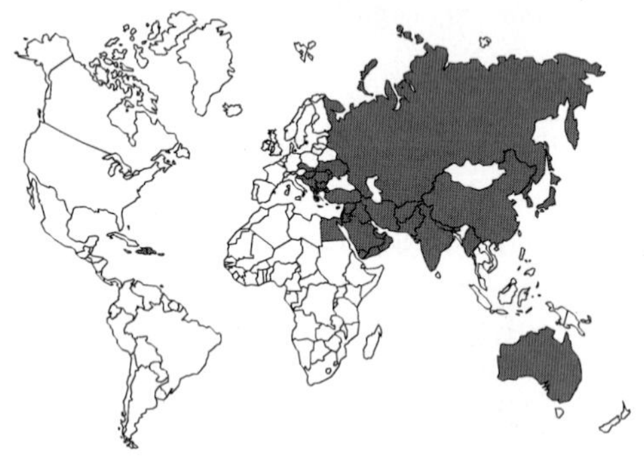

Fig. 2.66.

This trematode has a wide distribution throughout Asia and the Mediterranean that is very similar to that of *Haplorchis yokogawai* although it has not been observed in Australia (Pearson, 1964).

Location in Host

Small intestine.

Parasite Identification

Haplorchis taichui differs from the other species of *Haplorchis* found in the cat in that the ventral sucker is covered with a small number (12 to 16) of large spines (25 to 30 μm long) rather than with hooks as in *Haplorchis pumilio* or many small spines as in *Haplorchis yokogawai.*

The species *Haplorchis taichui* is a small fluke that is rather wide, 0.45 to 0.89 mm long by 0.21 to 0.32 mm wide. The eggs measure 24 to 28 μm by 12 to 15 μm.

Life Cycle

The life cycle was elucidated by the feeding of infected brackish-water mullet to human beings, dogs, and cats (Faust and Nishigori, 1926). The snail host in Taiwan is *Melania reiniana.* The fish hosts in Taiwan are members of the Cyprinidae, Siluridae, and Colitidae. In Palestine, Witenberg (1929) found the infected fish to be of the genera *Barbus, Tilapia,* and *Mugil.*

Clinical Presentation and Pathogenesis

Not reported, but thought to be asymptomatic.

Treatment

Probably praziquantel, but not reported.

Epizootiology

Cats become infected by eating raw fish. Other hosts that ingest infected raw fish are also likely to become infected. The normal natural hosts are probably piscivorous birds.

Hazards to Other Animals

None known; however, due to the requirements for two intermediate hosts, it is unlikely that an infected cat would pose a direct threat to other animals.

Hazards to Humans

Humans have been infected (Kliks and Tantachamrun, 1974) in Thailand by the ingestion of the infected fish intermediate hosts.

Control/Prevention

The prevention of the ingestion of raw fish.

REFERENCES

Faust EC, Nishigori M. 1926. The life cycles of two new species of Heterophyidae parasitic in mammals and birds. J Parasitol 13:91–128.

Kliks M, Tantachamrun T. 1974. Heterophyid (Trematoda) parasites of cats in North Thailand, with notes on a human case found at necropsy. Southeast Asian J Trop Med Publ Health 5:547–555.

Witenberg, G. 1929. Studies on the trematode family Heterophyidae. Ann Trop Med Parasitol 23:131–239.

Haplorchis sprenti Pearson, 1964

Etymology

Haplorchis = single testis and *sprenti* = for Dr. Sprent.

Synonyms

None.

History

This fluke was originally described from specimens collected from a water rat (*Hydromys chryogaster*), a domestic cat, a little black cormorant (*Phalacrocorax ater*), a little pied cormorant (*Phalacrocorax melanoleucus*), a pied cormorant (*Phalacrocorax sulcirostris*), a pelican (*Pelecanus conspicillatus*), herons, and egrets.

Geographic Distribution

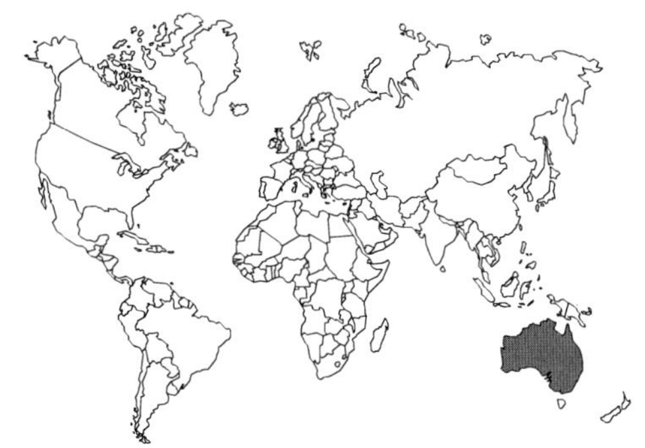

Fig. 2.67.

This trematode is found in Australia.

Location in Host

Small intestine.

Parasite Identification

Haplorchis sprenti is very similar to *Haplorchis yokogawai.* It differs mainly in the shape of the body, being pyriform with the length being 0.25 to 0.42 mm, and the width being 0.08 to 0.12 mm anteriorly and 0.09 to 0.17 mm posteriorly. The eggs measure 27 to 32 μm by 13 to 15.5 μm and contain a fully developed miracidium when laid.

Life Cycle

The life cycle was elucidated by the feeding of infected brackish-water fish to cats, rats, and chickens (Pearson, 1964).

Clinical Presentation and Pathogenesis

Not reported but thought to be asymptomatic.

Treatment

Probably praziquantel, but not reported.

Epizootiology

Cats become infected by eating raw fish. Other hosts that ingest infected raw fish are also likely to become infected. The normal natural hosts are probably piscivorous birds.

Hazards to Other Animals

None known; however, due to the requirements for two intermediate hosts, it is unlikely that an infected cat would pose a direct threat to other animals.

Hazards to Humans

Humans could be infected by the ingestion of the infected fish intermediate hosts.

Control/Prevention

The prevention of the ingestion of raw fish.

REFERENCES

Pearson JC. 1964. A revision of the subfamily Haplorchiinae Looss, 1899 (Trematoda: Heterophyidae). Parasitology 54:601–676.

Haplorchis parataichui Pearson, 1964

This trematode is very similar to *Haplorchis taichui.* It was obtained in Australia by feeding a fish (*Pseudomugil signifer*) collected from freshwater creeks in Brisbane to a cat (Pearson, 1964). The eggs are 24 to 28 μm long and 12 to 13 μm wide.

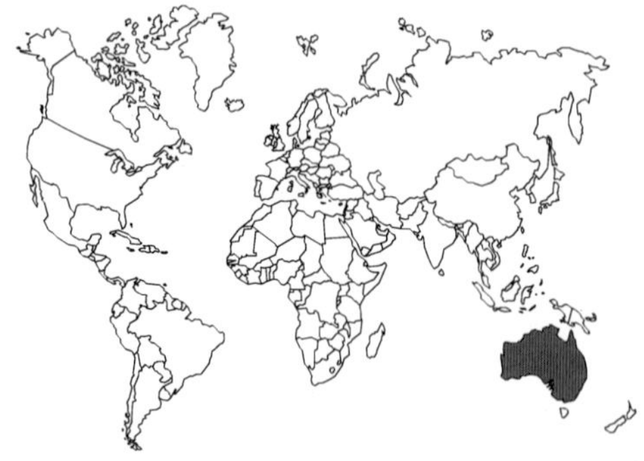

Fig. 2.68.

REFERENCES

Pearson JC. 1964. A revision of the subfamily Haplorchiinae Looss, 1899 (Trematoda: Heterophyidae). Parasitology 54:601–676.

Procerovum varium Onji and Nishio, 1916

Etymology

Procer = stretched out and *ovum* = uterus along with *varium* = varied.

Synonyms

Haplorchis sisoni Africa, 1938; *Haplorchis minutus* Kobayashi, 1942; *Haplorchis macrovesica* Kobayashi, 1942; *Haplorchis hoihowensis* Kobayashi, 1942; *Haplorchis cordatus* Kobayashi, 1942.

History

This species was originally recovered from a cat that was experimentally infected with metacercariae from infected fish (Onji and Nishio, 1924).

Geographic Distribution

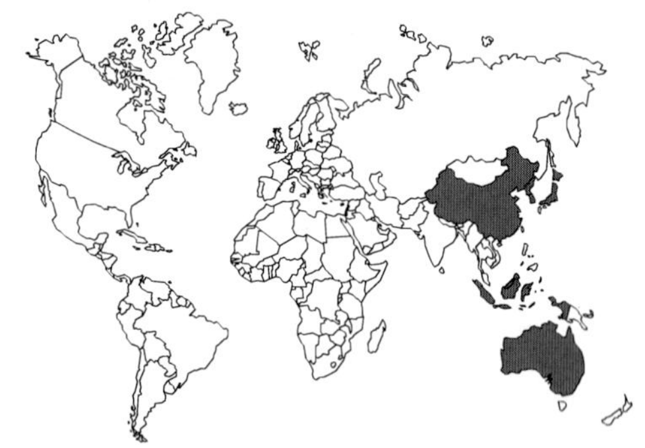

Fig. 2.69.

This trematode has been reported from Japan, China, the Philippines, Australia, and Malaysia (Pearson, 1964).

Location in Host

Small intestine.

Parasite Identification

Procerovum specimens differ from those of *Haplorchis* in that they possess a highly muscular ejaculatory duct called an expulsor. The species *Procerovum varium* can be differentiated from *Procerovum calderoni* by the presence of a much longer expulsor in the latter and by having small spines on the gonotyle.

This small pyriform trematode is 0.26 to 0.38 mm long and 0.13 to 0.16 mm wide. The eggs are 25 to 29 μm long by 12 to 14 μm wide.

Life Cycle

The life cycle was elucidated by the feeding of infected brackish-water mullet (*Mugil* species) to dogs and cats.

Clinical Presentation and Pathogenesis

Not reported but thought to be asymptomatic.

Treatment

Probably praziquantel, but not reported.

Epizootiology

Cats become infected by eating raw fish. Other hosts that ingest infected raw fish are also likely to become infected. The normal natural hosts include cats, pelicans (*Pelecanus conspicillatus*), egrets (*Egretta alba* and *Egretta intermedia*), the water rat (*Hydromys chyrsogaster*), herons (*Notophoyx novaehollandiae* and *Nycticorax caledonicus*), and a whistling eagle (*Haliastur sphenurus*).

Hazards to Other Animals

None known; however, due to the requirements for two intermediate hosts, it is unlikely that an infected cat would pose a direct threat to other animals.

Hazards to Humans

Humans probably could be infected by the ingestion of the infected fish intermediate hosts.

Control/Prevention

The prevention of the ingestion of raw fish.

REFERENCES

Onji Y, Nishio T. 1924. On the intestinal distomes. Chiba Igakki Zasshi 2:352–399.

Pearson JC. 1964. A revision of the subfamily Haplorchiinae Looss, 1899 (Trematoda: Heterophyidae). Parasitology 54:601–676.

Procerovum calderoni (Africa and Garcia, 1935) Price, 1940

This trematode is very similar to *Procerovum varium* but differs by having a larger expulsor and having only a few large spines on the gonotyle. It was originally described as *Monorchotrema calderoni* from a dog in the Philippines (Africa and Garcia, 1935). It was later redescribed as *Haplorchis calderoni* (Africa, 1938) from specimens collected from dogs, cats, and a human being. The metacercariae have been found in fish, including the brackish-water genera *Hebsetia, Hemirhamphus, Mugil,* and others. In 1940, Price transferred the species to the genus *Procerovum* (Price, 1940).

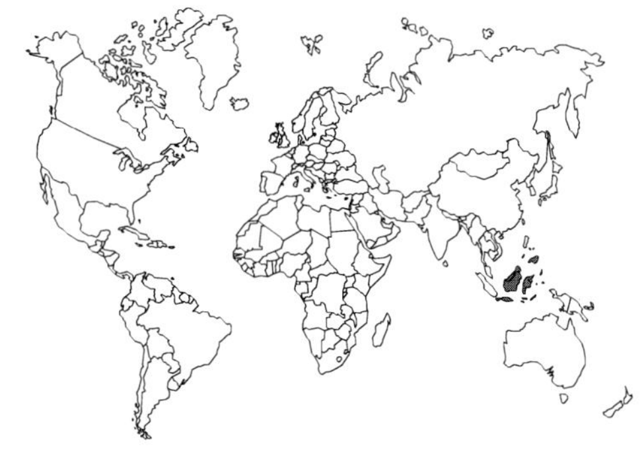

Fig. 2.70.

REFERENCES

Africa CM. 1938. Description of three trematodes of the genus *Haplorchis* (Heterophyidae), with notes on two other Philippine members of this genus. Philipp J Sci 66:299–307.

Africa CM, Garcia EY. 1935. Two more new heterophyid trematodes from the Philippines. Philipp J Sci 57:443–450.

Price EW. 1940. A review of the heterophyid trematodes, with special reference to those parasitic in man. Int Cong Microbiol Rep Proc 446–447.

Stellantchasmus falcatus Onji and Nishio, 1916

Etymology

Stella = star, *ant* = against, and *chasmus* = hollow along with *falcatus* = hooked.

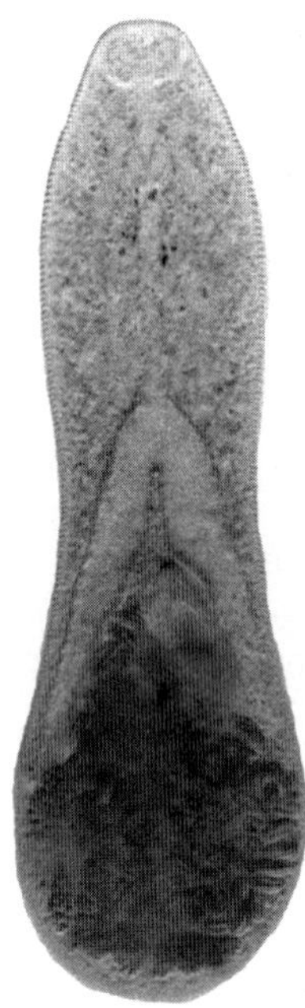

Fig. 2.71. *Stellantchasmus falcatus* from the small intestine of a domestic cat in Hawaii.

Synonyms

Diorchitrema pseudocirrata Witenberg, 1929; *Stellantchasmus formosanus* Katsuta, 1931; *Stellantchasmus amplicaecalis* Katsuta, 1932; and *Haplorchis pumilio* of Odening, 1962.

History

This species was originally described from cats that were experimentally infected by the feeding of fish containing metacercariae (Onji and Nishio, 1916). This trematode has since been recovered from naturally infected cats and other hosts.

Geographic Distribution

This trematode has been reported from Japan, Hawaii, China, the Philippines, Israel, Egypt, and Australia (Pearson, 1964).

Location in Host

Small intestine, mainly 6 to 18 inches from the junction with the stomach.

Parasite Identification

Stellantchasmus specimens differ from those of *Haplorchis* and *Procerovum* in that they possess two testes and possess an expulsor as in *Procerovum.*

This small pyriform trematode is 0.43 to 0.55 mm long and 0.19 to 0.34 mm wide (Fig. 2.71). The eggs are 21 to 23 µm long by 12 to 13 µm wide.

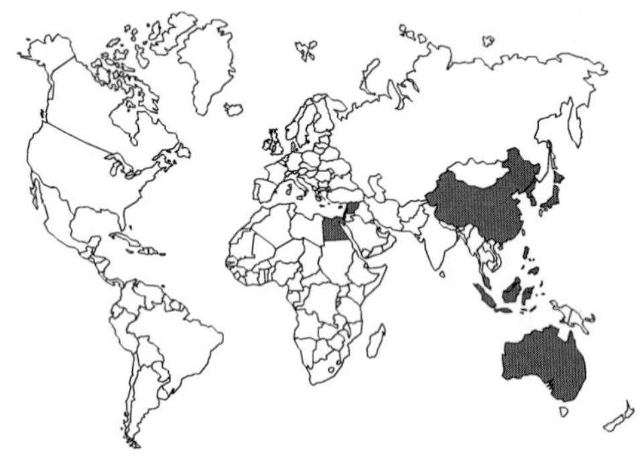

Fig. 2.72.

Life Cycle

The life cycle was elucidated by Martin (1958), Noda (1959), and Pearson (1960). The snail hosts include species of *Stenomelania, Melanoides,* and *Tarebia.* Fish that have been found to be infected include brackish and freshwater fish, *Mugil* and *Anabas* species; the larvae are found mainly within the skeletal muscle (Martin, 1958). The fully developed cysts are about 0.3 mm in diameter.

Clinical Presentation and Pathogenesis

Not reported but thought to be asymptomatic.

Treatment

Probably praziquantel, but not reported.

Epizootiology

Cats become infected by eating raw fish. Other hosts that ingest infected raw fish are also likely to become infected. The normal natural hosts include cats, nankeen night herons (*Nycticorax caledonicus*), and whistling eagles (*Haliastur sphenurus*).

Hazards to Other Animals

None known; however, due to the requirements for two intermediate hosts, it is unlikely that an infected cat would pose a direct threat to other animals.

Hazards to Humans

Humans have been infected with this species in Hawaii.

Control/Prevention

The prevention of the ingestion of raw fish.

REFERENCES

Martin WE. 1958. The life histories of some Hawaiian heterophyid trematodes. J Parasitol 44:305–323.

Noda K. 1959. The larval development of *Stellantchasmus falcatus* (Trematoda: Heterophyidae) in the first intermediate host. J Parasitol 45:635–642.

Onji Y, Nishio T. 1916. A new intestinal distome. Iji Shimbun 949:589–593.

Pearson JC. 1960. New records of trematodes from the cat. Aust Vet J 36:93.

Pearson JC. 1964. A revision of the subfamily Haplorchiinae Looss, 1899 (Trematoda: Heterophyidae). Parasitology 54:601–676.

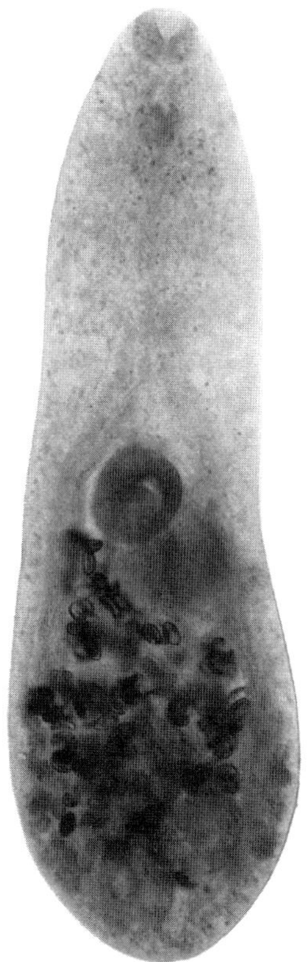

Fig. 2.73. *Heterophyes heterophyes* recovered from the intestine of a cat in Egypt. In this figure, it is difficult to appreciate the genital sucker except as a darkened area to the right and slightly posteriad to the ventral sucker.

Heterophyinae

There are two genera in cats that are within the subfamily Heterophyinae. The two genera are *Heterophyes* and *Heterophyopsis*. *Heterophyes* is characterized by the possession of a large genital sucker that is separated from the ventral sucker. It was the presence of this "third sucker" that caused *Heterophyes* to be one of the first genera of trematodes created from the old group the *Distoma* (two mouths) in the middle of the 1800s. *Heterophyopsis* differs from *Heterophyes* in that its testes lie one behind the other in the body rather than along side each other as they do in the case of *Heterophyes*.

Heterophyes heterophyes (von Siebold, 1852) Stiles and Hassall, 1900

Etymology

Hetero = different and *phyes* = form (named early in the study of trematodes to distinguish it from another fluke *Paragonimus* by Cobbold in 1866).

Synonyms

Heterophyes aegyptiaca Cobbold, 1866; *Mesogonimus heterophyes* Railliet, 1890; *Coenogonimus heterophyes* Looss, 1900; and *Cotylogonimus heterophyes* Lühe, 1900. In the Orient, *Heterophyes nocens* Onji and Nishio, 1915, was described, but it is now considered a subspecies of *Heterophyes heterophyes*.

History

This species was originally collected in 1851 by Bilharz from a human being in Egypt; the fluke was named *Distoma heterophyes* by von Siebold. The first report in cats is that of Looss (1902).

Geographic Distribution

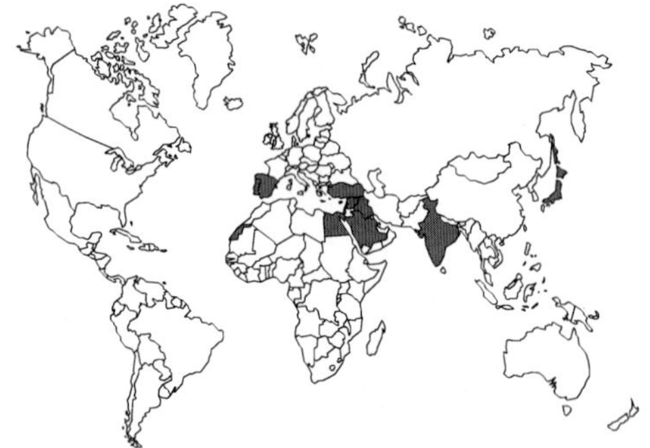

Fig. 2.74.

This trematode has been reported from Egypt, Israel, Kuwait, Greece, Turkey, and Spain (probably throughout the Mediterranean); as the subspecies *Heterophyes heterophyes nocens,* it has been reported from cats in Japan (Miyazaki, 1991). It has also been reported on rare occasions from West Africa and India (Malek, 1980).

Location in Host

Middle and upper portion, jejunum and duodenum of the small intestine (Tarachewski, 1987).

Parasite Identification

Specimens of the genus *Heterophyes* have a large genital sucker. The adult trematodes are found embedded in the villi and measure about 1 mm by 0.5 mm. The spines on the genital sucker of *Heterophyes heterophyes* number 50 to 80 and are digitate, looking like small leafless trees. The eggs are yellow brown, contain a miracidium, and have an average size of 27 μm by 16 μm.

Life Cycle

The life cycle in Egypt involves the snail *Pironella conica* and the brackish-water fish host *Mugil cephalus.* In Asia, the life cycle involves snails, *Certhideopsilla cingulata,* that live in the mouths of rivers and various brackish-water fish hosts, including *Mugil cephalus, Liza haematocheila, Acanthogobius flavimanus, Glossogobius giuris,* and *Tridentiger obscurus.* The metacercariae are found within the muscle of the fish hosts.

Clinical Presentation and Pathogenesis

An examination of the histopathology of the intestine of infected cats revealed that the parasites were closely associated with the villi (Hamdy and Nicola, 1980). At the sites of infection, the villi were swollen, the columnar epithelium was destroyed, and there was swelling of the underlying submucosa. There was a local cellular reaction, and the Peyer's patches were hyperplastic. Immature flukes were found in lymphoid follicles and in Peyer's patches. Mature flukes were also found within mesenteric lymph nodes. However, no clinical signs were described.

Treatment

Probably praziquantel, but not reported.

Epizootiology

Cats become infected by eating raw fish as do other piscivorous animals.

Hazards to Other Animals

None known; however, due to the requirements for two intermediate hosts, it is unlikely that an infected cat would pose a direct threat to other animals.

Hazards to Humans

Numerous humans have been infected with this parasite. In 1933, Khalil found 53 of 60 school children infected in an area close to the Suez Canal; in 1983, it was found in 14 of 65 cats in Egypt (Abo-Shady et al., 1983). Infection rates in Japan have also reached levels as high as 30 percent; however, more recently, infection levels in humans in Japan are less than 1 percent.

Control/Prevention

The prevention of the ingestion of raw fish.

REFERENCES

Abo-Shady AF, Ali MM, Abdel-Magied S. 1983. Helminth parasites of cats in Dakahlia, Egypt. J Egypt Soc Parasitol 13:129–133.

Hamdy EI, Nicola E. 1980. On the histopathology of the small intestine in animals experimentally infected with *H. heterophyes.* J Egypt Med Assoc 63:179–184.

Looss A. 1902. Notizen zur Helminthologie egyptens. V. Eine Revision der Fasciolidengattung *Heterophyes* Cobb. Centralblatt bakt. Orig. I. 32:886–891.
Malek EA. 1980. Snail-Transmitted Parasitic Diseases. Vols I and II. Boca Raton, Fla: CRC Press. 334 and 324 pp.
Miyazaki I. 1991. Helminthic Zoonoses. Fukuoka, Japan: International Medical Foundation of Japan. 494 pp.
Tarachewski H. 1987. Experiments on habitat selection of *Heterophyes* species in different definitive hosts. J Helminthol 61:33–42.

Heterophyes aequalis Looss, 1902

Etymology

Hetero = different and *phyes* = form, along with *aequalis* = equal, referring to the equivalent sizes of the ventral and oral suckers. The name distinguishes it from *Heterophyes dispar,* which was named at the same time and which supposedly had a ventral sucker much larger in diameter than the oral sucker.

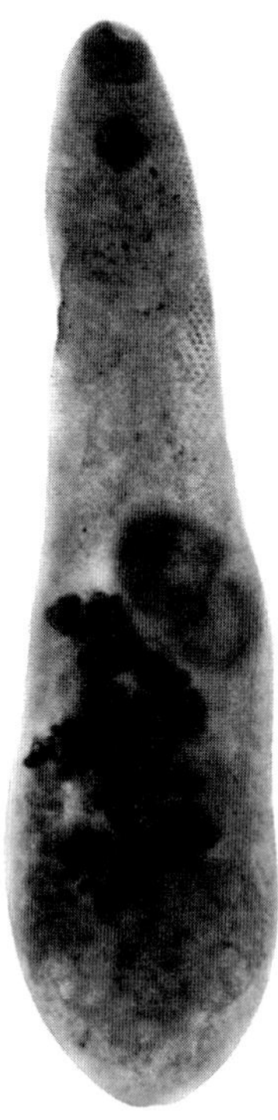

Fig. 2.75. *Heterophyes aequalis* recovered from a cat in Cairo, Egypt. The separate genital sucker on this species is more apparent than in Fig. 2.73.

Synonyms

Heterophyes dispar Looss, 1902 (according to Kuntz and Chandler, 1956).

History

This species was originally described from naturally infected cats in Egypt.

Geographic Distribution

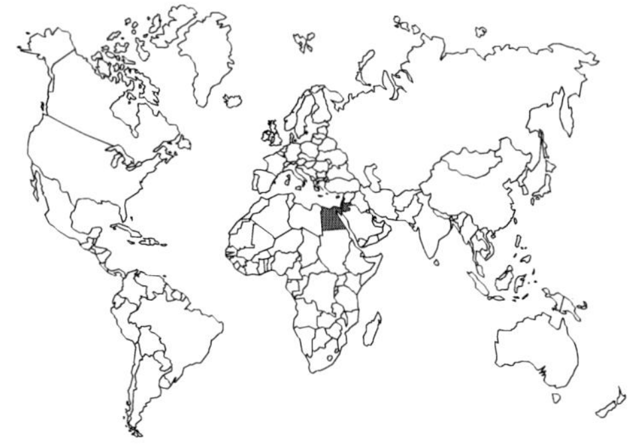

Fig. 2.76.

Egypt and Israel.

Location in Host

Small intestine, mainly the terminal portion of the intestinal tract (Taraschewski, 1987).

Parasite Identification

Specimens of *Heterophyes aequalis* are characterized by having a few, 15 to 35, rodlets surrounding the genital sucker versus the 50 to 80 digitate rodlets present on that of *Heterophyes heterophyes.* The flukes from cats range in length from 0.5 to 1.4 (rarely 1.6) mm with a width of 0.25 to 0.5 mm. The ventral sucker is typically 0.06 to 0.18 mm in diameter. The yellowish brown–shelled eggs are 23-25 μm long by 14-16 μm wide.

Life Cycle

The life cycle involves metacercariae encysted in *Mugil, Epinephelus, Lichia,* and *Barbus* fish. Cats become infected by the ingestion of these marine, brackish-water, or freshwater fish.

Clinical Presentation and Pathogenesis

Not reported but thought to be asymptomatic.

Treatment

Probably praziquantel, but not reported.

Epizootiology

Cats become infected by eating raw fish. Other hosts that ingest infected raw fish are also likely to become infected. The host that has been described for this parasite is the cat with adults sometimes being found in dogs.

Hazards to Other Animals

None known; however, due to the requirements for two intermediate hosts, it is unlikely that an infected cat would pose a direct threat to other animals.

Hazards to Humans

Humans probably could be infected by the ingestion of the infected fish intermediate hosts.

Control/Prevention

The prevention of the ingestion of raw fish.

REFERENCES

Kuntz RE, Chandler AC. 1956. Studies on Egyptian trematodes with special reference to the heterophyids of mammals. I. Adult flukes, with descriptions of *Phagicola longicollis* n. sp., *Cynodiplostomum namrui* n. sp., and a *Stephanoprora* from cats. J Parasitol 42:445–459.

Taraschewski H. 1987. Experiments on habitat selection of *Heterophyes* species in different definitive hosts. J Helminthol 61:33–42.

Heterophyopsis continua (Onji and Nishi, 1916) Tubangui and Africa, 1938

Etymology

Hetero = different and *phyopsis* = late form (referring to the testes being behind each other) along with *continua* = continuous, referring to the expanded nature of the uterus.

Synonyms

Heterophyes continua Onji and Nishi, 1916; *Heterophyes expectans* Africa and Garcia, 1935, *Pseudoheterophyes continua major* in a new genus created by Yamaguti (1939).

History

This species was originally described from a naturally infected tern, *Colymbus arcticus pacificus,* in Japan. It was also collected from a cat that was experimentally infected through eating the infected tissue of a fish, *Mugil cephalus.*

Geographic Distribution

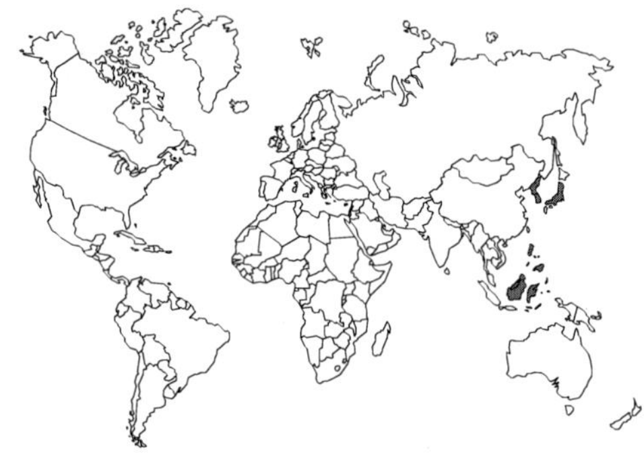

Fig. 2.77.

Cats in Japan and Korea (Eom et al., 1985) and in the Philippines (Tubangui and Africa, 1938).

Location in Host

Small intestine.

Parasite Identification

Specimens of *Heterophyopsis continua* differ from species of *Heterophyes* in that the testes of *Heterophyopsis* species are tandem (i.e., one is in front of the other), rather than being beside each other as in *Heterophyes.* The flukes collected from Korean cats measure 1.8 to 2.3 mm in length and 0.26 to 0.28 mm in width. The eggs are 25 × 15 μm.

Life Cycle

The life cycle involves metacercariae encysted in the brackish-water fish, *Mugil, Lateolabrax, Acanthogobius,* and *Clupanodon.* Cats become infected by the ingestion of these fish in which the metacercariae are encysted within the musculature.

Clinical Presentation and Pathogenesis

Signs in cats have not been reported. Signs have been reported with humans infected with these trematodes, but they were also hosts to other parasitic helminths, which confuses the assignment of signs specifically to this parasite.

Treatment

Probably praziquantel. Praziquantel (15 mg/kg followed by the administration of a purgative 30 g of magnesium sulfate in order to collect the worms) has been used successfully in the treatment of humans infected with this trematode (Seo et al., 1984).

Epizootiology

Cats become infected by eating raw fish. Other hosts that ingest infected raw fish are also likely to become infected, although it would appear that the rat is not a susceptible host.

Hazards to Other Animals

Dogs and other animals have been infected; however, due to the requirements for two intermediate hosts, it is unlikely that an infected cat would pose a direct threat to other animals.

Hazards to Humans

Humans in Japan and along the southern coast of Korea have been infected with this parasite by the ingestion of metacercariae in brackish-water fish (Seo et al., 1984).

Control/Prevention

The prevention of the ingestion of raw fish.

REFERENCES

Eom ES, Son SY, Lee JS, Rim HJ. 1985. Heterophyid trematodes (*Heterophyopsis continua, Pygidiopsis summa,* and *Heterophyes heterophyes nocens*) from domestic cats in Korea. Korean J Parasitol 23:197–202.

Seo BY, Lee SH, Chai JY, Hong SJ. 1984. Studies on intestinal trematodes in Korea. XIII. Two cases of natural human infection by *Heterophyopsis continua* and the status of metacercarial infection in brackish water fishes. Korean J Parasitol 22:51–60.

Tubangui MA, Africa CM. 1938. The systematic position of some trematodes reported from the Philippines. Philipp J Sci 66:117–127.

Yamaguti S. 1939. Studies on the helminth fauna of Japan. Part 27. Trematodes of Mammals. II. Jap J Med Sci, Bact, Parasitol 1:131–151.

Metagoniminae

The Metagoniminae subfamily of the Heterophyidae is characterized by having a fusion of the genital and ventral sucker into an organ called by some the genito-acetabulum. This ventral genital sucker is found displaced from the midline of the body in the genus *Metagonimus,* which aids in the recognition of this genus of heterophyid flukes.

Metagonimus yokogawai (Katsurada, 1912) Katsurada, 1912

Etymology

Meta = posterior and *gonimus* = genitalia along with *yokogawai* for Dr. Yokogawa.

Synonyms

Heterophyes yokogawai Katsurada, 1912; *Loxotrema ovatum* Kobayashi, 1912; *Metagonimus ovatus* Yokogawa, 1913; *Loossia romanica* Ciurea, 1915; *Loossia parva* Ciurea, 1915; *Loossia dobrogiensis* Ciurea, 1915.

History

This fluke was originally described as *Heterophyes yokogawai* by Katsurada, but later, the same author renamed the worm *Metagonimus yokogawai.* The original description was based on material obtained by Dr. Yokogawa from human beings and from experimentally infected cats and dogs in Taiwan.

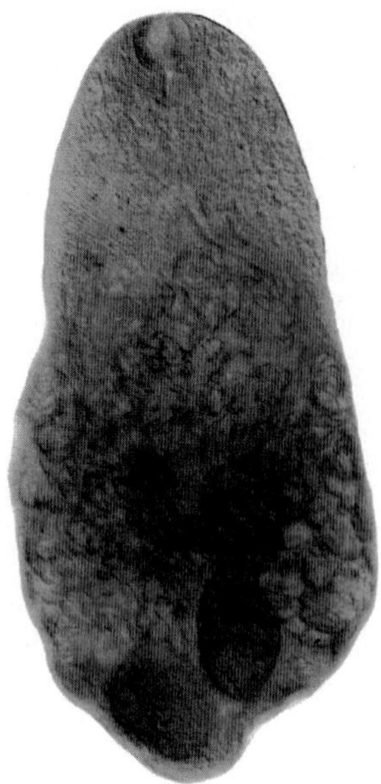

Fig. 2.78. *Metagonimus yokogawai* collected from a dog in Japan in 1919 by Dr. Yokogawa. Note the paired testes in the posterior of the body. The displaced genito-acetabulum is difficult to observe in this figure.

Geographic Distribution

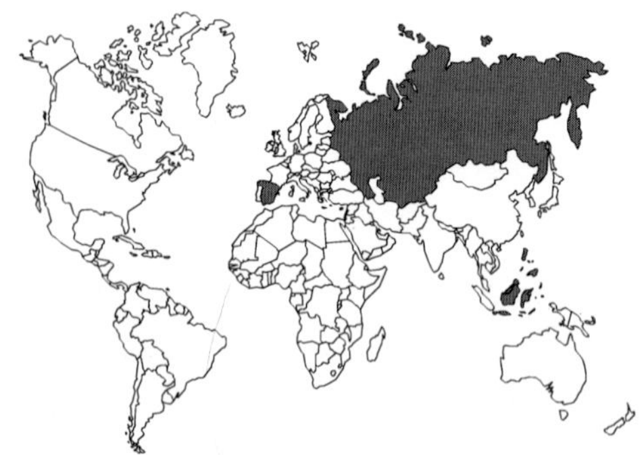

Fig. 2.79.

This is the most common heterophyid trematode in the Far East. It has also been reported from Siberia and the Balkans and from human beings in Spain.

Location in Host

Small intestine.

Parasite Identification

Members of the genus *Metagonimus* can be identified by the position of the ventral sucker and genital opening, which are fused and displaced to the right of the midline of the body. The testes are close together at the posterior of the body where one is slightly anteriad to the other. The ventral sucker is larger than the oral sucker. The adults of *Metagonimus yokogawai* are 1 to 1.5 mm long with eggs that are 26 to 28 μm by 15 to 17 μm.

Life Cycle

The miracidium within the egg, like that of *Heterophyes heterophyes,* does not hatch upon contact with water but, rather, only after it is infected by the appropriate freshwater snail (e.g., *Semisulcospira libertina*). The cercariae that are produced have long tails with thin dorso-ventral tail fins. The cercariae infect fish between the scales, and metacercariae develop predominantly within the muscles. Freshwater fish that have been shown to be intermediate hosts include *Plectoglossus altivelis, Odontobutis obscurus, Salmo perryi,* and *Tribolodon hakonensis.* Animals become infected when they ingest the raw flesh of these fish.

Clinical Presentation and Pathogenesis

Shallow ulcers may be present in the mucosa of the jejunum where parasites live within the villus epithelium. There is a shortening of the villus length and adhesions formed between villi. During the first 5 to 15 days after infection, there is a decrease in the number of goblet cells present in the areas around the trematodes; this number then returns to normal levels (Kim et al., 1983). Heavy infestations are likely to cause small-bowel diarrhea.

Treatment

Praziquantel.

Epizootiology

Cats become infected by eating raw fish. Other hosts that ingest infected raw fish are also likely to become infected.

Hazards to Other Animals

Dogs can be infected through the ingestion of infected raw fish; however, due to the requirements for two intermediate hosts, it is unlikely that an infected cat would pose a direct threat to other animals.

Hazards to Humans

Human beings have been infected with this parasite on numerous occasions and are the host from which the parasite was first recovered. People, like cats, obtain their infections by the ingestion of raw fish.

Control/Prevention

The prevention of the ingestion of raw fish.

REFERENCES

Kim BW, Lee JB, Cho SY. 1983. Attitude of goblet cells in small intestine of experimental cat metagonimiasis. Chung-Ang J Med 8:243–251.

Rho IH, Kim SI, Kang SY, Cho SY. 1984. Observation on the pathogenesis of villous changes in early phase of experimental metagonimiasis. Chung-Ang J Med 9:67–77.

Metagonimus takahashii Suzuki, 1930

This parasite is very similar to *Metagonimus yokogawai.* The egg of *Metagonimus takahashii* in the stool is larger than that of *Metagonimus yokogawai;* that of *Metagonimus takahashii* is 28.5 to 34 µm by 17.5 to 20.5 µm. Also, the cercaria is larger, and the second intermediate hosts are carp rather than the fish used by *Metagonimus yokogawai.* Cats, dogs, and human beings have been naturally infected with this parasite.

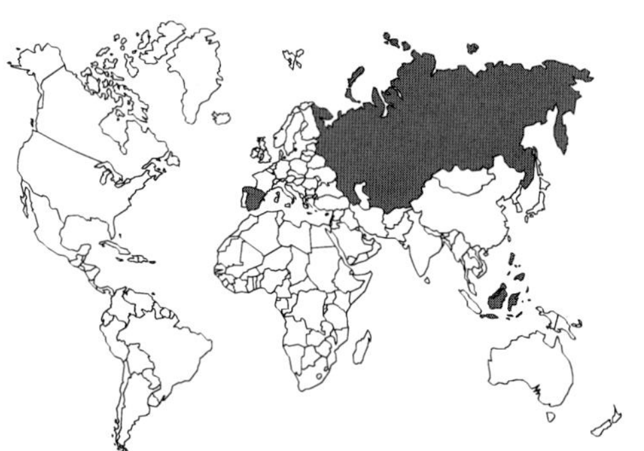

Fig. 2.80.

Dexiogonimus ciureanus Witenberg, 1929

This genus differs from *Metagonimus* in that the testes appear to be symmetrically situated in the posterior of the body rather than diagonally as in *Metagonimus.* This trematode (Fig. 2.82) has been recorded as infecting dogs and cats in Israel and other parts of the Middle East (Witenberg, 1929, 1934). The natural host appears to be gulls.

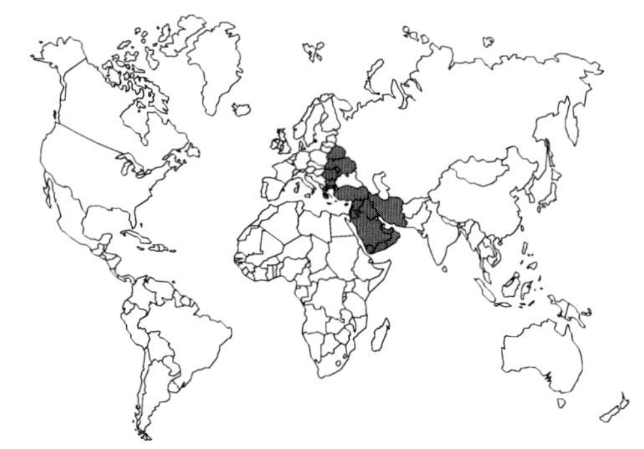

Fig. 2.81.

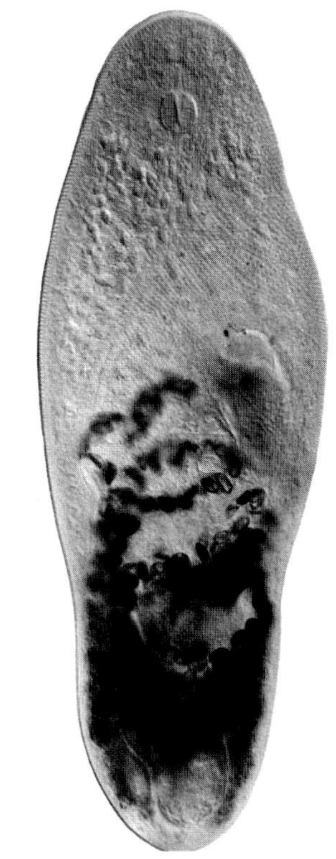

Fig. 2.82. *Dexiogonimus ciureanus* collected from a cat in Turkey. In this specimen, the body has the overall shape of the sole of a foot, which was part of the original description of this parasite.

REFERENCES
Witenberg G. 1929. Studies on the trematode family Heterophyidae. Ann Trop Med Parasitol 23:131–239.
Witenberg G. 1934. Parasitic worms of dogs and cats in Palestine. Vet Rec 14:232–239.

Stictodoriinae

This subfamily of heterophyids is characterized by having a rather elongate body and an anterior sucker that is subterminal. In this group, the testes are not terminally located in the body.

Stictodora sawakinensis Looss, 1899

The genus *Stictodora* (*sticto* = punctate; *dora* = skin) and species *sawakinensis* (from Sawakin) were described by Looss (1899) for specimens collected from gulls. Specimens of *Stictodora sawakinensis* and *Stictodora thaparai* Witenberg, 1953, have been described from cats in Egypt and Israel (Kuntz and Chandler, 1956; Witenberg, 1953). Specimens of *Stictodora* differ from those of *Metagonimus* in that the ventral sucker is reduced and combined with the genital opening and is not readily apparent. The testes are also further anteriad in the body of this trematode (Fig. 2.84).

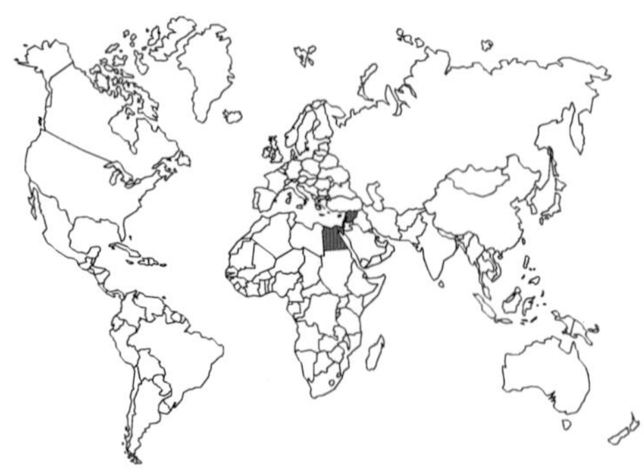

Fig. 2.83.

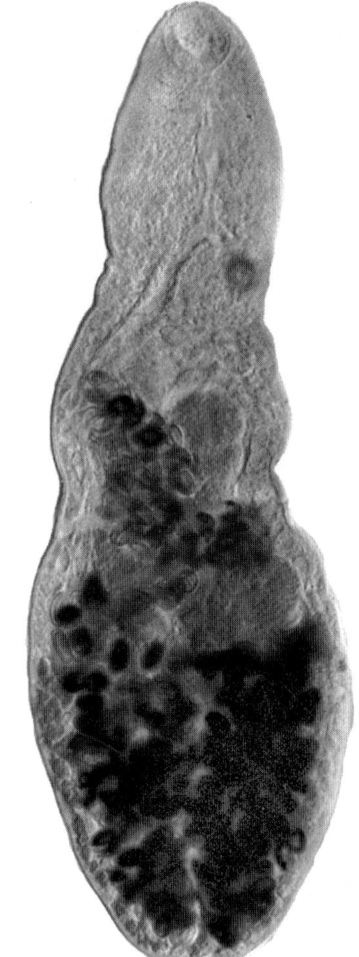

Fig. 2.84. *Stictodora sawakinensis* collected from a gull in Sawakin, Egypt, by Dr. Looss.

REFERENCES
Kuntz RE, Chandler AC. 1956. Studies on Egyptian trematodes with special reference to the heterophyids of mammals. I. Adult flukes, with descriptions of *Phagicola longicollis* n. sp., *Cynodiplostomum namrui* n. sp., and a *Stephanoprora* from cats. J Parasitol 42:445–459.
Looss A. 1899. Weitere BeitrÑge sur Kenntniss der Trematoden-Fauna Aegyptens, zugleich Versuch einer natürlichen Gliederung des Genus *Distomum* Retzius. Zool Jahrb 12:521–784.
Witenberg, G. 1953. Notes on *Galactosomum* and related genera (Trematode: Heterophyidae). Thapar Commemorative Volume, pp 293-300.

MICROPHALLIDAE

The microphallids are a group of trematodes wherein the adults are very similar in appearance to a heterophyid. However, these trematodes differ from the heterophyids in that the cercariae do not have eyespots and typically utilize crustaceans rather than fish as the second intermediate host.

Microphalloides vajrasthirae Waikagul, 1983

This trematode was recovered from a cat from a province in Central Thailand (Waikagul, 1983). This small fluke is about 0.75 mm long and just slightly narrower than it is long. The anterior end is gently rounded, while the posterior end is rather square. The testes are in the posterior part of the body where they are found to be widely spaced at the lateral margins of the body. The eggs are small, being only about 20 µm long. It is suspected, based on work performed by others with related species, that the cat became infected by the ingestion of a crab containing the metacercarial stages.

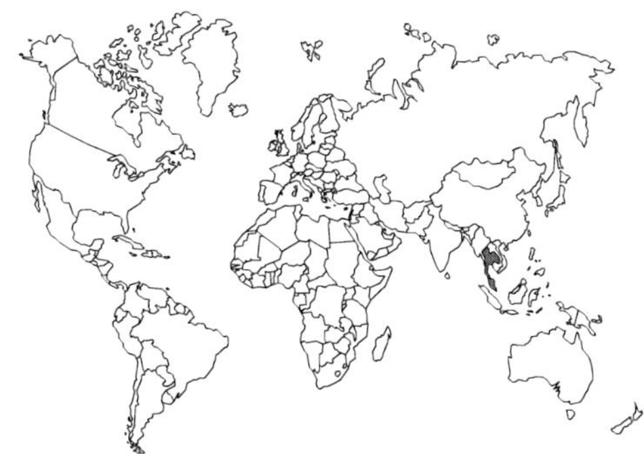

Fig. 2.85.

REFERENCES

Waikagul J. 1983. *Microphalloides vajrasthirae* n. sp. (Digenea: Microphallidae) from the small intestine of cat in Thailand. Southeast Asian J Trop Med Publ Health 14:260–263.

PLAGIORCHIDAE

The plagiorchids are characterized by having well-developed oral and ventral suckers, an ovary just posterior to the ventral sucker, and testes at the beginning of the posterior of the body that are situated diagonally from each other (Fig. 2.86). The typical plagiorchid has three hosts in it life cycle. The first host being a snail that produces a cercaria that typically has two suckers of the same size, an insect or a second snail that serves as the second intermediate host, and a final host.

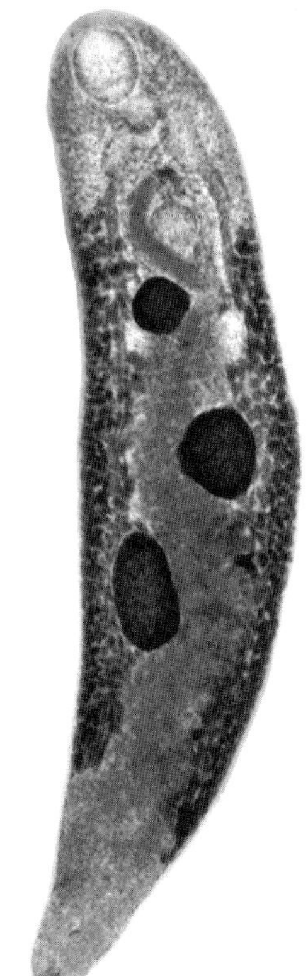

Fig. 2.86. *Plagiorchis micracanthos* from a bat, *Myotus sodalis,* in Kentucky. Note the large anterior and ventral suckers, the ovary about one-fourth of the body length from the anterior end, the two large oblique testes occurring in the second third of the body, and the lateral vitellaria.

Plagiorchis massino Petrov and Tikhonov, 1927

This fluke was originally described from dogs and cats in Armenia and Kazakistan. It has also been reported from a single cat found infected in Newfoundland, Canada (Smith and Threllfall, 1973). The life cycle probably involves a snail as the first intermediate host and an insect or a snail as the second intermediate host. The cats became infected by ingesting the second intermediate host.

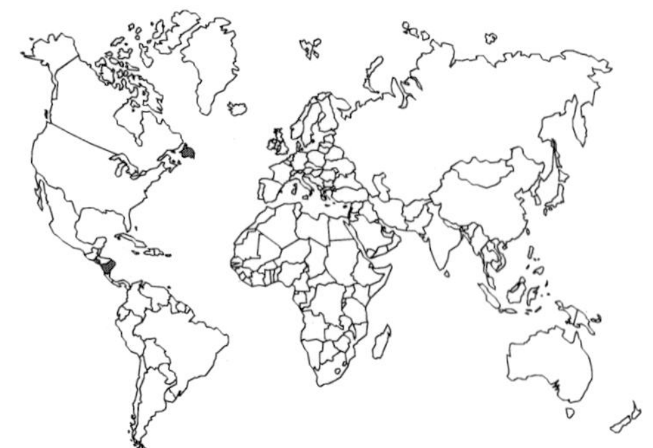

Fig. 2.87.

REFERENCES

Smith FR, Threllfall W. 1973. Helminths of some mammals from Newfoundland. Am Midl Nat 90:215–218.

NANOPHYETIDAE

These small flukes are found in the intestinal tract of numerous mammals. There are large anterior and ventral suckers. The testes are symmetrical, large, and in the hindbody. The cercarial stage that comes from the snail has a stylet and a short tail. The cercariae penetrate the skin of the fish, and the larval stages are found in the tissues of the fish. The final host becomes infected by the ingestion of the fish host.

One member of this family, *Nanophyetus salmincola,* is of additional importance in veterinary medicine because it has been shown to be the vector of the agent causing salmon poisoning in dogs on the west coast of the United States. It does not appear that the cat plays any major role in this story, but it is possible for a cat to develop patent infections if it is fed infected fish. The details of the biology and treatment of this infectious rickettsial agent can be found in many of the textbooks on microbiology and infectious disease, so these details have not been presented here.

Nanophyetus salmincola Chapin, 1928

Etymology

Nano = posterior and *phyetus* = genitalia along with *salmincola* = for the salmonid second hosts.

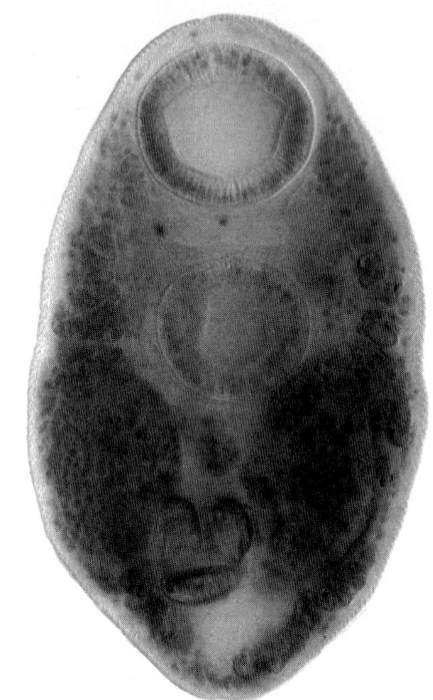

Fig. 2.88. *Nanophyetus salmincola* from the small intestine of an experimentally infected cat collected in Washington, D.C., in the 1920s. Note the two very large suckers and the large ovaries that are present on both sides of the body.

Synonyms

Chapin, 1926, first described this fluke as *Nanophyes salmincola.* He later (1928) changed the name to *Nanophyetus salmincola.* A synonym or sister species from the Siberian coast is *Nanophyetus schikhobalowi* Skrjabin and Podiapolskaia, 1931. Another synonym is *Distomulum oregonensis* Ward and Mueller, 1926. The genus *Nanophyetus* is also considered by some to be synonymous with the genus *Troglotrema.*

History

The fluke was noted be associated with salmon-poisoning disease in dogs because salmon that did not contain metacercariae did not transmit the disease to dogs (Donham et al., 1926). The infectious agent was later identified to be *Neorickettsia helminthoeca.* This rickettsia is passed from dog to dog within the body of the fluke.

Geographic Distribution

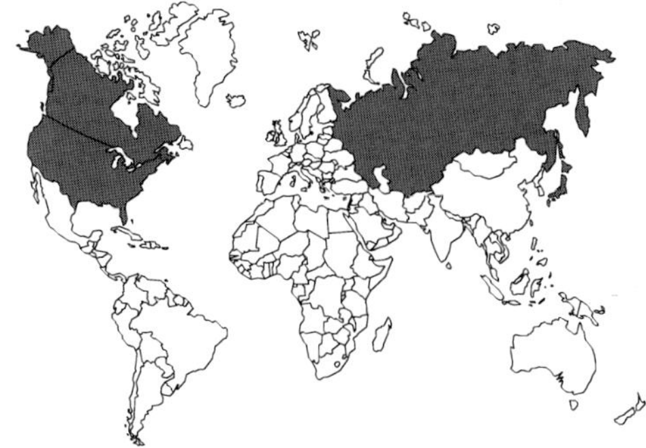

Fig. 2.89.

This trematode is found distributed around the northern Pacific Rim, mainly in various species of canids. The cat does not appear to be a major host of this parasite (Schlegel et al., 1968).

Location in Host

Small intestine.

Parasite Identification

Members of the genus *Nanophyetus* are small flukes, about 1 mm long. There is a muscular pharynx. The genital opening is just posteriad to the ventral sucker, with the ovary being at about the same level as the ventral sucker. The testes are large and are opposite each other in the middle of the hindbody.

The adult flukes may be anywhere from 0.8 mm to 2.5 mm in length. The eggs, 87 μm to 97 μm in length by 38 to 55 μm wide, are light brown, operculate, and not embryonated when passed in the feces.

Life Cycle

The miracidium within the egg hatches and swims by means of its cilia. The miracidium develops into a redia within the body of the freshwater snail *Oxytrema silicula.* Ultimately, cercariae are produced. The cercariae are microcercous (i.e., have a very small tail) and are grouped together by strands of mucus, which probably help them come into contact with the surface of a fish swimming by. The cercariae penetrate the skin of fish at the site of contact. The fish hosts utilized are members of the salmon family that become parasitized during the freshwater portion of their life cycle. After infection, the metacercariae are found to develop predominantly within the kidneys and muscles of the fish. The metacercariae are capable of persisting in the tissues of the fish for almost 2 years after they return to the sea and after this period are capable of transmitting the causative agent of salmon-poisoning disease to dogs. Mammals and birds become infected when they ingest raw salmon. The flukes mature into adults with eggs in 6 to 10 days after the fish has been eaten.

Clinical Presentation and Pathogenesis

Lesions in cats infected with *Nanophyetus salmincola* have not been described. Hoeppli (1926) examined the parasite-induced damage to the intestinal mucosa of the dog and believed it to be highly pathogenic; however, Hoeppli's studies were performed before the discovery of the rickettsial cause of this disease.

Treatment

Probably praziquantel, but not reported.

Epizootiology

Cats become infected by eating raw fish. In the wilds of Oregon, many other hosts are infected (Schlegel et al., 1968). The most important hosts in the wild are probably the raccoon, coyote, lynx, spotted skunk, and even birds (e.g., the hooded merganser).

Hazards to Other Animals

The rickettsia can be lethal to dogs that have ingested fish containing the rickettsial-bearing trematode. If infected with the trematode, cats need to be treated to prevent the parasite from being able to complete its life cycle.

Hazards to Humans

Human beings have been found infected with this parasite in Siberia. It is also possible that the rickettsial agent may cause disease in human beings.

People, like cats, obtain their infections by the ingestion of raw fish.

Control/Prevention

The prevention of the ingestion of raw fish.

REFERENCES

Chapin EA. 1926. A new genus and species of trematode, the probable cause of salmon-poisoning in dogs. North Am Vet 7:36–37.

Chapin EA. 1928. Note. J Parasitol 14:60.

Donham CR, Simms BT, Miller FW. 1926. So-called salmon poisoning in dogs. Progress report. JAVMA 71:215–217.

Hoeppli R. 1926. Anatomische veranderungen des Hundarms, hervorgerufen durch *Nanophyes salmincola* Chapin. Arch Schiffs Tropen-Hyg 30:396–399.

Schlegel MW, Knapp SE, Millemann RE. 1968. "Salmon poisoning" disease. V. Definitive hosts of the trematode vector, *Nanophyetus salmincola*. J Parasitol 54:770–774.

TREMATODES OF THE PANCREATIC DUCT, GALLBLADDER, AND BILE DUCT

Several trematodes are regularly found in the ducts that empty into the small intestine from the liver and the pancreas. One parasite, which is regularly found in the pancreatic duct, has been reported from the cat. This trematode, *Eurytrema procyonis*, is a member of the dicrocoelids. Most of the other dicrocoelid trematodes are parasites of the gallbladder and bile ducts. The dicrocoelid trematodes are one of two groups of trematodes that are found in the bile ducts and gallbladder; the other group is the opisthorchids. The dicrocoelids tend to utilize arthropods as their second intermediate host, and opisthorchids utilize fish. Both parasites cause similar hepatic disease.

DICROCOELIDAE

The dicrocoelids are delicate, elongate, and quite beautiful trematodes that are located in the bile ducts, gallbladder, or pancreatic ducts. The adults are characterized by testes that tend to be rather anteriorly placed, vitellaria that are localized in the lateral portions of the middle of the body, and a uterus filled with eggs that tends to fill most of the posterior portion of the body. The egg when passed in the feces is thick shelled and embryonated. In the life cycle of this parasite, the egg is eaten by a land snail. Within the snail the cercariae develop and possess a stylet. The cercariae that leave the snail must then typically enter an arthropod host. Some of the dicrocoelids, such as

Pancreas
- DICROCOELIDAE
  - *Eurytrema procyonis* Denton, 1942

Gallbladder and bile ducts
- DICROCOELIDAE
  - *Euparadistomum pearsoni* Talbot, 1970
  - *Euparadistomum buckleyi* Singh, 1958
  - *Euparadistomum heiwschi* Buckley and Yeh, 1958
  - *Platynosomum concinnum* (Braun, 1901) Purvis, 1933
- OPISTHORCHIDAE
  - *Amphimerus pseudofelineus* (Ward, 1901) Barker, 1911
  - *Clonorchis sinensis* (Cobbold, 1875) Looss, 1907
  - *Opisthorchis felineus* (Rivolta, 1884) Blanchard, 1895
  - *Opisthorchis viverrini* (Poirier, 1886) Stiles and Hassall, 1896
  - *Opisthorchis chabaudi* Bourgat and Kulo, 1977
  - *Paropisthorchis caninus* Stephens, 1912
  - *Metorchis conjunctus* (Cobbold, 1860) Looss, 1899
  - *Metorchis albidus* (Braun, 1893) Looss, 1899
  - *Metorchis orientalis* Tanabe, 1919
  - *Parametorchis complexum* (Stiles and Hassal, 1894) Skrjabin, 1913
  - *Pseudamphistomum truncatum* (Rudolphi, 1819) Lühe, 1909

Fig. 2.90. Trematodes of the pancreatic duct, gallbladder, and bile ducts.

Platynosomum concinnum, utilize paratenic hosts to transfer the snail from the arthropod to the mammalian final host.

Eurytrema procyonis Denton, 1942

Etymology

Eury = wide and *trema* = trematode along with *procyonis* for the original raccoon host.

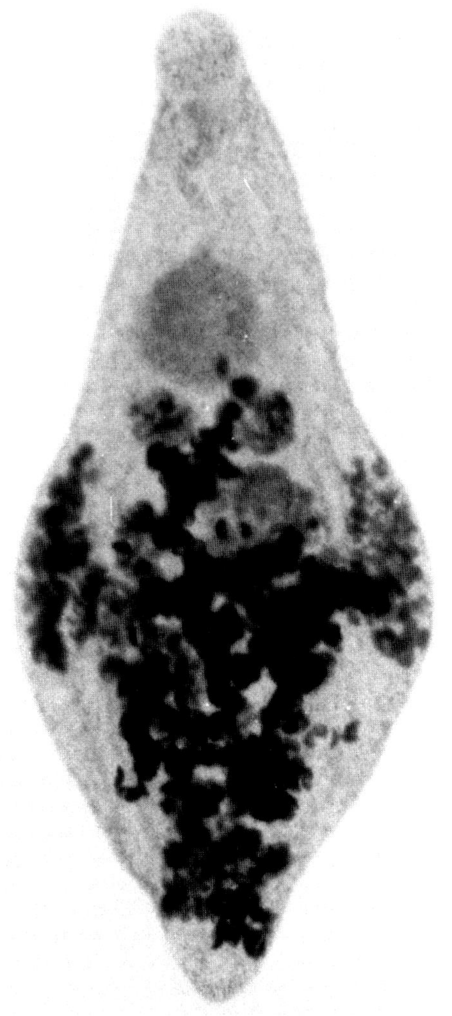

Fig. 2.91. *Eurytrema procyonis* recovered from the pancreatic duct of a cat in New Jersey. Note the lateral vitellaria, the testes that are anterior to midbody, the large anterior and ventral suckers, and the uterus filled with eggs that extends posteriad between the vitellaria to fill the body with dark eggs.

Synonyms

Eurytrema vulpis Stunkard, 1947; *Concinnum procyonis* of Schell, 1985.

History

This fluke was originally described from specimens recovered from the pancreatic duct of a raccoon in Texas (Denton, 1942). Burrows and Lillis (1960) discovered the same parasite in the pancreatic ducts of two cats in New Jersey.

Geographic Distribution

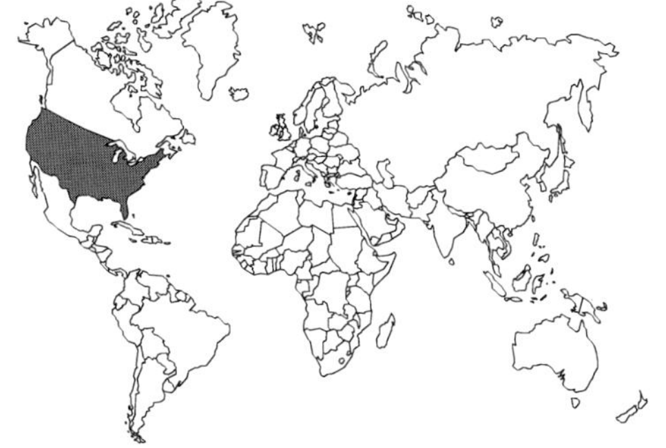

Fig. 2.92.

This species of *Eurytrema* has only been reported from the eastern United States of America. In a survey of 290 cats from St. Louis, Missouri, 31 were found to be infected with this parasite (Fox et al., 1981). A survey of 36 cats within a 250-mile radius of Fort Knox, Kentucky, revealed that 5 of these cats had pancreatic flukes (Sheldon, 1966).

Location in Host

Pancreatic duct; in one of the cases described by Burrows and Lillis, the cat had over 300 of these flukes in the pancreatic duct and an additional 67 flukes in the bile ducts and gallbladder.

Parasite Identification

This fluke is 1.7 to 2.5 mm in length, and 0.73 to 1.3 mm wide at midbody. There is a well-developed ventral sucker that is about one-fourth of the body length towards the posterior end, and the testes are large, paired, and just posteriad to the ventral sucker. There is a cirrus present behind the genital pore that opens anterior to the ventral sucker. The eggs are 45 to 53 μm long by 29 to 36 μm wide.

Life Cycle

The life cycle of this trematode is only incompletely described. Embryonated eggs are eaten by a land snail, *Mesodon thyroidus.* The cercariae develop within sporocysts within this snail, and when developed, the cercariae have very short tails. The sporocysts, containing numerous cercariae, are extruded from the snail. Viable cercariae are still present within the extruded sporocysts after 5 days. It is believed that the second intermediate host is most likely an arthropod (Denton, 1944).

Clinical Presentation and Pathogenesis

Cats infected can develop pancreatic atrophy and fibrosis (Anderson et al., 1987); the inflammatory pancreatic disease can lead to clinical signs of weight loss and intermittent vomiting. The pancreatic ducts become thickened, and the main duct can be enlarged with numerous flukes. Infected cats may show a reduction in the protein and carbonate content of pancreatic fluid, as well as an overall reduction in the volume of fluid produced. (Fox et al., 1981).

Treatment

Probably praziquantel, but not reported.

Epizootiology

It is not known how cats become infected. It is most likely that they are accidentally ingesting some arthropod that supports the development of the metacercarial stage.

Hazards to Other Animals

Raccoons and foxes are quite often infected with this parasite.

Hazards to Humans

There have been no records as to the infection of human beings with this parasite. If a person were to ingest the arthropod host, he or she could perhaps develop an infection.

Control/Prevention

This cannot be done until the life cycle has been elucidated. One of the naturally infected cats was a 4.5-year-old spayed female American indoor-outdoor cat (Anderson et al., 1987). It is not known how this cat became infected or how the infection could have been prevented.

REFERENCES

Anderson WI, Georgi ME, Car BD. 1987. Pancreatic atrophy and fibrosis associated with *Eurytrema procyonis* in a domestic cat. Vet Rec 120:235–236.

Burrows RB, Lillis WG. 1960. *Eurytrema procyonis* Denton, 1942 (Trematoda: dicrocoelidae), from the domestic cat. J Parasitol 45:810–812.

Denton JF. 1942. *Eurytrema procyonis,* n. sp. (Trematodea: Dicrocoelidae) from the raccoon, *Procyon lotor.* Proc Helminthol Soc Wash 9:31–32.

Denton JF. 1944. Studies on the life history of *Eurytrema procyonis* Denton, 1942. J Parasitol 30:277–286.

Fox JN, Mosley JG, Vogler GA, Ausitn JL, Reber HA. 1981. Pancreatic function in domestic cats with pancreatic fluke infection. JAVMA 178:58–60.

Sheldon WG. 1966. Pancreatic flukes (*Eurytrema procyonis*) in domestic cats. JAVMA 148:251–253.

Euparadistomum pearsoni Talbot, 1970

Etymology

Eupara = wide and *distomum* = two mouths along with *pearsoni* = for Dr. Pearson.

Synonyms

None.

History

This fluke was recovered from cats in Papua New Guinea. It was originally described as *Euparadistomum* sp. (Talbot, 1969) but then recognized as a new species. Other species of *Euparadistomum* have been described from cats, and a number of species have been described from reptiles. It may be that reptiles are the typical hosts of this group of trematode parasites.

Geographic Distribution

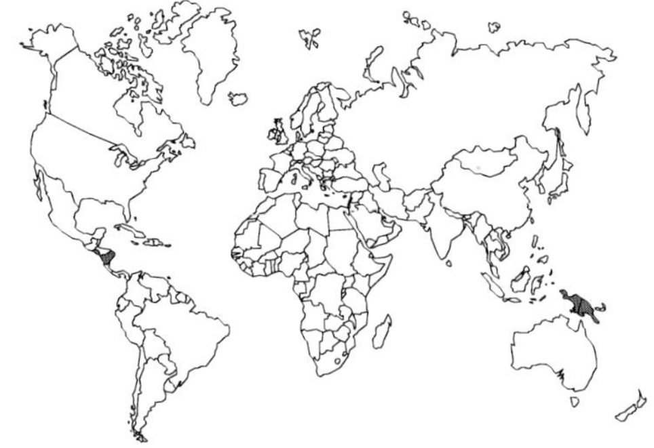

Fig. 2.93.

New Guinea.

Location in Host

Gallbladder, none in the bile ducts.

Parasite Identification

This fluke is quite discoid in appearance with a color that is pinkish gray when alive. The diameter of the body is about 5 mm. The ventral sucker is centrally placed and has a diameter of 1 to 1.3 mm; the oral sucker is slightly smaller than the ventral sucker. The testes are anterior to the ventral sucker, and each is about one-fourth the diameter of the ventral sucker. The small ovary is at the posterior margin of the ventral sucker. The genital opening is between the oral and ventral suckers. The eggs are operculate, with yellow to brown eggshells, measuring 35 to 52 μm in length by 18 to 26 μm in width.

Life Cycle

Not known. It is suspected that the intermediate host is an arthropod.

Clinical Presentation and Pathogenesis

Signs in infected cats have not been described if they are present.

Treatment

Probably praziquantel, but not reported.

Epizootiology

It is not known how cats become infected. It is most likely that they are accidentally ingesting some arthropod that supports the development of the metacercarial stage. Of course, it may be as in *Platynosomum* (below) in which there is a reptile as the third intermediate host.

Hazards to Other Animals

None known.

Hazards to Humans

There have been no records as to the infection of human beings with this parasite. If a person were to ingest the arthropod host, he or she could perhaps develop an infection.

Control/Prevention

This cannot be done until the life cycle has been elucidated.

REFERENCES

Talbot N. 1969. Trematodes of the gall bladder of cats in Port Moresby, New Guinea. Aust Vet J 45:206.

Talbot N. 1970. On *Euparadistomum pearsoni* n. sp. (Trematode: Dicrocoelidae) from the gall bladder of the domestic cat in Papua. J Helminthol 44:89–96.

Euparadistomum buckleyi Singh, 1958 and *Euparadistomum heiwschi* Buckley and Yeh, 1958

Two other species of *Euparadistomum* have been reported from cats. *Euparadistomum heiwschi* Buckley and Yeh, 1958, was described using specimens collected from the gallbladder of a cat in Kenya (Buckley and Liang-Sheng, 1958). *Euparadistomum buckleyi* Singh, 1958, was recovered from a cat in Madras, India (Rajavelu and Raja, 1988). Five other species of *Euparadistomum* are parasites of lizards, bats, opossums, birds, and the fox (Talbot, 1970). A sixth species, *Euparadistomum cercopithicai,* is a parasite of the gallbladder of the talapoin monkey in Guinea, Africa (Fig. 2.94).

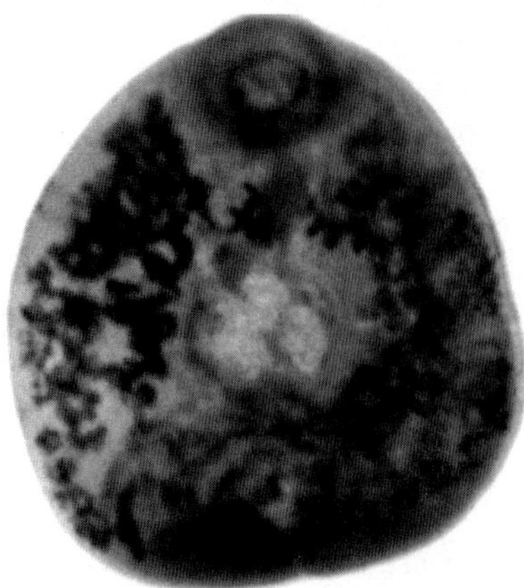

Fig. 2.94. *Euparadistomum cercopithicai* n. sp. from the gallbladder of a talapoin monkey in Africa. Although difficult to discern on the photograph, the large ventral sucker and the lateral vitellaria visible on the left side of the specimen are characteristic of this genus of dicrocoelids.

REFERENCES

Buckley JJC, Liang-Sheng Y. 1958. On *Euparadistomum heischi* n. sp. from the liver of a domestic cat on Pate Island, Kenya, and a new sub-family Euparadistominae (Dicrocoelidae). J Helminthol 32:81–88.

Rajavelu G, Raja EE. 1988. On helminth parasites in domestic cat in Madras. Cheiron 17:11–14.

Talbot N. 1970. On *Euparadistomum pearsoni* n. sp. (Trematodea: Dicrocoelidae) from the gall bladder of the domestic cat in Papua. J Helminthol 44:89–96.

Platynosomum concinnum (Braun, 1901) Purvis, 1933

Etymology

Platy = flat and *nosomum* = disease along with *concinnum* = graceful or harmoniously arranged.

Synonyms

Dicrocoelium lanceolatum var. *symmetricum* Baylis, 1918; *Concinnum concinnum* (Braun, 1901) Bhalerao, 1936; *Platynosomum concinnum* Kossack, 1910.

History

The genus *Platynosomum* was described by Looss in 1907 for a species recovered from a bird (*Cicaetus gallicus*). A fluke from the civet cat was described by Braun (1901) as *Dicrocoelium concinnum* and was transferred to the subgenus *Concinnum* by Bhalerao (1936). Later, the subgenus *Concinnum* was given generic rank (Yamaguti, 1958). Kossack (1910) described a fluke from a cat, *Felis minuta,* that he named *Platynosomum concinnum.* Purvis (1931 and 1933) examined specimens of what he considered to be *Platynosomum concinnum* that were recovered from cats in Malaysia, and after making his observations, Purvis believed that *Platynosomum concinnum* was identical with *Platynosomum planicipitis* (Cameron, 1928). It would appear that if the species *concinnum* is the same species as that described by Kossack as *Platynosomum concinnum,* that the name *Platynosomum concinnum* would be the name with priority because this is the name that was used as part of the original description.

Geographic Distribution

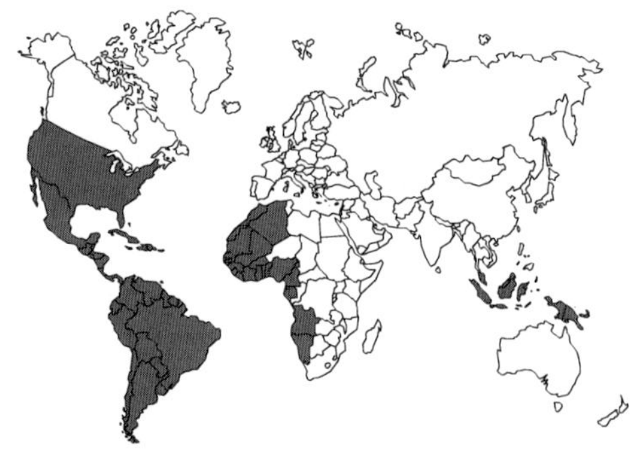

Fig. 2.95.

The tropics, including Malaysia, Hawaii, West Africa, South America, the Caribbean, and areas surrounding the Gulf of Mexico, including the southeastern United States and the Florida Keys (Bielsa and Greiner, 1985).

Location in Host

Gallbladder and bile ducts; rarely in the small intestine.

Parasite Identification

Platynosomum concinnum adults are about 5 mm long by 2 mm wide (Fig. 2.96). The suckers are about equal in size, with the ventral sucker being about one-fourth of the body length from the anterior end. The vitellaria are located mainly at midbody, and the genital opening is at or anterior to the branching point of the intestinal ceca. The testes and ovary are comparatively larger than in species of *Eurytrema.* The eggs are operculate and measure 34 to 50 μm by 20 to 35 μm (Fig. 2.97). A comparison of diagnostic methods revealed that a formalin-ether sedimentation technique was much more sensitive than either a sugar or zinc-sulfate flotation for the diagnosis of infections with this parasite (Palumbo et al., 1976).

Life Cycle

The life cycle has been incompletely described (Maldonado, 1945; Eckerlin and Leigh, 1962). Cercariae with very short tails (i.e., microcercous cercariae) develop in sporocysts within the terrestrial snail *Subulina octona.* The sporocysts leave the snail and are eaten by terrestrial isopods, "pill bugs." The metacercariae in the isopods do not infect cats, but if ingested by a lizard, frog, or toad, the encysted forms are found in the common bile duct and gallbladder of these animals. Cats become infected through the ingestion of the lizard or amphibian third-intermediate host.

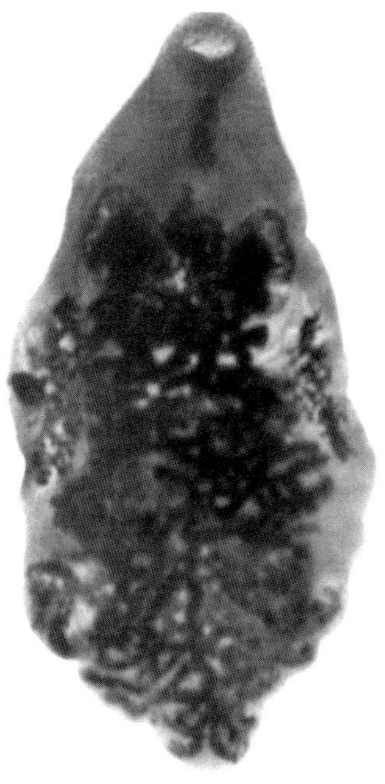

Fig. 2.96. *Platynosomum concinnum* adult collected from the bile duct of a cat in West Hollywood, Florida. Note the vitellaria along the lateral margins at midbody, the paired anterior testes in the anterior third of the body, and the extensive uterus filled with eggs.

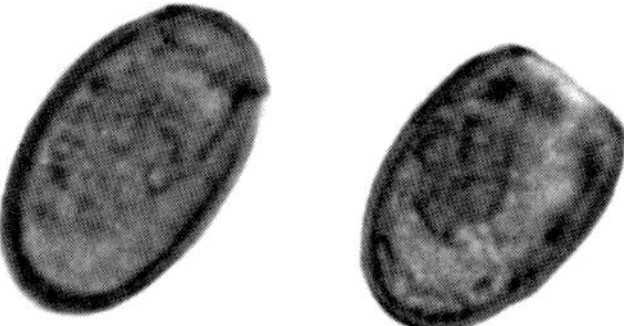

Fig. 2.97. Eggs of *Platynosomum concinnum* from the feces of a naturally infected cat from the Florida Keys. (Photograph supplied by Dr. Robert Foley)

Clinical Presentation and Pathogenesis

Cats infected with large numbers of these parasites can present with severe disease due to the blockage of the biliary system (Robinson and Ehrenford, 1962). Clinical signs have been described in eight infected cats in the Bahamas. The cats did not thrive and had occasional bouts of diarrhea, depression, and anorexia. On examination, the cats had severe weight loss, mild jaundice of the mucous membranes, and mild hepatic enlargement. If the condition progressed to complete biliary obstruction, there was severe diarrhea and vomiting with marked jaundice. At necropsy, severe jaundice was obvious, and the liver was a greenish yellow. The bile ducts were markedly dilated with thickened walls (Ikede et al., 1971). In histological sections, the trematodes could be observed within the dilated bile ducts (Fig. 2.98).

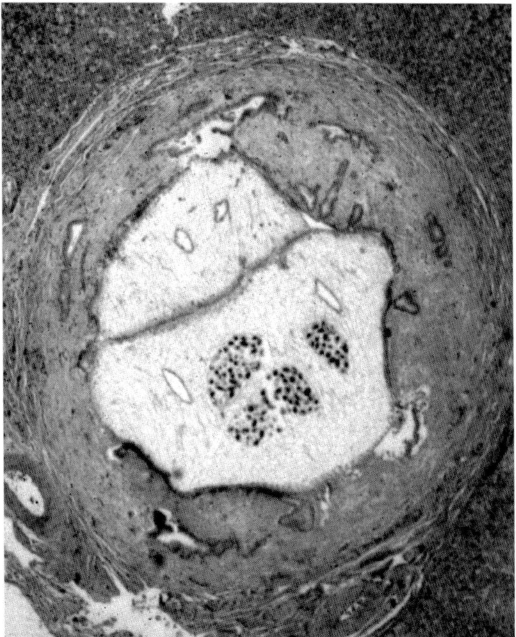

Fig. 2.98. Section of the liver showing the presence of *Platynosomum concinnum* flukes within a dilated bile duct.

Experimental infection of cats was induced by feeding them liver from infected toads, *Bufo marinus* (Taylor and Perri, 1977). Eggs were detected in the feces of several cats as early as 2 months after infection, and all cats were shedding eggs in their feces by 12 weeks after infection. No clinical signs were observed in cats given 125 metacercariae. However, in cats given about 1,000 infective stages, clinical signs were noted in a number of animals. The signs included lethargy, abdominal distension, inappetence, weight loss, and an enlarged liver. There were increased numbers of circulating eosinophils in all infected cats and increases in both alanine and aspartate aminotransferase activities. Histologically, there was severe adenomatous hyperplasia of the bile duct epithelium with periductal inflammation. The cats continued to shed eggs in their feces for 1.5 years after the initial exposure, which was when the study was terminated.

Treatment

Praziquantel at a dose of 20 mg/kg has markedly reduced the number of eggs shed by infected cats. Similarly, nitroscanate at 100 mg/kg also markedly reduced the numbers of eggs being shed by infected cats. Although cats often produced negative samples several weeks after treatment, they very often again shed eggs in their feces a number of weeks after having stopped shedding (Evans and Green, 1978). It has been reported to one author (D.D. Bowman) that treatment of infected cats in Florida with severe hepatic disease using praziquantel at a dosage of 40 mg/kg resulted in the death of a compromised cat.

Epizootiology

Cats are not the only hosts of this parasite. It has also been reported from opossums (*Didelphis marsupialis*) and from the civet (*Viverra zibetha*). Mice have been experimentally infected (Eckerlin and Leigh, 1962).

Hazards to Other Animals

None known.

Hazards to Humans

There have been no records as to the infection of human beings with this parasite. If a person were to ingest the lizard, he or she could perhaps develop an infection.

Control/Prevention

Prevent the ingestion of infected lizards, toads, and frogs.

REFERENCES

Bhalerao GD. 1936. Studies on the helminths of India. Trematoda I. J Helminthol 14:163–180.

Bielsa LM, Greiner EC. 1985. Liver flukes (*Platynosomum concinnum*) in cats. J Am Hosp Assoc 21:269–274.

Braun M. 1901. Ein neues *Dicrocoelium* aus der Gallenblase der Zibethkatze. Centralbl Bakt Parasitenk Infekt 30:700–702.

Cameron TWM. 1928. On some parasites of the rusty cat (*Felis planiceps*). J Helminthol 6:87–98.

Eckerlin RP, Leigh WH. 1962. *Platynosomum concinnum* Kossack, 1910 (Trematoda: Dicrocoelidae) in South Florida. J Parasitol 48(suppl.):49.

Evans JW, Green PE. 1978. Preliminary evaluation of four anthelmintics against the cat liver fluke, *Platynosomum concinnum*. Aust Vet J 54:454–455.

Ikede BO, Losos GJ. Isoun TT. 1971. *Platynosomum concinnum* infection in cats in Nigeria. Vet Rec 89:635–638.

Kossack W. 1910. Neue Distomem. Centralbl Bakt Parasitenk Infekt 56:114-120.

Looss A. 1907. Ueber einige sum Teil neue Distomen der europäischen Fauna. Centralbl Bakt Parasitenk Infekt 43:604–613.

Maldonado JF. 1945. The life history and biology of *Platynosomum concinnum* Kossack, 1910 (Trematoda: Dicrocoelidae). Puerto Rico J Publ Health Trop Med 21:17–60.

Palumbo NE, Taylor D, Perri SF. 1976. Evaluation of fecal technics for the diagnosis of cat liver fluke infection. Lab Anim Sci 26:490–493.

Purvis GB. 1931. The species of *Platynosomum* in felines. Vet Rec 11:228–229.

Purvis GB. 1933. The excretory system of *Platynosomum concinnum* (Braun, 1901); syn. *P. concinnum* (Kossack, 1910); and *P. planicipitis* (Cameron, 1928). Vet Rec 13:565.

Robinson VB, Ehrenford FA. 1962. Hepatic lesions associated with liver fluke (*Platynosomum concinnum*) infection in a cat. Am J Vet Res 23:1300–1303.

Taylor D, Perri SF. 1977. Experimental infection of cats with the liver fluke *Platynosomum concinnum*. Am J Vet Res 38:51–54.

Yamaguti S. 1958. Systema Helminthum, The Digenetic Trematodes of Vertebrates. New York, NY: Interscience.

OPISTHORCHIDAE

The opisthorchids make up a group of trematode parasites that are found in the bile ducts and gallbladder of several classes of vertebrates. There are seven different genera of these trematodes that are found in cats. Some of the species found in cats, *Clonorchis sinensis,* and species of *Opisthorchis* are also important parasites of humans in certain parts of the world and a great deal is written about these parasites in human parasitology texts. The first opisthorchid was, however, found in a cat by Rivolta (1884). The life cycle of the opisthorchids involves a fish as the second intermediate host, and therefore, cats around the world are commonly infected with this group of parasites. The opisthorchids, like the dicrocoelids, usually have the vitellaria confined to bands along the lateral edges of the body. Unlike the dicrocoelids, the testes of the opisthorchids are found in the posterior of the body. Usually, one testis is anterior to the other rather than being alongside each other; in the dicrocoelids, the testes are typically next to each other.

The characters differentiating the seven genera are as follows. The genus *Amphimerus* differs from the genus *Opisthorchis* in that the vitellaria are divided into an anterior and posterior group with the posterior group extending into the posterior portion of the body to the level of the posterior testis. Also, in the genus *Amphimerus,* unlike in the genera *Clonorchis* and *Opisthorchis,* the ventral sucker is larger than the oral sucker. The genus *Clonorchis* is characterized by having testes that are highly branched. The vitellaria of this trematode are restricted to the sides of the body anterior to the testes. The genus *Opisthorchis* is very similar to *Clonorchis,* but differs in that the testes are not branched. The genus *Paropisthorchis* is characterized by having the ventral sucker and genital pore located on a pedunculated structure that extends out from the ventral surface of the body. Specimens of *Metorchis* differ from those of *Opisthorchis, Clonorchis, Amphimerus,* and *Paropisthorchis* in that the uterus is more bunched together, "rosettiform," with branches that encircle the ventral sucker. *Metorchis* species also tend to be broader than the *Opisthorchi*s relatives. The testes of *Metorchis, Parametorchis,* and *Pseudamphistomum* tend to be more spheroid than those of *Clonorchis* and *Opisthorchis,* although branching does occur in some species. The vitellaria of *Metorchis* are confined to the lateral margins of the body, while in the genus *Parametorchis,* the vitellaria from the lateral sides become confluent anteriorly. In specimens of *Pseudamphistomum* the posterior end of the body is squared off, giving the ventral surface of the body the appearance of being a pseudo hold-fast structure.

REFERENCES

Rivolta S. 1884. Sopra una specie di *Distoma* nel gatto e nel cane. Giur Anat Fisiol Patol Animali 16:20–28.

Amphimerus pseudofelineus (Ward, 1901) Barker, 1911

Etymology

Amphi = on both sides and *merus* = part (referring to the break in the vitellaria) along with *pseudo* = false and *felineus* = cat host; differentiating it from *Opisthorchis felineus* which had already been described from cats in Europe.

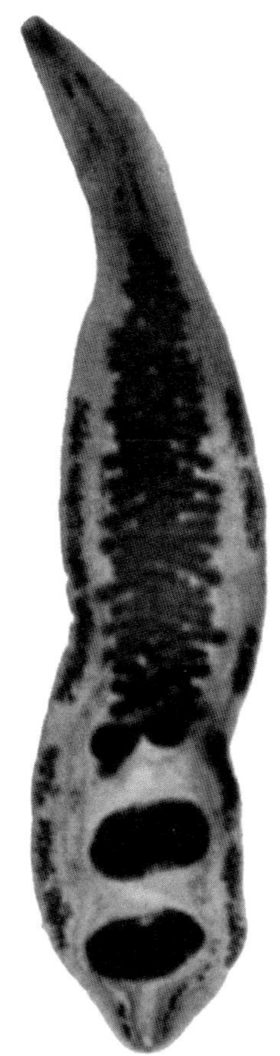

Fig. 2.99. *Amphimerus pseudofelineus* recovered from the bile duct of a cat in Temple, Texas, by Dr. D.M. Bandy.

Synonyms

Opisthorchis guyaquilensis Rodriguez et al., 1949.

History

This trematode was originally described from a cat in Nebraska. Barker (1911) differentiated the genus *Amphimerus* from that of *Opisthorchis,* and he transferred the species *pseudofelineus* to the new genus.

Geographic Distribution

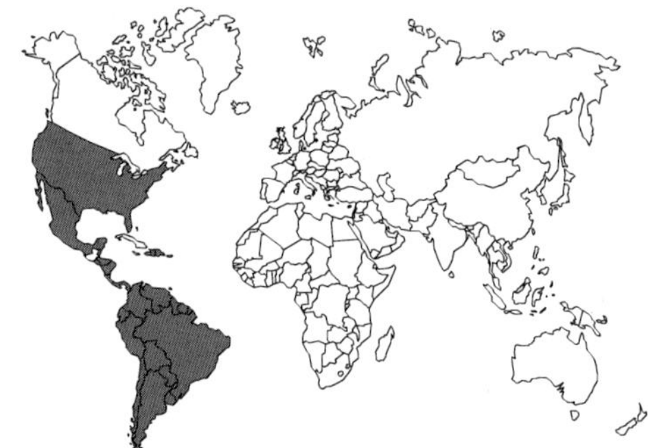

Fig. 2.100.

The Americas; besides the original description from Nebraska, *Amphimerus pseudofelineus* has been described from cats from Illinois and Michigan and experimentally from Manitoba, Canada. Human infections with *Opisthorchis guyaquilensis* in Ecuador were later identified as *Amphimerus psuedofelineus.* Miyazaki (1991) states that about 10 species have been found in the Americas and that all may potentially infect humans. In a similar fashion, it may be that all are capable of occurring in cats.

Location in Host

Gallbladder and bile ducts; occasionally in the small intestine.

Parasite Identification

Amphimerus pseudofelineus adults are very similar to those of *Opisthorchis.* The major difference is that the vitelline glands situated along the side of the body are divided on each side into anterior and posterior clusters at the level of the ovary. Also, the vitellaria extend more posteriad within the lateral field.

The adults measure about 16 to 24 mm in length. The eggs are similar to those of other opisthorchids measuring 27 by 15 μm.

Life Cycle

The life cycle has been incompletely described (Evans, 1963). A cat was fed 700 g of freshwater fish fillets from suckers, *Catostomus commersonii,* collected from Lake Manitoba. The examination of the cat 51 days after the last feeding revealed the *Amphimerus pseudofelineus* within the bile ducts.

Clinical Presentation and Pathogenesis

Infection of cats can result in severe cirrhosis of the liver ultimately resulting in death (Levine et al., 1956; Rothenbacher and Lindquist, 1963). In chronic cases the liver can be enlarged with a granular-appearing surface. Cut sections of the liver appear fibrotic with a distinct yellow-brown mottling. The larger bile ducts may contain a dark-brown exudate. Bile duct epithelium becomes thickened and fibrotic. Clinical signs reflect progression in liver dsyfunction with anorexia, weight loss, diarrhea, periodic vomiting, and icterus, with hepatomegally initially, then microhepatica.

Treatment

Praziquantel is likely to prove successful in eliminating these trematodes.

Epizootiology

Cats are not the only hosts of this parasite. It has also been reported from coyotes in the United States and as *Opisthorchis guayaquilensis* in dogs in Ecuador and in cats and opossums, *Didelphis marsupialis,* in Panama. A related species, *Amphimerus lancea,* has been reported from freshwater porpoises in Brazilian waters.

Hazards to Other Animals

None known.

Hazards to Humans

There have been records of human infections with this parasite in Ecuador where 4 percent of the human beings and 3 percent of the dogs in a village were found to be infected (Rodriguez et al., 1949). It is believed that the infections were obtained by the ingestion of raw fish.

Control/Prevention

Prevent the ingestion of raw fish.

REFERENCES

Barker FD. 1911. The trematode genus *Opisthorchis* R. Blanchard, 1895. Stud Zool Lab Univ Nebr 103:513–561.

Evans WS. 1963. *Amphimerus pseudofelineus* (Ward, 1901) (Digenea: Opisthorchidae) and its second intermediate host in manitoba. Can J Zool 41:649–651.

Levine ND, Beamer PD, Maksic D. 1956. Hepatitis due to *Amphimerus pseudofelineus* in a cat. J Parasitol 42(suppl.):37.

Miyazaki I. 1991. Helminthic Zoonoses. Fukuoka, Japan: International Medical Foundation of Japan. 494 pp.

Rodriguez JD, Gomez LF, Montalvan CJA. 1949. El *Opisthorchis guayaquilensis* (una nueva especie de *Opisthorchis* encontrada en el Ecuador). Rev Ecua Hig Med Trop 6:11–24.

Rothenbacher H, Lindquist WD. 1963. Liver cirrhosis and pancreatitis in a cat infected with *Amphimerus pseudofelineus*. JAVMA 143:1099–1105.

Clonorchis sinensis (Cobbold, 1875) Looss, 1907

Etymology

Clon = branched and *orchis* = testis along with *sinensis* = representing China.

Synonyms

Distoma sinens Cobbold, 1875; *Distoma spathulatum* Leuckart, 1876; *Distoma endemicum* Jima, 1886. Also, some have included the members of the genus *Clonorchis* within the genus *Opisthorchis*.

History

This trematode was originally described from the bile passages of a Chinese carpenter working in Calcutta, India. It was described in Japan in 1883 and was recognized as being endemic in south China in 1908 by Heanley. Cats were first noted to be infected in Japan (Ijima, 1887).

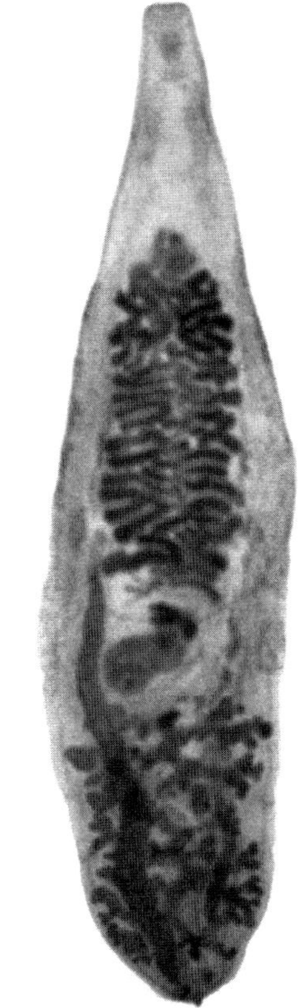

Fig. 2.101. *Clonorchis sinensis* from the gall bladder of a cat in China. Note the highly branched testes in the posterior of the body and the restriction of the uterus between the ventral sucker and the ovary. The vitellaria are not very distinct in this specimen.

Geographic Distribution

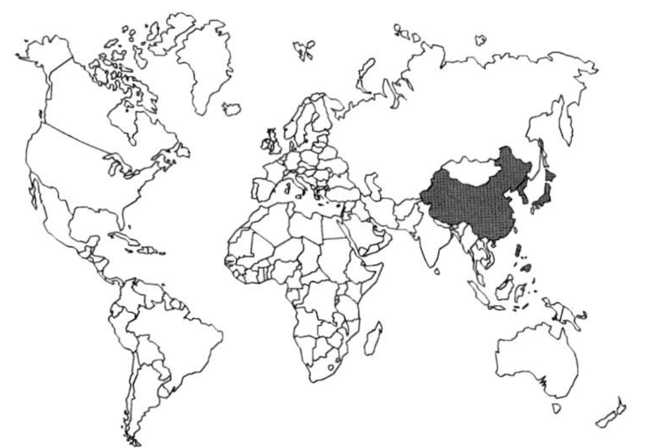

Fig. 2.102.

This fluke is found in Japan, Korea, Taiwan, China, and North Korea. The infection seems to be present in freshwater fish surrounding the areas bordering on the China Sea.

Location in Host

Gallbladder and bile ducts; occasionally in the pancreatic duct or the small intestine.

Parasite Identification

Clonorchis sinensis differs from specimens of *Opisthorchis* in that it has highly branched testes. The highly branched testes separate *Clonorchis* from the other genera of opisthorchid trematodes. The adults are 10 to 25 mm long and 3 to 5 mm wide. The eggs are yellowish brown with a distinct operculum. There is often a slight protuberance on the end of the egg opposite the operculum. The eggs measure 28 to 35 μm long by 12 to 19 μm wide.

Life Cycle

Cats were first used to show that a freshwater fish intermediate host was a required part of the life cycle (Kobayashi, 1915). About 80 species of fish have been identified as hosts; most of the piscine hosts are in the family Cyprinidae. A few years later, the snail hosts were identified and are now recognized as species of *Parafossarulus, Bulimus, Semisulcospira, Alocinma,* and *Melanoides.* The eggs of *Clonorchis sinensis* hatch only if they are ingested by the appropriate snail host.

After an animal ingests an infected fish, the young trematode migrates to the bile duct through the ampulla of Vater. It then takes about 1 month for the trematodes to reach maturity. The trematodes have been found to live as long as 12 years and 3 months in cats (Miyazaki, 1991).

Clinical Presentation and Pathogenesis

Ultimately the host develops cirrhosis of the liver. The changes in the liver have been divided in humans into three basic stages. The first stage consists primarily of proliferation of the biliary-tract epithelium. In the second stage the surrounding liver tissue is compressed by the growing connective tissue around the bile ducts. In the third stage, there is significant cirrhosis and destruction of the liver parenchyma. It is believed that an infection with only a few flukes will seldom induce more than the first stages of the disease. Similar progression of disease is thought to occur in infected cats.

Treatment

Praziquantel is likely to prove successful in eliminating these trematodes from many treated cases.

Epizootiology

Cats are a major host of this pathogen. In some areas of China and Vietnam, up to one-third of the feline population might be shedding eggs of this parasite in their feces. In areas where fish are consumed raw, this can have a major impact on the human population by the maintenance of the parasite in the surrounding fish population.

Hazards to Other Animals

Dogs and other fish-eating mammals can also be infected with this parasite.

Hazards to Humans

Large numbers of human beings are infected with this parasite in the geographical regions where it is found. Surveys in Korea and Vietnam have found prevalence rates above 15 percent in some populations (Chung et al., 1991; Kieu, et al., 1992).

Control/Prevention

Prevent the ingestion of infected raw, dried, or pickled fish; these latter methods are not necessarily going to kill the metacercarial stage of the trematode.

REFERENCES

Chung DI, Kim YI, Lee KR, Choi DW. 1991. Epidemiological studies of digenetic trematodes in Yongyan County, Kyungpok Province. Kisaengchunghap Chapchi 29:325–338.

Ijima I. 1887. Notes on *Distoma endemiocum,* Baelz. J Coll Sci, Imp Univ, Tokyo 1:47–59 [Cited in Grove DI. 1990. A History of Human Helminthology. Wallingford, UK: CAB Inter.]

Kieu TL, Bronshtein AM, Sabgaida TP. 1992. Clonorchiasis in the People's Republic of Vietnam. 2. The clinico-parasitological examination of a focus and a trial of praziquantel treatment. Med Parazitol Mosk 4:7–11.

Kobayashi H. 1915. On the life history and morphology of *Clonorchis sinensis.* Centralbl Bakt Parasitenk Infekt 75:299–318.

Miyazaki I. 1991. Helminthic Zoonoses. Fukuoka, Japan: International Medical Foundation of Japan. 494 pp.

Opisthorchis felineus (Rivolta, 1884) Blanchard, 1895

Etymology

Opistho = posterior and *orchis* = testis along with *felineus* = representing the feline host.

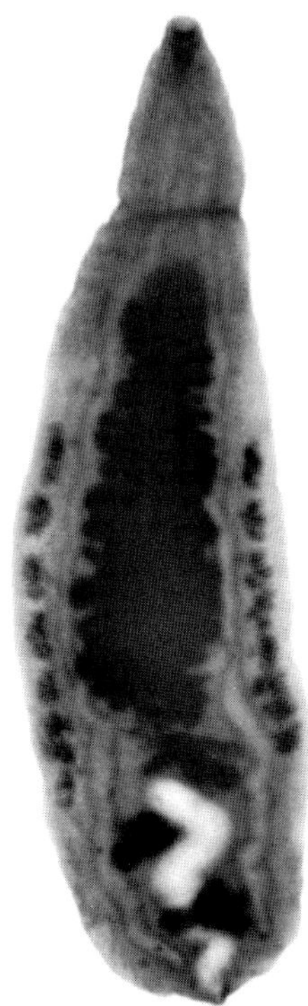

Fig. 2.103. *Opisthorchis felineus* from a cat. Note the slightly branched testes and the vitellaria that extend only to the anterior of the most anteriad testis.

Synonyms

Distoma felineum Rivolta, 1884; *Distoma sibiricum* Winogradoff, 1892.

History

This trematode was originally described from the bile passages of a cat in Italy (1884). In 1892, it was found in nine human beings in Siberia.

Geographic Distribution

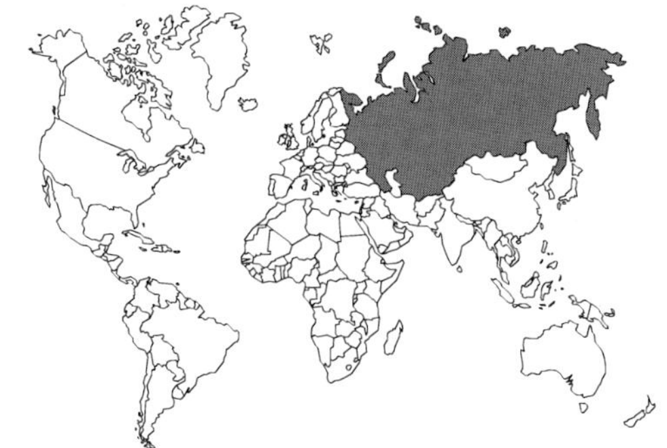

Fig. 2.104.

Opisthorchis felineus is found in Siberia, areas drained by the Danube in Europe, and the Volga in Russia.

Location in Host

Gallbladder and bile ducts; occasionally in the pancreatic duct or the small intestine.

Parasite Identification

Opisthorchis felineus is similar to *Clonorchis sinensis,* the most obvious difference is the difference in the amount of branching of the testes. Those of *Clonorchis* are highly branched, while those of *Opisthorchis* are lobed. The adults of *Opisthorchis felineus* differ from those of *Opisthorchis viverrini* mainly in larval development and morphology; however, the eggs of *Opisthorchis felineus* are 30 by 11 μm, while those of *Opisthorchis viverrini* are 27 by 15 μm. Specimens of the genus *Metorchis* have much wider bodies and spherical testes. In the genus *Parametorchis,* the flukes have vitellaria that become confluent in the anterior body. In specimens of *Pseudamphistomum* the posterior end of the body is squared off, giving the ventral surface of the body the appearance of being a pseudo hold-fast structure.

Life Cycle

The life cycle is very similar to that of *Clonorchis sinensis.* The eggs hatch only after they are ingested by the appropriate snail (*Bithynia leachi*). Ultimately a cercaria develops that has eyespots and a large tail fin. The cercaria penetrates a freshwater fish, typically of the carp family, between the scales and encysts as a metacercaria within the muscles. Cats become infected by eating infected fish. Once eaten, the fluke migrates through the ampulla of Vater into the bile ducts where it matures (Vogel, 1934).

Clinical Presentation and Pathogenesis

Little attention has been given to the pathological manifestations that take place within the feline host. It is expected that the changes will be similar to those observed in human beings infected with this parasite. Besides cirrhosis due to periportal fibrosis, there have also been reports of bile stones forming around eggs, causing cholecystitis.

As the periportal fibrosis continues, there will be the development of edema and ascites.

Treatment

Praziquantel is likely to prove successful in eliminating these trematodes from many treated cases.

Epizootiology

Cats are a major host of this pathogen. Throughout Europe, Siberia, and the Ukraine, infections of cats with *Opisthorchis felineus* are not uncommon. In some parts of the parasite's range, the infection is maintained mainly in the human population, and improved sanitation among the human hosts will reduce the transmission of the parasite. Other hosts that have been reported to support the development of this parasite include dogs, foxes, pigs, martens, wolverines, polecats, gray seals, and bearded seals.

Hazards to Other Animals

Dogs and other fish-eating mammals can also be infected with this parasite.

Hazards to Humans

Large numbers of human beings are infected with this parasite in the geographical regions where it is found.

Control/Prevention

Prevent the ingestion of infected raw, dried, or pickled fish; drying and pickling are not necessarily going to kill the metacercarial stage of the trematode.

REFERENCES

Vogel H. 1934. Der Entwicklungszyklus von *Opisthorchis felineus* (Riv.) nebst Bemerkungen über Systematik und Epidemioloie. Zoologica 33:1–103.

Opisthorchis viverrini (Poirier, 1886) Stiles and Hassall, 1896

Opistho = posterior and *orchis* = testis along with *viverrini* representing the host from which it was originally described, *Felis viverrus.*

The adult *Opisthorchis viverrini* is morphologically very similar to and almost indistinguishable from *Opisthorchis felineus;* there are, however, morphological differences in the larval stages. This trematode is a common problem in Thailand, where in some villages infections in human populations may be as high as 94 percent (Upatham et al., 1982). The infection also occurs in Laos, Malaysia, and India. In Thailand, cats are found infected with this parasite even in areas where human infections are uncommon (Sadun, 1955); in 1965, 60 percent of cats sampled in the northeastern part of the country were infected. The second intermediate host is a freshwater fish, and the infection is obtained by eating raw fish. Infections in humans have led to carcinoma of the bile ducts (Wykoff et al., 1966). Fecal examinations have shown that infected cats shed from 358 to 3,509 eggs per adult worm per day; 16 naturally infected cats were found to harbor an average of 99 worms per cat (Wykoff and Ariyaprakai, 1966).

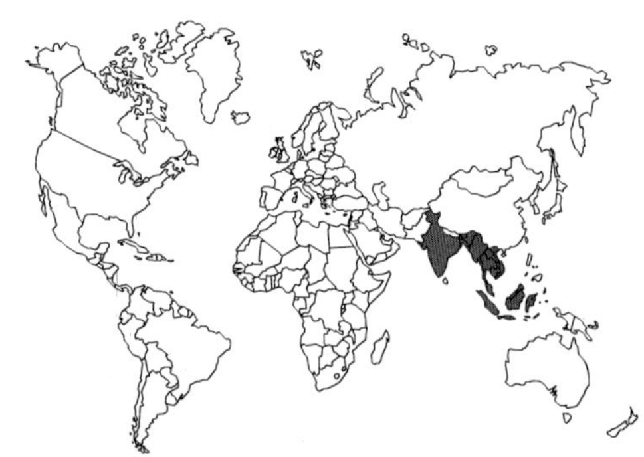

Fig. 2.105.

REFERENCES

Sadun EH. 1955. Studies on *Opisthorchis viverrini* in Thailand. Am J Hyg 62:81–115.

Upatham ES, Viyanant V, Kurathong S, Brockelman WY, Menaruchi A, Saowakontha S, Intarakhao C, Vajrasthira S, Warren KS. 1982. Morbidity in relation to intensity of infection in opisthorchiasis viverrin: study of a community in Khon Kaen, Thailand. Am J Trop Med Hyg 31:1156–1163.

Wykoff DE, Ariyaprakai K. 1966. *Opisthorchis viverrini* in Thailand—egg production in man and laboratory animals. J Parasitol 52:631.

Wykoff DE, Chittaysothorn K, Winn MM. 1966. Clinical manifestations of *Opisthorchis viverrini* infections in Thailand. Am J Trop Med Hyg 15:914–918.

Opisthorchis chabaudi Bourgat and Kulo, 1977

Opisthorchis chabaudi was described from specimens collected from an experimentally infected cat in Togo, Africa (Bourgat, 1977). The cats were infected with metacercariae from frogs that had been experimentally infected with cercariae from naturally infected snails. The typical definitive host of this parasite in Togo is not known.

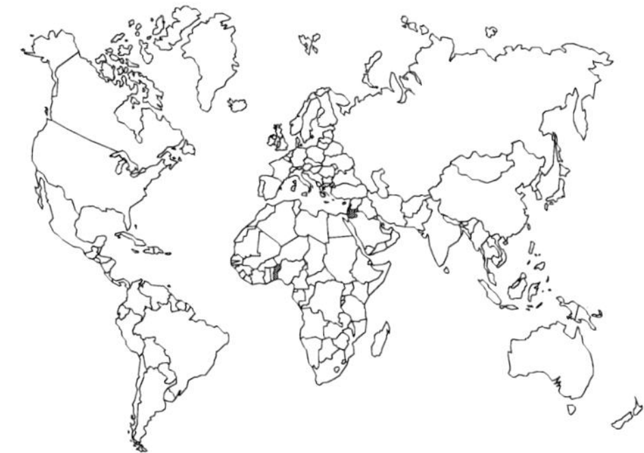

Fig. 2.106.

REFERENCES

Bourgat R, Kulo SD. 1977. Recherches expérimentales sur le cycle biologique d'*Opisthorchis chabaudi* n. sp. Description de l'adulte. Ann Parasitol 52:615–622.

Paropisthorchis caninus Stephens, 1912

Paropisthorchis caninus was described from material collected from a dog in India that was in the museum of the Liverpool School of Tropical Medicine (Stephens, 1912). It has been considered by some a synonym of a parasite described as *Distoma caninus* (Lewis and Cunningham, 1872). However, others have considered it a valid genus. It differs from other opisthorchids in that the ventral sucker and genital opening appear to be pedunculate (i.e., protruding from the body). This parasite was described once from a cat in India that was found dead on the side of a road and that had enlarged bile ducts and fibrosis of the liver (Bhatia et al., 1959).

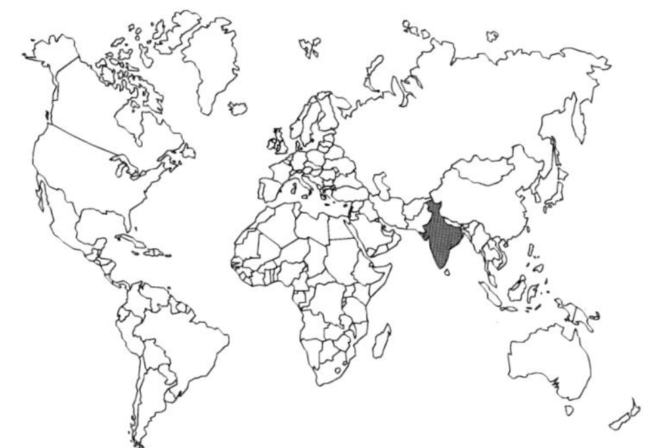

Fig. 2.107.

REFERENCES

Bhatia BB, Sood SM, Pande BP. 1959. An opisthorchid trematode from the domestic cat (*Felis catus domesticus*) with a report on three other helminths. In Vet J 36:528–531.

Stephens JWW. 1912. *Paropisthorchis caninus* the liver-fluke of the Indian non-descript dog. Ann Trop Med Parasitol 6:117–128.

Metorchis conjunctus (Cobbold, 1860) Looss, 1899

Etymology

Meta = posterior and *orchis* = testis along with *conjunctus* = joined.

Synonyms

Distoma conjunctum Cobbold, 1860; *Parametorchis noveboracensis* Hung, 1926; *Parametorchis intermedius* Price 1929; *Parametorchis canadensis* Price, 1929; *Parametorchis manitobensis* Allen and Wardle, 1934.

History

This trematode was originally described using specimens from the biliary ducts of a red fox that died in the Gardens of the British Zoological Society in London. Cameron (1944) examined the taxonomy of the genus *Metorchis* and stated that he believed there to only be three species: *Metorchis conjunctus* in North America, *Metorchis albidus* (Braun, 1893) Looss, 1899, in Europe and around the Mediterranean, and *Metorchis felis* Hsü, 1934, in Asia (*Metorchis felis* is considered here as a synonym of *Metorchis orientalis* Tanabe, 1919).

Geographic Distribution

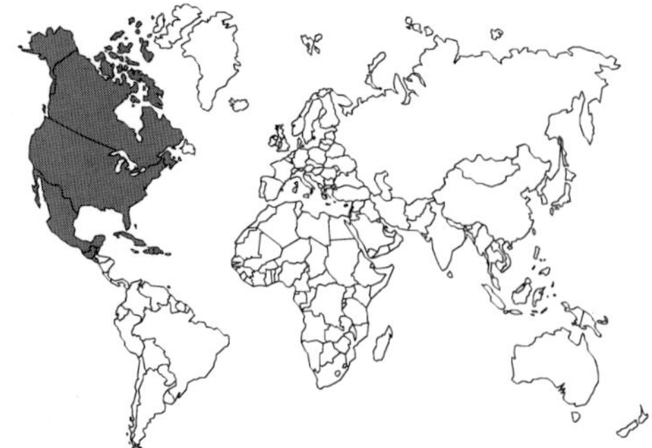

Fig. 2.108.

North America; most reports are from Canada and the northern parts of the United States. Under the name *Parametorchis noveboracensis,* the parasite was reported from a cat in Ithaca, New York (Hung, 1926), and it has been reported from a dog in South Carolina (Jordan and Ashby, 1957).

Location in Host

Bile ducts.

Parasite Identification

Specimens of *Metorchis* differ from those of *Amphimerus, Opisthorchis,* and *Clonorchis* in that the uterus is more bunched together, "rosettiform," than in *Opisthorchis* and has branches that encircle the ventral sucker. *Metorchis* species also tend to be broader than the opisthorchin relatives. The vitellaria of *Metorchis* are confined to the lateral margins of the body while in the genus *Parametorchis,* the vitellaria from the lateral sides become confluent anteriorly. In specimens of *Pseudamphistomum* the posterior end of the body is squared off, giving the ventral surface of the body the appearance of being a pseudo hold-fast structure.

Adult flukes measure from 1 to 6.6 mm in length with widths of 0.6 to 2.6 mm. The oral sucker is about the same size as the ventral sucker. The testes are situated in the third quarter of the body, tandem or slightly oblique, and tend to be round in outline. The eggs are yellowish brown, with a distinct operculum, and measure 22 to 32 μm long by 11 to 18 μm wide. The eggs contain an embryo when laid.

Life Cycle

Cameron (1944) examined the life cycle using material from Quebec, Canada. The snail hosts include specimens of *Anicola limosa.* The snail becomes infected when it ingests the egg. The cercaria is about 0.9 mm long, has a tail fin and eyespots, and has a potential life outside the snail of 60 to 72 hours. The cercariae enter and encyst in the muscles of freshwater fish (the common sucker, *Catostomus commersoni*), mainly the lateral muscles extending from the dorsal fin to the tail. In experimentally infected cats, eggs were found in the feces beginning 4 weeks after infection, and the flukes have been found capable of living in cats for at least 5 years.

Clinical Presentation and Pathogenesis

Watson and Croll (1981) reported the clinical changes in cats experimentally infected with *Metorchis conjunctus.* Cats given 200 metacercariae did not develop signs of infection, although they did display a marked eosinophilia and increased serum alanine aminotransferase and leucine aminopeptidase levels. In cats given 300 metacercariae, there were significant clinical signs that developed around patency (which in these studies was 17 days after infection). The cats occasionally developed icterus, bloody urine, and severe diarrhea that disappeared and then recurred over the next few months. The eosinophilia became much less obvious in chronic infections. Primary infections did not seem to prevent the establishment of secondary infections with this parasite. Hyperplasia of the biliary epithelium was the main pathology described in naturally infected cats from Ontario, Canada. (Mills and Hirth 1968).

Disease due to natural infections has been described. Axelson (1962) described lesions in the liver and bile ducts of a cat that also presented with lymphoma. Large numbers of flukes were present, with around 200 being in the gallbladder. The bile ducts were markedly enlarged, with signs of chronic cholangiohepatitis. Another case was described by Essex and Bollman (1930) where cirrhosis formed in a 5-year-old Persian cat from Rochester, Minnesota, due to a mixed infection with *Opisthorchis pseudofelineus* and *Metorchis complexus* (the photograph of the specimen clearly shows the vitellaria and indicates that this was actually an infection with *Metorchis conjunctus*). The cat became emaciated and developed ascites and jaundice. At necropsy, there was a hard, enlarged, grayish liver with no nodules on the surface. The walls of the bile ducts were thickened. The bile contained numerous trematode eggs. There was extensive hyperplasia of the entire biliary duct system and few normal hepatic cells in any histologic section of the liver.

Treatment

Praziquantel is likely to prove successful in eliminating these trematodes from many treated cases.

Epizootiology

Other hosts, including the red fox and the wolf, *Canis lupus,* have been found infected with this parasite (Wobeser et al., 1983). Other hosts include the raccoon, the gray fox, mink, and dogs. The range of the parasite seems to be restricted by the range of the snail intermediate host.

Hazards to Other Animals

Dogs and other fish-eating mammals can also be infected with this parasite.

Hazards to Humans

Cameron (1944) states that the eggs of this parasite were observed in the feces of a human being in Saskatchewan, Canada.

Control/Prevention

Prevent the ingestion of infected raw, dried, or pickled fish; drying and pickling are not necessarily going to kill the metacercarial stage of the trematode.

REFERENCES

Axelson RD. 1962. *Metorchis conjunctus* liver fluke infestation in a cat. Can Vet J 3:359–360.

Cameron TWM. 1944. The morphology, taxonomy, and life history of *Metorchis conjunctus* (Cobbold, 1860). Can J Res 22:6–16.

Essex HE, Bollman JL. 1930. Parasitic cirrhosis of the liver in a cat infected with *Opisthorchis pseudofelineus* and *Metorchis complexus.* Am J Trop Med 10:65–70.

Hung SL. 1926. A new species of fluke, *Parametorchis noveboracensis,* from the cat in the United States. Proc US Natl Mus 69:1–2.

Jordan HE, Ashby WT. 1957. Liver flukes (*Metorchis conjunctus*) in a dog from South Carolina. JAVMA 141:239–240.

Mills JHL, Hirth RS. 1968. Lesions caused by hepatic trematode, *Metorchis conjunctus,* Cobbold, 1860. A comparative study in carnivora. J Small Anim Pract 9:1–6.

Watson TG, Croll NA. 1981. Clinical changes caused by the liver fluke *Metorchis conjunctus* in cats. Vet Pathol 18:778–785.

Wobeser G, Runge W, Stewart RR. 1983. *Metorchis conjunctus* (Cobbold, 1860) infection in wolves (*Canis lupus*), with pancreatic involvement in two animals. J Wildl Dis 19:353–356.

Metorchis albidus (Braun, 1893) Looss, 1899

This fluke (Fig. 2.109) was described by Braun (1893) from the liver of the house cat. The species was transferred to the genus *Metorchis* by Looss in 1899. It has also been reported from foxes,

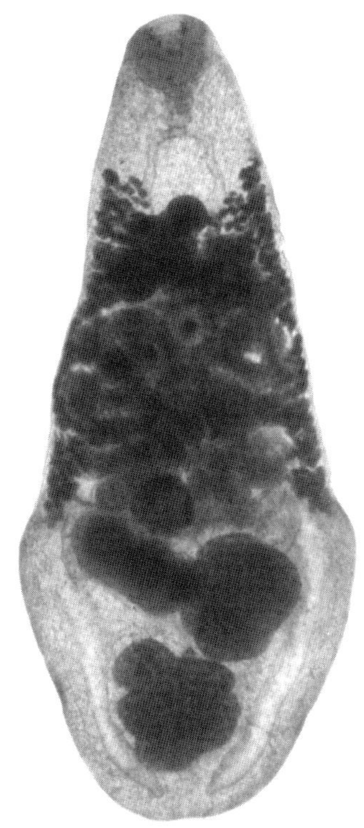

Fig. 2.109. *Metorchis albidus* from the liver of a cat in Königsberg, Germany. Note the spatulate shape of the body of this specimen. It is stated that the body of *Metorchis conjunctus* is more linguiform in shape. In the case of *Metorchis albidus* and *Metorchis conjunctus,* the vitellaria extend anterior to the uterine coils. This does not occur in the case of *Metorchis orientalis.*

dogs, and gray seals. There have been other reports in cats.

This species has been recovered from a cat in France used for teaching at the college of veterinary medicine in Alfort (Thiery, 1953). There was very little pathology associated with the infection of this animal. Histopathology on a cat from around Copenhagen, Denmark, revealed the infection with *Metorchis albidus* to have caused progressive icterus and cholangitis (Nielsen and Guidal, 1974).

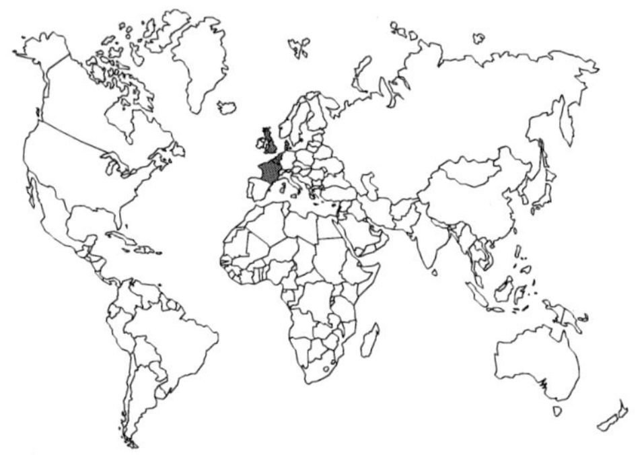

Fig. 2.110.

REFERENCES

Nielsen JCL, Guidal JA. 1974. Distomatose hos en kat forårsaget af ikten *Metorchis albidus* (Braun 1893) Loos 1899 (En kasuistisk meddelelse). Nord Vet Med 26:467–470.

Thiery G. 1953. Un parasite méconnu du chat: *Metorchis albidus*. Rec Med Vet 129:356–358.

Looss A. 1899. Weitere Beiträge zur Kenntnis der Trematodenfauna Aegyptens, zugleich Versuch einer natürlichen Gliederung des Genus *Distomum* Retzius. Zool Jahrb Syst 12:521-784.

Metorchis orientalis Tanabe, 1919

Metorchis orientalis (*Metorchis albidus* Hsü, 1934, is considered here to be a synonym) is probably the equivalent of *Metorchis albidus* and *Metorchis conjunctus* in Asia. It was originally described from a dog and cat in Japan and has since been described from Manchuria, China, and Formosa. The snail *Bulimus stiatulus* serves as the first intermediate host, and freshwater cyprinoid fish serve as the second intermediate hosts.

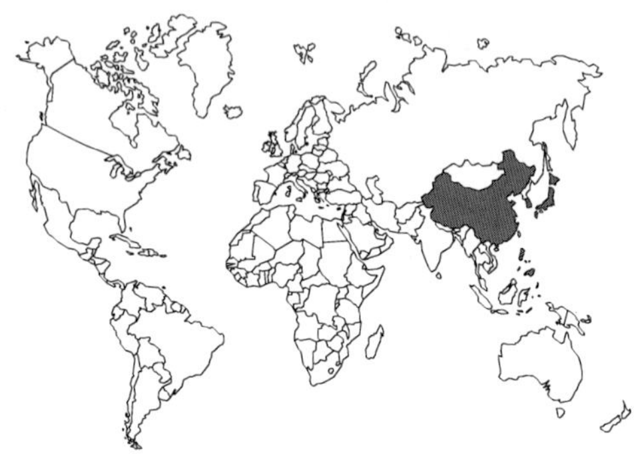

Fig. 2.111.

Parametorchis complexum (Stiles and Hassall, 1894) Skrjabin, 1913

Etymology

Para = near, *meta* = posterior and *orchis* = testis (thus, near *Metorchis*) along with *complexum* for the complex coiling of the uterus at the level of the acetabulum.

Synonyms

Distoma complexum Stiles and Hassal, 1894.

History

Parametorchis complexum was described from trematodes collected from cats in New York, Baltimore, and Washington, D.C. (Stiles and Hassall, 1894).

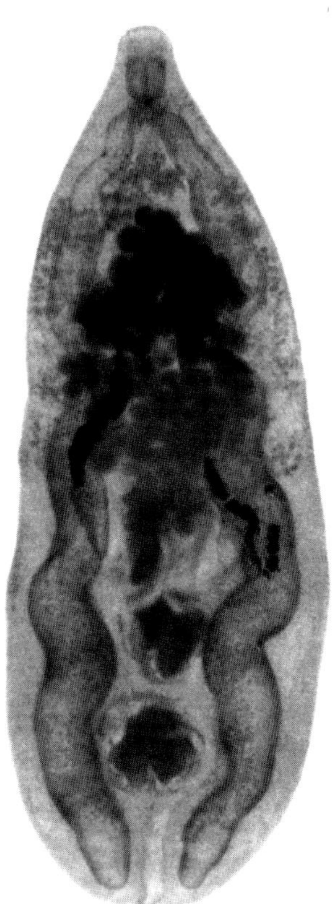

Fig. 2.112. *Parametorchis complexum* collected from a raccoon in Virginia. Although the vitellaria are rather light in this preparation, they can be observed to extend along the lateral sides of the trematode and to come together anterior to the dark, egg-filled uterus that fills the middle of the second fourth of the body.

Geographic Distribution

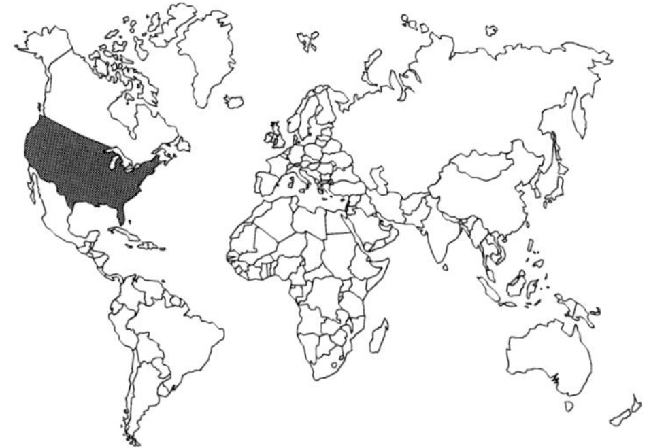

Fig. 2.113.

Northeastern United States; it was reported in 1965 from two cats in New Jersey (Burrows and Lillis, 1965).

Location in Host

Bile ducts.

Parasite Identification

Specimens of *Parametorchis* differ from those of *Metorchis* in that the vitelline glands on both sides of the body become confluent anterior to the ventral sucker.

Adult flukes measure from 5 to 7 mm in length with widths of 1.5 to 2 mm. The oral sucker is about the same size as the ventral sucker. The testes are situated in the third quarter of the body, tandem or slightly oblique, and tend to be lobate (3 to 8 lobes) in outline. The eggs measure 24 μm long by 12 μm wide.

Life Cycle

Not described.

Clinical Presentation and Pathogenesis

Not described.

Treatment

Praziquantel is likely to prove successful in eliminating these trematodes from many treated cases.

Epizootiology

Other hosts have not been described as infected with this parasite, including raccoons. It would appear that carnivores in Russia are infected with a related species.

Hazards to Other Animals

Not known.

Hazards to Humans

It is possible that humans could become infected if they were to ingest the infected intermediate host.

REFERENCES

Burrows RB, Lillis WG. 1965. Trematodes of New Jersey dogs and cats. J Parasitol 51:570–574.

Stiles CW, Hassall A. 1894. Notes on parasites—21. A new species of fluke (*Distoma* [*Dicrocoelium*] *complexum*) found in cats in the United States, with bibliographic and diagnoses of allied forms. Vet Mag 1:413–432.

Pseudamphistomum truncatum (Rudolphi, 1819) Lühe, 1909

This parasite has been described from the bile ducts of cats in Europe and India. The small trematode, 2 mm long, is found within the bile ducts. The parasite appears very similar to species of *Metorchis* and *Parametorchis* with the major difference being that the posterior end of the body appears abbreviated, "truncated," producing the appearance of a posterior sucking disk; hence the name meaning false amphistome. The life cycle was examined, and it was shown that it required a piscine intermediate host (Ciurea, 1917). There has been very little published on the disease or pathology induced by these worms.

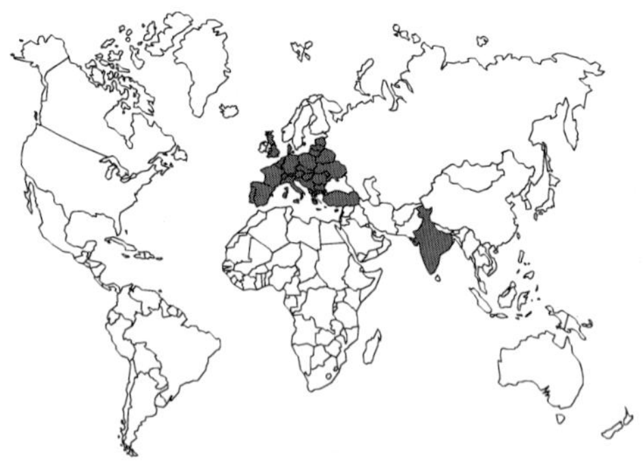

Fig. 2.114.

REFERENCES

Ciurea I. 1917. Die Auffindung der Larven von *Opisthorchis felineus, Pseudamphistomum danubiense* und *Metorchis albidus* und die morphologische Entwicklungung diser Larven zu den geschlechtsreifen Würmer. Ztschr Infk Haust 18:301–333.

ORCHIPEDIDAE
Orchipedum isostoma (Rudolphi, 1819)
TROGLOTREMATIDAE
Troglotrema mustelae Wallace, 1932

Fig. 2.115. Trematodes of the nasal fossae, or sinuses.

TREMATODES OF THE NASAL FOSSAE

Some trematodes normally live as adults in the nasal sinuses of their hosts (Fig. 2.115). There is every reason to believe that cats are capable of becoming infected with these trematodes if they eat infected intermediate hosts. However, there are no reports of this having occurred naturally.

ORCHIPEDIDAE

Orchipedum isostoma (Rudolphi, 1819)

Orchipedum isostoma has been shown in Africa to develop to adults in the frontal sinuses of cats fed crabs containing metacercariae. There was no discussion of the signs that may have developed in the infected cats.

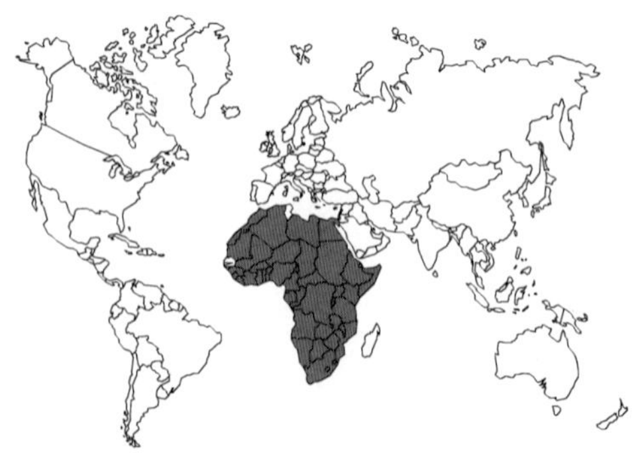

Fig. 2.116.

TROGLOTREMATIDAE

Troglotrema mustelae Wallace, 1932

Troglotrema mustelae was described by Wallace (1932), who showed that the cercariae have very short tails and become entrapped together in the water in balls of mucus. The metacercariae develop in the fins of freshwater catfish, *Ameiurus* species, and mature to the adult stage in carnivores, including the cat, in 5 days after having ingested a fish. A similar trematode, *Troglotrema acutum,* has been reported from the nasal sinuses of carnivores in Europe; this trematode has been reported to cause injury to the bones of the skull (Vogel and Voelker, 1978).

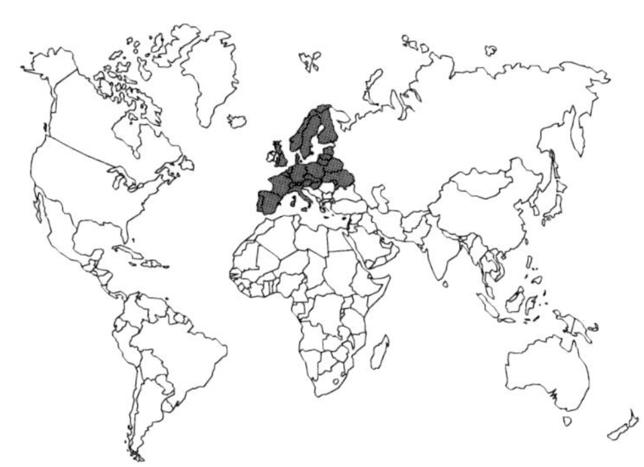

Fig. 2.117.

REFERENCES

Vogel H, Voelker J. 1978, Uber den Lebenszyklus von *Troglotrema acutum.* Tropenmed Parasitol 29:385–405.

Wallace FG. 1932. The life history of *Troglotrema mustelae* n. sp. J Parasitol 19:164.

TREMATODES OF THE LUNGS

Some trematodes develop to maturity in the lungs of their mammalian hosts (Fig. 2.118). The majority of these trematodes are in the genus *Paragonimus.* There are many different species within this genus. Miyazaki (1991) recognizes 28 species with 21 in Asia, 2 in Africa, and 5 from the Americas. All of these trematodes are parasites of the lungs as adults. Also, all are probably capable of developing within the cat. However, not all have been reported from the cat, with only 12 of the species being reported from this host. Typically cats become infected with these trematodes by the ingestion of an infected crustacean. The adults of *Paragonimus* are large, robust trematodes with thick bodies that are covered with spines. Typically they are found in cysts within the lungs that may contain anywhere from 1 to 10 adult flukes. These trematodes are capable of causing serious disease in the infected host. Again, as with the opisthorchids, some of these trematodes, especially *Paragonimus westermani,*

TROGLOTREMATIDAE
- *Paragonimus westermani* (Kerbert, 1878) Braun, 1899
- *Paragonimus pulmonalis* (Baelz, 1880) Miyazaki, 1978
- *Paragonimus miyazakii Kamo,* Nishida, Hatsushika, and Tomimura, 1961
- *Paragonimus heterotremus* Chen and Hsia, 1964
- *Paragonimus siamensis* Miyazaki and Wykoff, 1965
- *Paragonimus skrjabini* Chen, 1960
- *Paragonimus ohirai* Miyazaki, 1939
- *Paragonimus kellicotti* Ward, 1908
- *Paragonimus mexicanus* Miyazaki and Ishii, 1968
- *Paragonimus inca* Miyazaki, Mazabel, Grados, and Uyema, 1975
- *Paragonimus peruvianus* Miyazaki, Ibáñez, and Miranda
- *Paragoinimus caliensis* Little
- *Paragonimus amazonicus* Miyazaki, Grados, and Uyema
- *Paragonimus africanus* Voelker and Vogel, 1965
- *Paragonimus uterobilateralis* Voelker and Vogel, 1965

Fig. 2.118. Trematodes of the lungs.

cause serious disease in people, and therc is a great deal of literature on the subject in texts of human parasitology. An excellent concise summary of the different species causing disease in humans that is based on first-hand knowledge is found in Miyazaki's text *Helminthic Zoonoses*.

REFERENCES

Miyazaki I. 1991. Helminthic Zoonoses. Fukuoka, Japan: International Medical Foundation of Japan. 494 pp.

TROGLOTREMATIDAE

Paragonimus westermani (Kerbert, 1878) Braun, 1899

Etymology

Para = side-by-side and *gonimus* = gonads along with *westerman* for Dr. Westerman the curator of the Zoo in Amsterdam who submitted the original specimens to Dr. Kerbert for identification.

Synonyms

Distoma westermani Kerbert, 1878; *Distoma ringeri* Cobbold, 1880; *Distoma pulmonum* Baelz, 1881; *Distoma pulmonis* Kiyona, 1881; *Mesogonimus westermani* Railliet, 1890; *Polysarcus westermanni* Lühe, 1899.

History

Paragonimus westermani specimens that were recovered from Indian tigers that died in zoos in Amsterdam and Hamburg were described as *Distoma westermani.* At the same time parasites were observed by Drs. Manson, Ringer, and Cobbold that were described as a new species *Distoma ringeri.* Braun in 1899 created the genus *Paragonimus* in which he placed *Paragonimus westermani.*

Geographic Distribution

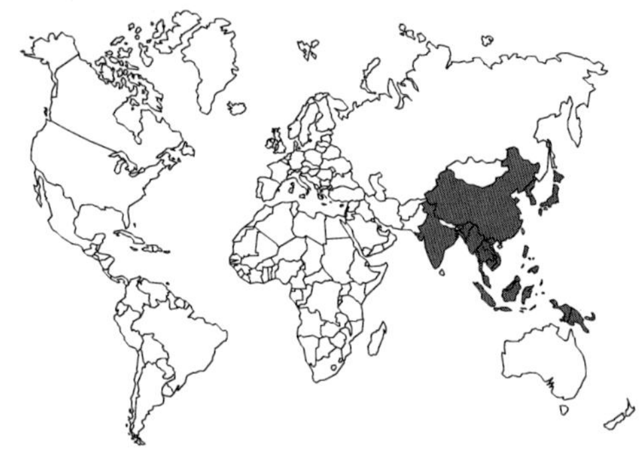

Fig. 2.120.

Paragonimus westermani is found in southeastern Siberia, Japan, and Korea through China, Taiwan, and the Philippines, through Indonesia, Malaysia, and Thailand, and into India and Sri Lanka.

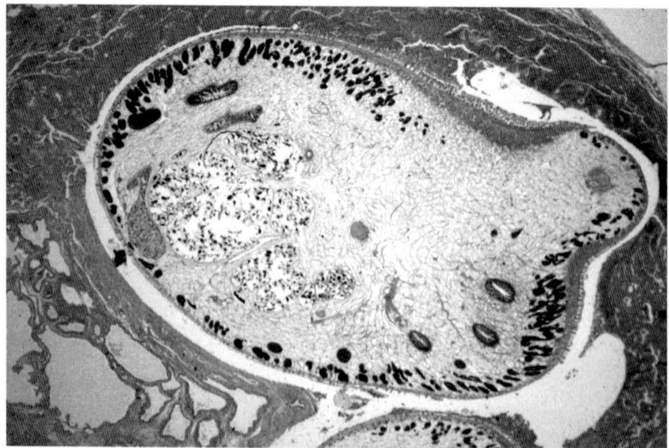

Fig. 2.119. *Paragonimus westermani* in the lung of a rhesus monkey. Sections through two adults can be observed in this cyst. (The one adult is just visible at the bottom edge of the photograph.)

Location in Host

In cysts in the lungs.

Parasite Identification

Species of *Paragonimus* are 7 to 12 mm long, 4 to 8 mm wide, and quite thick (i.e., 4 to 6 mm). *Paragonimus westermani* differs from other species of *Paragonimus* in Asia in that specimens of *Paragonimus pulmonalis* reproduce parthenogenetically and have no sperm in the seminal receptacle; specimens of *Paragonimus miyazakii* are more slender than *Paragonimus westermani* and *Paragonimus pulmonalis,* have a ventral sucker that is slightly larger than the oral sucker, and have more lobes on the ovary and testis; specimens of *Paragonimus heterotremus* have an oral sucker that is about twice the diameter of the ventral sucker (in most species they are approximately the same size); specimens of *Paragonimus skrjabini* tend to be more elongate with a tapered posterior end, and the ventral sucker is somewhat anteriad; specimens of *Paragonimus ohirai* are characterized by having the spines on the body surface appearing in groups or clusters rather than being singularly spaced.

The eggs of *Paragonimus westermani* have a brown shell, a distinct operculum, and occasionally a knob on the abopercular end; eggs range from 70 to 100 μm in length by 39 to 55 μm in width.

In Korea, work has been performed that has shown that ELISAs using both crude and purified antigens of *Paragonimus westermani* show promise for the identification of infections in cats (Lee and Chang, 1987; Choi et al., 1987). Specific antibody levels were significantly increased by 2 to 3 weeks after infection, and they remained elevated for up to 6 months. After treatment, specific antibody returned to baseline levels.

Life Cycle

The adult flukes lay eggs that are coughed up with sputum and then swallowed to be passed in the feces. After the feces enter fresh water, it takes about 2 weeks for the eggs to mature and for the miracidia to hatch. The free-swimming miracidia infect a species of snail within the genera *Brotia* or *Semisulcospira.* The second intermediate hosts are freshwater crabs (*Sinopotamon, Candidiopotamon, Sundathelphusa, Parathelphusa, Geohelphusa,* and *Ranguna*) and crayfish (*Cambaroides*). The second intermediate hosts typically become infected when they eat an infected snail that harbors cercariae that are characterized by a very short tail and a pronounced stylet associated with the oral sucker. The metacercariae of *Paragonimus westermani* are slightly smaller than those of *Paragonimus pulmonalis,* measuring about 0.35 mm in diameter; the metacercariae are found in the gills and the muscles. When ingested, the metacercariae migrate through the intestinal wall into the abdominal cavity. After several days in the abdominal cavity, the worms migrate through the diaphragm into the lungs where they develop to adult worms, typically in pairs. Infections become patent in 65 to 90 days, and in humans, patent infections have been maintained for up to 20 years. Pigs have been shown to serve as paratenic hosts, and it is possible that small rodents may also serve in this fashion. In these hosts, the young flukes are found distributed throughout the muscle tissues.

Clinical Presentation and Pathogenesis

Infections in cats produce signs that are markedly less severe than infections in human beings or other primates with similar numbers of worms (Yokogawa et al., 1960). Initially the young flukes appear to migrate about the abdominal cavity at random, causing hemorrhagic lesions in the liver and intestinal wall. Also, there are marked hemorrhagic lesions in the diaphragm, and at 20 to 30 days after infection, holes appear in the tendinous portion and at the edge of the muscular portions of the diaphragm, which indicates the passage of larger flukes. Experimentally infected cats have died of hemorrhage into the pleural cavity. The lung parenchymal nodules that develop in cats are more clearly circumscribed than those that develop in humans. In cats with heavy natural infections, there is extensive injury to the lung parenchyma and the pleura and enlargement of the lymphatic tissues. The pleura becomes thickened and fibrotic, and the lungs develop atelectasis and fibrosis. Eggs become widely scattered in the lung tissues and are present in the lymph nodes of the pleural cavity (Kau and Wu, 1936 [from

Yokogawa et al., 1960]). Cats infected with *Paragonimus westermani* may also have small numbers of eggs in other tissues, including the cerebrum, cerebellum, and myocardium (Shigemi, 1957 [from Yokogawa et al., 1960]).

Paragonimus westermani differs from *Paragonimus pulmonalis* in that more than a single worm is required for the production of fertilized eggs. Thus, if a cat is infected with a single metacercaria of *Paragonimus westermani,* the young fluke will not mature and will often continue to migrate around in the pleural cavity laying eggs that are not capable of developing mature miracidia (Miyazaki, 1991). This might mean that cats with single worm infections are more likely to develop lesions in ectopic sites.

Treatment

A cat from mainland China was treated with praziquantel for *Paragonimus westermani.* The cat was passing 11,390 eggs per gram of feces prior to treatment; it was treated with 100 mg of praziquantel per kilogram daily for 2 days. No eggs were detected in the feces of the cat 15 and 30 days after treatment (Cao et al., 1984). Experimentally infected cats have also been successfully treated with praziquantel (Choi et al., 1987).

Epizootiology

Numerous mammals are capable of being infected with *Paragonimus westermani.* The host that harbors the largest numbers of parasites is the tiger. In a survey performed in Sumatra, Indonesia, all of 10 tigers that were examined were infected, and 1 tiger had a total of 1,596 flukes in its lungs (Kwo and Miyazaki, 1968). Other hosts that have been naturally infected include dogs, foxes, pigs, raccoon dogs, various members of the cat family, civets, mongooses, and crab-eating macaques.

Hazards to Other Animals

If mammals ingest the infected crab, there is a possibility that larval flukes will penetrate the intestinal wall and migrate into the abdominal cavity. In permissive hosts, the flukes will go on to develop in the lungs, while in other hosts the flukes will persist in the abdominal cavity as in the swine paratenic host. In all these hosts, there is the possibility for associated pathology.

Hazards to Humans

Many human beings are infected with this parasite; infections are obtained by eating raw or undercooked crabs or meat of the swine paratenic host. Symptoms from the lung lesions can be severe. Similarly, the migration of worms to ectopic locations, such as the brain, can cause severe pathology. Cats are considered a major source of eggs in the environment.

REFERENCES

Cao WJ, He LY, Zhong HL, Xu ZS, Bi YC, Yu GT, Zhang QC, Li KC, Yang EV, She G, Li HJ. 1984. Paragonimiasis: treatment with praziquantel in 40 human cases and in 1 cat. Drug Res 34:1203–1204.

Choi WY, Yoo JE, Nam HW, Choi HR. 1987. Purification of antigenic proteins of *Paragonimus westermani* and their applicability to experimental cat paragonimiasis. Korean J Parasitol 24:177–186.

Kwo EH, Miyazaki I. 1968. *Paragonimus westermani* (Kerbert, 1878) from tigers in North Sumatra, Indonesia. J Parasitol 54:630.

Lee OR, Chang JK. 1987. ELISA of paragonimiasis in cat by crude and purified antigens of *Paragonimus westermani.* Korean J Parasitol 24:187–193.

Miyazaki I. 1991. Helminthic Zoonoses. Fukuoka, Japan: International Medical Foundation of Japan. 494 pp.

Yokogawa S, Cort WW, Yokogawa M. 1960. *Paragonimus* and Paragonimiasis. Exp Parasitol 10:81–205.

Paragonimus pulmonalis (Baelz, 1880) Miyazaki, 1978

Etymology

Para = side-by-side and *gonimus* = gonads along with *pulmonalis* for the location in the lung.

Synonyms

Distoma pulmonale Baelz, 1883.

History

Paragonimus pulmonalis was resurrected as a separate species by Miyazaki (1978). Miyazaki reported that *Paragonimus pulmonalis* was a triploid organism that reproduced by parthenogenesis, while *Paragonimus westermani* was diploid and reproduced sexually. Baelz, while he was a professor at the Tokyo Medical School in Japan, first saw the eggs of this parasite in 1880 in patients with pulmonary tuberculosis. Several years later, he realized that he was dealing with a trematode.

Geographic Distribution

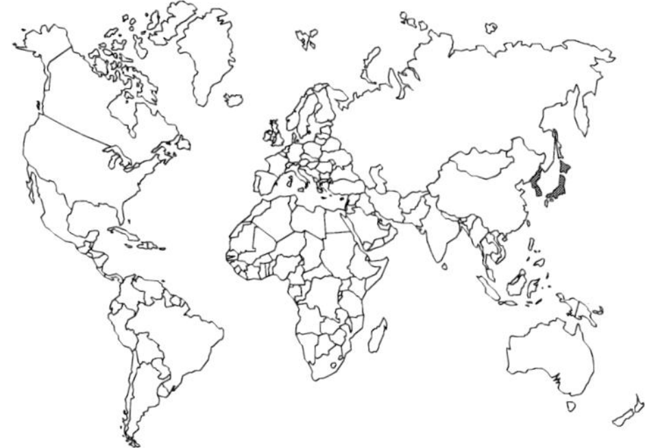

Fig. 2.121.

Paragonimus pulmonalis is found in Japan, Korea, and Taiwan. Miyazaki (1991) believes that *Paragonimus pulmonalis* is restricted to low-lying areas, while *Paragonimus westermani* is found in the mountainous areas of Japan and Taiwan.

Location in Host

In cysts in the lungs.

Parasite Identification

Species of *Paragonimus* are 7 to 12 mm long, 4 to 8 mm wide, and quite thick (i.e., 4 to 6 mm). For differentiation of the Asian species see *Paragonimus westermani.*

The eggs have a brown shell, a distinct operculum, and occasionally a knob on the abopercular end; eggs range from 85 to 100 μm in length by 40 to 58 μm in width and tend to be larger on the whole than those of *Paragonimus westermani.*

Life Cycle

The life cycle of *Paragonimus pulmonalis* is similar to that of *Paragonimus westermani,* with several marked distinctions. The second intermediate hosts are the freshwater crabs *Eriocheir japonicus* and *Eriocheir sinensis* and the freshwater crayfish *Cambaroides similis. Paragonimus pulmonalis* adults are parthenogenetic, and they do not, therefore, require a mate within a cyst in order to produce viable offspring. Thus, the tendency to localize in extrapulmonary sites is less than with other *Paragonimus* species.

Clinical Presentation and Pathogenesis

The signs are similar to those of *Paragonimus westermani;* the major difference is that these worms are capable of producing eggs when single in cysts. Infection of kittens with single metacercaria produced infections in 14 of 20 animals (Fan and Chiang, 1970). In 11 of the 14 cats that developed infections, the worms matured to egg-producing adults; in the remaining 3 animals the flukes remained immature.

Treatment

It has not been tried, but it is very likely that praziquantel would be a very successful treatment.

Epizootiology

Adults of *Paragonimus pulmonalis* has been reported from the lungs of dogs and cats and as larvae from the muscle of pigs; it has not been found in raccoon dogs or foxes (Miyazaki, 1991). Adults of this parasite have also been recovered from a tiger in Korea.

Hazards to Other Animals

If mammals ingest the infected crab, there is a possibility that larval flukes will penetrate the intestinal wall and migrate into the abdominal cavity. In permissive hosts, the flukes will go on to develop in the lungs, while in other hosts the flukes will persist in the abdominal cavity as in the swine paratenic host. In all these hosts, there is the possibility for associated pathology.

Hazards to Humans

Many human beings are infected with this parasite; infections are obtained by eating raw or undercooked crabs or meat of the swine paratenic host. Symptoms from the lung lesions can be severe. Similarly, the migration of worms to ectopic locations, such as the brain, can cause severe pathology. Cats are considered a major source of eggs in the environment.

REFERENCES

Fan PC, Chiang CH. 1970. Exposure of kittens and puppies to single metacercariae of *Paragonimus westermani* from Taiwan. J Parasitol 56:48–54.

Miyazaki I. 1991. Helminthic Zoonoses. Fukuoka, Japan: International Medical Foundation of Japan. 494 pp.

Paragonimus miyazakii Kamo, Nishida, Hatsushika, and Tomimura, 1961

Etymology

Para = side-by-side and *gonimus* = gonads along with *miyazakii* = for Dr. Miyazaki's lifelong efforts in the study of paragonimiasis.

Synonyms

None.

History

Paragonimus miyazakii was described based on specimens recovered from a weasel in Japan and initially considered to possibly be *Paragonimus kellicotti.* Kamo et al. (1961) found a different metacercaria of a *Paragonimus* type and after growing the flukes to maturity experimentally showed that it was a new species.

Geographic Distribution

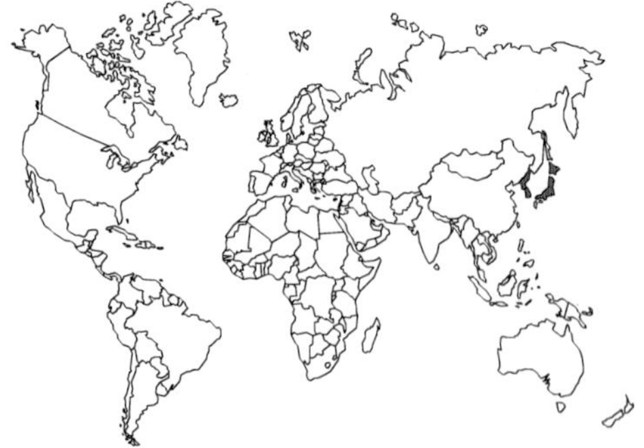

Fig. 2.122.

Japan.

Location in Host

In cysts in the lungs.

Parasite Identification

Species of *Paragonimus* are 7 to 12 mm long, 4 to 8 mm wide, and quite thick (i.e., 4 to 6 mm). For differentiation of the Asian species see *Paragonimus westermani.*

The eggs have a thin brown shell, a distinct operculum, and occasionally a knob on the abopercular end; eggs range from 75 μm in length by 43 μm in width and tend to be larger on the whole than those of *Paragonimus westermani.*

Life Cycle

The life cycle is similar to that of *Paragonimus westermani.* The first intermediate host is the snail *Bithynella nipponica.* The second intermediate host is a freshwater crab, *Geothelphusa dehaani,* in which the metacercariae are found in blood vessels around the heart. The metacercariae of *Paragonimus miyazakii* are larger than those of the other Asian species of *Paragonimus,* being about 0.5 mm in diameter. In cats fed 40 to 50 metacercariae, patent infections developed 51 to 52 days after infection (Tomimura et al., 1964 [cited in Miyazaki, 1991]).

Clinical Presentation and Pathogenesis

The presentation of infection in cats appears similar to that of *Paragonimus westermani.* In human hosts, outbreaks have tended to induce pleural rather than pulmonary manifestations.

Treatment

Probably praziquantel.

Epizootiology

Infected mammalian hosts other than the cat include dogs, weasels, sables, pigs, raccoon dogs, and badgers. These hosts are becoming infected by the ingestion of infected crabs.

Hazards to Other Animals

If mammals ingest the infected crab, there is a possibility that larval flukes will penetrate the intestinal wall and migrate into the abdominal cavity. In permissive hosts, the flukes will go on to develop in the lungs, while in other hosts the flukes will persist in the abdominal cavity as in the swine paratenic host. In all these hosts, there is the possibility for associated pathology.

Hazards to Humans

Human outbreaks have occurred with this infection due to the ingestion of raw or inadequately cooked crabs. The first known outbreak of infection with this parasite occurred in 1974 and was characterized by a large number of patients who had signs of fluke infection within the pleural cavity without eggs being present in the sputum.

REFERENCES

Kamo H, Nishida H, Hatsushika R, Tomimura T. 1961. On the occurrence of a new lung fluke, *Paragonimus miyazakii* n. sp. in Japan. (Trematoda: Troglotrematidae). Yonago Acta Medica 5:43–52.

Miyazaki I. 1978. Two types of the lung fluke which has been called *Paragonimus westermani* (Kerbert, 1878). Med Bull Fukuoka Univ 5:251–263.

Miyazaki I. 1991. Helminthic Zoonoses. Fukuoka, Japan: International Medical Foundation of Japan. 494 pp.

Paragonimus heterotremus Chen and Hsia, 1964

Etymology

Para = side-by-side and *gonimus* = gonads along with *heterotremus* referring to the different-sized oral and ventral suckers.

Synonyms

Paragonimus tuanshanensis Chung, Ho, Cheng, and Tsao, 1964.

History

This fluke was first found in rats in China. That same year, another group of workers described *Paragonimus tuanshanensis.*

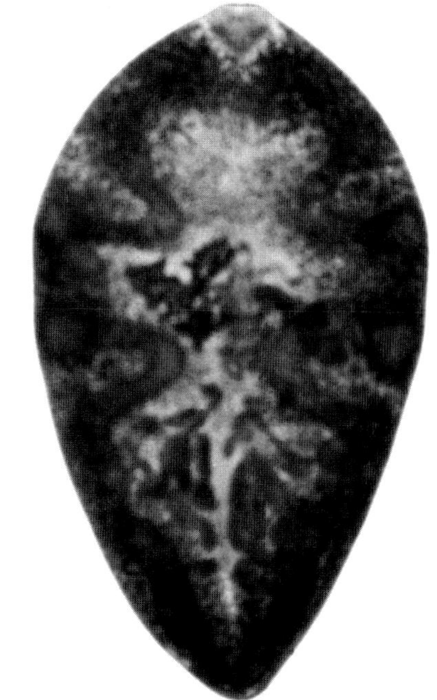

Fig. 2.123. *Paragonimus heterotremus* from the lung of a cat in Thailand. Note the large oral sucker.

Geographic Distribution

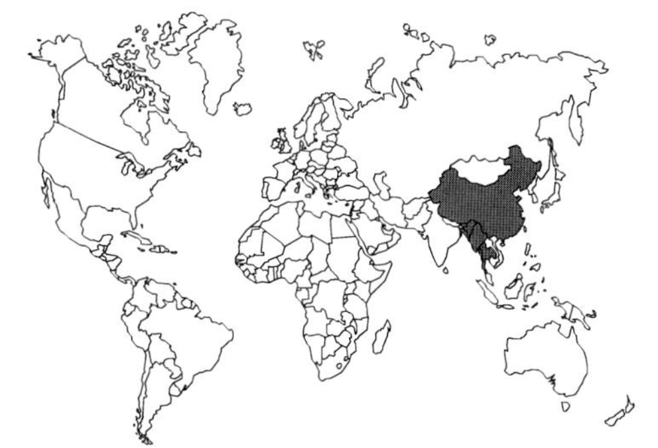

Fig. 2.124.

China, Thailand, and Laos.

Location in Host

In cysts in the lungs.

Parasite Identification

Species of *Paragonimus* are 7 to 12 mm long, 4 to 8 mm wide, and quite thick (i.e., 4 to 6 mm). *Paragonimus heterotremus* differs from other species of *Paragonimus* in Asia in that the oral sucker is larger than the ventral sucker.

The eggs have a brown shell, a distinct operculum, and occasionally a knob on the abopercular end; eggs are about 86 μm in length by 48 μm in width.

Life Cycle

The life cycle is basically the same as that of *Paragonimus westermani.* A snail intermediate host identified in China is *Tricula gregoriana.* The crab hosts that are used are *Ranguna smithiana* and *Parathelphus dugasti* in Thailand and *Sinopotamon* in China. The metacercariae are found in the liver, muscles, and gills of these crabs and are rather small (i.e., about 0.25 mm in diameter).

Clinical Presentation and Pathogenesis

Probably similar to the other species of *Paragonimus.* The death of a cat naturally infected with 13 of these flukes has been reported (Miyazaki and Vajrasthira, 1967).

Treatment

Probably praziquantel.

Epizootiology

Hosts include cats, dogs, leopards, rats, and bandicoots.

Hazards to Other Animals

If mammals ingest the infected crab, there is a possibility that larval flukes will penetrate the intestinal wall and migrate into the abdominal cavity. In permissive hosts, the flukes will go on to develop in the lungs, while in other hosts the flukes will persist in the abdominal cavity as in the swine paratenic host. In all these hosts, there is the possibility for associated pathology.

Hazards to Humans

Human beings have been infected with this trematode. Besides the typical pulmonary lesions, flukes have been recovered from subcutaneous tissues (Miyazaki and Harinasuta, 1966).

REFERENCES

Miyazaki I, Harinasuta T. 1966. The first case of human paragonimiasis caused by *Paragonimus heterotremus* Chen et Hsia, 1964. Ann Trop Med Parasitol 60:509–514.

Miyazaki I, Vajrasthira S. 1967. Occurrence of the lung fluke *Paragonimus heterotremus* Chen et Hsiua, 1964, in Thailand. J Parasitol 53:207.

Paragonimus siamensis Miyazaki and Wykoff, 1965

Paragonimus siamensis has been recovered from cats and freshwater crabs in Thailand (Miyazaki and Wykoff, 1965). This parasite has also been found in cats in the Philippines (Cabrera and Vajrathira, 1973). The metacercarial stage of this trematode is larger than that of *Paragonimus heterotremus.*

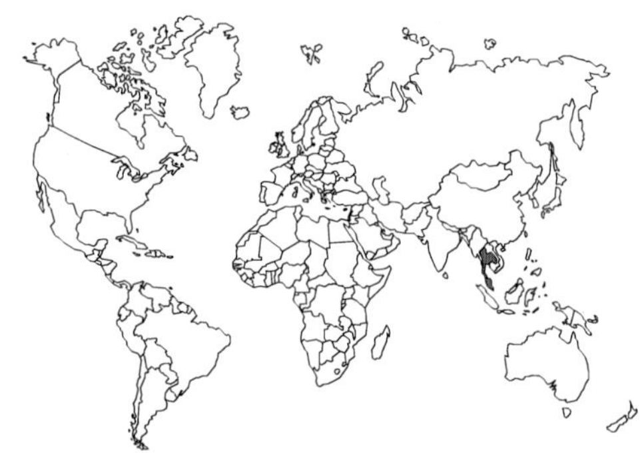

Fig. 2.125.

REFERENCES

Cabrera BD, Vajrathira S. 1973. Endemicity of *Paragonimus siamensis* Miyazaki and Wykoff 1965, the second species of lung flukes found in the Republic of the Philippines. J Philipp Med Assoc 49:385–398.

Miyazaki I, Wykoff DE. 1965. On a new lung fluke *Paragonimus siamensis* n. sp. found in Thailand (Trematoda: Troglotrematidae). Jap J Parasitol 14:251.

Yaemput S, Dekumyoy P, Visiassuk K. 1994. The natural first intermediate host of *Paragonimus siamensis* (Miyazaki and Wykoff, 1965) in Thailand. Southeast Asia J Trop Med Publ Health 25:284–290.

Paragonimus skrjabini Chen, 1960

Etymology

Para = side-by-side and *gonimus* = gonads along with *skrjabini* for Dr. Skrjabin, a Russian helminthologist.

Synonyms

Paragonimus szechuanensis Chung and Tsao, 1962.

History

Paragonimus skrjabini was described from a civet, *Paguma larvata,* in China. Chung and Tsao (1962) found the same worm in a cat and described it as a separate species.

Geographic Distribution

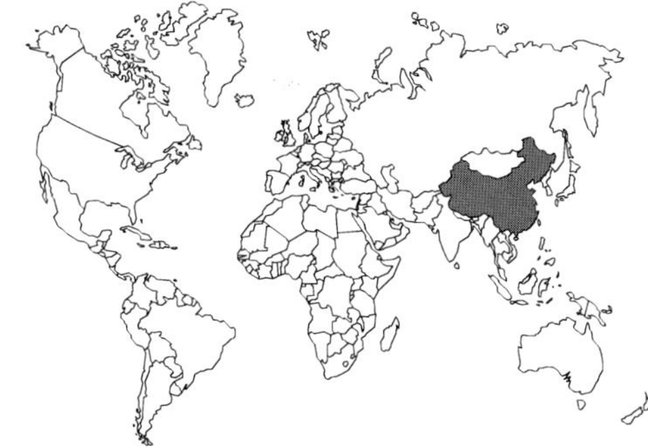

Fig. 2.126.

China.

Location in Host

In cysts in the lungs.

Parasite Identification

Species of *Paragonimus* are 7 to 12 mm long, 4 to 8 mm wide, and quite thick (i.e., 4 to 6 mm). Differentiation of the Asian species of *Paragonimus* is discussed under *Paragonimus westermani.*

The eggs have a brown shell, a distinct operculum, and occasionally a knob on the abopercular end; eggs average 80 by 48 μm.

Life Cycle

Similar to that of *Paragonimus westermani.* The snail hosts are species of *Tricula* and *Akiyoshia,* and the crab hosts are species of *Sinopotamon.*

Clinical Presentation and Pathogenesis

Not described in cats.

Treatment

Probably praziquantel.

Epizootiology

Hosts include civets, cats, and dogs.

Hazards to Other Animals

If mammals ingest the infected crab, there is a possibility that larval flukes will penetrate the intestinal wall and migrate into the abdominal cavity. In permissive hosts, the flukes will go on to develop in the lungs, while in other hosts the flukes will persist in the abdominal cavity as in the swine paratenic host. In all these hosts, there is the possibility for associated pathology.

Hazards to Humans

Human infections with *Paragonimus skrjabini* often present with flukes in ectopic locations, especially in subcutaneous tissues.

REFERENCES

Chen HT. 1960. Taxonomic consideration of *Paragonimus,* including morphological notes on *P. skrjabini.* Acta Zoologica Sinica 12:27–36.

Chung HL, Tsao WC. 1962. *Paragonimus westermani* (Szechuan variety) and a new species of lung fluke—*Paragonimus szechuanensis.* Part I. Studies on morphological and life history of paragonimiasis szechuanensis—a new clinical entity. Chin Med J 81:419–434.

Paragonimus ohirai Miyazaki, 1939

Paragonimus ohirai is found in Japan, Okinawa, Korea, Taiwan, and China, where it tends to be distributed around the mouths of rivers. The life cycle is typical of the other species of *Paragonimus.* The final hosts are rats and other mammals, including the cat; infections in humans are rare. The snail hosts tend to be localized in the regions in which they are found, as are the brackish-water crab hosts. These flukes differ from the other Asian species of *Paragonimus* in that the spines on the body occur in clusters rather than being single.

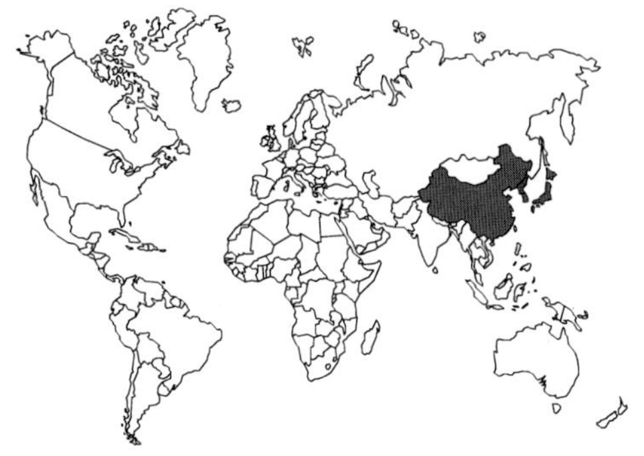

Fig. 2.127.

Paragonimus kellicotti Ward, 1908

Etymology

Para = side-by-side and *gonimus* = gonads along with *kellicotti* for Dr. Kellicott of Ohio State University, who described specimens of this parasite from the lungs of a dog and sent them to Dr. Ward for further identification.

Synonyms

None, although initially it was thought that it might be *Paragonimus westermani* introduced into North America.

History

This parasite was first observed by a Mr. W.A. Kirkland of the Zoology Laboratory of the University of Michigan, who found these trematodes in a cat from Ann Arbor, Michigan. The material was passed onto Dr. Ward, who several years later (1908) described the parasite as *Paragonimus kellicotti.*

Geographic Distribution

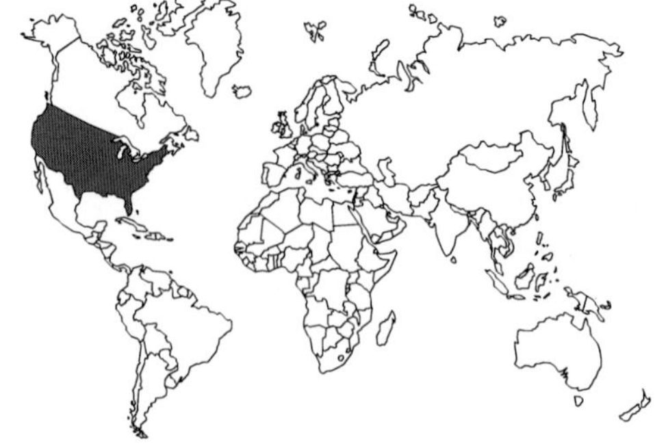

Fig. 2.128.

Distributed throughout the Mississippi and Great Lakes drainage systems of North America (Fig. 2.129).

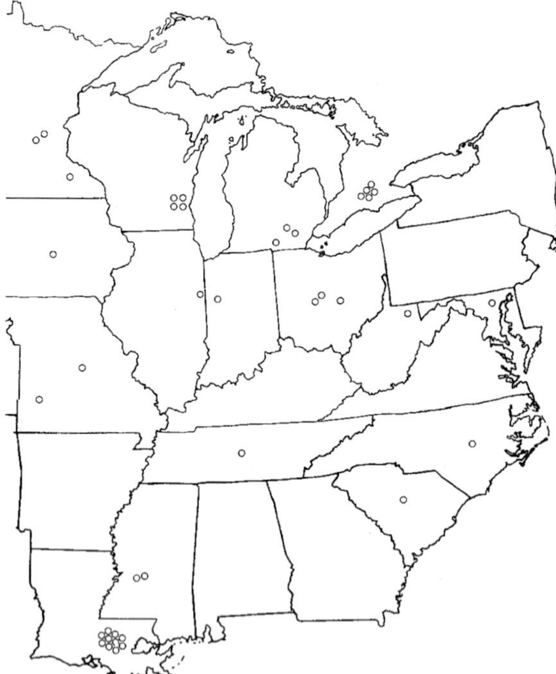

Fig. 2.129. Geographical distribution of *Paragonimus kellicotti* in naturally infected cats in the United States.

Location in Host

In cysts in the lungs.

Parasite Identification

Paragonimus adults are about a centimeter long (Fig. 2.130). Specimens of *Paragonimus kellicotti* overall appear to be a little longer and a little more slender than specimens of *Paragonimus westermani.* The major distinguishing characteristic between the adults of these two species, which both have single spines on the body surface, is the finer branching of the ovary in *Paragonimus kellicotti.* The metacercariae of these two flukes also differ; the metacercariae of *Paragonimus kellicotti* have a thin internal cyst wall, while those of *Paragonimus westermani* are much thicker (Ishii, 1966).

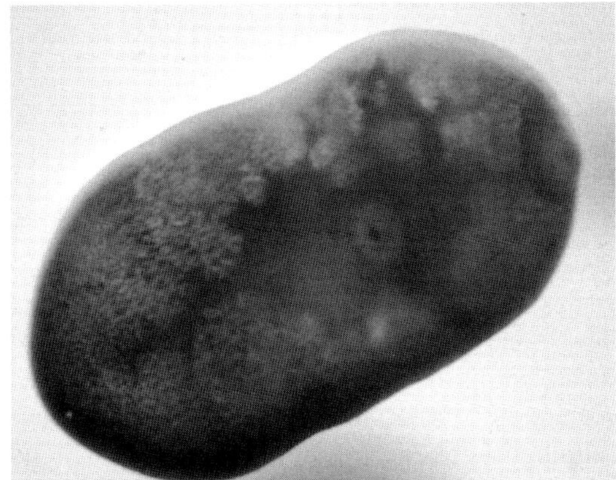

Fig. 2.130. Adult *Paragonimus kellicotti* recovered from the lung of a cat.

The eggs (Fig. 2.131) have a brown shell, a distinct operculum, and occasionally a knob on the abopercular end, and they are very similar in size and shape to those of *Paragonimus westermani.*

Life Cycle

The eggs of *Paragonimus kellicotti* are in a single-celled stage when passed in the feces. Once the eggs enter fresh, aerated water, they begin to develop and ultimately, depending on temperature, produce a ciliated miracidium. The miracidium lives 1 to 3 days and seeks out and penetrates a young snail host, *Pomatiopsis lapidaria,* which is an amphibious and nocturnal snail. Within the snail, the miracidium develops to a sporocyst within the lymphatic system. Ultimately, first- and second-generation stages, rediae, are produced, the latter containing the cercariae. The cercariae emerge from the snails in the evening or at night and are capable of living in water for 1 to 2 days; the cercariae penetrate the snail in the thin chitin on the undersurface of the tail (Ameel, 1934). In freshwater crayfish of the genera *Cambarus* and *Orconectes,* the cercariae develop into metacercariae within the pericardium. The metacercariae are somewhat resistant to environmental extremes; they have been maintained in crayfish at 7°C for 19 days and shown to be infective and can persist free in water at 12° to 20°C for 10 days.

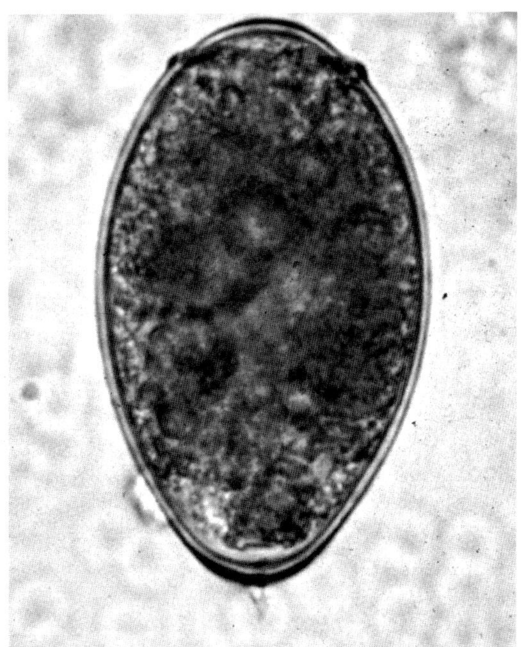

Fig. 2.131. Egg of *Paragonimus kellicotti* in the feces of a cat.

In a cat that ingests metacercariae, the young flukes rapidly penetrate the intestinal tract and enter the peritoneal cavity (Stromberg and Dubey,

1978). The young flukes migrate about in the peritoneal cavity for a week to 10 days and then migrate through the diaphragm into the pleural cavity. Penetration of the lung begins around 10 to 14 days after infection, and most worms have succeeded in forming pairs within the lungs by 3 weeks after infection. Most of the flukes take up residence in the caudal lobes of the lung, and more flukes were found in the right lung than in the left lung. It has also been shown that if a single young fluke is present, a metacercaria ingested 2 months later is capable of finding and pairing with the fluke that is already present in the cat (Sogandares-Bernal, 1966). The cysts in the lungs of cats often contain only two flukes; however, as many as six flukes may be present in some cysts. According to Wallace (1931), more than two flukes per cyst is not uncommon in the natural host, the North American mink. Cats are most likely to become infected by the ingestion of metacercariae in crawfish; however, it has been shown that rats can serve as paratenic hosts of *Paragonimus kellicotti* (Ameel, 1934), and it is possible that cats are infected by the ingestion of infected rodents. It has also been postulated that due to the appearance of possible paragonimiasis in kittens of an infected queen that were only a few months of age, transmammary transmission of the juvenile flukes might be possible if the queen is infected while pregnant (Bowman et al., 1991); however, examination of four kittens born 67 days after the infection of the queen revealed no stages of *Paragonimus kellicotti* in the tissues (Dubey et al., 1978b). Cats begin to shed eggs 5 to 7 weeks after infection.

Clinical Presentation and Pathogenesis

Clinical signs in experimentally infected cats are typically quite mild. There is occasional coughing, although bouts of paroxysmal coughing and dyspnea due to pneumothorax from rupture of lung cysts has been described (Dubey et al., 1978b). Marked eosinophilia in peripheral blood has been described, especially 3 weeks after infection, which is when the worms would first enter the lungs. Radiographs of early lesions will reveal indistinct nodular densities containing small air cavities and having irregular, sharply defined margins; older cysts are typical air-filled pneumatocysts (Fig. 2.132), although cats often present with ill-defined interstitial nodular densities (Pechman, 1976, 1984).

Beginning about 1 week after infection, cats develop an eosinophilic pleuritis that may be associated with areas where flukes have attempted to penetrate or actually penetrated the lung tissue (Hoover and Dubey, 1978). The young flukes within the lung are surrounded by intense eosinophilic inflammation, necrotic tissue, and cellular infiltrates. There is also hyperplasia of the

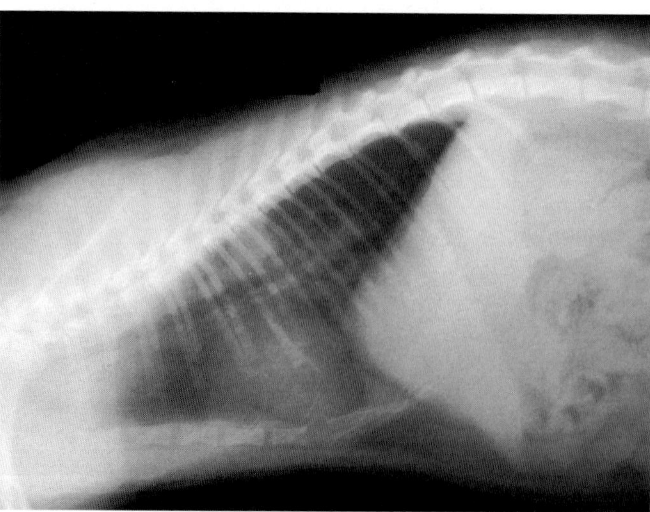

Fig. 2.132. Radiograph of young cyst of *Paragonimus kellicotti* in an experimentally infected cat. Note the indistinct edges to the observed parasitic opacity.

bronchiolar glands, type II pneumocytes, and the smooth muscles of the bronchioles and alveolar ducts. As the cysts continue to mature, they cause atelectasis of the adjacent tissue; the hyperplasia of the peribronchiolar glands becomes pronounced. Finally, collagenous connective tissue forms a well-developed wall around the fluke-containing cyst (Figs. 2.133 and 2.134). This capsular wall is richly vascularized, and eggs that remain in the lung become surrounded by multinucleate giant cells (Lumsden and Soganderes-Bernal, 1970).

Treatment

Albendazole has been used to treat cats with experimental (50 to 100 mg/kg for 14 to 21 days) and natural (25 mg/kg twice a day for 11 to 24 days) infections (Dubey et al., 1978a; Hoskins et al., 1981). In the case of the naturally infected cats, treatment was successful in 8 of the 10 treated animals. Praziquantel has been used to treat infections of *Paragonimus kellicotti* in experimentally infected cats (23 mg/kg three times each day for 3 days) with excellent results (Bowman et al., 1991). There was a marked improvement in

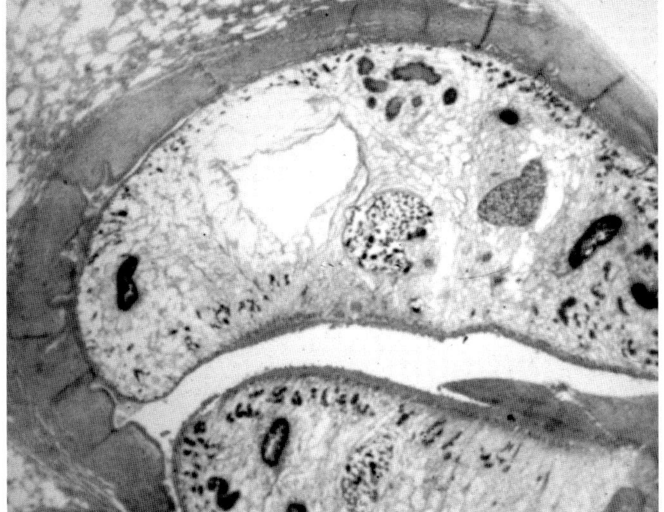

Fig. 2.133. Section through a cyst of *Paragonimus kellicotti* in the lungs of a cat; sections through two adult trematodes. Note the thick fibrous capsule.

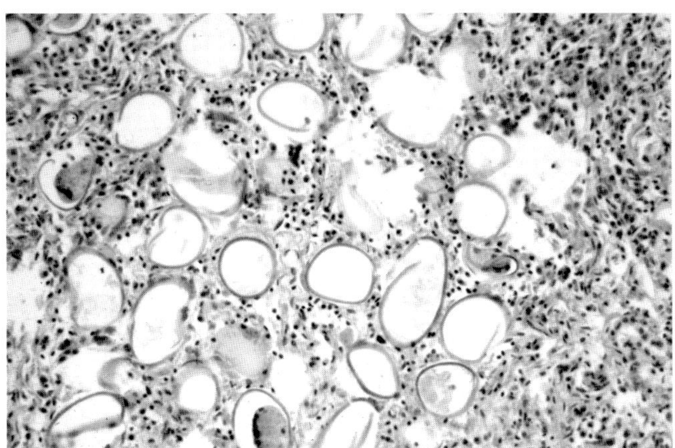

Fig. 2.134. Section through a cyst of *Paragonimus kellicotti* in the lungs of a cat (higher magnification than Fig. 2.133). Note the large number of eggs embedded in the tissue.

the lungs of these cats as evidenced by radiography within 11 days after treatment.

Epizootiology

Numerous mammals are capable of being infected with *Paragonimus kellicotti.* Dogs are commonly infected. The natural host appears to be the mink. The raccoon seems to be rather refractory to infection.

Hazards to Other Animals

Other animals appear likely to develop infection and disease similar to that seen in the cat, but only if they ingest the infected crayfish. Thus, the infected cat is not a direct threat to other uninfected animals.

Hazards to Humans

Until recently, there was only a single report of infection in humans with this trematode (Beaver et al., 1984). This infection occurred in a German laborer who had eaten crayfish. After returning to Germany, the infection was diagnosed. Recently a 21-year-old man in Ohio developed hemoptysis following ingestion of undercooked local crayfish (Procop et al., 2000). Treatment with praziquantel was successful and uneventful.

REFERENCES

Ameel DJ. 1934. *Paragonimus,* its life history and distribution in North America and its taxonomy (Trematoda:Troglotrematidae). Am J Hyg 19:279–317.

Beaver PC, Jung RC, Cupp EW. 1984. Clinical Parasitology, 9th ed. Philadelphia, Pa: Lea and Febiger. 825 pp.

Bowman DD, Frongillo MK, Johnson RC, Beck KA, Hornbuckle WE, Blue JT. 1991. Evaluation of praziquantel for treatment of experimentally induced paragonimiasis in dogs and cats. Am J Vet Res 52:68–71.

Dubey JP, Hoover EA, Stromberg PC, Toussant MJ. 1978a. Albendazole therapy for experimentally induced *Paragonimus kellicotti* infection in cats. Am J Vet Res 39:1027–1031.

Dubey JP, Stromberg PC, Toussant MJ, Hoover EA, Pechman RD. 1978b. Induced paragonimiasis in cats: clinical signs and diagnosis. JAVMA 173:734–742.

Hoover EA, Dubey JP. 1978. Pathogenesis of experimental pulmonary paragonimiasis in cats. Am J Vet Res 39:1827–1832.

Hoskins JD, Malone JB, Root CR. 1981. Albendazole therapy in naturally occurring feline paragonimiasis. J Am Hosp Assoc 17:265–269.

Ishii Y. 1966. Differential morphology of *Paragonimus kellicotti* in North America. J Parasitol 52:920–925.

Lumsden RD, Sogandares-Bernal F. 1970. Ultrastructural manifestations of pulmonary paragonimiasis. J Parasitol 56:1095–1109.

Pechman RD. 1976. The radiographic features of pulmonary paragonimiasis in the dog and cat. J Am Vet Radiol Soc 17:182–191.

Pechman RD. 1984. Newer knowledge of feline bronchopulmonary disease. Vet Clin North Am Small Anim Pract 14:1007–1019.

Procop GW, Marty AM, Scheck DN, Mease DR, Maw GM. 2000. North American paragonimiasis: a case report. Acta Cytologica 44: 75–80.

Sogandares-Bernal F. 1966. Studies on American paragonimiasis. IV. Observations on the pairing of adult worms in laboratory infections of domestic cats. J Parasitol 52:701–703.

Stromberg PC, Dubey JP. 1978. The life cycle of *Paragonimus kellicotti* in cats. J Parasitol 64:998–1002.

Wallace FG. 1931. Lung flukes of the genus *Paragonimus* in American mink. JAVMA 31:225–234.

Ward HB. 1908. Data for the determination of human entozoa II. Trans Am Microsc Soc 28:177–202.

Paragonimus mexicanus Miyazaki and Ishii, 1968

Etymology

Para = side-by-side and *gonimus* = gonads along with *mexicanus,* referring to the geographical location of this parasite.

Synonyms

Paragonimus peruvianus Miyazaki, Ibáñez, and Miranda, 1968; *Paragonimus ecuadorensis* Voelker and Arzube, 1979.

History

This trematode was originally found in an opossum, *Didelphis marsupialis,* captured in Mexico. It has been found in other animals and in humans.

Geographic Distribution

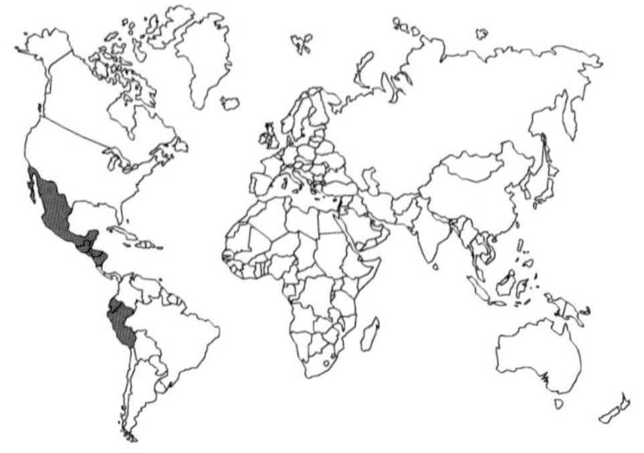

Fig. 2.135.

Mexico, Central America, and the western coast of South America, including Ecuador and Peru.

Location in Host

In cysts in the lungs.

Parasite Identification

Specimens of *Paragonimus mexicanus* are similar to the other species of *Paragonimus* possessing single cuticular spines (Tongu et al., 1995).

The eggs of the American species of *Paragonimus,* other than those of *Paragonimus kellicotti,* have eggshells that are undulated rather than smooth. The size of the eggs average 79 by 48 μm. In other aspects the eggs are quite similar morphologically to the other species.

Life Cycle

The first intermediate hosts of this parasite are species of snails of the genus *Aroapyrgus.* The second intermediate hosts are freshwater crabs of the genera *Pseudothelphusa, Ptychophallus, Potamocarcinum,* and *Hypolobocerca.* In the crab, the metacercaria has no cyst stage, and it moves freely about in the liver tissue of the crab. This species has been shown to have metacercarial stages that persist in the tissues of rats as paratenic hosts and that are capable of developing to the adult stage upon the ingestion of the rats by cats.

Clinical Presentation and Pathogenesis

Clinical signs similar to those of *Paragonimus kellicotti.*

Treatment

Probably praziquantel.

Epizootiology

Numerous mammals are capable of being infected with *Paragonimus mexicanus;* including cats, jaguars, dogs, foxes, raccoons, coatimundis, skunks, and three species of opossums.

Hazards to Other Animals

Other animals appear likely to develop infection and disease similar to that seen in the cat, but only if they ingest the infected crayfish. Thus, the infected cat is not a direct threat to other uninfected animals.

Hazards to Humans

Human infections with this parasite have been reported in Mexico, Central America, Ecuador, and Peru, where people are known to eat raw crabs (Brenes et al., 1983).

REFERENCES

Brenes RR, Little MD, Raudales O, Múñoz G, Ponce C. 1983. Cutaneous paragonimiasis in man in Honduras. Am J Trop Med Hyg 32:376–378.

Tongu Y, Hata H, Orido Y, Pinto MR, Lamoth-Argumedo R, Yokogawa M, Tsuji M. 1995. Morphological observations of *Paragonimus mexicanus* from Guatemala. Jap J Parasitol 44:365–370.

Paragonimus inca Miyazaki, Mazabel, Grados, and Uyema; *Paragonimus peruvianus* Miyazaki, Ibáñez, and Miranda; *Paragonimus caliensis* Little; and *Paragonimus amazonicus* Miyazaki, Grados, and Uyema

Other species of *Paragonimus* have been described in South America. *Paragonimus inca* has been described from felids in Peru. *Paragonimus peruvianus* has been recovered from cats, and it has been shown that praziquantel (10 mg/kg/day for 10 days) causes the death of worms in the experimentally infected feline host (Ibáñez and Jara, 1992). *Paragonimus caliensis* and *Paragonimus amazonicus* have been described from opossums. These trematodes are similar to *Paragonimus mexicanus* in that the eggshells are undulated unlike specimens from other parts of the world.

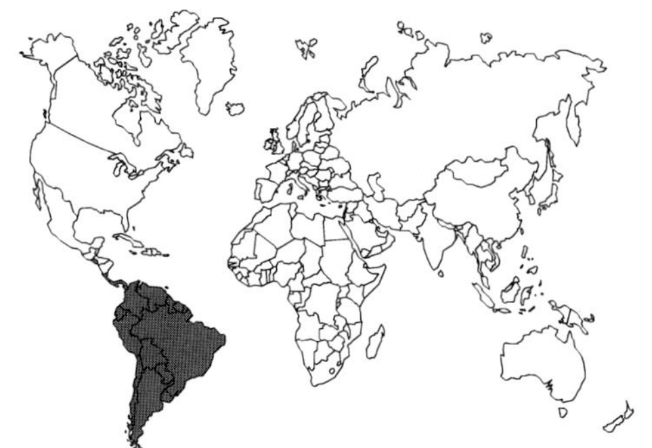

Fig. 2.136.

REFERENCES
Nicanor Ibáñez H, Cesar Jara C. 1992. Experimental paragonimiasis: therapeutical tests with praziquantel—final report. Mem Inst Oswaldo Cruz 87(suppl.):107.

Paragonimus africanus Voelker and Vogel, 1965, and *Paragonimus uterobilateralis* Voelker and Vogel, 1965

These two species of *Paragonimus* have been described from Africa. *Paragonimus africanus* was described in the Cameroon from the mongoose, *Crossarchus obscurus,* and the dog and human beings; cats were experimentally infected. *Paragonimus uterobilateralis* was described from the swamp mongoose, *Atilax paludinosus,* in Liberia, the dog in the Cameroon, and human beings in Liberia, Cameroon, and Nigeria; cats have not been described as being infected with this species. The eggs of *Paragonimus africanus* measure 92 by 48 μm, while those of *Paragonimus uterobilateralis* are smaller (i.e., 68 μm by 41 μm).

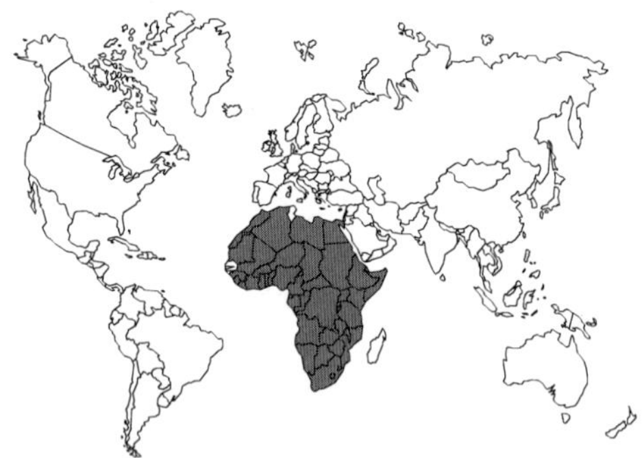

Fig. 2.137.

Eggs of an unidentified species of *Paragonimus* were found in a fecal sample from a cat in the Durban area of South Africa (Proctor and Gregory, 1974). The eggs measured 68–76 μm by 44–48 μm. There was no apparent attempt to perform a clinical examination or to treat the cat.

REFERENCES
Proctor EM, Gregory MA. 1974. An ultrastructural study of ova of *Paragonimus* species from human and cat feces. S Afr Med J 48:1947–1948.

TREMATODES OF THE BLOOD VESSELS

A single group of trematodes parasitize the blood vessels of cats and other mammals. These are the schistosomes. There are three species of schistosomes that are of major importance in human medicine, *Schistosoma mansoni, Schistosoma haematobium,* and *Schistosoma japonicum.* Only one of these three species, *Schistosoma japonicum,* is capable of developing in a wide range of hosts, which includes the cat. In the Americas, the indigenous schistosome parasite of raccoons, opossums, and other wild mammals, *Heterobilharzia americana,* is capable of infecting the cat experimentally. *Ornithoturkestanica* is a parasite of cattle in the Middle East and southern Russia; it has on rare occasions been reported from cats in these areas.

SCHISTOSOMATIDAE

Schistosoma japonicum (Katsurada, 1904) Stiles, 1905

Etymology

Schisto = split and *soma* = body along with *japonicum,* referring to the geographical region in which it was first found.

Synonyms

Schistosomum japonicum Katsurada, 1904; *Schistosoma cattoi* Blanchard, 1905.

History

This parasite was first discovered by Dr. Katsurada in the portal vein of a cat; a single male

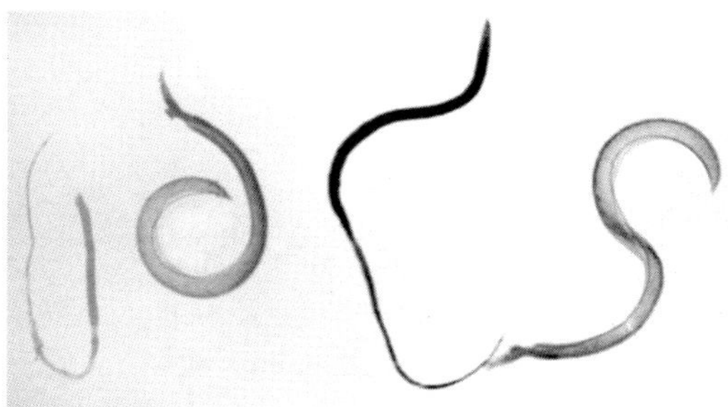

Fig. 2.138. *Schistosoma japonicum.* Four adults recovered from an experimentally infected cat. The two females are the thinner flukes that, in the blood vessel, are held within the gynecophoral canal of the male. These may be the worst pictures of *Schistosoma japonicum* ever published.

worm was recovered. Not long after, 32 male and female worms were found by this worker in the veins of another cat that was noticed to have a swollen abdomen. In this same year, a female was found in the portal vein of a human being; the first indication of this parasite's medical importance. This was also the first schistosome for which the life cycle was described; it was described by Drs. Miyairi and Suzuki.

Geographic Distribution

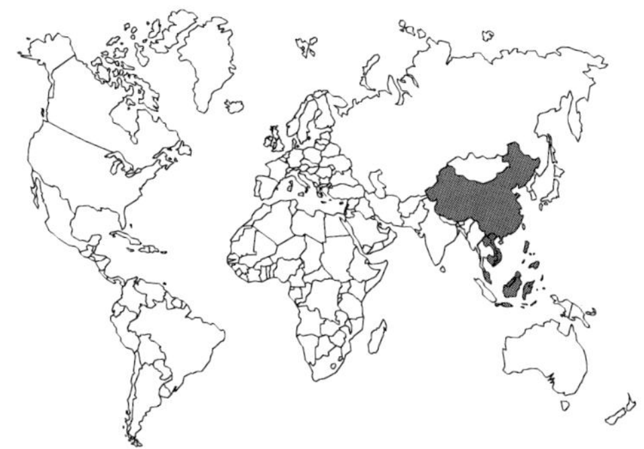

Fig. 2.139.

Japan, the Yangtze basin of China, Taiwan, Indonesia, Malaysia, and the Philippines.

Location in Host

In the portal veins.

Parasite Identification

The adults of *Schistosoma japonicum,* like those of other schistosomatids, occur as separate sexes. Males are about 15 mm long, and females are about 20 mm long. Both sexes are very elongate organisms compared with other trematodes; about 90 percent to 95 percent of the total body length is posterior to the ventral sucker, and the worms are no more than 1 mm in width. The male is stouter than the female, and the ventral body surface posterior to the ventral sucker has lateral inflations throughout its length that roll towards the midline and form a groove, the gynecophoral canal. The female is held within this groove of the male throughout most of her adult life. The male has seven testes just posterior to the ventral sucker. The female has an elongate uterus that appears as a single chain of eggs and takes up most of the anterior half of her body.

The eggs of this species of *Schistosoma* are nearly spherical. The thin eggshell is light yellow and lacks an operculum. On one end of the shell a small bump or process is often visible. The eggs are 70–100 μm long by 50–65 μm wide, and they contain a fully developed miracidium when passed in the feces.

Life Cycle

Within 15 minutes to an hour after a *Schistosoma japonicum* egg enters fresh water, the developed miracidium hatches from the eggshell. The released miracidium then penetrates a snail of the genus *Oncomelania.* Within the snail, the miracidium develops through several stages to produce cercariae; the cercariae produced by a single miracidium will all be of the same sex when they become adults. The cercaria is characterized by its possession of a forked tail. The final host is infected by the cercaria penetrating the skin. After going through the skin, the tail is lost, and the so-called schistosomulum makes its way into the vascular system and is carried to the lung. The growing flukes then make their way to the liver and ultimately to the mesenteric veins where they develop. The females begin to lay eggs 5 to 6 weeks after infection of the final host.

Clinical Presentation and Pathogenesis

There are no descriptions of clinical illness in cats with this infection, which suggests that it may be asymptomatic given the large numbers of cats that are probably infected.

Treatment

Praziquantel is probably the drug of choice.

Epizootiology

Numerous mammals are capable of being infected with *Schistosoma japonicum.* Other hosts besides the cat include human beings, cattle, horses, dogs, pigs, goats, and rats.

Hazards to Other Animals

Other animals appear likely to develop infection and disease similar to those seen in the human, but only if the infective cercariae penetrate the skin. Thus, the infected cat is not a direct threat to other uninfected animals.

Hazards to Humans

Numerous human beings are infected with this parasite, and serious disease and perhaps death can result from the infection.

Table 2.2. Intermediate hosts and geographic distribution of the trematode parasites of the domestic cat

Family and species	Intermediate host	Geographical distribution
Clinostomatidae		
Clinostomum falsatum	Freshwater fish	South Africa
Clinostomum kalappahi	Freshwater fish	India
Clinostomum abdoni	Freshwater fish	Philippines
Cyathocotylidae		
Mesostephanus milvi	Brackish-water fish	Japan, India, Africa
Prohemistomum vivax	Brackish- and freshwater fish	Middle East
Diplostomatidae		
Alaria marcianae	Frogs, paratenic mammals	North America
Cynodiplostomum azimi	Frogs	Middle east
Fibricola minor	Frogs	Australia
Pharyngostomum cordatum	Toads, reptiles, shrews	Europe, Africa, China
Echinostomatidae		
Echinochasmus perfoliatus	Freshwater fish	Europe, Middle and Far East
Echinochasmus breviviteilus	Freshwater fish	Middle east
Echinochasmus liliputanus	Freshwater fish	Middle east
Episthmium caninum	Freshwater fish	India
Stephanoprora denticulatoides	Freshwater fish	Europe
Artyfechinostomum sufrartyfex	Snail, frogs	India
Isthmiophora melis	Frogs	North America
Echinoparyphium	Frogs	Tasmania
Heterophyidae		
Apophallus donicus	Freshwater fish	Europe
Apophallus venustus	Freshwater fish	North America
Apophallus muehlingi	Brackish-water fish	Europe
Ascocotyle ascolonga	Brackish-water fish	Middle East
Ascocotyle longicollis	Brackish-water fish	Middle East
Ascocotyle minuta	Brackish-water fish	Middle East
Ascocotyle angrense	Freshwater fish	Brazil
Ascocotyle longa	Brackish-water fish	Americas
Ascocotyle pachycystis	Brackish-water fish	North America
Ascocotyle arnoldoi	Brackish-water fish	South America
Centrocestus caninus	Freshwater fish	Taiwan
Pygidiopsis genata	Brackish-water fish	Europe, Middle East, Asia
Pygidiopsis summa	Brackish-water fish	Asia
Pygidiopsoides spindalis	Brackish-water fish	North America
Cryptocotyle lingua	Saltwater fish	North America
Cryptocotyle concavum	Brackish-water fish	Russia
Cryptocotyle quinqueangularis	Brackish-water fish	Europe, North Africa, North America
Euryhelmis squamula	Newt, toads	Europe, North America
Euryhelmis monorchis	Frogs	North America
Euryhelmis pacifica	Salamanders	North America
Galactosomum fregatae	Brackish-water fish	West Indies, India
Haplorchis pumilio	Freshwater fish	Middle East, Asia, Australia
Haplorchis yokogawai	Brackish-water fish	Middle East, Asia
Haplorchis taichui	Brackish-water fish	Middle East, Asia
Haplorchis sprenti	Brackish-water fish	Australia
Haplorchis parataichui	Freshwater fish	Australia
Procerovum varium	Brackish-water fish	Australia
Procerovum calderoni	Brackish-water fish	Philippines
Stellantchasmus falcatus	Brackish- and freshwater fish	Middle East, Asia, Australia, Hawaii

(continued)

Table 2.2. (Continued)

Family and species	Intermediate host	Geographical distribution
Heterophyes heterophyes	Brackish-water fish	Mediterranean, India, Japan
Heterophyes aequalis	Salt, brackish, and freshwater fish	Middle East
Heterophyopsis continua	Brackish-water fish	Japan, Korea
Metagonimus yokogawai	Freshwater fish	Asia, Spain, Balkans
Metagonimus takahashii	Freshwater fish	Asia
Dexiogonimus ciureanus	Brackish-water fish	Middle East
Stictodora sawakinensis	Brackish-water fish	Middle East
Stictodora thapari	Brackish-water fish	Middle East
Microphallidae		
Microphalloides vajrasthirae	Crab	Thailand
Plagiorchidae		
Plagiorchis massino	Snail	Eurasia, Canada
Nanophyetidae		
Nanophyetus salmincola	Freshwater fish	Northern Pacific coast
Dicrocoelidae		
Eurytrema procyonis	Arthropod	North America
Euparadistomum pearsoni	Arthropod	New Guinea
Euparadistomum buckleyi	Arthropod	Siberia, Europe
Euparadistomum heiwschi	Arthropod	Africa
Platynosomum concinnum	Lizards, frogs, toads	South Pacific, West Africa, Caribbean
Opisthorchidae		
Amphimerus pseudofelineus	Freshwater fish	Americas
Clonorchis sinensis	Freshwater fish	Asia
Opisthorchis felineus	Freshwater fish	Siberia, Europe
Opisthorchis viverrini	Freshwater fish	Thailand
Opisthorchis chabaudi	Frogs	Africa
Paropisthorchis caninus	Freshwater fish	India
Metorchis conjunctus	Freshwater fish	North America
Metorchis albidus	Freshwater fish	Europe
Metorchis orientalis	Freshwater fish	Asia
Parametorchis complexum	Freshwater fish	North America
Pseudamphistomum truncatum	Freshwater fish	Europe, India
Orchipedidae		
Orchipedum isostoma	Crabs	Africa
Troglotrematidae		
Troglotrema mustelae	Freshwater fish	North America
Paragonimus westermani	Freshwater crabs	Asia
Paragonimus pulmonalis	Freshwater crabs and crayfish	Japan, Korea, Taiwan
Paragonimus miyazakii	Freshwater crabs	Japan
Paragonimus heterotremus	Freshwater crabs	China
Paragonimus siamensis	Freshwater crabs	Thailand
Paragonimus skrjabini	Freshwater crabs	China
Paragonimus ohirai	Brackish-water crabs	Asia
Paragonimus kellicotti	Freshwater crayfish	North America
Paragonimus mexicanus	Freshwater crabs	Mexico, Central and South America
Paragonimus inca	Freshwater crabs	Peru
Paragonimus peruvianus	Freshwater crabs	Peru
Paragonimus caliensis	Freshwater crabs	Colombia
Paragonimus amazonicus	Freshwater crabs	Peru
Paragonimus africanus	Freshwater crabs	Africa
Paragonimus uterobilateralis	Freshwater crabs	Africa
Schistosomatidae		
Heterobilharzia americana	Skin penetration	North America
Ornithobilharzia turkestanica	Skin penetration	Eurasia
Schistosoma japonicum	Skin penetration	Asia

3 THE CESTODES

With Notes on the Few Acanthocephala Reported from Cats

The cestodes or tapeworms comprise a large assemblage of parasites that as adults are found in the intestinal tract of vertebrates. Most typically, the tapeworms are acquired by the final host ingesting an intermediate host that contains a larval stage of the tapeworm. There are 14 orders of cestodes currently recognized (Khalil et al., 1994). Most of these 14 orders are found in sharks, rays, fish, reptiles, and birds, with only a few being found in mammals. The cat is a final host to only two orders of these tapeworm parasites, the Pseudophyllidea and the Cyclophyllidea. Within the Pseudophyllidea are the two genera *Diphyllobothrium* and *Spirometra.* Within the Cyclophyllidea are the genera *Mesocestoides* of the Mesocestoididae, *Dipylidium, Joyeuxiella,* and *Diplopylidium* of the Dipylidiidae, and *Taenia* and *Echinococcus* of the Taeniidae. There have been rare reports of other cyclophillidean tapeworms in the cat, including *Choanotaenia* of the Dilepididae.

The adult tapeworm is characterized by having a long ribbon-like body that is divided into segments containing the sexual organs and eggs. This collection of segments is called a strobila. Some tapeworms are very small and have strobila composed of only a few segments (e.g., *Echinococcus*), while some tapeworms become very long and have strobila composed of many segments (e.g., *Diphyllobothrium*). The head of the tapeworm is typically equipped with a holdfast organ that is often termed a bothridia, bothria, or scolex. The holdfast may be armed with spines or tentacles and may or may not have muscular suckers. The anterior of the scolex may also have a central anteriad portion, the rostellum, which may be equipped with hooks of various types. In some groups, the rostellum can be retracted. The segments of the body typically each bear both male and female reproductive organs and ultimately produce eggs that require fertilization. In some cases, the eggs are shed from the tapeworm's segment while the segment is still attached to the strobila within the host (as with *Diphyllobothrium* and *Spirometra*), while in other cases, the segments become large sacks of eggs that are shed into the environment (as is the case with *Dipylidium* and *Taenia*). The eggs of tapeworms typically contain a larva that has six hooklets that are used for locomotion when ingested by the proper intermediate host. Some eggs are passed with the larvae already developed (*Taenia* and *Dipylidium*), while others are passed in a state that requires additional development in the external environment (*Spirometra*). Some eggs have opercula, and some eggs do not.

With a group as large as the Cestoda, there are, of course, exceptions to almost every "typical" plan. Thus, three orders of tapeworms, the Gyrocotylidea, Amphilinidea, and Caryophyllidea, have no external segmentation. These three orders are parasites of fish and turtles. The larva in the egg of the Amphilinidea and Gyrocotylidea has 10 hooks rather than 6 hooks. There is a tapeworm parasitic in wading birds, *Dioecocestus* in the Cyclophyllidea, that has separate male and female strobila. Also, even though almost all adult parasites are found in the intestine, there are exceptions; those of the Amphilinidea are found in the body cavities of their final hosts. One tapeworm of rodents and humans, *Rodentolepis straminea* (syns., *Hymenolepis nana* and *Vampirolepis nana*), is capable of direct development in the vertebrate host.

The tapeworm parasites of cats have two major life-cycle types. In the first type, the pseudophyllidean parasites utilize an aquatic environment for the early stages of the life cycle. Thus, there is a swimming larval stage in the life cycle that

Table 3.1—Tapeworms of the cat, how it is infected, and the geographical distribution of the parasites

Parasite	Larval stage ingested by cat	Host containing larval stage ingested by cat	Significant areas of geographical distribution
PSEUDOPHYLLIDEA			
Diphyllobothriidae			
Diphyllobothrium latum	Plerocercoid	Fish	Northern Europe, Japan; imported to northern North America and Chile
Spirometra erinaceieuropae	Sparganum (Plerocercoid)	Amphibia, reptiles, rodents	Worldwide
Spirometra mansonoides	Sparganum (Plerocercoid)	Amphibia, reptiles, rodents, birds	Americas
CYCLOPHYLLIDEA			
Mesocestoididae			
Mesocestoides lineatus	Tetrathyridium	Amphibia, reptiles, rodents, birds	Worldwide
Dipylidiidae			
Dipylidium caninum	Cysticercoid	Flea larva	Worldwide
Diplopylidium acanthotetra	Cysticercoid	Lizard	Southern Europe, Middle East
Diplopylidium nölleri	Cysticercoid	Lizard	Southern Europe, Middle East
Joyeuxiella pasqualei	Cysticercoid	Lizard	Southern Europe, Middle East, Asia
Joyeuxiella fuhrmanni	Cysticercoid	Lizard	Africa
Joyeuxiella echinorhyncoides	Cysticercoid	Lizard	Africa
Dilepididae			
Choanotaenia atopa	Cysticercoid	Invertebrate	Kansas, USA
Taeniidae			
Taenia taeniaeformis	Strobilocercus	Rodent	Worldwide
Echinococcus multilocularis	Alveolar hydatid	Rodent	Holarctic

infects aquatic invertebrates. Later in their life cycle, these pseudophyllidean parasites utilize various vertebrate paratenic hosts such as fish, amphibians, reptiles, and mammals to facilitate the transfer of the larvae to the carnivorous final host (Table 3.1). In the second life-cycle type, the cyclophyllidean parasites of cats utilize the terrestrial environment for the larval stages of the life cycle. The larvae of *Dipylidium* are found in fleas, and the larvae of *Joyeuxiella* and *Diplopylidium* are found in amphibia and reptiles. The larvae of *Taenia* and *Echinococcus* are found in mammalian hosts. The host in which the initial larval development of *Mesocestoides* occurs has not been found (it is presumed to be an invertebrate), but the later larval stages are found in vertebrates. In all cases, the cat becomes infected by ingesting a host that contains the larval stage of the parasite that grows to adulthood within the host's intestinal tract.

Cats can also serve as the intermediate host of certain tapeworms. Within the Pseudophyllidea, cats have been found to be infected with the larval stage of *Spirometra,* called a sparganum. Within the Cyclophyllidea, cats have been infected with larval stages of members of the Mesocestoididae and the Taeniidae. The larval stage of the Mesocestoididae is the tetrathyridium. The larval stage of the Taeniidae that has been found in cats is a coenurus of the *Taenia* species that is parasitic as an adult in dogs.

Cats have been reported on occasion to be the final host of another phylum of parasites, the Acanthocephala. There have been very few reports of the Acanthocephala in cats, and in almost all cases, the reports have been the results of necropsy results from surveys. Thus, the Acanthocephala did not seem to warrant a chapter of its own. This phylum has no affinities with the tapeworms and is placed in this chapter only for convenience.

REFERENCES

Khalil LF, Jones A, Bray RA (eds). 1994. Key to the Cestode Parasites of Vertebrates. Wallingford, UK: CAB International. 751 pp.

PSEUDOPHYLLIDEA

The Pseudophyllidea is a group of tapeworms whose adults are most commonly found in fish. The group is characterized by having a scolex that usually is armed with two bothria, slits on the dorsal and ventral aspect. The genital pores in this group are located medially on each segment. The majority of genera in this order are found in fish, but one family, the Diphyllobothriidae, is found mainly as adults in reptiles, birds, and mammals (such as whales, cetaceans, and pinnipeds). The typical life cycle involves a crustacean as the first intermediate host and a fish as the second intermediate host. Cats are hosts to two genera of these parasites in the adult stage, *Diphyllobothrium* and *Spirometra. Diphyllobothrium* is found as adults in fish-eating birds and mammals. *Spirometra* differs from *Diphyllobothrium* in that the second intermediate host tends to be a terrestrial or semiterrestrial vertebrate and the adults are mainly in cat-like carnivores.

DIPHYLLOBOTHRIIDAE

Diphyllobothrium latum (Linnaeus, 1758) Cobbold, 1858

Etymology

Di = two; *phyllos* = leaf, and *bothrium* = groove; along with *latum* from the Latin *Lumbrici lati,* which was the term the Romans used to describe all tapeworms (as opposed to *Lumbrici teretes* for the earthworm).

Synonyms

Taenia lata Linnaeus, 1758; *Taenia vulgaris* Linnaeus, 1758; *Taenia membranacea* Pallas, 1781; *Taenia tenella* Pallas, 1781; *Taenia dentata* Batsch, 1786; *Taenia grisea* Pallas, 1796; *Bothriocephalus latus* (Linnaeus, 1758) Bremser, 1819; *Dibothrium latum* (Linnaeus, 1758) Diesing, 1830; *Bothriocephalus balticus* Küchemnmeister, 1855; *Bothriocephalus cristatus* Davaine, 1874; *Bothriocephalus taenioides* Léon, 1916; *Dibothriocephalus minor* Cholodlowsky, 1916; *Diphyllobothrium americanus* Hall and Wigdor, 1918; *Dibothrium serratum* Diesing, 1850; *Diphyllobothrium fuscum* (Krabbe, 1865); *Diphyllobothrium luxi* (Rutkevich, 1937); *Diphyllobothrium parvum* Stephens, 1908; *Diphyllobothrium stictus* Talysin, 1932; *Diancyrobothrium taenioides* Bacigalupo, 1945.

History

In 1592 Dunus was the first to recognizably describe *Diphyllobothrium latum;* this description was confirmed by Plater in 1602, who differentiated it from the *Taenia* species (beef and pork tapeworms) of humans (cited in Grove, 1990). Braun (1883) found that the fish contained the stage that transmits the parasite to humans. Braun fed plerocercoids from fish to cats, dogs, and medical students. The role of the copepod as the first intermediate host was elucidated by Janicki (1917) and Rosen (1917).

Geographic Distribution

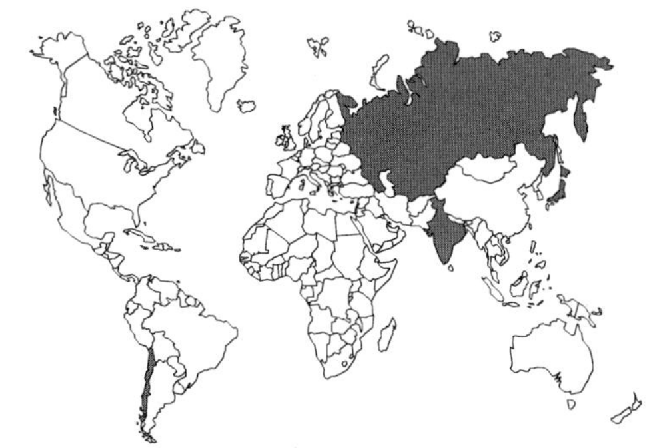

Fig. 3.1.

Diphyllobothrium latum has been reported to occur in humans throughout the world—Finland, Scandinavia, the Baltic states, the former Soviet Union, France, and Switzerland. It is believed to have expanded its range at some point with human travels to Israel, central Africa, and Siberia. It was brought by Europeans to the Americas where foci were established in Canada, the Great Lakes of North America (although no longer present in most of the central United States) (Peters et al., 1978), and Chile in South America (Torres et al., 1991). The worm in Japan may have been brought by Europeans or may represent a separate species, *Diphyllobothrium nihonkaense* Yamane, Kamo, Bylund, and Wikgren, 1986. It has also been reported on occasion from the Philippines and Taiwan. Infection in the domestic cat should parallel that in the human. Infection by a *Diphyllobothrium latum* has been reported in domestic cats in Scotland (Hutchison, 1957), Russia (Vereta, 1986), India (Chandler, 1925), Japan (Tanaka et al., 1985), Philippines (Tongson and San Pablo, 1979), and Chile (Torres et al., 1990).

Location in Host

Diphyllobothrium latum adults are found in the small intestine of the cat. "The function of the scolex is to anchor the early strobila to the host gut wall. In the older worm, maintenance of position in the host gut is effected by muscular tonus, by pressure of the powerfully muscular strobila against the gut wall; the scolex serves little purpose, adheres only loosely to the gut wall, and any increase in its size and development is not to be expected." (Wardle and Green, 1941).

Parasite Identification

Diphyllobothrium latum is referred to as a diphyllobothriid tapeworm or as a pseudophyllidean tapeworm. Common names include "the broad tapeworm" and "the broadfish tapeworm." The scolex of *Diphyllobothrium latum* lacks hooks and suckers but instead possesses two shallow, longitudinal grooves called bothria (Khalil et al., 1994). The scolex is 2.5 mm long and 1 mm wide. (Figs. 3.2 and 3.3).

Each proglottid of the *Diphyllobothrium latum* tapeworm possesses a centrally located, rosette-shaped uterus (Fig. 3.4) and associated uterine pore through which its eggs are released (Faust, 1952). This tapeworm continuously releases eggs until it becomes exhausted of its uterine contents. The terminal segments become senile rather than gravid and detach in chains rather than individually. This tapeworm may have as many as 3,000 or more proglottids and may range in length from 2 to 12 m. It is probable that this tapeworm does not attain this considerable length in the domestic cat.

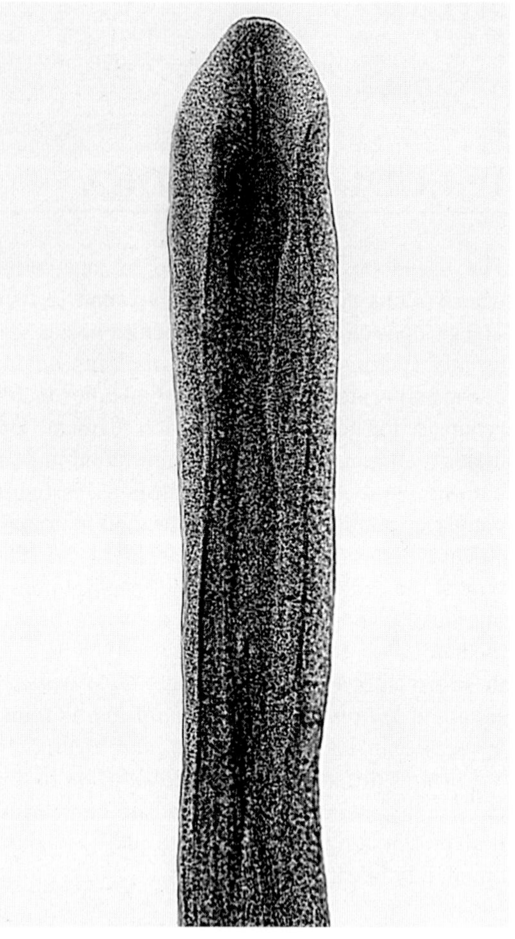

Fig. 3.2. Bothrium of *Diphyllobothrium latum* showing the finger-like nature of the holdfast.

The egg of *Diphyllobothrium latum* resembles the egg of a digenetic trematode; that is, it is oval and possesses a distinct operculum at one pole of the shell. The eggs are light brown and have dimensions that average 67–71 μm by 40–51 μm. The eggs tend to be rounded at one end. The operculum is present on the end opposite the rounded pole. The eggs are unembryonated when passed in the feces. The eggs can be distinguished from those of the pseudophyllidean tapeworms of the genus *Spirometra,* which also have a similar morphology in that the operculum is ellipsoidal in shape, while the eggshell of the *Spirometra* species tends to appear irregular because of the uneven curvature of the eggshell (Miyazaki, 1991).

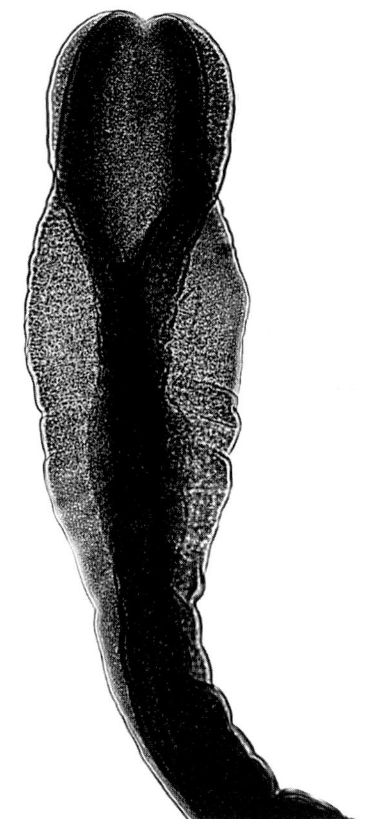

Fig. 3.3. Another view of the bothrium of *Diphyllobothrium latum,* showing the holdfast twisted, giving it a wider appearance.

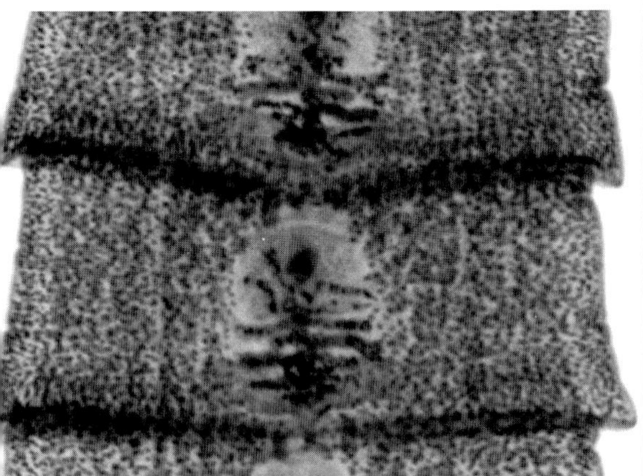

Fig. 3.4. Gravid segments of *Diphyllobothrium latum* showing the branching uterus.

Life Cycle

Humans serve as the principal definitive hosts for *Diphyllobothrium latum,* although many other mammals that eat freshwater fish (e.g., the cat, dog, bear, and pig) may harbor the adult cestodes. In areas where human infection is rare or no longer present, infection of the fish intermediate hosts also becomes reduced or disappears, suggesting that wild mammalian hosts are not sufficient to maintain the cycle in many environments (Beaver et al., 1984). However, in areas of Russia where the infection is endemic, up to 90 percent of cats may be infected (Shamarina et al., 1980).

Unembryonated eggs pass through the uterine pore of each of the adult cestode's gravid proglottids. The eggs are discharged to the external environment with the feces. In fresh water, the first developmental stage, the ciliated coracidium, emerges from the egg and is eaten by the first intermediate host, an aquatic copepod (a crustacean). This copepod may be of the genera *Cyclops* or *Diaptomus.* The second developmental stage, the worm-like procercoid stage, develops within the copepod. When the procercoid is ingested by the second intermediate host (e.g., a fish such as a freshwater fish), the procercoid develops into a plerocercoid within the musculature of the fish.

Cats become infected with *Diphyllobothrium latum* by eating the fish, and the plerocercoid develops to a mature tapeworm in the small intestine. Examination of the intestines of a kitten 13 hours after being fed plerocercoids recovered from fish revealed the worms at distances of 7, 11, 12, 13, and 16 inches from the pylorus in a gut measuring 33 inches between pylorus and ileocecal valve; after 25 hours in another kitten, 17 worms were found between 7.5 and 36 inches behind the pylorus in a gut measuring 56 inches from pylorus to ileocecal valve (Wardle, 1933). In dogs, the first eggs are passed between 18 and 20 days after ingestion of the plerocercoid, and in some dogs, worms are a meter and a half long by 30 days after infection is initiated (Wardle and Green, 1941). In human beings, the worms may remain alive and active for several years or even decades, but the patent period in the cat has not been determined. With *Diphyllobothrium latum,* there is no clear distinction between mature and gravid proglottids, with maturation occurring sometimes anterior to less developed proglottids (Faust, 1952). Also, ultimate gravid proglottids are not "shed" in the feces as actively motile sacks of eggs as with *Dipylidium caninum* and *Taenia taeniaeformis,* but instead, as groups of segments become "spent," they detach from the strobila and are shed as strands of variable length.

Clinical Presentation and Pathogenesis

As with many of the feline tapeworms, cases of diphyllobothriasis are apparently asymptomatic. Pet owners may observe chains of "spent" or empty proglottids in the cat's feces. Humans with this parasite demonstrate the same poorly defined symptoms as they do when infected with other tapeworms (vague abdominal discomfort, diarrhea, nausea and weakness). In humans, this parasite may produce a serious megaloblastic anemia. Virtually all of the cases have been in Finnish people. The cestode does absorb large amounts of vitamin B_{12}, and affected humans also have an impaired ability to absorb this vitamin (von Bonsdorff, 1978). Pernicious anemia has not been reported in cats or any other domesticated or wild animals; however, the experimental infection of dogs with *Diphyllobothrium latum* has induced decreased red cell numbers and decreases in total hemoglobin (Wardle et al., 1937).

Diagnosis

Identification of characteristic eggs and "spent" proglottids as those of *Diphyllobothrium latum* is necessary for the practical requirements of controlling this cestode. The eggs of *Diphyllobothrium latum* are operculated and resemble the eggs of *Spirometra* species and many of the digenetic trematodes.

Gross inspection with or without a hand lens is usually sufficient for the identification of proglottids of *Diphyllobothrium latum.* Identification is based on the appearance of each proglottid's centrally located, rosette-shaped uterus and its associated genital pore. In cases of intact tapeworms recovered at necropsy, identification can also be made utilizing the characteristic appearance of the scolex with its slit-like bothria.

Treatment

Praziquantel must be administered at an elevated dose to be effective against *Diphyllobothrium latum.* A single dose of 35 mg/kg body weight eliminated all *Diphyllobothrium latum* from infected dogs (Sakamoto, 1977).

Epizootiology

Cats become infected when they eat raw or undercooked fish.

Hazards to Other Animals

In addition to cats, suitable hosts include a wide variety of various terrestrial and marine fish-eating carnivores (dogs, bears, mongooses, mink foxes, seals, and sea lions) in many parts of the world. The stage passed in the feces of cats requires a period of development in fresh water; thus, infected cats pose no direct threat to other animals.

Hazards to Humans

Human beings are considered to be the normal definitive hosts for *Diphyllobothrium latum.* Because *Diphyllobothrium latum* is a human tapeworm and because it may be transmitted to both wild and domesticated animals, it is considered to be a zooanthroponosis. The infected cat poses no direct threat to its owner or to any other individuals that may handle the cat or its feces.

Control/Prevention

Prophylaxis involves the freezing or cooking of fish. At no time should cats be fed raw fish. Such habits may lead to infections with the infective plerocercoid stages of *Diphyllobothrium latum,* and if possible, cats should not be allowed to roam freely or to scavenge dead fish (Hendrix and Blagburn, 1983). Precautions should be taken against raw human sewage reaching fresh water lakes in endemic areas; this has been a major cause of the infection of the stock of fish in lakes and rivers (von Bonsdorff, 1978).

REFERENCES

Beaver PC, Jung RC, Cupp EW. 1984. Clinical Parasitology. 9th edition. Philadelphia, Pa: Lea and Febiger. 825 pp.

Braun M. 1883. *Bothriocephalus latus* und seine Herkunft. Arch Pathol Anat Physiol lin Med (Virchow) 92:364–366.
Chandler AC. 1925. The helminthic parasites of cats in Calcutta and the relation of cats to human helminthic infections. J Parasitol XX:213–227.
Faust EC. 1952. Some morphologic characters of *Diphyllobothrium latum.* Anals Inst Med Trop 9:1277–1300.
Grove DI. 1990. A History of Human Helminthology. Wallingford, UK: CAB International. 848 pp.
Hendrix CM, Blagburn BL. 1983. Common gastrointestinal parasites. Vet Clin North Am 13:627-646.
Hutchison WM. 1957. The incidence and distribution of *Hydatigera taeniaeformis* and other intestinal helminths in Scottish cats. J Parasitol 43:318–321.
Janicki, C. 1917. Observations su quelques espèces de poissons afin d'arriver à connaître plus à fond le contenu de leour estomac et pour trover des stades encore inconnus de plerocercoide. Bull Soc Neuch Sci Nat 42:22–29.
Khalil LF, Jones A, Bray RA. 1994. Keys to the Cestode Parasites of Vertebrates. Wallingford, UK: CAB International. 751 pp.
Miyazaki I. 1991. Helminthic Zoonoses. Japan, Tokyo: Intl Med Found. 494 pp.
Peters L, Calvis D, Robertson J. 1978. *Diphyllobothrium latum* currently present in northern Michigan? J Parasitol 68:999–1003.
Rosen F. 1917. Recherches sur le développement des Cestodes. I. Le cycle évolutif des Bothriocéphales. Etudes sur l'origine des cestodes et leurs états larvaires. Bul Soc Neuch Sci Nat 43:1–55.
Sakamoto T. 1977. The anthelmintic efficacy of Droncit on adult tapeworms of *Hydatigera taeniaeformis, Mesocestoides corti, Echinococcus multilocularis, Diphyllobothrium erinacei,* and *D. latum.* Vet Med Rev 1:64–74.
Shamarina AG, Kazantseva NA, Zavgorodnyaya NF, Balkov YM. 1980. The role of waterbodies in the spread of human diphyllobothriasis and opisthorchiasis in the Perm region. Biol Resu vodo sapad Urala, 145–147.
Tanaka H, Watanabe M, Ogawa Y. 1985 Parasites of stray dogs and cats in the Kanto region, Honshu, Japan. J Vet Med, Japan 771:657–661.
Tongson MS, San Pablo FG. 1979. A study on the prevalence of gastro-intestinal worms of cats in metropolitan Manila. Philipp J Vet Med 18:1–15.
Torres P, Ruiz E, Rebolledo C, Mira A, Cubillos V, Navarrete N, Gesche W, Montefusco A, Valdés L, Alberdi A. 1990. Parasitism in fish and human riverside communities from Huillinco and Natri Lakes (Great Island of Chiloé), Chile. Bol Chil Parasitol 45:47–55.
Torres P, Cubillos V, Gesche W, Rebolledo C, Montefusco A, Miranda JC, Arenas J, Mira A, Nilo M, Abello C. 1991. Difilobotriasis en salmonidos introducidos en lagos del sur de Chile: aspectos patologicos, relatcion don infeccion humana, animales domestics y aves piscivoras. Arch Med Vet 23:165–183.
Vereta LE. 1986. Helminths of cats in Moscow and epizootic aspects of some helminthiases. Bull Vsesoy Inst Gelmint, KI Skryabina 42:20–26.
von Bonsdorff B. 1978. The broad tapeworm story. Acta Med Scand 204:241–247.
Wardle RA. 1933. Significant factors in the plerocercoid environment of *Diphyllobothrium latum* (Linn.). J Helminthol 11:25–44.
Wardle RA, Green NK. 1941. The rate of growth of the tapeworm *Diphyllobothrium latum* (L.). Can J Res 19:245–251.
Wardle RA, Gotschall MJ, Horder LJ. 1937. The influence of *Diphyllobothrium latum* infestation upon dogs. Trans Roy Soc Can 31:59–69.

Other Species of *Diphyllobothrium* and Related Genera

Besides other species of *Diphyllobothrium* that occur in marine mammals and fish-eating birds are species representative of other genera: These genera include *Ligula, Digramma, Hexagonoporus, Diplogonoporus, Baylisiella,* and *Plicobothrium. Diplogonoporus grandis* of whales of the genus *Balaenoptera* has been reported in Peru and Japan from humans who have had a history of eating raw fish, and it is assumed that this is how they obtained the infection. Rare human infections with several other species representing some of the other genera have also been reported. Thus, it would be likely that infection with species other than *Diphyllobothrium latum* is possible in coastal areas where cats have access to marine fish.

Spirometra Species

The taxonomy of the genus *Spirometra* is very confused for reasons ranging from inadequate descriptions to assumptions made that specimens of larval forms recovered from intermediate or paratenic hosts in Asia are the same as those recovered from related hosts in Europe. It is also apparent that authors had initially tried to assume that the same final host would indicate specimens of the same species. For those interested in reading about the history of this confusion, it is recommended that they examine the section on *Spirometra* in Wardle and McLeod (1952).

For the purpose of the text that follows, two major species of *Spirometra* are recognized. *Spirometra erinaceieuropaei* (Rudolphi, 1819) is discussed as the representative of specimens mainly from Europe and Asia, although this species has also been reported from the Americas. *Spirometra mansonoides* Mueller, 1935, is considered to represent specimens that are mainly from the Americas. This classification is likely to be less than perfect; however, it represents a beginning that can be used to allow information to be gained on these parasites. In recent years, very little attention has been given to the actual identity of the species of *Spirometra* present in cats in any given area, and it is hoped that further examination of specific characters will allow the identification of the important species infecting cats.

Four other species have been described from felids. One species is *Spirometra felis,* which was described by Southwell (1928) for specimens recovered from *Felis tigris* and *Felis pardus* in the Calcutta Zoological Gardens; Southwell believed them the same as the *Spirometra felis* described as *Bothriocephalus felis* by Creplin (1825) from a domestic cat. A second species, *Spirometra decipiens,* was originally described from a "cat-like" animal in Brazil by Diesing (1850). Chandler (1925) supposedly "rediscovered" *Spirometra decipiens* in a domestic cat and a *Felis nebulosa* in the Calcutta Zoological Gardens. In Uruguay, Wolffhügel and Vogelsang (1926) described *Spirometra decipiens* from forms obtained by feeding dogs larvae from frogs, and these authors claimed they were the same as *Spirometra longicolle* from a *Felis jaguarondi* in Argentina. Faust et al. (1929) recovered specimens identified as *Spirometra decipiens* from a cat, a leopard, and a dog in China and obtained the same form by feeding larvae from frogs to dogs. Saleque et al. (1990) described a case of *Spirometra* in a cat in India that was not assigned to any certain species. Two other species have been reported from nondomestic cats in the Americas. *Spirometra gracile* was described from small specimens recovered from *Felis macrura* in Brazil. *Spirometra urichi* was recovered from an ocelot in Trinidad and described by Cameron (1936).

REFERENCES

Cameron TWM. 1936. Studies on the endoparasitic fauna of Trinidad. III. Some parasites of Trinidad carnivora. Can J Res 14:25–38.

Chandler AC. 1925. The helminthic parasites of cats in Calcutta and the relation of cat to human helminthic infections. Ind J Med Res 13:213–220.

Creplin FCH. 1825. Observactiones de entozois. Gryphiswaldiae. 86 pp.

Diesing KM. 1850. System helminthum 2. Vienna, Austria.

Faust EC, Campbell HE, Kellogg CR. 1929. Morphological and biological studies on the species of *Diphyllobothrium* in China. Am J Hyg 9:560–583.

Saleque A, Juyal PD, Bhatia BB. 1990. *Spirometra* sp. in a domestic cat in India. Vet Parasitol 35:273–276.

Southwell T. 1928. Cestodes of the order Pseudophyllidea recorded from India and Ceylon. Ann Trop Med Parasitol 22:419–448.

Wardle RA, McLeod JA. 1952. The Zoology of Tapeworms. New York, NY: Hafner Publishing Company (facsimile, 1968 printing).

Wolffhügel K, Vogelsang EG. 1926. *Dibothriocephalus decipiens* (Diesing) y su larva *Sparganum reptans* en el Uruguay. Rev Med Vet, Montevideo Jg 2: 433–434.

Spirometra erinaceieuropaei (Rudolphi, 1819)

Etymology

Spiro = spiral and *metra* = uterus (referring to the spiral-shaped uterus as opposed to the rosette-shaped uterus in *Diphyllobothrium*) and *erinaceieuropaei* for the European hedgehog (genus = *Erinaceus*) from which the larval stage was originally recovered and named.

Synonyms

The following list of synonyms is taken from Schmidt (1986), who did not recognize the genus *Spirometra* but considered it a synonym of *Diphyllobothrium: Bothriocephalus decipiens* Railliet, 1866; *Bothriocephalus felis* Creplin, 1825; *Bothriocephalus maculatus* Leuckart, 1848; *Bothriocephalus mansoni* (Cobbald, 1882) Blanchard, 1888; *Bothriocephalus liguloides* (Diesing, 1859); *Bothriocephalus sulcatus* Molin, 1858; *Dibothrium serratum* Diesing, 1850; *Dibothrium mansoni* Ariola, 1900; *Diphyllobothrium fausti* Vialli, 1931; *Dubium erinaceieuropaei* Rudolphi, 1819; *Ligula mansoni* Cobbold, 1882; *Ligula pancerii* Polonio, 1860; *Ligula ranarum* Gastaldi, 1854; *Ligula reptans* Diesing, 1850; *Sparganum affine* Diesing, 1854; *Sparganum ellipticum* Molin, 1858; *Sparganum mansoni* (Cobbold, 1882) Stiles and Taylor, 1902; *Sparganum philippinensis* Tubangui, 1924; *Spar-*

ganum proliferum Ijima, 1905; *Sparganum reptans* Diesing, 1854; *Spirometra decipiens* Faust, Campbell, and Kellogg, 1929; *Spirometra erinacei* Faust, Campbell, and Kellogg, 1929; *Spirometra houghtoni* Faust, Campbell, and Kellogg, 1929; *Spirometra okumurai* Faust, Campbell, and Kellogg, 1929; *Spirometra raillieti* (Ratz, 1913) Wardle, McLeod, and Stewart, 1947; *Spirometra ranarum* Meggitt, 1925; *Spirometra reptans* (Diesing, 1850) Meggitt, 1924; *Spirometra tangalongi* (MacCallum, 1921).

History

In 1819, Rudolphi described a larval tapeworm recovered from a European hedgehog as the species *erinaceieuropaei.* Faust et al. (1929) recovered larval stages from a Chinese hedgehog (*Erinaceus dealbatus*) and reared the adult stage by feeding this form to dogs. These authors believed this form identical to that described by Rudolphi from the European hedgehog. While this was occurring, Dr. Patrick Manson in 1882 recovered 12 tapeworm larvae, spargana, during an autopsy in Amoy, China, and this type of larval worm came to be known as Manson's sparganum, or *Sparganum mansoni.* In 1917, Yoshida obtained adult worms by feeding sparganids obtained from humans to dogs. Joyeux and Houdemer (1928) described *Spirometra mansoni* (as *Diphyllobothrium mansoni*) using sparganids obtained from different animals in Southeast Asia. Odening (1982) reexamined the biology of the European form. Work of Fukumoto et al. (1992) on the isoenzyme patterns of *Spirometra erinaceieuropaei* from Japan and Australia indicated that these two forms were similar.

Geographic Distribution

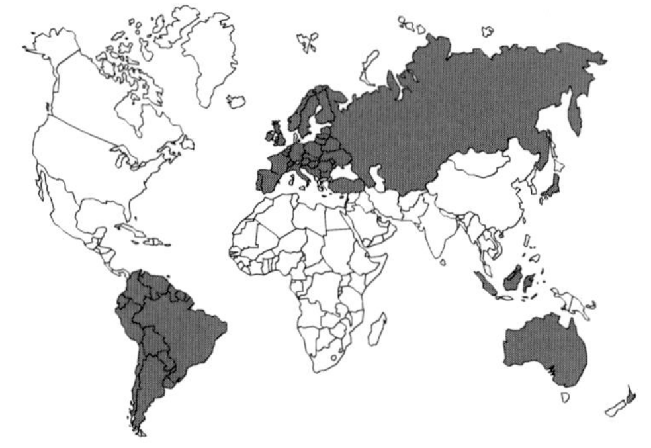

Fig. 3.5.

Spirometra mansoni has been reported on numerous occasions from the orient (Fujinami et al., 1983; Tang, 1935 (sparganosis in the cat); Wu, 1938; Rhode, 1962; Shanta et al., 1980). Schmidt et al. (1975) found *Spirometra* in cats from Taiwan and the Philippines; Tongson and San Pablo (1979) also reported *Spirometra mansoni* from the Philippines. It has been reported from the Americas (Mueller et al., 1975; Torres and Figueroa, 1982). *Spirometra mansoni* has also been reported in cats from Hawaii (Olsen and Hass, 1976) and Puerto Rico (Acholonu, 1977). Australia can also be considered to be within the range of *Spirometra mansoni* (Gregory and Munday, 1976; Thompson et al., 1993). Reports from Europe include those of Odening (1982) and Manfredi and Felicita (1993).

Location in Host

Adult worms are found in the small intestine. Cats can on occasion be infected with the plerocercoid larval stage (see the section Feline Sparganosis, below).

Parasite Identification

The strobila of this tapeworm is about 1 m long and less than 1 cm in width. The bothria is similar to that of *Diphyllobothrium.* The uterus of *Spirometra* species appears spiral as the uterine loops from the posterior to the anterior pile up on each other; the uterus of *Diphyllobothrium* appears to have a rosette formation. Each proglottid has separate openings of the cirrus and vaginal pore that are in the anterior portion of each segment, while the uterine pore is the posterior of each segment. In contrast, the cirrus and vaginal pores of *Diphyllobothrium* are fused into a single pore. Also, the cirrus sac and seminal vesicle are fused together in *Spirometra.*

The proglottids of *Spirometra erinaceieuropaei* contain a uterus that is not expanded terminally into a U-shaped portion as is the case with *Spirometra mansonoides.*

The egg of *Spirometra* resembles the egg of a digenetic trematode; that is, it is oval and possesses a distinct operculum at one pole of the shell. The eggs are oval and yellow-brown and have dimensions that average 60 μm by 36 μm. The eggs have an asymmetric appearance and tend to be pointed at one end. On eggs that are ruptured, a distinct operculum is visible. The eggs are unembryonated when passed in the feces. It is possible that cats will go for extended periods with negative fecal samples that will be followed by periods when eggs are present in the feces.

Life Cycle

It is reported that the Asian and African forms of *Spirometra erinaceieuropaei* typically prefer the dog as the final host (Mueller, 1974). The life cycle has been completed experimentally through all stages in the laboratory (Lee et al., 1990). The egg that is passed in the feces is not embryonated. After a few days in the water, a ciliated larva with six hooklets typical of tapeworms (called a coracidium) hatches and swims about. This larva is ingested by copepods of the genus *Mesocyclops* and *Eucyclops,* and within the body cavities of these minute crustaceans, a small larval stage called a procercoid develops. Once the larva is 15 days old, it is infective to tadpoles. When the stage in the infected tadpole, which is called a plerocercoid, is 15 days old, it is capable of infecting murine paratenic hosts. After cats are orally infected with plerocercoids, eggs appear in the feces in 15 to 18 days.

Odening (1982) compiled the literature on the prepatent period and life expectancy of *Spirometra erinaceieuropaei* using observations of experimental infections with plerocercoids obtained from hosts from Poland, Burma, Japan, North America, Thailand, and Russia. He found the prepatent period in cats to be between 10 and 25 days and found that the worms in cats lived between 178 to 763 days, or about 6 months to 2.5 years. Odening also reported that the shedding of eggs and proglottids appeared to occur in cycles where the cats would shed eggs for about a month and then would undergo a similar period where they did not shed eggs. The necropsy of cats in the "negative phase" revealed that only the scolex and anterior body were present during this period, and it was felt that this occurred if even more than one tapeworm from the same initial infection were present (i.e., that somehow the shedding of the "spent" proglottids became synchronized).

Clinical Presentation and Pathogenesis

Most of the reports of infection with *Spirometra* species in domestic cats have been results from parasitologic surveys or fecal assays. There has been very little reported on the signs associated with infection, so it may be assumed that infection is often without clinical signs in the cat.

Treatment

Oral, subcutaneous, or intramuscular administration of praziquantel at 30 mg/kg body weight to cats experimentally infected with *Spirometra erinaceieuropaei* cleared all animals of their infections (Fukase et al., 1992). Treatment of 22 cats with naturally acquired infections by the intramuscular or subcutaneous administration of 34 mg/kg body weight eliminated the cestodes from the treated animals. Note: this treatment is with dosages of praziquantel that are greater than those required to treat intestinal dipylidiasis and taeniasis in cats.

Epizootiology

Dogs and cats serve as major hosts of the adults of *Spirometra erinaceieuropaei.* Cats become infected when they eat infected prey. The plerocercoids are present in amphibia, reptiles, and small mammals. Thus, the infection would be expected in cats that hunt. Uga and Yatomi (1992) reported that a survey of cats in Japan revealed that there were almost no cases where cats were infected with both *Spirometra erinaceieuropaei* and with *Dipylidium caninum.* Experimental infection of cats with larval stages from both parasites revealed that only adults of *Spirometra erinaceieuropaei* developed in cats given larvae of both types; this result suggests that somehow infection with this species prevented the development of *Dipylidium caninum* through some form of competition.

Hazards to Other Animals

The hazard posed by the stage passed in the feces of the cat is minimal because it requires a period of development in water to produce the larval stage infectious to copepods. However, infected cats are shedding eggs into the environment that might infect copepods that would then pose a threat to any animal that might be drinking unfiltered water. Thus, infected cats should be treated even if they show no untoward signs from their infection.

Hazards to Humans

Humans have been reported to be infected with both the larval stage and the adult stage of this parasite.

Infection with the larval stage of *Spirometra* is termed "sparganosis," and for a summary of the human cases of sparganosis the reader is referred to texts on human parasitology (Beaver et al., 1984; Gutierrez, 1990). Humans may become infected in three ways. One way is by the accidental ingestion of the aquatic crustacean *Cyclops* infected with procercoids. These procercoids migrate to the subcutaneous tissues and develop to plerocercoids. A second way humans become infected with sparganosis is by the ingestion of plerocercoids within the second intermediate host. These plerocercoids are found in the connective tissue of the muscles, particularly of the abdomen and hindlimbs and under the peritoneum, pericardium, and pleura of the second intermediate host. When these plerocercoids are ingested by humans, they migrate to the various tissue sites and reestablish in the human. A third way humans become infected with sparganosis is by the application of poultices. When infected frog or snake flesh is used as a wound dressing or applied to the eyes, the plerocercoids may migrate to these sites. The plerocercoids migrate subcutaneously, producing inflammation, urticaria, edema, and eosinophilia. Spargana are often found in the periorbital area, in the subcutaneous tissues, and in the muscles. The most probable source of infection is contaminated drinking water (Taylor, 1976).

There have been five cases where humans have been infected with the adult stage of this parasite (Suzuki et al., 1982).

Control/Prevention

Prevention would require that cats be dissuaded from hunting, which is liable to be impossible. Thus, it will be necessary to perform fecal examinations on cats living in areas where this parasite is present. Because of the nature of this parasite to undergo periods when it doesn't shed eggs in the feces, it may be necessary to perform more than one fecal examination each year to ensure that a cat is free of this parasite.

REFERENCES

Acholonu AD. 1977. Some helminths of domestic fissipeds in Ponce, Puerto Rico. J Parasitol 63:-757–758.

Beaver PC, Jung RC, Cupp EW. 1984. Clinical Parasitology. 9th edition. Philadelphia, Pa: Lea and Febiger.

Faust EC, Campbell HE, Kellogg CR. 1929. Morphological and biological studies on the species of *Diphyllobothrium* in China. Am J Hyg 9:560–583.

Fujinami F, Tanaka H, Ohshima S. 1983. Prevalence of protozoan and helminth parasites in cats for experimental use obtained from Kanto Area, Japan. Exp Anim 32:133–137.

Fukase T, Suzuki M, Igawa H, Chinone S, Akihama S, Itagaki H. 1992. Anthelmintic effect of an injectable formulation of praziquantel against cestodes in dogs and cats. J Jap Vet Med Assoc 45:408–413.

Fukumoto S, Tsuboi T, Hirai K, Phares CK. 1992. Comparison of isozyme patterns between *Spirometra erinacei* and *Spirometra mansonoides* by isoelectric focusing. J Parasitol 78:735–738.

Gregory GG, Munday BL. 1976. Internal parasites of feral cats from the Tasmanian Midlands and King Island. Aust Vet J 52:317–320.

Gutierrez Y. 1990. Diagnostic Pathology of Parasitic Infections with Clinical Correlations. Philadelphia, Pa: Lea and Febiger. 532 pp.

Joyeux C, Houdemer E. 1928. Recherches sur la faune helminthologique d l'Indochine (cestodes et trématodes). Ann Parasitol Hum Comp 6:27–58.

Lee SH, We JS, Sohn WM, Hong ST, Chai JY. 1990. Experimental life history of *Spirometra erinacei.* Kor J Parasitol 28:161–173.

Manfredi MT, Felicita A. 1993. Recenti rilievi epidemiologici sui cestodi del cane e del gatto. Prax Vet Milano 14:5–7.

Mueller JF. 1974. The biology of *Spirometra.* J Parasitol 60:3–14.

Mueller JF, Miranda Fróes O, Fernández T. 1975. On the occurrence of *Spirometra mansonoides* in South America. J Parasitol 61:774–775.

Odening K. 1982. Zur Strobilaperiodizität von *Spirometra* (Cestoda: Diphyllobothriidae). Angew Parasitol 24:14–27.

Olsen OW, Hass WR. 1976. A new record of *Spirometra mansoni,* a zoonotic tapeworm, from naturally infected cats and dogs in Hawaii. Hawaii Med J 35:261–263.

Rhode K. 1962. Helminthen aus Katzen un Junden in Malaya; Bermerkungen zu ihrer epidemiologischen Bedeutung für Menschen. Ztsch Parasitenk 22:237–244.

Rudolphi CA. 1819. Entozoorum synopsis cui accedeunt mantiss duplex et indices locupletissimi. Berolini. 811 pp.

Schmidt GD. 1986. Handbook of Tapeworm Identification. Boca Raton, Fla: CRC Press. 675 pp.

Schmidt GD, Fuerstein V, Kuntz RE. 1975. Tapeworms of domestic dogs and cats in Taiwan with remarks on *Spirometra* spp. BS Chauhan Comm Vol 41–46.

Shanta CS, Wan SP, Kwong KH. 1980. A survey of the endo- and ectoparasites of cats in and around Ipoh, West Malaysia. Malay Vet J 7:17–27.
Suzuki N, Kumazawa H, Hosogi H, Nakagawa O. 1982. A case of human infection with the adult of *Spirometra erinacei* (Rudolphi, 1819) Faust, Campbell and Kellogg, 1929. Jap J Parasitol 31:23–26.
Tang CC. 1935. A survey of helminth fauna of cats in Foochow. Pek Nat Hist Bull 10:223–231.
Taylor RL. 1976. Sparganosis in the United States. Report of a case. Am J Clin Pathol 66:560–564.
Thompson RCA, Meloni BP, Hopkins RM, Deplazes P, Reynoldson JA. 1993. Observations on the endo- and ectoparasites affecting dogs and cats in aboriginal communities in the north-west of Western Australia. Aust Vet J 70:268–270.
Tongson MS, San Pablo FG. 1979. A study on the prevalence of gastrointestinal worms of cats in metropolitan Manila. Philip J Vet Med 18:1–15.
Torres P, Figueroa L. 1982. Infeccion por *Spirometra mansoni* (Cestoda, Pseudophyllidea) en el sur de Chile. Bol Chileno Parastiol 37:72–73.
Uga S, Yatomi K. 1992. Interspecific competition between *Spirometra erinacei* (Rudolphi, 1819) and *Dipylidium caninum* (Linnaeus, 1758) in cats. Jap J Parasitol 41:414–419.
Wu K. 1938. Helminthic fauna in vertebrates of the Hangchow area. Pek Nat Hist Bull 12:1–8.
Yoshida S. 1917. The occurrence of *Bothriocephalus liguloides* Leuckart, with special reference to its development. J Parasitol 3:171–176.

Spirometra mansonoides Mueller, 1935

Etymology

Spiro = spiral and *metra* = uterus (referring to the spiral-shaped uterus as opposed to the rosette-shaped uterus in *Diphyllobothrium*) and *mansonoides* because it was "like" *Spirometra mansoni,* the synonym that Mueller used as representing *Spirometra erinaceieuropaei.*

Synonyms

Diphyllobothrium mansonoides, Mueller, 1935.

History

Faust et al. (1929) created a subgenus called *Spirometra* within the genus *Diphyllobothrium.* Mueller (1935) described *Diphyllobothrium mansonoides* using specimens recovered from dogs and cats in the area around Syracuse, New York. In 1937, Mueller raised *Spirometra* to generic rank, and hence, *Diphyllobothrium mansonoides* became *Spirometra mansonoides.*

Geographic Distribution

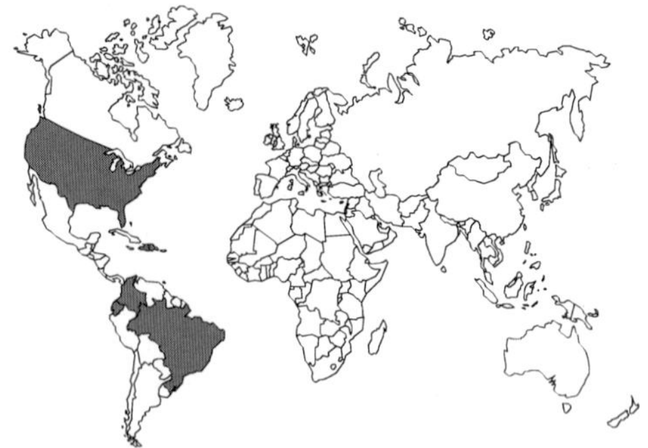

Fig. 3.6.

Spirometra mansonoides is considered a parasite of the eastern United States that extends into parts of South America where it has been reported from Colombia, Ecuador, and Brazil (Fernandez, 1978; Lillis and Burrows, 1964; Mueller et al., 1975; Ogassawara and Benassi, 1980.).

Location in Host

The adults of *Spirometra mansonoides* are found within the small intestine of the feline host.

Parasite Identification

Mueller (1935) provided the original description of this tapeworm. At that time he stated that the maximum length of the strobila was 60 cm with a maximum width of 7 mm. Following almost 40 years of study, he later determined that in a large dog, this tapeworm may attain a length of 1.5 m with a maximum width of a centimeter or more (Mueller, 1974). The margins of this tapeworm are serrate. The strobila appears to be delicate in the neck region and robust posteriorly. Like the adult *Diphyllobothrium latum, Spirometra mansonoides* selectively absorb large quantities of vitamin B_{12} (Marchiondo et al., 1989). This absorption gives the adult tapeworms a characteristic pinkish color (Mueller, 1974). This tapeworm is unique due to the fact that while attached in the host's intestine, the mature proglottids often separate along the longitudinal axis for a short distance.

The scolex of *Spirometra mansonoides* lacks suckers but instead possesses two shallow longitudinal grooves called "bothria" (Mueller, 1935). It varies in diameter from 0.2 mm to almost 0.5 mm

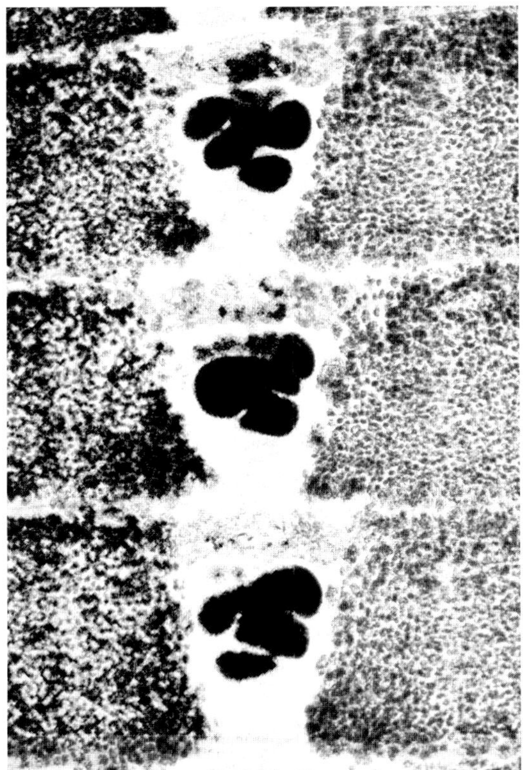

Fig. 3.7. Gravid segments of *Spirometra mansonoides* showing the compact anterior of the uterus in this genus.

with bothria approximately 1 mm in length. The bothria are shallow, broad, and flat bottomed. Each proglottid of *Spirometra* possesses a centrally located spiraled uterus and associated uterine pore through which eggs are released (Fig. 3.7). The uterus is composed of two sections: an anterior series of heavy "outer" coils and a posterior series of narrow "inner" coils. These two regions are joined by a narrow duct that will accommodate only three or four eggs. The uterine and genital apertures open on the ventral surface of the proglottid. The tapeworm characteristically releases the eggs until it becomes exhausted of its uterine contents. Segments are not discharged into the feces until groups of segments have shed all their eggs and are passed as "spent" segments (Kirkpatrick and Sharninghausen, 1983). The uterus in each proglottid of *Spirometra mansonoides* terminates in the anterior of the proglottid in a distinct U-shaped uterus packed full of eggs. This distinct uterine formation does not occur in *Spirometra erinaceieuropaei.*

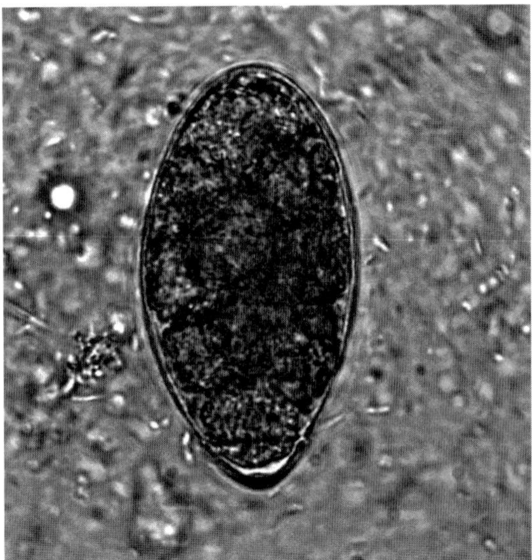

Fig. 3.8. Egg of *Spirometra mansonoides.* (Specimen courtesy of Dr. Raab, Florida, USA)

The egg of *Spirometra* resembles the egg of a digenetic trematode; that is, it is oval and yellow-brown and possesses a distinct operculum at one pole of the shell (Fig. 3.8). The eggs have dimensions that average 60 μm by 36 μm. *Spirometra* eggs have an asymmetric appearance and tend to be pointed at one end. There may be a slight bump on the abopercular end. The eggs are unembryonated when passed in the feces. It is possible that cats will go for extended periods with negative fecal samples that will be followed by periods when eggs are present in the feces.

Life Cycle

Domestic and wild felids serve as the principal definitive hosts for *Spirometra mansonoides,* although dogs and raccoons may harbor the adult cestodes; Mueller believed the natural host in the Americas was probably the bobcat, *Lynx rufus.* Unembryonated eggs pass through the uterine pore of each of the adult cestode's gravid proglottids. The eggs are discharged to the external environment with the cat's feces. In the presence of aeration at room temperature, the eggs develop to the infective stage and can then be stored at 4°C for at least a year without any significant decreases in viability. Eggs are induced to hatch by exposure to direct sunlight and cold temperature shock. In fresh water, the first developmental stage, the ciliated coracidium emerges from the egg and is eaten by the first intermediate host, a freshwater crustacean of the genus *Cyclops.* The second developmental stage, the procercoid, develops within the copepod. When the procercoid is ingested by the second intermediate host, a frog, water snake, or rodent, the procercoid develops into a plerocercoid or sparganum, the third developmental stage. These white, ribbon-like spargana are found primarily in subcutaneous sites. Cats become infected with *Spirometra mansonoides* by preying on frogs, water snakes, fish, birds, or rodents containing the infective plerocercoids. Within 10 to 30 days, the tapeworm develops to the mature stage in the cat's small intestine. Some of the plerocercoids may develop in the wall of the intestine, and Mueller hypothesized that they may eventually migrate back into the lumen of the gut to begin an infection with the adult tapeworm. The adult tapeworm may survive for as long as 3.5 years in the cat (Mueller, 1974). The prepatent period can be as short as 10 days.

Cats can be infected with the larval form of *Spirometra mansonoides* (described below under Feline Sparganosis).

Clinical Presentation and Pathogenesis

Most of the reports of infection with *Spirometra* species in domestic cats have been from results from parasitologic surveys or from results of fecal assays. Mueller (1938) described the signs of infection of adult worms in cats as being marked. The infected animal loses weight but remains hungry. The wall of the intestine of the infected cat becomes thickened, particularly in the layers of circular muscles. If a cat is given an anthelminthic, recovery is rapid—unless the animal has been infected for a long period, causing stunted growth in which case deworming fails to result in the animal reaching target weight. If nursing kittens become infected, there is a marked retardation in growth. Mueller believed that a severe anemia developed in infected cats, but no specific parameters were reported to substantiate this claim. One cat infected with adult *Spirometra* in the United States did exhibit an intermittent watery diarrhea of 2 months duration that resolved following therapy (Kirkpatrick and Sharninghausen, 1983).

Treatment

It is expected that treatment of cats with *Spirometra mansonoides* with praziquantel at the elevated dosage of 30 to 35 mg/kg body weight would cause the elimination of these parasites as it does *Spirometra erinaceieuropaei* (Fukase et al., 1992).

The *Spirometra* in a domestic cat reported by Kirkpatrick and Sharninghausen (1983) was likely to be *Spirometra mansonoides.* This tapeworm was refractory to treatment with albendazole (25 mg/kg BID for 6 consecutive days) and with 1,500 mg of niclosamide following an overnight fast. A single treatment of the cat with 100 mg of bunamidine hydrochloride appeared to remove the worms from this cat based on a postmortem performed a month later after death due to other causes. Bunamidine (Scolaban) is administered orally to cats at a rate of 25 to 50 mg/kg body weight up to a maximum of 600 mg. The tablets should not be broken, crushed, mixed with food, or dissolved in liquid because bunamidine irritates the oral mucosa. Bunamidine should be administered on an empty stomach, and food should be withheld for 3 hours following medication. Treatment with bunamidine should not be repeated within 14 days. It should not be concurrently administered with butamisole, to unweaned kittens, or to cats with cardiac or hepatic disease. Cats should not be allowed to exercise or become excited immediately after treatment with bunamidine. Vomiting, diarrhea, and ventricular fibrillation are the most frequent side effects (Sakamoto, 1977).

Epizootiology

Cats become infected when they eat water snakes, tadpoles, other amphibians, and small mammals (e.g., rats and mice containing the infective plerocercoid stage). Domestic and wild felids serve as the principal definitive hosts for *Spirometra mansonoides,* although dogs and raccoons may harbor the adult cestodes (Mueller, 1974). In a survey of animals from Louisiana, plerocercoids were found in two amphibian, eight reptilian, and three mammalian species. The mammalian species included the opossum, the raccoon, and the gray fox (Corkum, 1966).

Hazards to Other Animals

The egg passed in the feces of the cat is not directly infectious to other hosts. The hazard to other animals is mainly in the form of the plerocercoid that can be obtained from the drinking of water containing copepods infected with the procercoid stage.

Hazards to Humans

The procercoids of *Spirometra mansonoides* are of public health significance as a cause of sparganosis in human beings in the United States; most of the American cases in humans have occurred in the southeastern United States. Mueller and Coulston (1941) had spargana from experimentally infected mice surgically implanted in their arms to show that the sparganum of *Spirometra mansonoides* was capable of persisting in humans. The introduced spargana were about 2 mm long, and when the larvae were recovered from the investigators 3 to 4 months later, the spargana were 12 to 60 mm long. One was fed to a cat, and the cat developed a patent infection. Mueller et al. (1963a, b) reported on the first naturally acquired human case of sparganosis in the United States. There have been rare cases of sparganosis that are apparently of the *Spirometra erinaceieuropaei* type and a second form of proliferating sparganosis reported from humans in Florida, but these seem to be the exception rather than the majority of cases. Mueller (1974) believed the plerocercoid stage is rather characteristic for each of the two species: that of *Spirometra mansonoides* is thin and elongate, while that of the *Spirometra erinaceieuropaei* type is massive and rather fragile; the growth factors produced by the two species also appear to have different effects on mice and rats (Mueller, 1972). There have been over 50 cases of human sparganosis reported in the United States, and for further information, readers are referred to Taylor (1976) and the texts by Beaver et al. (1984) and Gutierrez (1990).

Control/Prevention

At no time should cats be allowed to ingest frogs, water snakes, or rodents. Such habits may lead to infections with the infective plerocercoid stages of *Spirometra.* Cats should not be allowed to roam freely or to scavenge carcasses. Predation and carrion feeding may lead to parasitism if prey animals such as frogs, water snakes, rodents, or their carcasses contain the infective plerocercoid stages (Hendrix and Blagburn, 1983).

REFERENCES

Beaver PC, Jung RC, Cupp EW. 1984. Clinical Parasitology. 9th edition. Philadelphia, Pa: Lea and Febiger.

Corkum KC. 1966. Sparganosis in some vertebrates of Louisiana and observations on a human infection. J Parasitol 52:444–448.

Faust EC, Campbell HE, Kellogg CR. 1929. Morphological and biological studies on the species of *Diphyllobothrium* in China. Am J Hyg 9:560–583.

Fernandez TE. 1978. Reporte del *Diphyllobothrium* (*Spirometra*) en el Ecuador. Rev Ecuator Hig Med Trop 31:93–97.

Fukase T, Suzuki M, Igawa H, Chinone S, Akihama S, Itagaki H. 1992. Anthelmintic effect of an injectable formulation of praziquantel against cestodes in dogs and cats. J Jap Vet Med Assoc 45:408–413.

Gutierrez Y. 1990. Diagnostic Pathology of Parasitic Infections with Clinical Correlations. Philadelphia, Pa: Lea and Febiger. 532 pp.

Hendrix CM, Blagburn BL. 1983. Common gastrointestinal parasites. Vet Clin North Am: Small Anim Pract 13:627–645.

Kirkpatrick CE, Sharninghausen F. 1983. *Spirometra* sp. in a domestic cat in Pennsylvania. J Am Vet Med Assoc 183:111–112.

Lillis WG, Burrows RB. 1964. Natural infections of *Spirometra mansonoides* in New Jersey cats. J Parasitol 50:680.

Marchiondo AA, Weinstein PP, Mueller JF. 1989. Significance of the distribution of ^{57}Co-Vitamin B_{12} in *Spirometra mansonoides* (Cestoidea) during growth and differentiation in mammalian intermediate and definitive hosts. Int J Parasitol 19:119–124.

Mueller JF. 1935. A *Diphyllobothrium* from cats and dogs in the Syracuse region. J Parasitol 21:114–122.

Mueller JF. 1937. A repartition of the genus *Diphyllobothrium.* J Parasitol 23:308–310.

Mueller JF. 1938. The life history of *Diphyllobothrium* mansonoides *Mueller,* 1935, and some considerations with regard to sparganosis in the United States. Am J Trop Med 18:41–58.

Mueller JF. 1972. Failure of oriental spargana to immunize the hypophysectomized rat against the sparganum growth factor of *Spirometra mansonoides.* J Parasitol 58:872–875.

Mueller JF. 1974. The biology of *Spirometra.* J Parasitol 60:3–14.

Mueller JF, Coulston F. 1941. Experimental human infection with the sparganum larva of *Spirometra mansonoides* (Mueller, 1935). Am J Trop Med 21:399–425.

Mueller JF, Hart EP, Walsh WP. 1963a. First reported case of naturally-occurring human sparganosis in New York State. NY State J Med 63:715–718.

Mueller JF, Hart EP, Walsh WP. 1963b. Human sparganosis in the United States. J Parasitol 49:294–296.

Mueller JF, Miranda Fróes O, Fernández T. 1975. On the occurrence of *Spirometra mansonoides* in South America. J Parasitol 61:774–775.

Ogassawara S, Benassi S. 1980. *Spirometra mansonoides* Mueller, 1935, em animal da especie felina no estado de Sao Paulo. Arq Inst Biol Sao Paulo 47:43–46.

Sakamoto T. 1977. The anthelmintic efficacy of Droncit on adult tapeworms of *Hydatigera taeniaeformis, Mesocestoides corti, Echinococcus multilocularis, Diphyllobothrium erinacei,* and *D. latum.* Vet Med Rev 1:64–74.

Taylor RL. 1976. Sparganosis in the United States. Am J Clin Pathol 66:560–564.

Feline Sparganosis

Cats can also serve to support the plerocercoid larval stage of *Spirometra* species; they act in this case as the paratenic hosts rather than the final hosts of the infection. Infection with this larval stage often goes by the name "sparganosis." Plerocercoids or spargana are white, ribbon-like structures that usually occur subcutaneously in the tissues of the second intermediate host. These larval tapeworms may reach several centimeters in length. Like the adult tapeworms, the spargana selectively absorb large quantities of vitamin B_{12}, giving the head of the larva a characteristic pinkish color. Mueller (1974) stated that the appearance of the plerocercoid of *Spirometra erinaceieuropaei* is more robust than that of the slender plerocercoid of *Spirometra mansonoides.* Another form of spargana that has been reported from humans is a plerocercoid that seems to reproduce inside the host and has been called sparganum proliferum or the proliferating sparganum. A case of proliferating sparganosis has been reported from a cat from Florida.

Cats infected with the plerocercoids of *Spirometra erinaceieuropaei* have been reported in China (Tang, 1935), in Japan (Uga et al., 1986), and in a cat from Taiwan that was purchased in Cambodia and brought to the United States (Schmidt et al., 1968). Uga et al. (1986) found that 10 of 1,880 cats were infected with this parasite in the Hyogo Prefecture of Japan, with cats harboring between 1 and 166 spargana each. The average length of the plerocercoids was 11.5 cm (2.0–28.0 cm), and they had the thickened body with a distinct cup-shaped groove in the scolex described by Mueller (1974) for the plerocercoids of *Spirometra erinaceieuropaei.* Some of these plerocercoids were fed to dogs that developed patent infections with *Spirometra erinaceieuropaei.* From the cats, the plerocercoids were recovered from the inguinal and cervical regions, from the fatty tissue around the kidneys, on the chest, and in both femoral regions. All the cats harboring the plerocercoids were also found to be infected with the adults of *Spirometra erinaceieuropaei;* however, only 0.5 percent of the cats in the survey harbored plerocercoids, while 39 percent of the cats in the survey harbored the adult tapeworm. There have been no studies describing the clinical signs of infection in cats or the attempted treatment of the infections with either anthelminthics or via surgical removal of the worms.

There have been rare reports of humans infected with plerocercoids that seem to proliferate unchecked in the tissues of the human host. Some of these cases have been from Japan, one has been from Florida, and one from Venezuela (Beaver and Rolon, 1981; Moulinier et al., 1982). There has been one such case reported from a cat in Florida where proliferating plerocercoids were found in the abdominal cavity of a 6-year-old, male, domestic long-haired cat that had lived its entire life in Florida. The cat developed a painful abdomen over a 2-month period, at the end of which it was noted to have a palpable abdominal mass and was euthanatized. Necropsy revealed that the spleen, liver, and stomach wall had numerous plerocercoids that appeared to be budding.

The plerocercoids of *Spirometra mansonoides* are capable of persisting in the tissues of cats, as was noted by Mueller (1938), who reported the presence of an active larva being recovered from a cyst on the external wall of the duodenum of a cat from Rome, New York. Cats can be infected with spargana by feeding procercoids to young kittens. The cysts appear in the flat muscles of the body wall or under the skin (Mueller, 1974). There has been very little description of the clinical signs associated with potential plerocercoid infection in cats.

REFERENCES

Beaver PC, Rolon FA. 1981. Proliferating larval cestode in a man in Paraguay. A case report and review. Am J Trop Med Hyg 30:635–637.

Moulinier R, Martinez E, Torres J, Noya O, de Noya BA, Reyes O. 1982. Human proliferative sparganosis in Venezuela. Report of a case. Am J Trop Med Hyg 31:358–363.

Mueller JF. 1938. The life history of *Diphyllobothrium mansonoides* Mueller, 1935, and some considerations with regard to sparganosis in the United States. Am J Trop Med 18:41–58.

Mueller JF. 1974. The biology of *Spirometra*. J Parasitol 60:3–14.

Schmidt RE, Reid JS, Garner FM. 1968. Sparganosis in a cat. J Small Anim Pract 9:551–553.

Tang CC. 1935. A survey of helminth fauna of cats in Foochow. Pek Nat Hist Bull 10:223–231.

Uga Sm Goto M, Matsumura T, Kagei N. 1986. Natural infection of sparganum mansoni in cats captured in Hyogo Prefecture, Japan. Jap J Parastiol 35:153–159.

CYCLOPHYLLIDEA

The order Cyclophyllidea is characterized by having a scolex that typically bears four suckers. The genital openings are lateral, except in the case of the Mesocestoididae. This order of tapeworms contains almost all the major tapeworms found in domestic animals and man. Most of the other orders of tapeworms, with the exception of some members of the Pseudophyllidea, are parasites of fish, amphibia, and reptiles.

MESOCESTOIDIDAE

The Mesocestoididae are parasites in the small intestine of mammals, rarely birds (Rausch, 1994). Two genera, *Mesocestoides* and *Mesogyna*, are recognized within this family. The adult is characterized mainly by the possession of a scolex that bears four muscular suckers, but no rostellum, and segments that contain medial sexual openings. In the mature proglottid, the eggs are contained in a single thick-walled parauterine organ. The life cycle of the members of this family is not known, but what is known based on our knowledge of *Mesocestoides* is that it appears that there are two intermediate hosts in the life cycle. The first intermediate host has been assumed to be an arthropod. The second intermediate host can be a reptile or small mammal that contains a larval stage, called a tetrathyridium, which is a solid-bodied larva that has a scolex similar to that of the adult worm. Cats can serve as the final host for *Mesocestoides,* in which case the adult worms are present in the small intestine. Cats can also be infected with the tetrathyridial stage of this parasite.

REFERENCES

Rausch RL. 1994. Family Mesocestoididae Fuhrmann, 1907. In Keys to the Cestode Parasites of Vertebrates, ed LF Khalil, A Jones, and RA Bray. Wallingford, UK: CAB International.

Mesocestoides lineatus (Goeze, 1782) Railliet, 1893

Etymology

Meso = in between and *cestoides* is for cestode; this genus has characteristics that are rather between those of the Pseudophyllidea and the Cyclophyllidea, especially the presence of a four-suckered holdfast accompanying a strobila that has the openings of the reproductive system on the center of the ventral surface of the proglottid rather than along the margins of the proglottid.

Synonyms

Taenia vulpina Schrank, 1788; *Taenia pseudocucumerina* Bailliet, 1863; *Taenia pseudoelliptica* Bailliet, 1863; *Mesocestoides ambiguus* Joyeux and Baer, 1932; *Mesocestoides variabilis* Mueller, 1927; *Taenia canis lagopodis* Rudolphi, 1810; *Taenina cateniformis* Gmelin, 1750; *Mesocestoides elongatus* Leuckart, 1879; *Mesocestoides litteratus* (Batsch, 1786); *Mesocestoides longistriatus* Setti, 1879; *Mesocestoides mesorchis* Cameron, 1925; *Mesocestoides caestus* Cameron, 1925; *Mesocestoides latus* Mueller, 1927; *Mesocestoides utriculifer* (Walter, 1866); *Mesocestoides tenuis* Meggitt, 1931; *Mesocestoides manteri* Chandler, 1942; *Mesocestoides kirbyi* Chandler, 1944; *Mesocestoides jonesi* Ciodia, 1955; *Mesocestoides carnivoricolus* Grundmann, 1956; *Mesocestoides bassarisci* MacCullum, 1921; *Mesocestoides angustatus* (Rudolphi, 1819).

History

In 1863, Vaillant described a tapeworm as *Mesocestoides ambiguus* from a genet in North Africa. It was noted at this time that the parasite was unusual because it possessed four suckers and medial reproductive openings. However, although the characteristics defining the genus have never been questioned, no criteria to define species have emerged as readily acceptable to most workers in this field. Thus, numerous species began to appear in the literature. In 1932, Witenberg, in a review of the genus, recognized only one species, *Mesocestoides lineatus,* and he discounted or synonymized 24 described species. Other workers (e.g., Chandler, 1942a, 1944; Ciordia, 1955; Voge, 1955; Grundmann, 1956) have created other species for specimens recovered from mammals, but it is difficult to ascertain what criteria are valid or should be accepted. Loos-Frank (1980) created the name *Mesocestoides leptothylacus* for the species of *Mesocestoides* commonly found in foxes in Europe, but it is hard to understand why another named specimen from foxes would not have priority. A second problem that has developed around the taxonomy and systematics of the genus *Mesocestoides* is due to the fact that the life cycle has not been entirely elucidated. Thus, the experimental infection of hosts with eggs from adult worms cannot be used to test host specificity of the species present in different carnivores. There is every reason to believe that there is more than one species occurring in mammals around the world and that many of the worms that infect cats are commonly parasites of other mammals such as other species of the feline family, wild canids, raccoons, opossums, and mustelids. However, this genus is in need of a careful revision based on the examination of type material.

The second life-cycle stage of *Mesocestoides lineatus,* called a tetrathyridium, is a stage that has been recovered from various amphibians, reptiles, birds, and mammals. This is a small solid-bodied worm with a holdfast (often inverted) that resembles that of the adult worm (Skrjabin and Schultz, 1926). Schultz (1926) and Henry (1927) showed that the larval stage in rodents could develop to adults in cats. Joyeux and Baer (1932) showed that larvae from snakes would develop in cats. Henry (1927) also showed that larvae recovered from the peritoneal cavity of cats could develop to adults if fed to other cats.

Geographic Distribution

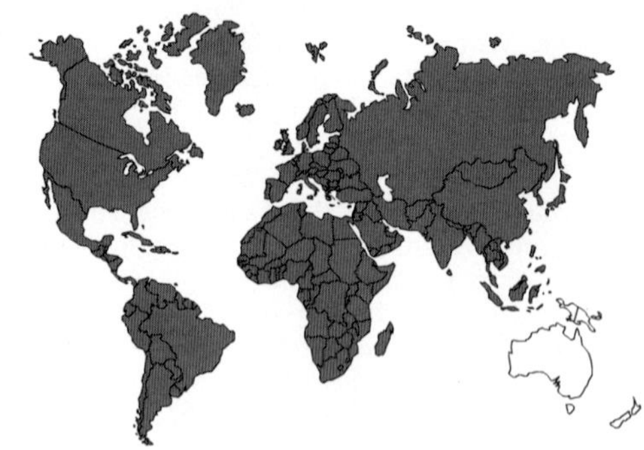

Fig. 3.9.

North and South America (Nolan and Smith, 1985; Loennberg, 1896), Europe (Persson, 1973; Brglez and Zeleznik, 1976; Hiepe et al., 1988; Martini and Poglayen, 1990), Middle East (Ismail et al., 1983; Dincer et al., 1980; Loos-Frank, 1990), Africa (Reid and Reardon, 1976), India (Meggitt, 1931), and Southeast Asia, Japan, and China (Cameron, 1925; Yamaguti 1959). It appears that *Mesocestoides* has not been reported from Australia.

Location in Host

The adults of *Mesocestoides lineatus* are found in the small intestine of the cat. The tetrathyridial larval stage is found on occasion in cats, usually within the peritoneal cavity although sometimes in the muscles (see the section Feline Tetrathyridiosis, below).

Parasite Identification

The gravid proglottids of *Mesocestoides lineatus* are smaller than those of *Dipylidium caninum* and *Taenia taeniaeformis* and are easily recognized by the large parauterine organ present in each segment. The parauterine organ contains the eggs of this worm that have the common hexacanth embryos of cestodes (Figs. 3.10 and 3.11). The anterior end of the worm has a scolex with four distinct suckers but bears neither a rostellum nor hooks (Fig. 3.12). The tapeworm has a neck that contains immature segments.

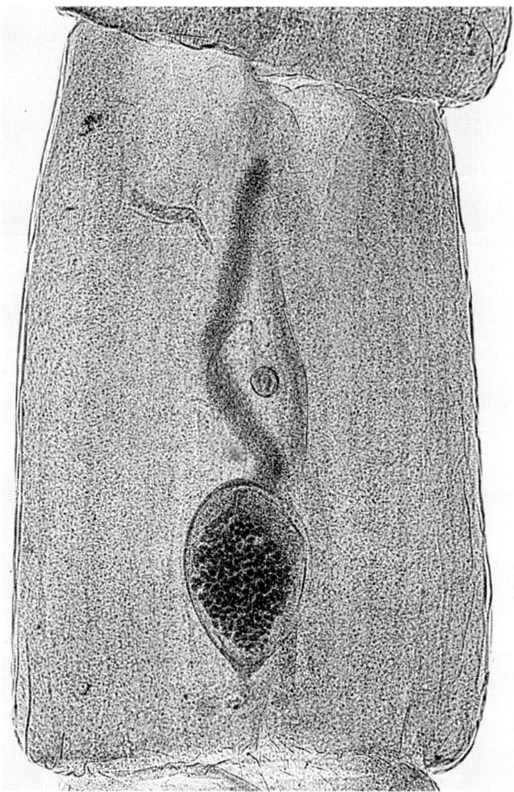

Fig. 3.10. Gravid segment of *Mesocestoides lineatus* showing the large parauterine organ filled with eggs.

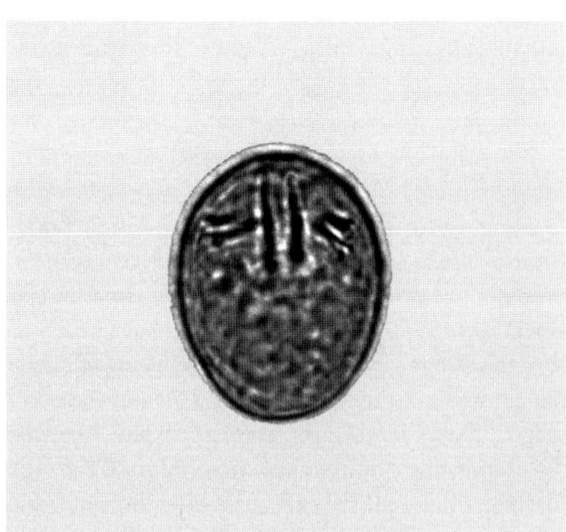

Fig. 3.11. Egg of *Mesocestoides lineatus* expressed from a gravid segment. Note the three pairs of hooklets typical of a tapeworm larva.

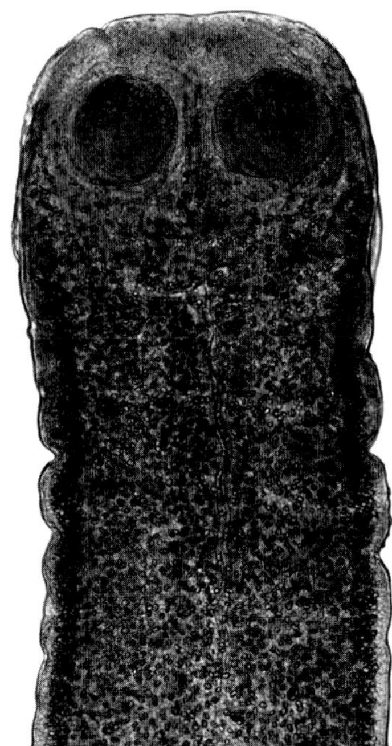

Fig. 3.12. Scolex of *Mesocestoides lineatus.* Note the total lack of a rostellum or hooks on the anterior end.

Life Cycle

The adult cestode sheds segments that are passed in the feces. Loos-Frank (1987) described the behavior of the proglottids shed in the feces and noted that "Gravid proglottids have a conspicuous behavior. On freshly produced feces they stand more or less upright and make slow waving movements with their elongated anterior part. After a few minutes they start crawling away from the feces and in moist conditions can be found quite a distance away from the pellets. In a meadow they were observed on grasses all around freshly deposited feces of a wild fox." She also described the fact that the strobilae of *Mesocestoides lineatus,* like those of *Spirometra mansonoides,* are often shed from worms in a host in a relatively cyclical manner wherein they may be shed for a month and then no segments are shed during the next month. Examination of the animals at necropsy revealed that these cestodes were shedding rather large portions of their strobilae during the periods of segment shedding, causing the populations of worms present to become markedly shortened. This is supported by the observations of Witenberg (1932) that there were often cestodes of varying stages of maturity recovered from infected animals.

The host of the development of the presumed first-stage larval form of *Mesocestoides lineatus* has not been described. Loos-Frank (1991) examined this question with Dr. Ebermann, who had experience with the infection of oribatid mites with other cestode larvae, and they tried, as have others, to reproduce the work of Soldatova (1944), who claimed that development occurred in a few of the mites that were fed on the eggs of this parasite. Other arthropod hosts that have been fed eggs without the development of tetrathyridia include the maggots of *Musca domestica* and *Calliphora* species and cockroaches. As have many other researchers, Loos-Frank (1991) also tried feeding the eggs directly to rodents, but the larvae did not develop; similarly Witenberg (1932) fed eggs to various lizards without the production of any tetrathyridia. Thus, what host serves as the first host of this parasite has never been determined, although it is believed to be some form of arthropod. The fact that the parasite is so universally found around the world would suggest that the first intermediate host must be relatively common.

The second larval stage, the tetrathyridium (Fig. 3.13), occurs in the peritoneal cavity and musculature of numerous animals including amphibia, reptiles, birds, and mammals (including the cat). Some animals can harbor large numbers of these larvae. Cats become infected with the adult tapeworm by the ingestion of an intermediate host that is infected with tetrathyridia. The tetrathyridia of *Mesocestoides lineatus* do not undergo asexual multiplication within the intermediate host (Conn, 1991; Kawamoto et al., 1986). When cats are infected with the tetrathyridial stage of *Mesocestoides lineatus,* each tetrathyridium develops into a single adult cestode (Loos-Frank, 1987). Using tetrathyridia taken from snakes and later maintained in the peritoneal cavities of mice, Kawamoto et al. (1986) demonstrated that after the larvae from mice were ingested by the cat, the majority of the tetrathyridium were shed, leaving only the scolices and necks attached to the mucosa of the intestine.

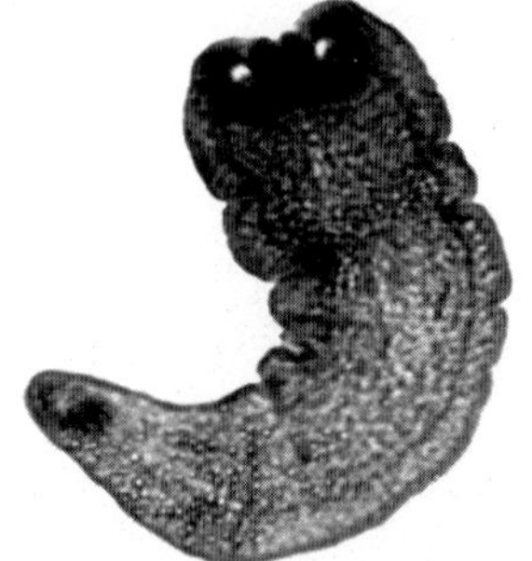

Fig. 3.13. Tetrathryidium of *Mesocestoides.* Note the suckers lacking a rostellum as in the adult and the elongate body. Tetrathyridia can become much longer than this example.

By 10 days after infection of the cats, the strobila had reached lengths of 23 to 52 cm, and gravid proglottids with eggs occupied about 20 percent of the terminal portion of the strobila. Shedding of proglottids began 21 days after the cats were infected. The larvae of a related species, *Mesocestoides vogae* (synonym = *Mesocestoides corti*), which was found in the peritoneal cavity of a population of fence lizards in southern California by Specht and Voge (1965), does undergo proliferation when inoculated into other hosts, such as the laboratory mouse; however, this is the only isolate of *Mesocestoides* that has displayed this property. This tapeworm also undergoes proliferation in the intestine of dogs and cats that are fed the tetrathyridial stage (Kawamoto et al., 1986), but it has never been determined that the cat or dog is the natural final host of this species of tapeworm.

When the cat ingests the tetrathyridial stage of *Mesocestoides lineatus,* the adult worms develop in about 2 to 3 weeks (Witenberg, 1932; Loos-Frank, 1987). Other authors have reported prepatent periods as long as 56 days (Joyeux and Baer, 1932; Schwartz, 1927). Witenburg believed that the longer prepatent periods occurred when the cat was not the typical natural host of the adult stage. Not all tetrathyridia ingested by cats develop to the adult stage; some migrate through the intestinal wall to continue as the tetrathyridial stage in cats (Henry, 1927; Reid and Reardon, 1976; Witenberg, 1932). The adults of *Mesocestoides lineatus* can probably live for around a year in the infected cat (Loos-Frank, 1987).

Clinical Presentation and Pathogenesis

Signs of infection with the adult stage of *Mesocestoides lineatus* in cats have never been described, and so it is presumed not to typically cause clinical signs.

Treatment

Praziquantel has been used to treat dogs experimentally infected with *Mesocestoides vogae* (synonym = *Mesocestoides corti*) and was found to be 100 percent efficacious at 5 mg/kg (Thomas and Gönnert, 1978). Dogs with *Mesocestoides vogae* have also been successfully treated with a dose of 2 mg/kg (Sakamoto et al., 1979). Nitaxzoxanide (at 100 mg/kg) was found to be 100 percent effective against *Mesocestoides lineatus* in cats naturally infected with this parasite.

Epizootiology

Numerous animals can be found infected with the tetrathyridial stage of *Mesocestoides lineatus.* These hosts include various amphibia, reptiles, rodents, opossums, and other mammals; Witenberg (1932) listed the many hosts of the tetrathyridial stage. Cats become infected by the ingestion of these hosts. In some areas, relatively large percentages of these hosts can be infected. The epizootiology is very poorly known, however, due to the lack of knowledge concerning the first host involved in the transmission of this parasite.

Hazards to Other Animals

There is no direct danger to other animals from the proglottids of *Mesocestoides lineatus* passed in the feces of cats. It is likely that the first intermediate host could be infected in an establishment, but that host is not currently known.

Hazards to Humans

Humans have been reported infected with *Mesocestoides lineatus.* The first report was in a girl in Texas who harbored the adult stage of this parasite (Chandler, 1942b), and there have now been six reported cases in humans in the United States (Schultz et al., 1992). There have been a number of reports in Japan where many of the infections are related to the eating of raw snake meat (Ohtomo et al., 1983). There have also been reports of the adult worms in humans in China and Korea (Jin et al., 1991; Eom et al., 1992).

Control/Prevention

Control would be through the prevention of hunting by cats. This will be exceedingly difficult due to the wide range of hosts that are capable of harboring the tetrathyridia.

REFERENCES

Brglez J, Zeleznik Z. 1976. Eine ubbersicht uber die Parasiten der Wildkatze (*Felis sylvestris* Schreber) in Slowenien. Z Jadgwiss 22:109–112.

Cameron TWM. 1925. The cestode genus *Mesocestoides* Vaillant. J Helminthol 3:33–44.

Chandler AC. 1942a. *Mesocestoides manteri* n. sp. from a lynx, with notes on other North American species of *Mesocestoides.* J Parasitol 28:227–231.

Chandler AC. 1942b. First case of human infection with *Mesocestoides.* Science 96:112.

Chandler AC. 1944. A new species of *Mesocestoides, M. kirbyi* from *Canis latrans.* J Parasitol 30:273.

Ciordia H. 1955. *Mesocestoides jonesi* n. sp. from the gray fox, with descriptions of the chromosome complement and a dicephalic specimen. J Tenn Acad Sci 30:57–63.

Conn DB. 1991. The rarity of asexual reproduction among *Mesocestoides* tetrathyridia (Cestoda). J Parasitol 76:453–455.

Dincer S, Cantoray R, Tasan E. 1980. Elazig sokak kedilerinde gorulen ic ce dis parasitler ile bunlarin yayilis oranlari uzerinde arastirmalar. Firat Univ Vet Fak Dergisi 5:7–15.

Eom KS, Kim SH, Rim HJ. 1992. Second case of human infection with *Mesocestoides lineatus* in Korea. Korean J Parasitol 30:147–150.

Grundmann AW. 1956. A new tapeworm, *Mesocestoides carnivoricolus,* from carnivores of the Great Salt Lake desert region of Utah. Proc Helmithol Soc Wash 23:26–28.

Henry A. 1927. *Tétrathyridium* et *Mesocestoides.* Bull Soc Cent Ned Vet 80:147–152.

Hiepe T, Buchwalder R, Kruger A, Schindler W. 1988. Untersuchungen zum endoparasitenbefall streunender Katzen unter besonderer Berucksichtigung der Helminthen. Wien Tierartzl Monatschr 75:499–503.

Ismail NS, Abdel-Hafez, Toor MA. 1983. Prevalence of gastrointestinal helminths in cats from northern Jordan. Pak Vet J 3:129–132.

Jin LG, Yi SH, Liu Z. 1991. The first case of human infections with *Mesocestoides lineatus* (Goeze, 1782) in Jilin Province. J Norman Bethune Univ Med Sci 4:360–361.

Joyeux C, Baer JG. 1932. Recherches sur les cestodes appartenant au genre *Mesocestoides* Villant. Bull Soc Pathol Exot 25:993–1010.

Kawamoto F, Fujioka H, Mizuno S, Kumada N, Voge M. 1986. Studies on the post-larval development of cestodes of the genus *Mesocestoides:* shedding and further development of *M. lineatus* and *M. corti* tetrathyridia *in vivo.* Int J Parasitol 16:323–331.
Loennberg E. 1896. Cestoden. In Hamburger Malhaenische Sammelreise. 10 pp. (Cited in Witenberg, 1932)
Loos-Frank B. 1980. *Mesocestoides leptothylacus* n. sp. und das nomenklatorische Problem in der Gattung *Mesocestoides* Vallant, 1863 (Cestoda). Tropenmed Parasitol 31:2–14.
Loos-Frank B. 1987. Shedding of gravid proglottids and destrobilation in experimental infections of foxes with *Mesocestoides leptothylacus* Loos-Frank, 1980 (Cestoda). J Helminthol 61:213–218.
Loos-Frank B. 1990. Cestodes of the genus *Mesocestoides* (Mesocestoididae) from carnivores in Israel. Isr J Zool 37:3–13.
Loos-Frank B. 1991. One or two intermediate hosts in the life cycle of *Mesocestoides* (Cyclophyllidea, Mesocestoididae)? Parasitol Res 77:726–728.
Martini M, Poglayen G. 1990. Etude sur la valeur de la coprologie chez les carnivores. Epidemiol et Sante Anim 18:123–133.
Meggitt FJ. 1931. On cestodes collected in Burma. II. Parasitology 23:250–263.
Nolan TJ, Smith G, 1985. Time series analysis of the prevalence of endoparasitic infections in cats and dogs presented to a veterinary teaching hospital. Vet Parasitol 59:87–96.
Ohtomo H, Hioki A, Ito A, Kagei N, Hayashi S. 1983. The 13th human case of the infection with *Mesocestoides lineatus* in Japan treated with Paromomycin sulfate. Jap J Antibiot 36:1490–1493.
Persson L. 1973. Spolmask och bandmask hos Stockholmskattor. Svensk Vet 25:214–216.
Reid WA, Reardon MJ. 1976. *Mesocestoides* in the baboon and its development in laboratory animals. J Med Primatol 5:345–352.
Sakamoto T, Kono I, Yasuda N, Kitano Y, Togoe T, Yamamoto Y, Iwashita M, Aoyama K. 1979. Studies on anthelmintic effects of praziquantel against parasites in animals. Bull Fac Agri, Kagoshima University 29:81–87.
Schultz RE. 1926. The twentieth helminthological expedition in USSR–in Novotscherkassk. (Cited in Witenberg, 1932)
Schultz LJ, Roberto RR, Rutherford GW, Hummert B, Lubell I. 1992. *Mesocestoides* (Cestoda) infection in a California child. Pediatr Infect Dis J 11:332–334.
Schwartz B. 1927. The life-history of tapeworms of the genus *Mesocestoides.* Science 66:17–18.
Skrjabin KI, Schultz RE. 1926. Affinités entre *Dithyridium* de souris et le *Mesocestoides lineatus* (Goeze, 1782) des carnivores. Ann Parasitol Hum Comp 4:68–73.
Soldatova AP. 1944. A contribution to the study of the developmental cycle of the cestode *Mesocestoides lineatus* (Goeze, 1782) parasitic in carnivorous mammals. Dokl Akad Nauk SSSR 45:310–312.
Specht D, Voge M. 1965. Asexual multiplication of *Mesocestoides* tetrathyridia in laboratory animals. J Parasitol 51:268–272.
Thomas H, Gönnert R. 1978. The efficacy of praziquantel against cestodes in cats, dogs and sheep. Res Vet Sci 24:20–25.
Vaillant L. 1863. Sur deux helminthes cestoides de la genette. Inst Paris 31:87–88
Voge M. 1955. North American cestodes of the genus *Mesocestoides.* Univ Calif Publ Zool 59:125–156.
Witenberg G. 1932. Studies on the cestode genus *Mesocestoides.* Arch Zool Ital 20:467–509.
Yamaguti S. 1959. Systema Helminthum. Volume II. The Cestodes of Vertebrates. New York, NY: Interscience Publishers.

Feline Tetrathyridiosis

Cats can serve as the second intermediate host of *Mesocestoides* species. It is not known if cats develop infections with this life-cycle stage of the parasite after ingestion of the first intermediate host containing the undescribed first larval stage or only after ingestion of the second intermediate host, which contains the tetrathyridium. There have been no clinical signs ascribed to this infection. In Norway, Berg and Andersen (1982) discovered two tetrathyridia about 7 to 8 cm long as incidental findings in a cat during an ovariohysterectomy.

It has been shown that the tetrathyridial stage of *Mesocestoides lineatus* can be collected from snakes and transferred to frogs, lizards, and mice (Joyeux and Baer, 1932; Kawamoto et al., 1986). Cats have been experimentally infected with the tetrathyridial stage of *Mesocestoides* during attempts to complete the life cycle. Henry (1927), Witenberg (1932), and Reid and Reardon (1976) infected cats with tetrathyridia recovered from the peritoneal cavity of cats or baboons and found that although some of the worms developed to the adult stage, some migrated through the intestinal wall and again took up residence as tetrathyridia within the peritoneal cavity.

Larvae from the cat tend to be free within the peritoneal cavity and range in length from 1 to 7 or 8 cm. The anterior end of the larva has a scolex with four suckers that may be inverted into the body of the larva. The scolex, especially in a small larva, is not often observed until the larva is processed and histological sections made. The tetrathyridia observed in the body of cats by Witenberg (1932) had rather long pointed tails and were about 2 to 7 cm long. The tetrathyridia observed by Loos-Frank (1980) free in the peritoneal cavity of rodents were about 1 to 1.5 mm long and did not possess the long tails observed by Witenberg on the larger larvae, although Witenberg also saw small, compact tetrathyridial forms about 1 to 1.5 mm long encysted in the omentum of cats.

When cats ingest the tetrathyridial stage, the majority of the posterior of the tetrathyridium is lost within the gastrointestinal tract, and the anterior portion, which migrates through the intestinal wall to the peritoneum, may regenerate the posterior body. The tetrathyridia recovered from cats apparently do not undergo asexual division within the peritoneal cavity (Conn, 1991). Dogs in the United States and Europe sometimes develop severe peritonitis that is due to an infection with an asexually dividing cestode that does not bear a scolex and that has been considered by some to be the larval stage of *Mesocestoides corti* (Barsanti et al., 1979), but Conn (1991) has questioned whether this form should be considered a tetrathyridial stage of *Mesocestoides*. Similarly, Conn felt that the identity of the more than 1,000 cestode larvae observed by Neumann (1896) in the abdominal cavity of a European cat were considered those of *Mesocestoides* without a good basis. Witenberg (1932) observed some very small forms encysted in the omentum of cats that were without scolices although they contained numerous calcareous corpuscles typical of tapeworm larvae.

REFERENCES

Barsanti JA, Jones BD, Bailey WAS, Knipling GD. 1979. Diagnosis and treatment of peritonitis caused by a larval cestode *Mesocestoides* spp. in a dog. Cornell Vet 69:45–53.

Berg C, Andersen K. 1982. Bendelormlarver, tetrathyridier, I bukhulen hos en norsk katt. Norsk Vet 94:563–565.

Conn DB, 1991. The rarity of asexual reproduction among *Mesocestoides* tetrathyridia (Cestoda). J Parasitol 76:453–455.

Henry A. 1927. *Tétrathyridium* et *Mesocestoides*. Bull Soc Cent Ned Vet 80:147–152.

Joyeux C, Baer JG. 1932. Recherches sur les cestodes appartenant au genre *Mesocestoides* Villant. Bull Soc Pathol Exot 25:993–1010.

Kawamoto F, Fujioka H, Mizuno S, Kumada N, Voge M. 1986. Studies on the post-larval development of cestodes of the genus *Mesocestoides:* shedding and further development of *M. lineatus* and *M. corti* tetrathyridia *in vivo*. Int J Parasitol 16: 323–331.

Loos-Frank B. 1980. The common vole, *Microtus arvalis,* as intermediate host of *Mesocestoides* (Cestoda) in Germany. Z Parasitenk 63:129–136.

Neumann LG. 1896. Notes sur des téniadés du chien et du chat. Mém Soc Zool Frame 9:171–184.

Reid WA, Reardon MJ. 1976. *Mesocestoides* in the baboon and its development in laboratory animals. J Med Primatol 5:345–352.

Witenberg G. 1932. Studies on the cestode genus *Mesocestoides*. Arch Zool Ital 20:467–509.

DIPYLIDIIDAE

The Dipylidiidae is a group of tapeworms that parasitize the small intestine of mammals in the adult stage. The adult forms tend to be relatively smaller and more fragile than the other forms found in cats. The terminal proglottids are shed with the feces, and instead of being contained in a uterine opening, the eggs are contained within the gravid proglottid in uterine capsules or "egg balls." The uterine capsules may contain several eggs or only one egg. The small scolex bears four suckers and a protrusible rostellum that is armed with several rows of hooks that are most typically rose-thorn shaped. The current classification of Jones (1994) recognizes three genera of tapeworms in this family: *Dipylidium, Diplopylidium,* and *Joyeuxiella*. Cats are host to all three. The first intermediate host of *Dipylidium caninum* is an arthropod, and it is assumed that the first host of *Diplopylidium* and *Joyeuxiella* is also an arthropod, but this has not been proven. In the case of *Dipylidium,* the arthropod is the only intermediate host, but in *Diplopylidium* and *Joyeuxiella,* there is a second intermediate host, which is a reptile.

REFERENCES

Jones A. 1994. Family Dipylidiidae Stiles, 1896. In Keys to the Cestode Parasites of Vertebrates, ed LF Khalil, A Jones, and RA Bray. Wallingford, UK: CAB International.

Dipylidium caninum (Linnaeus, 1758) Leuckart, 1863

Etymology

Di = two and *pylidium* = entrances plus *caninum* for the canine host.

Synonyms

Witenburg (1932) stated that "*Dipylidium* is probably the only species in the genus." He then goes on to list numerous synonyms including *Dipylidium canicum* Lopez-Neyra, 1927; *Dipylidium canium* cani Galli Valerio, 1898; *Dipylidium caracidoi* Lopez-Neyra, 1927; *Dipylidium cati* Neumann, 1896; *Dipylidium compactum* Milzner, 1926; *Dipylidium crassum* Milzner, 1926; *Dipylidium cucumerinum* (Block, 1782); *Dipylidium diffusum* Milzner, 1926; *Dipylidium gracile* Milzner, 1926; *Dipylidium halli* Tubangui, 1925; *Dipylidium longulum* Milzner, 1926; *Dipylidium porimamillanum* Lopez-Neyra, 1927; *Dipylidium sexcoronatum* Ratz, 1900; *Dipylidium walkeri* Sonhi, 1923. The one other species Witenberg thought might be valid was *Dipylidium buencaminoi* Tubangui, 1925, for very small specimens with very small eggs from a dog in Manila, Philippines. Venard (1938) thought there were three species of *Dipylidium,* described from specimens recovered from *Otocyon megalictis* in Somalia. *Dipylidium caninum, Dipylidium buencaminoi,* and *Dipylidium otocyonis* Joyeux, Baer, and Martin, 1936.

History

Dipylidium caninum has been known to man since the time of the ancient Babylonians (Venard, 1938). In 1758, Linnaeus recognized the parasite and named it *Taenia canina.* In 1863, Leuckart created the genus *Dipylidium,* but it was not until 1893 that it was described by Diamare. Early work on the life cycle was reported by Neveau-Lemaire (1936). This parasite is one of the most common parasites of domesticated dogs and cats.

Geographic Distribution

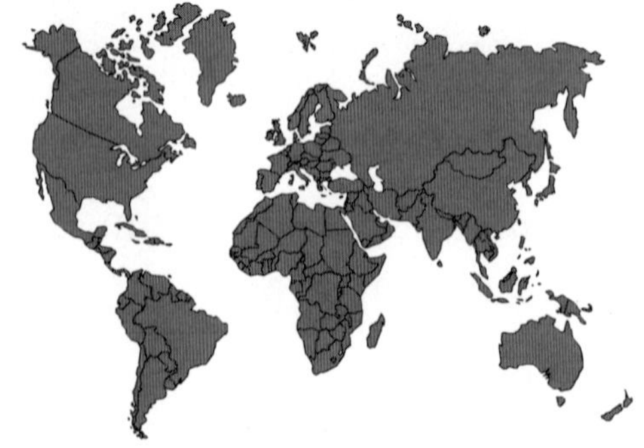

Fig. 3.14.

Dipylidium caninum is by far the most common tapeworm of cats in North America (Flick, 1973; Hitchcock, 1953; Lillis, 1967) and perhaps throughout the world (Arundel, 1970; Baker et al., 1989; Bearup, 1960; Boreham and Boreham, 1990; Chandler, 1925; Clarkson and Owen, 1959; Collins, 1973; Coman, 1972; Coman et al., 1981; Cowper, 1978; Dubey, 1960; Engbaek et al., 1984; Esle et al., 1977; Gadale et al., 1988–1989; Gregory and Munday, 1976; Hutchison, 1957; Kelly and Ng, 1975; Lewis, 1927a, b; McColm and Hutchison, 1980; Mirzayans, 1971; Moore and O'Callaghan, 1985; Niak, 1972; Nichol et al., 1981a, b; Poglayen et al., 1985; Ryan, 1976; Umeche and Ima, 1988).

Location in Host

The adult *Dipylidium caninum* is found anchored to the wall of the small intestine by its scolex, its holdfast organelle. In nature, the metacestode or larval stage of the parasite is found within the body cavity of *Ctenocephalides felis,* the cat flea, *Ctenocephalides canis,* the dog flea, *Pulex irritans,* the human flea, or more uncommonly within *Trichodectes canis,* the dog louse (Boreham and Boreham, 1990; Georgi, 1987; Pugh, 1987; Zimmermann, 1937).

Parasite Identification

The scolex of the adult *Dipylidium caninum* is tiny, measuring less than 0.5 mm in diameter. It possesses four muscular suckers that aid in attachment and locomotion. At the apex of the scolex is the rostellum, a dome-shaped projection. The rostellum of *Dipylidium caninum* is armed with four to seven rows of tiny, backward-facing, rose-thorn–like hooks and is retractable into the scolex (Figs. 3.15 and 3.16) (Witenberg, 1932). This tapeworm may attain a length of from 15 to 70 cm and be 2 to 3 mm wide with a white to a light reddish yellow color. The body is composed of 60 to 175 elliptical segments or proglottids (Boreham and Boreham, 1990). Each proglottid of this hermaphroditic tapeworm contains two sets of male reproductive organs and two sets of female reproductive organs with each set of genital apertures opening medially on the lateral edges of the proglottid (Fig. 3.17). Proglottids of *Dipylidium caninum* have two genital pores for fertilization, but no opening to allow

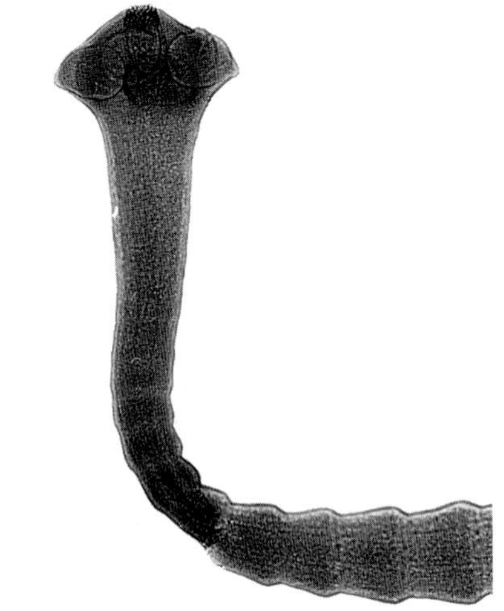

Fig. 3.15. Rostellum of *Dipylidium caninum* with the rostellum inverted.

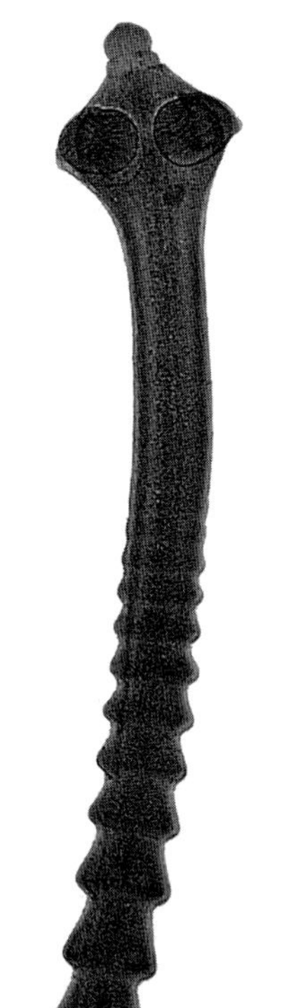

Fig. 3.16. Rostellum of *Dipylidium caninum* with the rostellum everted.

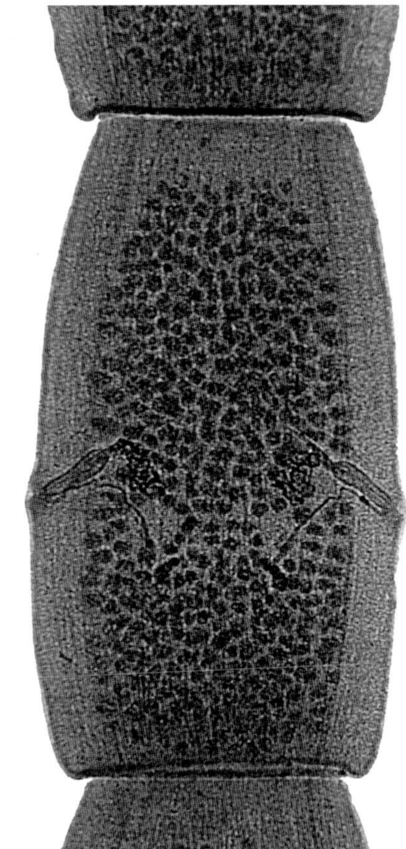

Fig. 3.17. Mature segment of *Dipylidium caninum* showing the two sets of genital organs with separate openings on each side of the proglottid.

eggs to escape. Because of these bilateral genital pores, *Dipylidium caninum* is often referred to as the "double-pored tapeworm." Eggs accumulate within each proglottid until the proglottid becomes packed like a ripe seed pod (Georgi, 1987). Gravid proglottids are creamy white, are 10 to 12 mm in length, and resemble cucumber seeds. Hence, *Dipylidium caninum* is also referred to as the "cucumber seed tapeworm" (Griffiths, 1978). Gravid tapeworm proglottids (Fig 3.18) are filled to capacity with egg capsules or egg packets (Fig. 3.19), each of which contain from 5 to 30 hexacanth embryos (Georgi, 1987).

The terminal tapeworm proglottids are often passed singly in the feces (Griffiths, 1978). Since the tapeworm proglottids possess both circular and longitudinal smooth musculature (Chitwood and Lichtenfels, 1973), they have the ability to

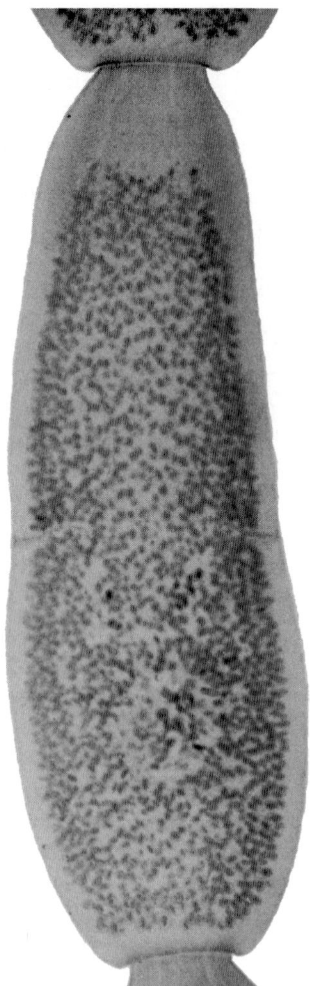

Fig. 3.18. Gravid segment of *Dipylidium caninum* showing the large number of contained egg capsules.

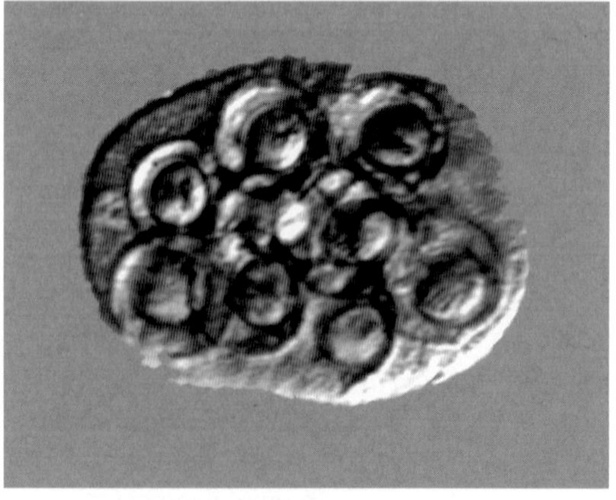

Fig. 3.19. Egg capsules of *Dipylidium caninum* as they appear in a sugar flotation.

move about the cat's perianal region, on the feces, on the bedding, or across any surface where they may be deposited (Griffiths, 1978). These proglottids will desiccate in the external environment. As they lose moisture, they shrivel up, often resembling uncooked rice grains (Boreham and Boreham, 1990).

Life Cycle

Due to its common occurrence, the life cycle of *Dipylidium caninum* is perhaps recounted by veterinarians more than any other parasite. As mentioned previously, the hermaphroditic adult parasite is found attached in the small intestine of the feline definitive host. The gravid terminal segments are passed in the feces of the cat. The larval stages of the cat flea (*Ctenocephalides felis*) savor these segments and will actively descend upon a freshly passed proglottid to eat it (Pugh, 1987). The flea larva has mandibulate mouth parts that allow it to ingest the eggs of *Dipylidium caninum.* The adult flea, however, is not able to ingest these proglottids due to its siphon-like mouth parts that restrict it to a totally liquid diet. Larvae of *Ctenocephalides canis, Pulex irritans,* and the dog louse, *Trichodectes canis,* are also capable of serving as intermediate hosts for *Dipylidium caninum.*

Within the intermediate host, the hexacanth embryo develops into a tailless cysticercoid. This is the stage that is infective to the feline definitive host. The ambient temperature determines the rate of development of the larval tapeworm. The flea becomes infected as a larva; however, the hexacanth embryo does not develop to an infective cysticercoid until the adult flea has emerged from its pupal case. In response to the host's body temperature, development is completed to the infective cysticercoid stage (Pugh, 1987). The flea may contain an average of 10 cysticercoids (range 2 to 82). The cat becomes infected by ingesting the flea during the grooming process.

Venard (1938) experimentally infected a cat with fleas infected with *Dipylidium caninum.* He recovered tapeworms from the cat 23 days later. Hinaidy (1991) also reported the prepatent period to be 2 to 4 weeks. Growth of *Dipylidium caninum* within the definitive host is dependent upon diet, age of the host, and health.

Clinical Presentation and Pathogenesis

Adult tapeworms cause little harm or inconvenience to the feline definitive host unless they are present in large numbers. In cats with severe infections, convulsions and epileptiform seizures occasionally occur (Boreham and Boreham, 1990). Heavy infections in young animals can produce nonspecific abdominal symptoms including constipation or diarrhea. The animal may exhibit an unthrifty, pot-bellied appearance. Intestinal obstruction may occur; however, this is rare. However, most clients are disgusted by the sight of proglottids of *Dipylidium caninum* crawling about the cat's haircoat, on the client's bedclothes, or on the recently passed feces of the cat.

Diagnosis

Identification of egg packets and proglottids as those of *Dipylidium caninum* is necessary for controlling this ubiquitous tapeworm. The client may irrefutably observe tapeworm segments crawling on or about the cat, yet the laboratory diagnostician may fail to demonstrate the characteristic eggs packets on fecal flotation. Egg packets within proglottids are best demonstrated by taking a gravid proglottid and teasing it open in a small amount of physiologic saline or tap water to disperse the characteristic egg packets.

Inspection with the naked eye or a hand lens is usually sufficient for the identification of segments of *Dipylidium caninum.* The characteristic cucumber seed shape coupled with the double-pored effect are pathognomonic indicators.

Pet owners often find dehydrated, shriveled objects in the vicinity of their cat's resting places. These desiccated objects bear little resemblance to segments of *Dipylidium caninum,* but if they are rehydrated in water, they will assume their former cucumber seed appearance.

Treatment

The anthelmintic with the broadest spectrum of cestocidal activity is praziquantel. A single oral or subcutaneous dose (5 mg/kg body weight) of this anthelmintic eliminates 100 percent of both immature and adult *Dipylidium caninum* from cats. An alternative cestocide is epsiprantel administered in a single oral dose of 5.5 mg/kg of body weight. An important adjunct to the treatment of dipylidiasis in cats is a vigorous flea control program. Whenever a dose of cestocidal medication is administered or dispensed, the cat's owner should be informed of the acute potential for reinfection via the flea intermediate host.

Epizootiology

Adult *Dipylidium caninum* parasitize the small intestine of many members of the Felidae and Canidae families. In addition to domestic cats and dogs, this cosmopolitan parasite may be found in foxes, dingoes, hyenas, wild cats, jungle cats, Indian palm cats, civet cats, and wild dogs (Boreham and Boreham, 1990).

Boreham and Boreham (1990) stated that almost nothing is known of the epizootiology of *Dipylidium caninum;* however, Georgi and Georgi (1992) stated that transmission potential is a function of the density of the flea intermediate host. Hinaidy (1991) examined 9,134 fleas in Austria and found that 2.3 percent of *Ctenocephalides felis* collected from cats and 1.2 percent of *Ctenocephalides felis* collected from dogs were found to be infected with cysticercoids of *Dipylidium caninum.* From *Ctenocephalides canis* collected from dogs, 3.1 percent were found to harbor cysticercoids. Fleas harbored anywhere from 1 to 162 cysticercoids with a mean of around 8 per infected flea. Male fleas tended to be infected slightly more often than female fleas, but they tended to harbor fewer cysticercoids.

A Danish survey revealed a higher prevalence of *Dipylidium caninum* in backyard cats, probably due to the ideal conditions for the survival of the flea intermediate host. A higher prevalence was found in female cats than in male cats. This was attributed to the care of the kittens (Engbaek et al., 1984). In the Republic of South Africa, *Dipylidium caninum* is marginally more common (24 percent) in adult cats and is the most common helminth in juvenile cats (21 percent) (Baker et al., 1989).

Uga and Yatomi (1992) reported that a survey of cats in Japan revealed that there were almost no cases where cats were infected with both *Dipylidium caninum* and *Spirometra erinaceieuropaei.* Experimental infection of cats with larval stages from both parasites revealed that somehow infection with *Spirometra erinaceieuropaei* prevented the development of *Dipylidium caninum* through some form of competition.

Hazards to Other Animals

Due to environmental transmission of fleas and the ease of ingestion during the grooming process, once *Dipylidium caninum* is diagnosed in any pet in a household, all cats and dogs within that environment should be treated.

Hazards to Humans

Veterinarians should be aware of the public health significance potential of *Dipylidium caninum.* If fleas containing the infective cysticercoid stage are ingested by a human, patent infections with this tapeworm may occur. Children are at an increased risk of infection owing to their close association with the family pet, and therefore, their increased risk of accidentally ingesting a flea. Although human infection with *Dipylidium caninum* is not common, neither is it a rare event. *Dipylidium caninum* is mildly pathogenic, producing nocturnal irritability, anorexia, and weight loss in infected children. Diagnosis is by finding the characteristic proglottids in the feces or in the perianal area. Most human cases, however, are asymptomatic for the patient, although they can be very traumatic for the parent who might come across segments while changing a diaper or in the child's undergarments or pajama. It must be emphasized that this condition is a rarity.

Control/Prevention

Rigorous on-animal and environmental flea control programs coupled with an effective cestocidal agent must be implemented to control *Dipylidium caninum* in the feline. It is also necessary to be certain to develop programs that handle all the canine and feline pets in the household.

REFERENCES

Arundel JH. 1970. Control of helminth parasites of dogs and cats. Aust Vet J 46:164–168.

Baker MK, Lange L, Verster A, van der Plaat S. 1989. A survey of helminths in domestic cats in the Pretoria area of Transvaal, Republic of South Africa. Part 1: The prevalence and comparison of burdens of helminths in adult and juvenile cats. J S Afr Vet Assoc 60:139–142.

Bearup AJ. 1960. Parasitic infection in cats in Sydney, with special reference to the occurrence of *Ollulanus tricuspis.* Aust Vet J 36:352–354.

Boreham RE, Boreham PFL. 1990. *Dipylidium caninum:* life cycle, epizootiology, and control. Comp Cont Educ Pract Vet 12(5):667–676.

Chandler AC. 1925. The helminthic parasites of cats in Calcutta and the relation of cats to human helminthic infections. J Parasitol 20:213–227.

Chitwood M, Lichtenfels JR. 1973. Identification of parasitic metazoa in tissue sections. Exp Parasitol 32:407–519.

Clarkson MJ, Owen LN. 1959. The parasites of domestic animals in the Bahama Islands. Ann Trop Med Parasitol 53:341–346.

Collins GH. 1973. A limited survey of gastro-intestinal helminths of dogs and cats. N Z Vet J 21:175–176.

Coman BJ. 1972. A survey of the gastro-intestinal parasites of the feral cat in Victoria. Aust Vet J 48:133–136.

Coman BJ, Jones EH, Driesen MA. 1981. Helminth parasites and arthropods of feral cats. Aust Vet J 57:324–327.

Cowper SG. 1978. Helminth parasites of dogs and cats and toxoplasmosis antibodies in cats in Swansea, South Wales. Ann Trop Med Parasitol 72:455–459.

Diamare V. 1893. Il genere *Dipylidium* Lt. Atti R Acad Sc Fis Mat Napoli Series Z 6:1–31.

Dubey JP. 1960. *Toxocara cati* and other intestinal parasites of cats. Vet Rec 79:506, 508.

Engbaek K, Madsen H, Larsen SO. 1984. A survey of helminths in stray cats from Copenhagen Denmark with ecological aspects. Z Parasitenkd 70:87–94.

Esle RW, Bagnall BG, Phaff JJG, Potter C. 1977. Endo- and ecto-parasites of dogs and cats: a survey from practices in the East Anglian Region BSAVA. J Small Anim Pract 18:731–737.

Flick SC. 1973. Endoparasites in cats: current practice and opinions. Feline Pract XX(4):21–34.

Gadale OI, Capelli G, Ali AA, Poglayen G. 1988–1989. Cat's intestinal helminths: first reports in Somali Democratic Republic. VIII Boll Sci Del Fac Zootec Vet 12–24.

Georgi JR. 1987. Tapeworms. Vet Clin North Am 17:1285–1305.

Georgi JR, Georgi ME. 1992. Canine Clinical Parasitology. Philadelphia, Pa: Lea and Febiger, pp 138–141.

Gregory GG, Munday BL. 1976. Internal parasites of feral cats from the Tasmanian midlands and King Island. Aust Vet J 52:317–320.

Griffiths HJ. 1978. In A Handbook of Veterinary Parasitology of Domestic Animals of North America, p 119. Minneapolis: University of Minnesota.

Hinaidy HK. 1991. Beitrag sur Biologie des *Dipylidium caninum.* 2. Mitteilung. J Vet Med B 38: 329–336.

Hitchcock DJ. 1953. Incidence of gastro-intestinal parasites in some Michigan kittens. North Am Vet 34:428–429.

Hutchison WM. 1957. The incidence and distribution of *Hydatigera taeniaeformis* and other intestinal helminths in Scottish cats. J Parasitol 43:318–321.
Kelly JD, Ng BKY. 1975. Helminth parasites of dogs and cats. II. Prevalence in urban environments in Australasia. Aust Vet Pract 6:89–100.
Leuckart R. 1863. Die Parasiten des Menschen und die von ihnen herrührenden Krankheiten. Leipzig, 1879–1886.
Lewis EA. 1927a. A study Welsh helminthology. J Helminthol 5:121–132.
Lewis EA. 1927b. A study of the helminths of dogs and cats of Aberystwyth, Wales. J Helminthol 5:171–182.
Lillis WG. 1967. Helminth survey of dogs and cats in New Jersey. J Parasitol 53:1082–1084.
McColm AA, Hutchison WM. 1980. The prevalence of intestinal helminths in stray cats in central Scotland. J Helminthol 54:255–257.
Mirzayans A. 1971. Incidence of gastrointestinal helminths of domestic cats in the Teheran area of Iran. J Parasitol 57:1296.
Moore E, O'Callaghan MG. 1985. Helminths of dogs and cats determined by fecal examination in Adelaide, South Australia. Aust Vet J 62:198–200.
Neveau-Lemaire M. 1936. Traité d'helminthologie médicule et vétérinaire. Paris. 1544 pp.
Niak A. 1972. The prevalence of *Toxocara cati* and other parasites in Liverpool cats. Vet Rec 91:534–536.
Nichol S, Ball SJ, Snow KR. 1981a. Prevalence of intestinal parasites in domestic cats from the London area. Vet Rec 109:252–253.
Nichol S, Ball SJ, Snow KR. 1981b. Prevalence of intestinal parasites in feral cats in some urban areas of England. Vet Parasitol 9:107–110.
Poglayen G, Traldi G, Capelli G, Genchi C. 1985. Fauna parassitaria gastro-intestinale del gatto nelle città di Bologna, Firenze e Milano. Parassitol 27:297–302.
Pugh RE. 1987. Effects on the development of *Dipylidium caninum* and on the host reaction to this parasite in the adult flea (*Ctenocephalides felis felis*). Parasitol Res 73:171–177.
Ryan GE. 1976. Gastro-intestinal parasites of feral cats in New South Wales. Aust Vet J 52:224–227.
Uga S, Yatomi K. 1992. Interspecific competition between *Spirometra erinacei* (Rudolphi, 1819) and *Dipylidium caninum* (Linnaeus, 1758) in cats. Jap J Parasitol 71:414–419.
Umeche N, Ima AE. 1988. Intestinal helminthic infections of cats in Calabar, Nigeria. Folia Parasitol 35:165–168.
Venard CE. 1938. Morphology, bionomics, and taxonomy of the cestode *Dipylidium caninum*. Ann NY Acad Sci 37:273–328.
Witenberg G. 1932. On the cestode subfamily Dipylidiinae Stiles. Z Parasitenk 4:541–584.
Zimmermann HR. 1937. Life-history studies on cestodes of the genus *Dipylidium* from the dog. Z Parasitenk 9:717–729.

Diplopylidium acanthotetra (Parona, 1886) Witenberg, 1932

Etymology

Diplo = double and *pylidium* = openings along with *acantho* = spined and *tetra* = four rows of hooks.

Synonyms

Witenberg (1932) reviewed the genus *Diplopylidium,* and he recognized four species of which only two were considered parasites of the domestic cat. The synonyms he recognized were *Diplopylidium fabulosum* Meggitt, 1927; *Diplopylidium quinquecoronatum* (Lopez-Neyra and Munoz-Medina, 1921); *Diplopylidium trinchesii* (Diamare, 1892); and *Diplopylidium triseriale* (Lühe, 1898).

History

The genus *Diplopylidium* was first described by Beddard in 1913, who noted the characteristics of the genus, that is that the openings of the male reproductive system are behind the openings of the female reproductive system. The species *Diplopylidium acanthotetra* was first described as a larval stage from a lizard, *Zamensis viridiflavus,* in Italy by Parona. Later the adult stage was found by Diamare, 1892, who described it as *Dipylidium trinchesii* but thought it to be the same species as that described as *Diplopylidium acanthotetra.* Later work on the life cycle convinced Witenberg that these were the same species.

Geographic Distribution

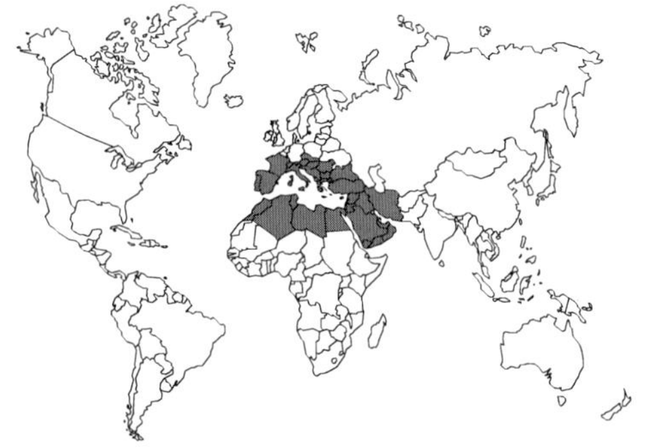

Fig. 3.20.

Diplopylidium acanthotetra has been reported from the Middle East, North Africa, and southern Europe (Daoud et al., 1988; El-Shabrawy and Imam, 1978; Haralampidis, 1977; Ismail et al., 1983; Roca and Lluch, 1988; Witenberg, 1932). In Egypt, El-Shabrawy and Imam (1978) reported that 51 out of 66 cats were host to cestode parasites, 22.5 percent harbored a single species, 45.1 percent had two species, while 32.4 percent were reported with three or more types of tapeworms: *Diplopylidium acanthotetra* was found in 16 cats (24.2 percent); *Diplopylidium nölleri* was found in 24 cats (36.4 percent); *Joyeuxiella pasqualei* was found in 21 cats (31.8 percent); *Dipylidium caninum* was found in 30 cats (45.5 percent); and *Taenia taeniaeformis* was found in 20 cats (30.3 percent).

Location in Host

The adult *Diplopylidium acanthotetra* is found in the small intestine of the feline host.

Parasite Identification

When compared with *Dipylidium* and *Joyeuxiella* species, *Diplopylidium* species are the smallest, only 4–12 cm, of these types of tapeworms found in the cat. The *Diplopylidium* holdfast possesses four suckers and a retractable rostellum armed with thorn-like hooks. The proglottids are shaped like cucumber seeds, possessing two complete sets of genital organs and bilateral genital pores. The genital pores of *Diplopylidium* lie anterior to the middle of the proglottid. Each egg capsule contains a single egg. *Diplopylidium acanthotetra* is characterized by having a short neck and hooks on the scolex that are larger than those of *Diplopylidium nölleri.*

Life Cycle

Very little has been described relative to the biology of this parasite. The cat sheds segments into the environment that contain eggs that are infectious. It is believed that the first intermediate host is some form of coprophagous insect, but this has never actually been proven for any member of this genus. The second larval stages are cysticercoids (small solid-bodied tapeworm larvae with an inverted scolex) that are found in reptiles. Cats become infected by the ingestion of the reptilian second intermediate host. Parrot and Joyeux (1920) fed cysticercoids to three cats, and two became infected. Tapeworms recovered 14 days after the feeding of the cysticercoids contained mature but no gravid proglottids. Tapeworms recovered 22 days after the feeding of the cysticercoids contained gravid proglottids.

Clinical Presentation and Pathogenesis

There have been no descriptions of signs in cats infected with this parasite, so it is thought to be without clinical signs.

Diagnosis

Little has been described on the actual diagnosis of infection with this tapeworm other than at necropsy. It would seem likely that proglottids are passed in the feces of the cat as occurs with *Dipylidium,* and it may be that occasionally free egg capsules containing a single egg may be observed in fecal samples. Each proglottid of *Diplopylidium* species possesses two genital pores for fertilization. The egg with its capsule is best demonstrated by taking a gravid proglottid and teasing it open in a small amount of physiologic saline or tap water to disperse the characteristic egg capsule with its single egg (Georgi, 1987).

Treatment

Praziquantel (Droncit) administered at 25 mg per animal at 6-week intervals has proven to be effective against *Joyeuxiella* species (Blagburn and Todd, 1986), tapeworms in the same family as *Diplopylidium acanthotetra.*

Epizootiology

Cats become infected by ingesting reptiles in dwellings and yards.

Hazards to Other Animals

Adult *Diplopylidium acanthotetra* have also been reported from civets.

Hazards to Humans

None.

Control/Prevention

Cats should not be allowed to roam freely or to scavenge carcasses. Predation may lead to infection with *Diplopylidium acanthotetra* if prey animals or carcasses containing cysticercoids are eaten.

REFERENCES

Beddard FE. 1913. Contributions to the anatomy and systematic arrangement of the Cestoidea. X. On two new species of tapeworm from *Genetta dongolana.* Proc Zool Soc Lond 549–579.

Blagburn BL, Todd KS. 1986. Exotic cestodiasis (*Joyeuxiella pasquaqlei*) in a cat. Feline Pract 16(2):8–11.

Daoud IS, Al-Tae ARA, Salman YJ. 1988. Prevalence of gastro-intestinal helminths in cats from Iraq. J Biol Sci Res 19:363–368.

Diamare V. 1892. Il genere *Dipylidium.* Lt Atti Accad Sc Napoli 6:1–31.

El-Shabrawy MN, Imam EA. 1978. Studies on cestodes of domestic cats in Egypt with particular reference to species belonging to genera *Diplopylidium* and *Joyeuxiella.* J Egypt Vet Med Assoc 38:19–27.

Georgi JR. 1987. Tapeworms. Vet Clin North Am 17:1285–1305.

Haralampidis ST. 1977. Contribution to the study of cat's parasites and their public health importance. Summary of Thesis. Hell Kteniatike 21:117–119.

Hendrix CM, Blagburn BL. 1983. Common gastrointestinal parasites. Vet Clin North Am 13:627–646.

Ismail NS, Abdel-Hafez SK, Toor MA. 1983. Prevalence of gastrointestinal helminths in cats from northern Jordan. Pak Vet J 3:129–132.

Parrot L, Joyeux C. 1920. Les cysticercoãdes de *Tarentola mauritanica* L. et les Ténias du chat. Bull Soc Pathol Exot 13:687–695.

Roca V, Lluch, J. 1988. L'helmintofaune des Lacertidae (Reptilia) de la zone thermomediterraneenne de l'est de 'Espagne. Aspects ecologiques. Vie et Milieu 38:201–205.

Witenberg G. 1932. On the cestode subfamily Dipylidiinae Stiles. Z Parasitenk 4:541–584.

Diplopylidium nölleri (Skrjabin, 1924) Lopez-Neyra, 1927

Etymology

Diplo = double and *pylidium* = openings along with *nölleri* for Dr. Nöller.

Synonyms

Witenberg (1932) reviewed the genus *Diplopylidium,* and he recognized four species of which only two were considered as parasites of the domestic cat. The synonym Witenberg recognized for *Diplopylidium nölleri* was *Diplopylidium monoophoroides* (Lopez-Neyra, 1927) Witenberg, 1932.

History

Diplopylidium nölleri was originally described as *Progynopylidium nölleri* by Skrjabin (1924) from a cat in Turkistan. The genus *Diplopylidium,* first described by Beddard in 1913, had priority over that proposed by Skrjabin. The name proposed for the genus by Skrjabin similarly recognized the same generic condition of this worm's morphology.

Geographic Distribution

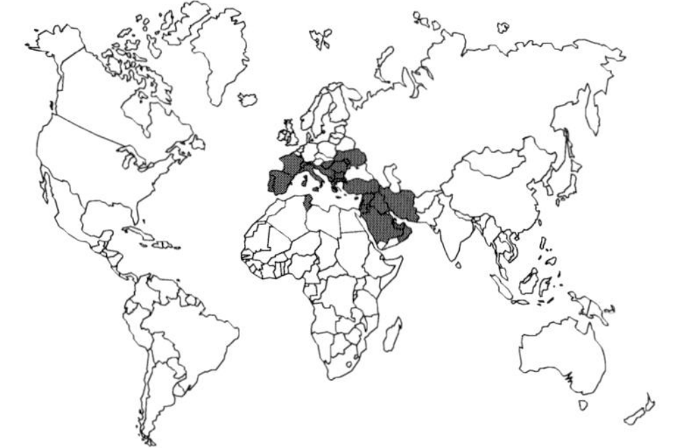

Fig. 3.21.

Diplopylidium nölleri has been reported from the Middle East and southern Europe (Abdul-Salam and Baker, 1990; Burgu et al., 1985; El-Shabrawy and Imam, 1978; Gadale et al., 1989; Haralampidis, 1977; Ismail et al., 1983; Witenberg, 1932). In some cases *Diplopylidium nölleri* was found commonly, being reported by Haralampidis (1977) in 71 of 123 cats in Greece and by El-Shabrawy and Imam in 24 of 66 cats in Egypt. In Jordan, Ismail et al. (1983) reported that 96 of 123 cats had *Dipylidium caninum,* 32 cats had *Diplopylidium acanthotetra,* and 24 cats had *Diplopylidium nölleri.* Geckos have been found infected with cysticercoids in Tanzania (Simonsen and Sarda, 1985).

Location in Host

The adult *Diplopylidium nölleri* is found in the small intestine of the feline host. Ismail et al.

(1983) stated that *Diplopylidium nölleri* is usually found in the very posterior of the small intestine, while *Diplopylidium acanthotetra* is found at the end of the first third of the small intestine. *Dipylidium caninum* was found in the posterior two-thirds of the small intestine, overlapping the posterior range of *Diplopylidium acanthotetra* and extending through the range of *Diplopylidium nölleri. Taenia taeniaeformis* was found by these authors mainly in the first third of the small intestine.

Parasite Identification

When compared with *Dipylidium* and *Joyeuxiella* species, *Diplopylidium* species are the smallest, only 4–12 cm, of these types of tapeworms found in the cat. The *Diplopylidium* holdfast possesses four suckers and a retractable rostellum armed with thorn-like hooks. The proglottids are shaped like cucumber seeds, possessing two complete sets of genital organs and bilateral genital pores. The genital pores of *Diplopylidium* lie anterior to the middle of the proglottid. Each egg capsule contains a single egg. *Diplopylidium nölleri* is characterized by having a long neck and hooks on the scolex that are smaller than 0.05 mm and those of *Diplopylidium acanthotetra.* The posterior, gravid segments of fresh specimens of *Diplopylidium nölleri* have a dark reddish brown coloration that distinguishes this parasite from specimens of *Diplopylidium acanthotetra, Dipylidium caninum,* and *Joyeuxiella* species that may be found within the intestine of a cat.

Life Cycle

Very little has been described relative to the biology of this parasite. The cat sheds segments into the environment that contain eggs that are infectious. It is believed that the first intermediate host is some form of coprophagous insect, but this has never actually been proven for any member of this genus. The second intermediate hosts, reptiles, contain cysticercoids (small solid-bodied tapeworm larvae with an inverted scolex). Cats become infected by the ingestion of the second intermediate host. Popov (1935) described the life cycle of a species of *Diplopylidium* that he described as *Diplopylidium skrjabini.* Two cats were infected with cysticercoids recovered from lizards, and 6 weeks later, they were found to harbor adult tapeworms in their intestines. At this time the adults were 4 to 5 cm long, and the posterior segments were darkly colored, being red rather than brown. It is very likely that these represent the same species as *Diplopylidium nölleri.*

Clinical Presentation and Pathogenesis

There have been no descriptions of signs in cats infected with *Diplopylidium nölleri,* so it is thought to be without clinical signs.

Diagnosis

Methods for the diagnosis of infection with this tapeworm other than at necropsy have not been described in any detail. It would seem likely that proglottids are passed in the feces of the cat as occurs with *Dipylidium,* and it may be that occasionally free egg capsules containing a single egg may be observed in fecal samples. Each proglottid of *Diplopylidium nölleri* possesses two genital pores for fertilization. The egg with its capsule is best demonstrated by taking a gravid proglottid and teasing it open in a small amount of physiologic saline or tap water to disperse the characteristic egg capsule with its single egg (Georgi, 1987).

Treatment

Praziquantel (Droncit) administered at 25 mg per animal at 6-week intervals has proven to be effective against *Joyeuxiella* species (Blagburn and Todd, 1986), tapeworms in the same family as *Diplopylidium nölleri.*

Epizootiology

Cats become infected by ingesting reptiles in dwellings and yards. Some surveys have shown that up to 16 of 55 examined geckos have cysticercoids in their body cavity (Simonsen and Sarda, 1985).

Hazards to Other Animals

There probably is no significant hazard from an infected cat because the larvae must pass through a first intermediate host, probably an arthropod. Thus, cats probably pose no significant hazard to other animals. Of course, as the number of pet reptiles increases, and because the first host is not known, there is the possibility of increasing the potential of large numbers of infected arthropods in areas where both cats and reptiles share the same living quarters. Dogs can be infected with this parasite (Ilescas Gomez et al., 1989).

Hazards to Humans

None.

Control/Prevention

Cats should not be allowed to roam freely or to scavenge carcasses. Predation may lead to infection with *Diplopylidium nölleri* if prey animals or carcasses containing cysticercoids are eaten (Hendrix and Blagburn, 1983).

REFERENCES

Abdul-Salam J, Baker K. 1990. Prevalence of intestinal helminths in stray cats in Kuwait. Pak Vet J 10:17–21.

Beddard FE. 1913. Contributions to the anatomy and systematic arrangement of the Cestoidea. X. On two new species of tapeworm from *Genetta dongolana*. Proc Zool Soc Lond 549–579.

Blagburn BL, Todd KS. 1986. Exotic cestodiasis (*Joyeuxiella pasqualei*) in a cat. Feline Pract 16(2):8–11.

Burgu A, Tinar R, Doganay A, Toparlak M. 1985. Ankara'da sokak kedilerinin ekto-ve endoparazitleri uzerinde bir arastirma. Vet Fak Derfiusi, Ankara Univ 32:288–300.

El-Shabrawy MN, Imam EA. 1978. Studies on cestodes of domestic cats in Egypt with particular reference to species belonging to genera *Diplopylidium* and *Joyeuxiella*. J Egypt Vet Med Assoc 38:19–27.

Gadale OI, Capeo G, Ali AA, Poglaayen G. 1989. Elminti intestinali del gatto. Prime segnalazioni nella Repubblica Democaratica Somala. Boll Sci Fac Zootech Vet Univ Nat Somala 8:13–24.

Georgi JR. 1987. Tapeworms. Vet Clin North Am 17:1285–1305.

Haralampidis ST. 1977. Contribution to the study of cat's parasites and their public health importance. Summary of Thesis. Hell Kteniatike 21:117–119.

Hendrix CM, Blagburn BL. 1983. Common gastrointestinal parasites. Vet Clin North Am 13:627–646.

Ilescas Gomez MP, Rodriguez-Osorio M, Granados-Tejerop D, Fernandez-Valdivia J, Gomez-Morales MA. 1989. Parasitoismo por helmintos en el perro (*Canis familiaris* L.) en la provincia de Granada. Rev Iber Parasitol 49:3–9.

Ismail NS, Abdel-Hafez SK, Toor MA. 1983. Prevalence of gastrointestinal helminths in cats from northern Jordan. Pak Vet J 3:129–132.

Popov P. 1935. Sue le dévelopment de *Diplopylidium skrjabini* n. sp. Ann Parasitol 13:322–326.

Simonsen P, Sarda PK. 1985. Helminth and arthropod parasites of *Hemidactylus mabouia* from Tanzania. J Herpetol 19:428–430.

Skrjabin KI. 1924. *Progynopylidium nölleri* nov. Gen., nov. Spec., ein neuer Bandwurm der Katze. Berl Tierartzl Wschr 32:420–422.

Witenberg G. 1932. On the cestode subfamily Dipylidiinae Stiles. Z Parasitenk 4:541–584.

Joyeuxiella pasqualei (Diamare, 1893) Fuhrmann, 1935

Etymology

Joyeuxiella for Dr. Joyeux and *pasqualei* for Dr. Pasquale.

Synonyms

Dipylidium pasqualei Diamare, 1893; *Joyeuxia pasqualei* (Diamare, 1893) Lopez-Neyra, 1927; *Dipylidium chyzeri* Ratz, 1897; *Dipylidium rossicum* Skrjabin, 1923; *Diplopylidium fortunatum* Meggitt, 1927; *Joyeuxia aegyptica* Meggitt, 1927; *Joyeuxia pasqualeiformis* Lopez-Neyra, 1928; *Joyeuxiella guilhoni* Troncy, 1970.

History

The genus *Joyeuxia* was created by Lopez-Neyra (1927) for *Dipylidium*-like tapeworms that had thorn-like hooks, one egg per uterine capsule, and a vagina opening posteriorly to the cirrus sac. Unfortunately, the name was already in use for a genus of sponge, and Fuhrmann (1935) emended the name to be *Joyeuxiella*. Witenberg (1932) recognized two valid species, *Joyeuxia pasqualei* and *Joyeuxia echinorhynchoides*. This author declared that any other species were insufficiently described or were identical to *Joyeuxia pasqualei*. Jones (1983) redescribed the genus and recognized three species: *Joyeuxiella pasqualei*, *Joyeuxiella fuhrmanni*, and *Joyeuxiella echinorhynchoides*. The description of *Joyeuxiella domestica* Deschmukh, 1990, from a domestic cat in Parhani, India, does not present features that would distinguish this species from *Joyeuxiella pasqualei*.

Geographic Distribution

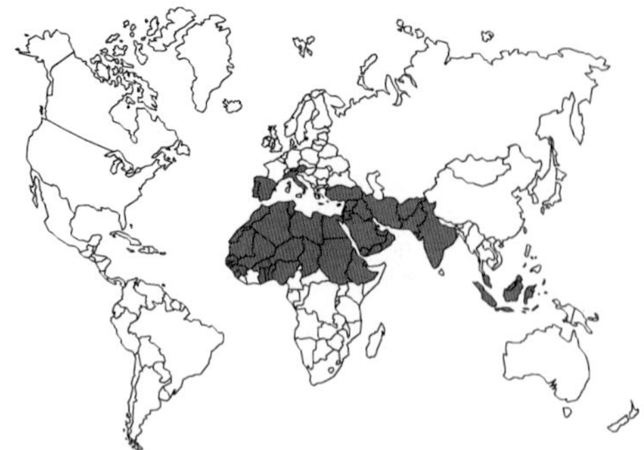

Fig. 3.22.

Specimens of *Joyeuxiella pasqualei* have been collected from cats in southern Europe (Austria, Spain, Italy, Hungary, and Southern Russia), the Middle East, northern Africa, and India (Agrawal and Pande, 1979; Jones, 1983; Supperer and Hinaidy, 1986; Witenberg, 1932). *Joyeuxiella pasqualei* has also been reported from Malaysia (Shanta et al., 1980) and New Guinea (Talbot, 1970). Specimens of *Joyeuxiella pasqualei* have been reported in the United States in cats that have traveled to foreign countries, that is, in a cat that was born in Nigeria (Linquist and Austin, 1981) and in a cat that had resided for some time in Saudi Arabia (Blagburn and Todd, 1986).

Location in Host

The adult *Joyeuxiella pasqualei* is found anchored to the mucosa just distal to the duodenum and at intervals throughout the small intestine (Blagburn and Todd, 1986).

Parasite Identification

The adult parasite is structurally similar to *Dipylidium caninum* and can be easily confused with it. This is a small to medium size tapeworm; however, it may attain a length of 30 cm. The scolex exhibits a retractable rostellum with crowns of recurved thorn-like hooks and four cup-like suckers. The gravid proglottids contain egg packets located both medially and laterally to the osmoregulatory canals. Specimens of the genus *Joyeuxiella* are distinguished from those of *Dipylidium* by the fact that the egg capsules of *Joyeuxiella* specimens each contain only a single hexacanth embryo covered by uterine material while the egg capsules of *Dipylidium* contain several embryos. Specimens of *Joyeuxiella* are mainly distinguished from those of *Diplopylidium* because the latter has some hooks that are of the claw-hammer shape of taeniid tapeworms rather than the rose-thorn shape of *Joyeuxiella.* Paired genital atria are located in the anterior half of the tapeworm segment. When dissected from gravid proglottids, *Joyeuxiella* egg packets contain single, hexacanth embryos surrounded by a covering of uterine material. Three pairs of hooklets are often visible within the hexacanth embryo (Blagburn and Todd, 1986).

The species of *Joyeuxiella* are distinguished by the shape of the rostellum, the location of the egg capsules relative to the longitudinal excretory vessels, and the locations of the testes relative to the vas deferens (Jones, 1983). *Joyeuxiella pasqualei* has a rostellum that is conical in shape, has eggs capsules median and lateral to the longitudinal excretory vessels, and has testes present anterior to the vas deferens. The rostellum of *Joyeuxiella fuhrmanni* is very similar in shape to that of *Joyeuxiella pasqualei,* but it has no testes anterior to the vas deferens, and the egg capsules are all median to the longitudinal excretory vessels. Specimens of *Joyeuxiella echinorhynchoides* have an elongate, cylindrical rostellum and egg capsules median to the longitudinal excretory canals.

Life Cycle

Segments of this cestode are shed in the feces. Witenberg (1932) reported that with *Joyeuxiella echinorhynchoides* the shedding was intermittent and that one infected cat shed 112, 74, 80, 155, 55, 90, 90, 123, 82, and 63 proglottids over a consecutive 10-day period. The first intermediate host of this parasite has not been determined. Witenberg (1932) was unable to infect fly maggots fed gravid proglottids, and Ortlepp (1933) was unable to infect dung beetles fed the gravid proglottids of *Joyeuxiella fuhrmanni.* The second intermediate host is a small reptile that contains a small (0.6 × 0.75 mm) solid-bodied cysticercoid larva that is found in the peritoneal cavity and liver, although occasionally in the muscles or under the skin (Witenberg, 1932); hosts include the house gecko, *Hemidactylus frenatus,* a ground-frequenting lizard, *Oblepharus boutoni* (Talbot, 1970), and other similar reptiles. Although cysticercoids identified as those of *Joyeuxiella pasqualei* have been reported from a small mammal, *Crocidura suaveolens,* it seems that the majority of larval stages are found in reptiles. The cat becomes infected by ingesting this reptilian second host. Work based on the experimental oral inoculation of kittens with 20 or 30 cysticercoids revealed that 5 and 10 days after the cats are infected the worms are immature and only about 0.3 cm long. In a cat that had been infected for 90 days, the worms had matured and measured between 16 and 28 cm long and had a total of around 200 to 300 segments (Agrawal and Pande, 1979).

Clinical Presentation and Pathogenesis

Normally, infections with adult tapeworms are not very harmful to cats. The site of attachment of the scolex of *Joyeuxiella pasqualei* to the mucosa has been described as having considerable mucosal damage with necrosis of surrounding villi (Agrawal and Pande, 1979). Cestode proglottids have been observed in the feces of infected cats (Lindquist and Austin, 1981; Blagburn and Todd, 1986).

Diagnosis

In one of the cases of infection with *Joyeuxiella pasqualei* in the United States, the client noted that the cat was shedding proglottids (Linquist and Austin, 1981). Each proglottid of *Joyeuxiella pasqualei* possesses two genital pores for fertilization and single eggs in egg capsules. The egg with its capsule is best demonstrated by taking a gravid proglottid and teasing it open in a small amount of physiologic saline or tap water to disperse the characteristic eggs. In cases of intact tapeworms recovered at necropsy, the characteristic appearance of the scolex with its four suckers and retractable rostellum identifies the tapeworms (Blagburn and Todd, 1986).

Treatment

Praziquantel (Droncit) administered at 25 mg per animal at 6-week intervals has proven to be effective in domestic cats (Blagburn and Todd, 1986); praziquantel has also been shown to be effective at 5 mg/kg body weight (Dorchies et al., 1980) and at 2.5 mg/kg body weight (Guralp et al., 1976). Drocarbil (Nemural) has also been reported to be effective (Lindquist and Austin, 1981).

Epizootiology

Cats become infected by ingesting reptiles in dwellings and yards.

Hazards to Other Animals

Adult *Joyeuxiella pasqualei* will also infect dogs, foxes, *Mustela nivalis, Felis sylvestris, Felis serval,* and probably other cat species. As with *Diplopylidium* species it is possible that if the unidentified first intermediate host is present in a household, pet reptiles might be infected with large numbers of the cysticercoid stage if they share living quarters with an infected cat.

Hazards to Humans

None.

Control/Prevention

Cats should not be allowed to hunt small reptiles in the areas where this parasite is prevalent.

REFERENCES

Agrawal RD, Pande BP. 1979. Cysticercoid of *Joyeuxiella pasqualei* in the wall-lizard and its experimental development in kitten. Ind J Helminthol 31:75–80.

Blagburn BL, Todd KS. 1986. Exotic cestodiasis (*Joyeuxiella pasqualei*) in a cat. Feline Pract 16(2):8–11.

Deshmukh AL. 1990. *Joyeuxiella domestica* sp. n. (Cestoda: Dipylidiidae) from the domestic cat, *Felis domesticus* (Carnivora), in India. Helminthology 27:233–238.

Dorchies P, Franc M, Lahitte JD, Berthonneau MC. 1980. Traitment du teniasis du chien et du chat par le praziquantel. Rev Med Vet 131:409–411.

Fuhrmann O. 1935. Rectification de nomenclature. Ann Parasitol 13:386.

Guralp N, Tigin Y, Oguz T, Tinar R, Burgu A. 1976. The effect of droncit on dog and cat tapeworms. Ankara Univ Vet Fak Derg 23:171–174.

Jones A. 1983. A revision of the cestode genus *Joyeuxiella* Fuhrmann, 1935 (Dilepididae: Dipylidiinae) Syst Parasitol 5:203–213.

Linquist WD, Austin ER. 1981. Exotic parasitism in a Siamese cat. Feline Pract 11:9–11.

Lopez-Neyra CR. 1927. Considérations sur le genre *Dipylidium* Leuckart. Bull Soc Pathol Exot 20: 434–440.

Ortlepp RJ. 1933. *Joyeuxia fuhrmanni* Baer, 1924, a hitherto unrecorded cestode parasite of the domesticated cat in South Africa. Onderstep J Vet Sci Anim Ind 1:97–98.
Shanta CS, Wan SP, Kwong KH. 1980. A survey of the endo- and ectoparasites of cats in and around Ipoh, West Malaysia. Malay Vet J 7:17–27.
Supperer R, Hinaidy HK. 1986. Parasitic infections of dogs and cats in Austria. Deutch Tierärtzl Wochenschr 93:383–386.
Talbot N. 1970. Helminth and arthropod parasites of the domestic cat in Papua and New Guinea. Aust Vet J 46:370–372.
Witenberg G. 1932. On the cestode subfamily Dipylidiinae Stiles. Z Parasitenk 4:541–584.

Joyeuxiella fuhrmanni (Baer, 1924) Fuhrmann, 1935, and *Joyeuxiella echinorhyncoides* (Sonsino, 1889) Fuhrmann, 1935

Cats are host to two other species of *Joyeuxiella* that are found mainly in Africa. *Joyeuxiella fuhrmanni* has been reported from South Africa, Zimbabwe, and the Congo (Baker et al., 1989; Jones, 1983). It has also been reported from cats in Turkey (Burgu et al., 1985) and in Palestine (Witenberg, 1932). *Joyeuxiella fuhrmanni* tends to be a smaller worm than *Joyeuxiella pasqualei*. *Joyeuxiella fuhrmanni* has a maximum length of 9 cm and often is only 2 to 3 cm in length. *Joyeuxiella echinorhyncoides* has been reported from cats in the Middle East and in India (Gupta, 1970; Jones, 1983). This parasite is recognized by its long rostellum.

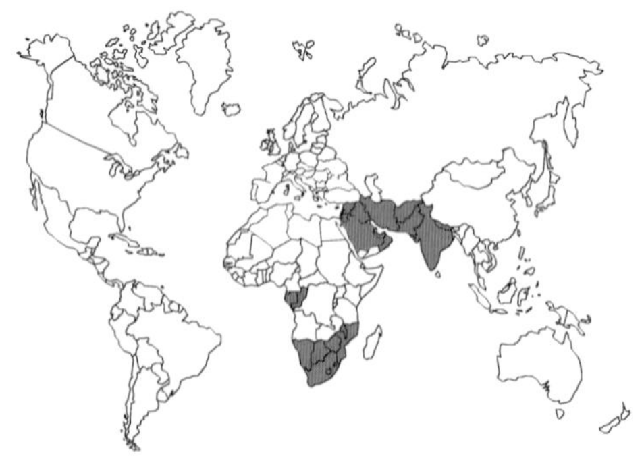

Fig. 3.23.

REFERENCES

Baker MK, Lange L, Verster A, van der Plaat S. 1989. A survey of helminths in domestic cats in the Pretoria area of Transvaal, Republic of South Africa. Part 1: The prevalence and comparison of burdens of helminths in adult and juvenile cats. J S Afr Vet Assoc 60:139–142.
Burgu A, Tinar R, Doganay A, Poparlak M. 1985. Ankara'da sokak kedilerinin ekto-ve endoparaizitleri uzerinde bir arastirma. Vet Fak Derg, Ankara Univ 32:288–300.
Gupta VP. 1970. A dilepidid cysticercoid from *Uromastix hardwickii* and its experimental development in pup. Curr Sci 39:137–138.
Jones A. 1983. A revision of the cestode genus *Joyeuxiella* Fuhrmann, 1935 (Dilepididae: Dipylidiinae). Syst Parasitol 5:203–213.
Witenberg G. 1932. On the cestode subfamily Dipylidiinae Stiles. Z Parasitenk 4:541–584.

DILEPIDIDAE

Choanotaenia atopa Rausch and McKown, 1994

The Dilepididae is a group of tapeworms with a scolex that has four suckers and an armed rostellum. The reproductive organs are usually single per proglottid. The group as a whole is typically found to parasitize birds and rodents. A large number of genera are considered members of this family of tapeworms. One species has been reported from cats (Rausch and McKown, 1994).

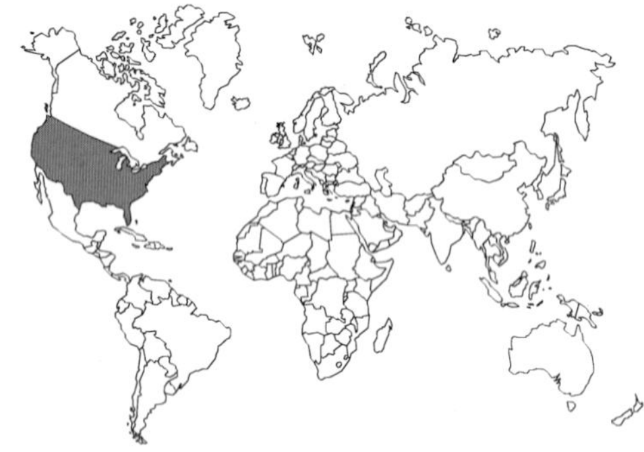

Fig. 3.24.

A cat from Manhattan, Kansas, was found to be passing the eggs of an unidentified tapeworm species. The eggs are rather thin shelled, subspherical, and 45 × 56 μm in diameter, with a visible hexacanth embryo. The cat was treated with drocarbil (18 mg/kg) about 4 months later, and the adult tapeworms recovered. The tapeworms passed by the cat had a maximum length of 7 cm. There were two rows of rostellar hooks and a total of 22 hooks per rostellum. The specimens were described as *Choanotaenia atopa,* and it was presumed that the normal host was a small rodent. It was thought that the cat had probably become infected by eating the insect or other invertebrate that serves as the intermediate host of this parasite.

REFERENCES

Rausch RL, McKown RD. 1994. *Choanotaenia atopa* n. sp. (Cestoda: Dilepididae) from a domestic cat in Kansas. J Parasitol 80:317–320.

TAENIIDAE

This family within the cyclophyllidean tapeworms is characterized by having segments that contain a uterus with a large central uterine body that has numerous side branches and a lateral genital opening. The family is made up of a group of large adult tapeworms that have scolices that each bear four muscular suckers. In almost all species there is a crown of two rows of hooks on the rostellum that have a typical "taeniid" shape, that is, they are shaped very similar to the head of a claw hammer, with one row of hooks being smaller than the other. The eggs of the taeniid are also characteristic; they have a dark brown shell that is formed from many small truncated blocks and contains a six-hooked larva when passed in the feces. The tapeworms of this family have a two-host life cycle, the first host being a mammal that ingests the egg wherein a larval stage develops. The second host is a mammal that ingests the first host. The adult stage develops within the small intestine of the second host. The stages in the first host have distinctive morphologies and have been given distinct names (i.e., "cysticercus," "strobilocercus," "coenurus," and "hydatid"). At various times the family has contained different numbers of genera because various workers have either split the species in this group into many genera or lumped the species into few genera. The classification used here is based on that of Rausch (1994) wherein only two genera are recognized, *Taenia* and *Echinococcus*. Cats can be parasitized with adults of a single species from each of these genera. The cat serves as the final host for *Taenia taeniaeformis*. Cats can also be infected with the larval stage of a taeniid tapeworm whose adult form is found in the dog. The larval form of this tapeworm is called a coenurus, and the disease produced is called feline coenurosis. Cats can also serve as a final host for *Echinococcus multilocularis,* although the fox is the more typical host.

REFERENCES

Rausch RL. 1994. Family Taeniidae Ludwig, 1886. In Keys to the Cestode Parasites of Vertebrates, ed LF Khalil, A Jones, and RA Bray. Wallingford, UK: CAB International.

Taenia taeniaeformis (Batsch, 1786) Wolffügel, 1911

Etymology

Taenia = tapeworm and *taeniaeformis* for the tapeworm form of the adult.

Synonyms

Taenia infantis Bacigalupo, 1922; *Hydatigera taeniaeformis* (Batsch, 1786) Lamarck, 1816; *Multiceps longihamatus* Morishita and Sawada, 1966.

History

This worm has been known for some time both as the adult found in the cat and in the segmented larval stage found in the liver of rodents, the strobilocercus. The larval stage was first described as *Cysticercus fasciolaris* Rudolphi, 1808. The genus *Hydatigera* was established for this larval form. In the attempt to divide the genus *Taenia* on the basis of various life cycle patterns, the species in the cat, *taeniaeformis,* was assigned to the genus *Hydatigera,* while other species were assigned to genera such as *Taenia, Multiceps,* and *Taeniarhynchus*. While this division of the genus has some merit, it has been questioned by Verster (1969) and by Rausch (1994), who felt that this division was unwarranted. Küchenmeister (1852) was the first to show that the larval stage in rodents could infect cats. Leuckart (1854) completed the entire life cycle, infecting rodents with eggs and cats with the larval stage in the laboratory.

Geographic Distribution

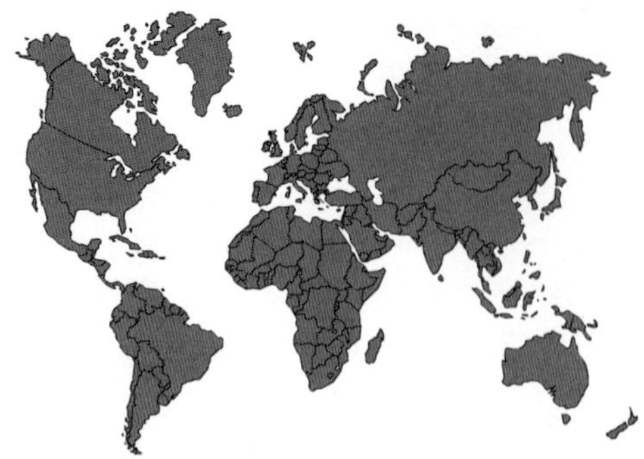

Fig. 3.25.

Taenia taeniaeformis is worldwide in its distribution, which parallels that of the domestic cat. Reports include the Americas (Alcaino et al., 1992; Esterre and Maitre, 1985; Nolan and Smith, 1995; Ogassawara et al., 1986); Europe (Hinaidy, 1991); northern Africa and the Middle East (Hasslinger et al., 1988; Ismail et al., 1983;); southern Africa (Verster, 1969); India (Singh and Rao, 1965); southeast Asia (Andrews, 1937; Tanaka et al., 1985); southern Pacific (Ng and Kelly, 1975; Tongson and San Pablo, 1979; Gregory and Munday, 1976).

Location in Host

The adult tapeworms tend to be located such that the scolex is within the first one-half of the small intestine (Miller, 1932). The scolex is often found attached to the mucosa, and the worms seem to move about because several attachment sites can be observed in the intestine of a cat that has been infected with only a single parasite.

Parasite Identification

Taenia taeniaeformis is the most robust of the tapeworm parasites found in the cat. This is also the only species of *Taenia* typically reported from the domestic cat around the world. The worm tends to be white, thick bodied, and around 15 to 60 cm in length. The scolex (Fig. 3.26) has two rows of hooks that have the typical claw-hammer shape of the Taeniidae (Fig. 3.27) There tends to be somewhere between 30 to 50 hooks per scolex.

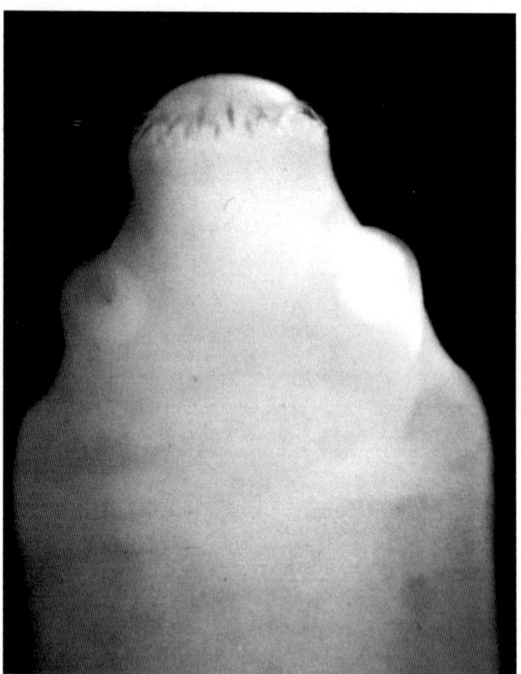

Fig. 3.26. *Taenia taeniaeformis* scolex of adult tapeworm.

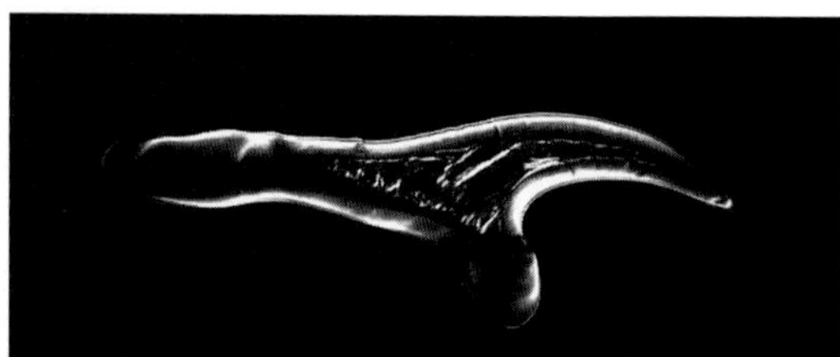

Fig. 3.27. Typical claw-hammer–shaped hook from the scolex of a taeniid tapeworm.

There is typically no neck (i.e., a portion of narrow segments) posterior to the scolex. Each of the mature segments (Fig 3.28) possesses a single lateral genital opening that randomly occurs on either one lateral side of a segment or the other. The terminal, gravid segments (Fig. 3.29) that are shed in the feces tend to be packed full of eggs. Eggs can easily be recognized as those of a *Taenia* through examination under a microscope, which reveals the typical brown-shelled taeniid eggs containing six-hooked larvae (Fig 3.30). The

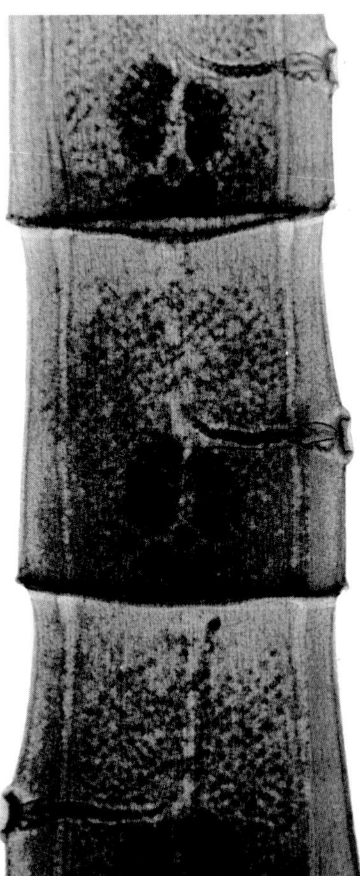

Fig. 3.28. Mature segment of a taeniid tapeworm showing the vitellaria at the bottom of the segment and the ovary just above them. The lateral pore containing the vagina and cirrus are on the right side of the center segment. The testes are dispersed throughout the parenchyma of the body.

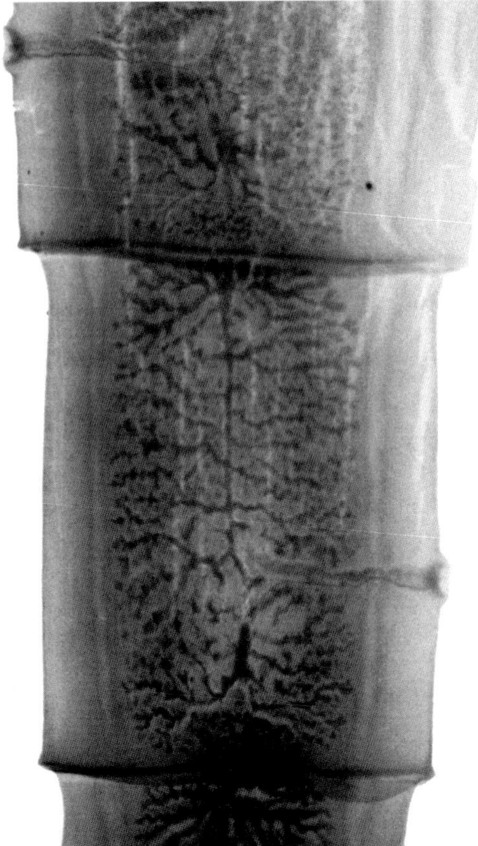

Fig. 3.29. Gravid segment of a taeniid tapeworm showing the highly branched uterus that is full of eggs.

eggs of *Taenia taeniaeformis* are spherical and measure between 31 to 36 μm in diameter.

There are many species of *Taenia* found in carnivores; Verster (1969) recognized 29 species and several of questionable validity. Many species are found in the dog as the final host, including *Taenia pisiformis, Taenia ovis,* and *Taenia multiceps.* Some species are found in human beings, *Taenia solium* and *Taenia saginata,* or large cats, including *Taenia gonyamai, Taenia ingwei, Taenia macrocystis,* and *Taenia omissa.* Other final hosts include hyenas, foxes, mustellids, and viverrids. The separation of the species is based on the size and shape of the hooks on the rostellum along with other characteristics, such as the type of larval stage and position of the genital ducts relative to the longitudinal excretory canals. *Taenia taeniaeformis* is considered to be most like the species found in mustellids and viverrids and was considered by Verster as the representative species for this group of species.

Life Cycle

Adult tapeworms live within the small intestine of the cat and shed the terminal segments into the feces. These segments are capable of exiting through the sphincter of a cat at times other than during the passage of feces, and they may be found crawling near the cat or on the cat's fur. The segments are capable of crawling considerable

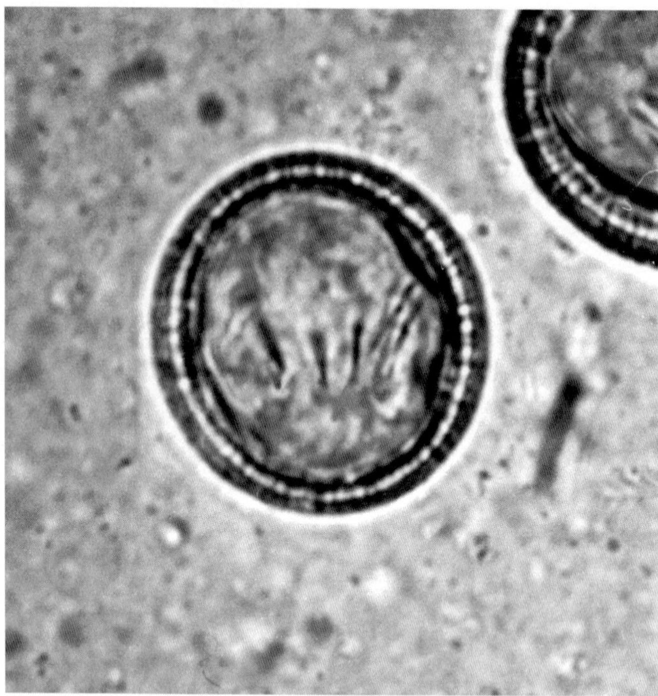

Fig. 3.30. Egg of *Taenia taeniaeformis* in feces. Note the thick wall and the six hooks on the contained embryo.

distances. The intermediate host is a small rodent in which the larvae migrate through the intestinal wall and develop to a strobilocercus stage in the rodent's liver (Fig. 3.31). The strobilocercus is a larval stage that has a terminal bladder and a rather long segmented body that is crowned with a scolex that looks very similar to that found on the adult form. It seems that the strobilocercus must attain an age of about 2 months before it is infective to a cat upon ingestion (Singh and Rao, 1965). Once a cat ingests the strobilocercus, the posterior portion of the larva is digested away, and then the anterior portion begins to develop (Hutchison, 1959). Patent infections develop in the cat between 32 to 80 days after strobilocerci are ingested (Williams and Shearer, 1981). Cats maintain patent infections for 7 months to greater than 34 months. Cats produce about three to four segments each day, although the majority of segments appear to contain only 500 eggs or less (maximum 12,180 eggs). Destrobilization may occur sporadically throughout the patent period without the termination of infection. It appears that cats can be infected again with adult tapeworms if reinfected with strobilocerci soon after their prior infections with the adult stage have terminated (Williams and Shearer, 1981). It has also been shown that cats can be superinfected with young tapeworms by being fed strobilocerci in the presence of existing mature worms (Miller, 1932).

Clinical Presentation and Pathogenesis

There are no signs associated with infection of *Taenia taeniaeformis* in cats that have been described, so it is considered to be without clinical signs.

Diagnosis

Infection in cats is diagnosed by finding the distinctive segments in the feces or by finding the eggs upon fecal flotation. The eggs of *Taenia taeniaeformis* are spherical and measure between 31 and 36 μm in diameter. To identify a segment, it can be crushed on a glass slide and examined for eggs. Sometimes, however, segments have shed most of their eggs, and they will contain very few eggs or perhaps none at all. In those areas where cats could also be potentially infected with

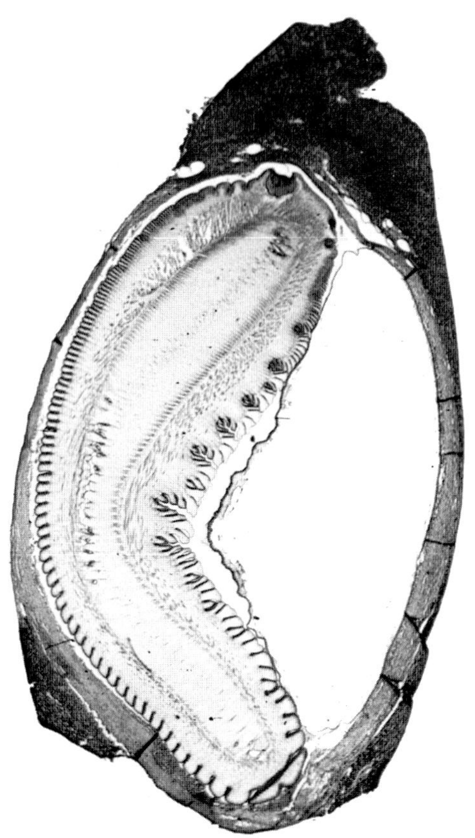

Fig. 3.31. A strobilocercus of *Taenia taeniaeformis*. Sections through two of the suckers on the anterior end can be noted on the top of the illustration.

Echinococcus multilocularis (see below), the shedding of segments in the feces will typically ensure that the cat is infected with *Taenia taeniaeformis* and not *Echinococcus multilocularis,* although it is possible for cats to be hosts of both parasites.

Treatment

Praziquantel (5 mg/kg body weight) and epsiprantel have both been shown to be efficacious in the treatment of *Taenia taeniaeformis* in cats. Similarly, febantel and fenbendazole are approved for the treatment of this parasite in most of the world. Mebendazole and nitroscanate are also products that have efficacy against *Taenia taeniaeformis* in cats.

Epizootiology

Murid and cricetid rodents are those most typically infected as intermediate hosts (e.g., *Mus musculus, Rattus norvegicus, Cricetus auratus, Meriones persicus, Microtus* species, and *Sciurus carolinenesis*). Rabbits in North America and Europe have been occasionally found to have strobilocerci in their livers (Verster, 1969), but this must be considered a less commonly utilized intermediate host than the rodent species. Interestingly, Abdul Salam and Baker (1990) found that of 103 stray cats in Kuwait that harbored more than 50 percent prevalence of infection with *Joyeuxiella pasqualei* and *Diplopylidium nölleri,* none of these cats were infected with *Taenia taeniaeformis, Dipylidium caninum,* or *Toxocara cati.*

Japanese workers are examining the difference in infectivity to the intermediate host of different field isolates of *Taenia taeniaeformis.* They found, by feeding eggs from adults derived from strobilocerci isolated from a red-backed vole (*Clethrionomys rufocanus bedfordiae*), strobilocerci failed to develop in rats, mice, and gerbils, although they did grow in experimentally infected voles. Other isolates from rats and voles grew in mice and rats but not in voles or gerbils (Nonaka et al., 1994). They further examined strains of *Taenia taeniaeformis* using the nucleotide sequence variations in the mitochondrial cytochrome c oxidase gene and found that this same vole strain differed from the others to a greater extent than would be expected by chance alone (Okamoto et al., 1995). Similarly, isolates, at least during the initial passages, seem to grow best in hosts from which they were originally isolated (Azuma et al., 1995).

Hazards to Other Animals

The eggs passed in the feces of cats are infective to many different species of rodent and potentially rabbits. The proglottids are highly motile and can move great distances from the site of fecal deposition. Also, proglottids are capable of leaving the cat by direct migration through the anal sphincter. Thus, if cats share households with pet rodents or lagomorphs, they may serve as a potential hazard to these animals if the cats are infected. Although large numbers of rodents have been experimentally infected for studies on the immunology and development of the strobilocercus (Perry et al., 1994), there have apparently been no reports on the disease that might occur in naturally infected animals.

Sambon (1924) described strobilocerci collected from the omentum and serous membranes of a gibbon from Java (*Hylobates leuciscus*). It now seems that this is a strobilocercus of *Taenia taeniaeformis,* although it is possible that it could be the larval stage of some related tapeworm. Blyumberg in 1886 (cited in Abduladze, 1964) supposedly recovered a strobilocercus from the brain of a cat; however, it seems highly likely that this was actually a misidentified coenurus (see the section Feline Coenurosis, below).

Hazards to Humans

Adults of *Taenia taeniaeformis* have been recovered from the intestines of humans. *Taenia taeniaeformis* was described once as *Taenia infantis* based on a single adult worm recovered from the intestine of a 5-year-old boy in Buenos Aires, Argentina (Bacigalupo, 1922). Morishita and Sawada (1966) recovered adult specimens of *Taenia taeniaeformis* from a 3-year-old girl (three adult worms) and a 55-year-old woman (three adult worms) after they were dewormed for reasons of abdominal discomfort and the presence of the eggs of *Ascaris lumbricoides* in the feces. These worms were originally described as *Multiceps longihamatus*. Another specimen collected from a 4-year-old girl (one adult worm) in Okinawa was described by these authors, and this was probably another case of intestinal infection with *Taenia taeniaeformis*. Spassky et al. (1966 [cited in Sterba and Barus, 1976]) determined that all these worms were the same as *Taenia taeniaeformis*. It is not known how any of these patients became infected. In the two cases where a single worm was passed spontaneously, it is possible that the adult worm may have actually been consumed by the child after the worm had been passed in the feces of a cat. However, in the other two cases it seems that the patients must have ingested the larval stage in the tissues of a rodent or rabbit.

A single case of human infection with a larval stage of *Taenia taeniaeformis* has been reported (Sterba and Barus, 1976). In this case, a 77-year-old man died of unrelated causes, and the necropsy revealed that there were numerous serous cysts in the liver. One of these cysts was confirmed to contain a strobilocercus. Based on the relatively high prevalence of *Taenia taeniaeformis* around the world, the fact that there has only been a single human infection with this parasite would indicate that this parasite does not develop well in the human host.

REFERENCES

Abduladze KI. 1964. Essentials of Cestodology. Vol. IV. Taeniata of Animals and Man and Disease Caused by Them. Ed KI Skrjabin. [Translated from Russian—Israel Program for Scientific Translations, Jerusalem, 1970] 549 pp.

Abdul Salam J, Baker K. 1990. Prevalence of intestinal helminths in stray cats in Kuwait. Pak Vet J 10:17–21.

Alcaino H, Gorman T, Larenas I. 1992. Endoparasitological fauna of the domestic cat in an urban zone of the metropolitan region, Chile. Parasitologia al Dia 16:139–142.

Andrews MN. 1937. The helminth parasites of dogs and cats in Shanghai, China. J Helminthol 15:145–152.

Azuma H, Okamoto M, Oku Y, Kamiya M. 1995. Intraspecific variation of *Taenia taeniaeformis* as determined by various criteria. Parasitol Res 81:103–108.

Bacigalupo J. 1922. Sobre una nueva especie de Taenia, *Taenia infantis*. Semana Med 26:726.

Esterre P, Maitre MJ. 1985. Les affections parasitaires des mongastriques en Guadeloupe. Rev Elev Méd Vét Pays Trop 38:43–48.

Gregory GG, Munday BL. 1976. Internal parasites of feral cats from the Tasmanian midlands and Kings Island. Aust Vet J 52:317–320.

Hasslinger MA, Omar HN, Selim KE. 1988. The incidence of helminths in stray cats in Egypt and other Mediterranean countries. Vet Med Rev 59:76–81.

Hinaidy HK. 1991. Parasitosen und Antiparasitika bein Hund und Katze in österreich—Hinweise für den Kleintierpraktiker. Wien Tiararztl Mschr 78:302–310.

Hutchison WM. 1959. Studies on *Hydatigera* (*Taenia*) *taeniaeformis*. II. Growth of the adult phase. Exp Parasitol 8:557–567.

Ismail NS, Abdel Hafez SK, Toor MA. 1983. Prevalence of gastrointestinal helminths in cats from northern Jordan. Pak Vet J 3:129–132.

Küchenmeister GFH. 1852. Ueber die Umwandelung der Finnen Bandwürmer. Vierteljahr Schr Prakt Heilk Prag 33:106–158.

Leuckart R. 1854. Erzeugung des *Cysticercus fasciolaris* aus den Eiren der *Taenia crassicollis*. Gurlt's Mag ges Tierarzneikunde.

Miller HM. 1932. Superinfection of cats with *Taenia taeniaeformis*. J Prev Med 6:17–29.

Morishita K, Sawada I. 1966. On tapeworms of the genus *Multiceps* hitherto unrecorded from man. Jap J Parasitol 15:495–501.

Ng BKY, Kelly JD. 1975. Anthropozoonotic helminthiases in Australasia: Part 3: Studies on the prevalence and public health implications of helminth parasites of dogs and cats in urban environments. Int J Zoon 2:76–91.

Nolan TJ, Smith G. 1995. Time series analysis of the prevalence of endoparasitic infections in cats and dogs presented to a veterinary teaching hospital. Vet Parasitol 59:87–96.

Nonaka N, Iwaki T, Okamoto M, Ooi HK, Ohbayashi M, Kamiya M. 1994. Infectiveness of four isolates of *Taenia taeniaeformis* to various rodents. J Vet Med Sci 56:565–567.

Ogassawara S, Beneassi S, Larsson CE, Leme PTZ, Hagiwara MK. 1986. Prevalencia de infecções helminticas em gatos na cidade de São Paulo. Rev Fac Med Vet Zootec Univ S Paulo 23:145–149.

Okamota M, Bessho Y, Kamiya M, Kurosawa T, Horii T. 1995. Phylogenetic relationships within *Taenia taeniaeformis* variants and other taeniid cestodes inferred from the nucleotide sequence of the cytochrome c oxidase subunit I gene. Parasitol Res 81:451–458.

Perry RL, Williams JF, Carrig CB, Kaneene JB, van Veen TWS. 1994. Radiologic evaluation of the liver and gastrointestinal tract in rats infected with *Taenia taeniaeformis*. Am J Vet Res 55:1120–1126.

Rausch RL. 1994. Family Taeniidae Ludwig, 1886. In Keys to the Cestode Parasites of Vertebrates, ed LF Khalil, A Jones, and RA Bray. Wallingford, UK: CAB International.

Sambon LW. 1924. *Cysticercus fasciolaris* and cancer in rats. J Trop Med Hyg 27:124–174.

Singh BB, Rao BV. 1965. Some biological studies on *Taenia taeniaeformis*. Ind J Helminthol 18:151–160.

Sterba J, Barus V. 1976. First record of *Strobilocercus fasciolaris* (Taeniidae-larvae) in man. Folia Parasitol 23:221–226.

Tanaka H, Watanabe M, Ogawa Y. 1985. Parasites of stray dogs and cats in the Kanto region, Japan. J Vet Med Jap 771:657–661.

Tongson MS, San Pablo FG. 1979. A study on the prevalence of gastrointestinal worms of cats in metropolitan Manila. Philipp J Vet Med 18:1–15.

Verster A. 1969. A taxonomic revision of the genus *Taenia* Linnaeus, 1758 s. str. Onderstpoort J Vet Res 36:3–58.

Williams JF, Shearer AM. 1981. Longevity and productivity of *Taenia taeniaeformis* in cats. Am J Vet Res 42:2182–2183.

Feline Coenurosis

There have been several reports of cats developing neurologic disease due to the intracranial development of the larval stage of a tapeworm called a coenurus. The coenurus is a cyst-like structure, wherein the tapeworm undergoes asexual development in the intermediate host, and thus, each coenurus contains several scolices (Figs. 3.32 and 3.33). Each scolex in the coenurus is capable of developing into a separate adult tapeworm after the coenurus is ingested by the final host. The taeniid larva, which is called a cysticercus (e.g., the larval stage of *Taenia saginatta* with adults in humans and the cysticercus in the muscle of beef), forms a cyst that contains a single scolex. The strobilocercus of *Taenia taeniaeformis* of the cat, like the cysticercus, has a single scolex, but the scolex develops a long strobilate neck, and hence the term "strobilocercus." The taeniid larva of *Echinococcus* is called a hydatid, and this cyst contains hundreds to thousands of small scolices that are called protoscolices. Thus, the larval stages of different species of taeniid tapeworms have different morphologies, and therefore, there can be some designation of the larval type to a species that correlates with the adult form.

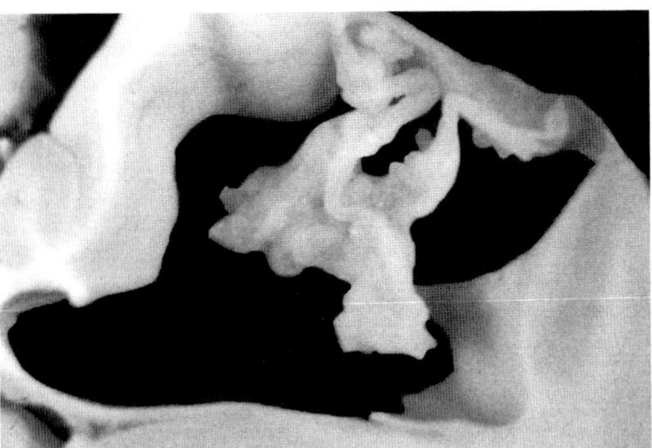

Fig. 3.32. Coenurus in the brain of a cat. This is from the case reported by Georgi et al. (1969).

The species of tapeworm that is expected to be that causing coenurosis in cats is *Taenia serialis*. The morphology of the coenurus from cats matches that of *Taenia serialis* in that the scolices within the coenurus are in a series or a linear arrangement. Also, cats have been reported to be infected only in the United States and Australia. In the United States, there are only two species of coenurus-forming tapeworms, *Taenia serialis,* which has a dog-lagomorph life cycle, and *Taenia mustelae,* which produces coenuri with few scolices that are found in small rodents and with adults in various mustelids. In Australia, the only coenurus-producing species that has been described is the imported *Taenia serialis.* In Europe, *Taenia multiceps,* which has a dog-sheep life cycle, is also present, but although this was imported into the United States, *Taenia multiceps* is no longer considered present in North America (Becklund, 1970).

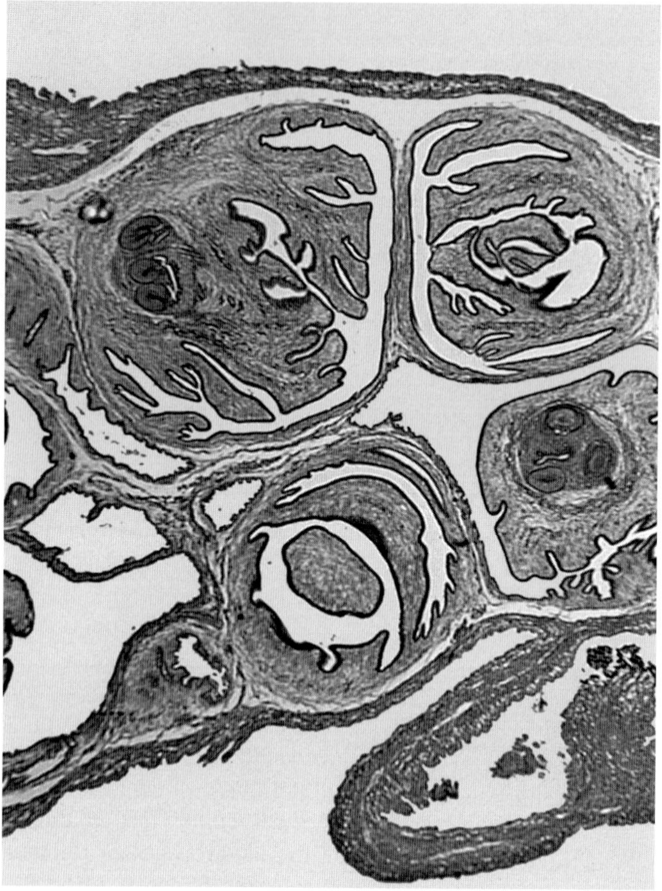

Fig. 3.33. Histologic section through a coenurus. Sections through two scolices can be identified by the sections through the suckers.

In North America, coenurosis has been reported from cats in New York (Georgi et al., 1969), Saskatchewan (Hayes and Creighton, 1978); Wyoming and Alaska (Kingston et al., 1984); California (Smith et al., 1988); and Missouri (Huss et al., 1994). The single case from Australia was from a cat referred to the university clinic in Werribee, Victoria (Slocombe et al., 1989). In all cases to date, the infection has proven fatal. Typically, cats have presented with neurological signs that progressively worsen over a period of 1 to 2 weeks to a point of severe neurologic disease. Examination of cats by X-ray computed tomography (Smith et al., 1988) and of the coenuri collected at necropsy has revealed large cysts that may measure 2 to 5 cm in diameter. The coenuri typically contain scolices, but in most cases they have been malformed or immature with hooks that have appeared abnormal or varied in size. In one case, the scolices were completely developed, and the hooks were comparable to those of *Taenia serialis* (Huss et al., 1994).

Taenia serialis has adults that are typically found in the intestine of dogs around the world. The intermediate hosts are lagomorphs, rabbits and hares, that ingest the eggs while feeding on grass. In the rabbits, the coenurus typically develops in the muscle fascia or subcutaneously, and the scolices are typically formed within 2 months after infection. It is difficult to know how old the various coenuri are that have been recovered from cats, but it is likely that the disease may have an acute onset soon after the larva takes up residence in the brain. Treatment could consist of surgical excision of the cyst or perhaps treatment with mebendazole, albendazole, or praziquantel.

REFERENCES

Becklund WH. 1970. Current knowledge of the gid bladder worm, *Coenurus cerebralis* (= *Taenia multiceps*), in North American domestic sheep, *Ovis aries*. Proc Helm Soc Wash 37:200–203.

Georgi JR, de Lahunta A, Percy DH. 1969. Cerebral coenurosis in a cat. Report of a case. Cornell Vet 59:127–134.

Hayes MA, Creighton SR. 1978. A coenurus in the brain of a cat. Can Vet J 19:341–343.

Huss BT, Miller MA, Corwin RM, Hoberg EP, O'Brien DP. 1994. Fatal cerebral coenurosis in a cat. JAVMA 205:69–71.

Kingston N, Williams ES, Bergstrom RC, Wilson WC, Miller R. 1984. Cerebral coenuriasis in domestic cats in Wyoming and Alaska. Proc Helm Soc Wash 51:309–314.

Slocombe RF, Arundel JH, Labuc R, Doyle MK. 1989. Cerebral coenuriasis in a domestic cat. Aust Vet J 66:92–93.

Smith MC, Bailey CS, Baker N, Kock N. 1988. Cerebral coenurosis in a cat. JAVMA 192:82–84.

Echinococcus multilocularis (Leuckart, 1863) Vogel, 1957

Etymology

Echino = spined and *coccus* = cyst along with *multilocularis* referring to the multicyst nature of the hydatid larval form.

Synonyms

Taenia alveolaris Klemm, 1883; *Echinococcus sibericensis* Rausch and Schiller, 1954; *Alveococcus multilocularis* (Leuckart, 1863) Abduladze, 1960.

History

Leuckart (1863) wrote that *Taenia echinococcus multilocularis* represented a form of hydatid cyst that pathologists had long recognized as different from the typical unilocular hydatid that is caused by the larvae of *Echinococcus granulosus*. It was not until the work of Rausch and Schiller (1951), Thomas et al. (1954), Fay (1973), and others in Alaska showed the relationship of the cyst occurring in human beings to the cycle that occurred in foxes and arvicolid rodents; sled dogs served to bring the adult forms into the human environment. Vogel (1955) showed that a similar cycle occurs in south Germany. Cats were first shown to be hosts to the adult stage of this parasite by Ambo et al. (1954 [cited in Kamiya et al., 1985]) on Rebun Island where the parasite had been introduced with foxes from the Kurile Islands.

Geographic Distribution

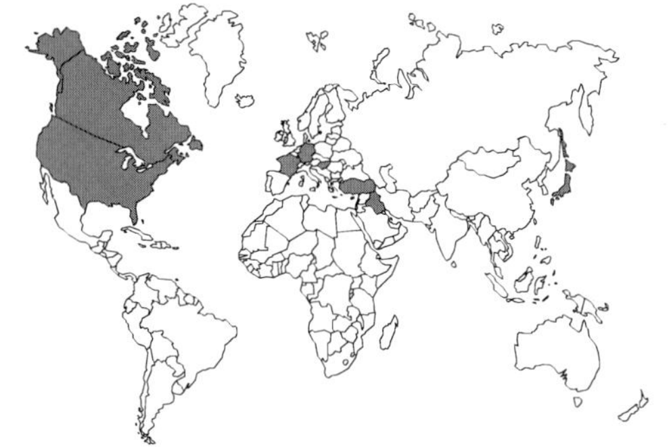

Fig. 3.34.

The distribution of *Echinococcus multilocularis* includes the northern areas of the world, including many of the tundra areas across North America and Eurasia; it was recently described in detail by Rausch (1995). *Echinococcus multilocularis* seems to be lacking in Greenland and Iceland. There are southern foci that are found in the central plains of North America, crossing the border between Canada and the United States, and in an area in southern Germany, eastern France, and parts of Switzerland and Austria. The range extends down into the Middle East, including Turkey and Iran, and it has been reported from Tunisia. The parasite exists naturally on the Sakahlin Island of Japan but was introduced to Rebun Island and Hokkaido where it has spread widely.

Cats have been shown to be natural hosts of this infection on several occasions. Adult *Echinococcus multilocularis* was described from cats in Saskatoon, Canada (Wobeser, 1972), and North Dakota (Leiby and Kritsky, 1972). In Europe, it has been described in cats from Baden-Württemburg, Germany (Eckert et al., 1974), the Saubian Alps, Germany (Zeyhle, 1982), and France (Deblock et al., 1989). In the Middle East, *Echinococcus multilocularis* has been reported from cats in Amman, Jordan (Morsy et al., 1980). In Japan, the parasite has been reported by Ambo (1954 [cited in Kamiya et al., 1985]) from Rebun Island and from Nemuro, Japan (Yagi et al., 1984 [cited in Kamiya et al., 1985]).

Parasite Identification

Adults of *Echinococcus* are all very small forms; the total length of all species is usually less than 1 cm, with typical sizes being 2 to 11 mm. Also, there are typically very few numbers of segments (ranges between two and seven in the strobilae) in these different species. The typical *Echinococcus multilocularis* has two rows of taeniid (claw-hammer–shaped) hooks on the scolex. The first row of hooks measures 25 to 34 μm in length, and the small hooks in the second row measure 20 to 31 μm in length. The body typically has two to six, although commonly five, segments. The total length of the body is typically 1.2 to 4.5 mm. The opening of the genital pore tends to be anterior to the middle of each segment.

There are three species of *Echinococcus* from which *Echinococcus multilocularis* needs to be differentiated. It appears that *Echinococcus granulosus* does not develop to the adult stage in the cat; thus, it is not expected that this species will be recovered from cats. However, the genital opening in *Echinococcus granulosus* is posterior to the middle of each segment in the gravid proglottid. *Echinococcus oligarthus* (Fig. 3.35) has been reported from wild felids in South and Central America and could perhaps develop in cats. The hooks on the scolex of *Echinococcus oligarthus* range from 28 to 60 μm in length, or about twice the size of those in *Echinococcus multilocularis*. Also *Echinococcus vogeli* in South and Central America is found typically as an adult in the bush dog, *Speothos venaticus*, and it is not known if the cat could serve as a host for this species. *Echinococcus vogeli* has hooks that are similar in length to those of *Echinococcus oligarthus*.

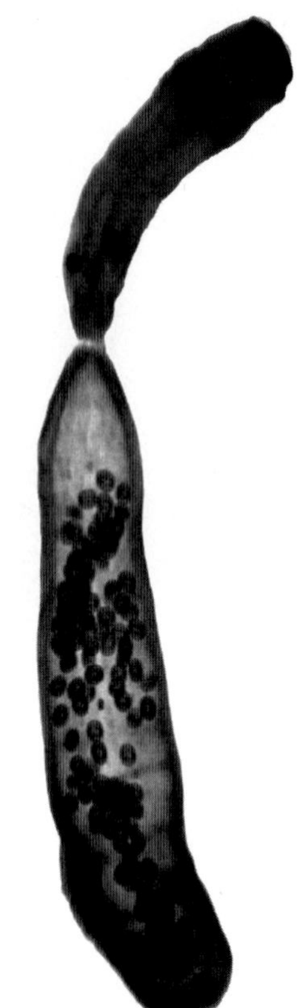

Fig. 3.35. Adult *Echinococcus oligarthus*. Although it cannot be observed at this magnification, the hooks on the rostellum are larger than those of *Echinococcus multilocularis*.

Life Cycle

Rausch (1995) described the natural cycle of *Echinococcus multilocularis* as involving the arctic fox and rodents typically of the genera *Microtus, Lemmus,* and *Clethriomys*. In other parts of the world, other fox species and coyotes typically serve as the final host. Around villages in the Arctic, cycles develop wherein dogs become infected with the adult tapeworm and then pose a threat to the humans living in the villages. Vogel (1960) suggested that a cycle involving cats and house mice might be present on farms in central Europe. Leiby and Kritsky (1972) suggested that this might be occurring on farms in North Dakota where cats and deer mice, *Peromyscus maniculatus,* were found naturally infected.

In general, the final host, the fox or dog, will produce eggs beginning 28 to 35 days after the ingestion of an infected rodent. These eggs are shed into the environment and are highly resistant to various environmental extremes (Hildreth et al., 1991). When the egg is ingested by a suitable rodent intermediate host, the six-hooked larva hatches from the egg, penetrates the intestinal wall, and is carried to the liver where it establishes the hepatic larval stage. The stage in the liver is termed an alveolar hydatid cyst (Figs. 3.36–3.38). The alveolar hydatid cyst serves to allow the asexual proliferation of the cestode in the intermediate host. The cyst contains a germinal membrane and develops hundreds to thousands of small stages, termed protoscolices, and each protoscolex is capable of developing into an adult worm. In the rodents, it takes about 60 days for the protoscolices to become infective, but it is possible that the

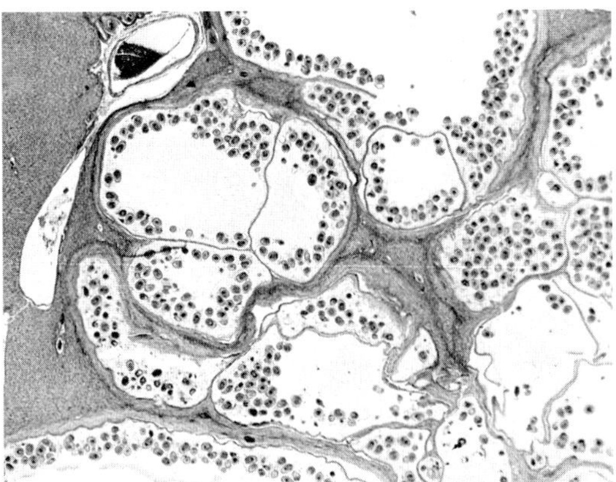

Fig. 3.36. *Echinococcus multilocularis.* A histologic section through an alveolar hydatid cyst in the liver of a rodent. Note the many chambers, each containing numerous protoscolices.

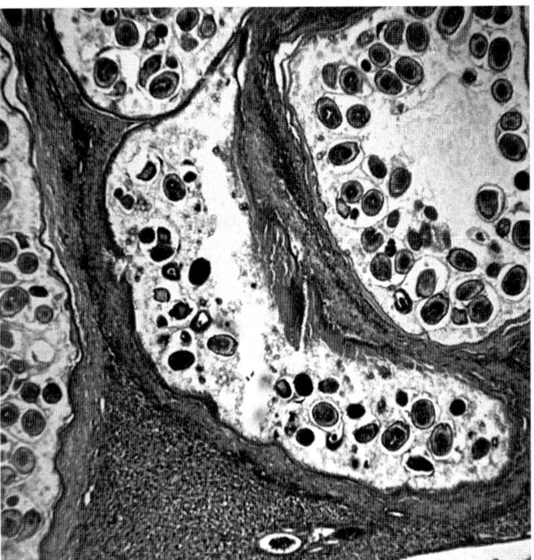

Fig. 3.37. *Echinococcus multilocularis.* A higher magnification of Fig. 3.36 showing the alveolar hydatid and the border of the different lacunae that contain the germinal membrane from which the protoscolices develop.

rapidly forming cyst can overwhelm rodents and kill them within weeks of infection (Hildreth et al., 1991). When infective protoscolices are ingested by a suitable final host, the protoscolices embed themselves within the crypts of Lieberkühn where they begin their development. The adults of *Echinococcus multilocularis* tend to localize in the posterior portion of the small intestine (Thompson and Eckert, 1983).

The cat is apparently a relatively poor host for *Echinococcus multilocularis.* Vogel (1957) succeeded in infecting five of six cats with *Echinococcus multilocularis* from southern Germany and noted that, compared with the worms in other hosts, those in the cats were smaller and produced fewer eggs. Thompson and Eckert (1983) infected two cats with the European strain and found that neither developed worms containing eggs. Zeyhle and Bosche (1982) inoculated 10 cats and two red foxes with protoscolices and found large numbers of cestodes in two cats, very few cestodes in six cats, and no cestodes in two of the cats. In comparing the worms from cats and from foxes infected at the same time, it was found that the worms from cats had an average of 106 eggs per gravid proglottid, while the worms from foxes had an average of 300 eggs per gravid proglottid. Crellin et al. (1980), using *Echinococcus multilocularis* from a red fox in Minnesota, found that infections developed in 12 dogs that were inoculated with protoscolices, while only 11 of 12 cats

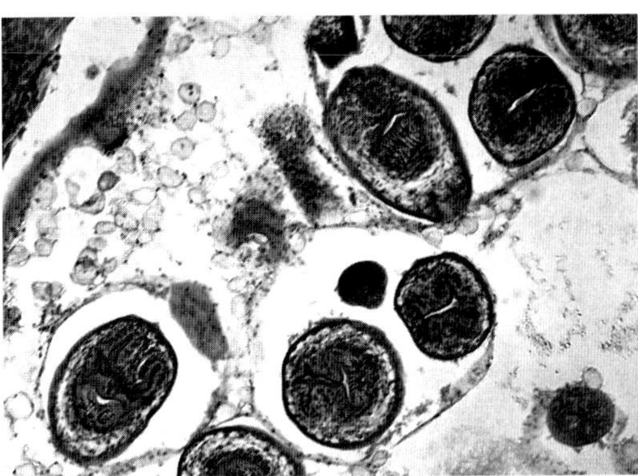

Fig. 3.38. *Echinococcus multilocularis.* Another higher magnification of Fig. 3.36 showing close-ups of protoscolices in which the suckers and the inverted rostellum with hooklets can be observed.

became infected. The dogs harbored more adults 21 days after infection (mean of 875) versus the number recovered from cats (mean of 102). Also, the worms recovered from dogs were longer. Kamiya et al. (1985), using *Echinococcus multilocularis* originally isolated from Alaska and maintained in rodents by intraperitoneal passage for 30 years, found that the worms developed poorly in cats relative to dogs. They recovered very few worms from the cats, and on day 30 of the study, the cat that was examined contained no worms at necropsy. Natural infections also indicate that the cat is probably a poor host. The prevalence of infection in cats is often low even when the levels of infection in surrounding foxes are quite high (Crellin et al., 1980; Wobeser, 1972). Often, there are few worms recovered from infected cats (Deblock et al., 1989; Wobeser, 1972), although Leiby and Kritsky (1972) recovered 26 gravid worms from one cat and about 500 worms (50 percent gravid) from a second cat in North Dakota.

Clinical Presentation and Pathogenesis

There are no signs associated with infection of *Echinococcus multilocularis* in cats that have been described. Foxes and dogs that have been observed to harbor even thousands of worms also show few signs.

Diagnosis

The eggs of *Echinococcus multilocularis* are typical taeniid eggs (i.e., they are surrounded by a brown eggshell and contain a six-hooked embryo). The eggs are 27 to 38 μm in width and are slightly ovoid in shape. In areas where cats could be hosts to either *Echinococcus multilocularis* or *Taenia taeniaeformis,* ante mortem diagnosis is difficult because the eggs are virtually indistinguishable by light microscopy. Thus, the risk is great of having an infection with *Echinococcus multilocularis* being misidentified as an infection with the more common *Taenia taeniaeformis*. The small proglottids of *Echinococcus* will not be recognized as such in the feces, and thus, if a cat routinely sheds eggs but never appears to shed segments, then an infection with *Echinococcus multilocularis* should be suspected.

Treatment

Praziquantel (5 mg/kg body weight) has been shown to be efficacious in the treatment of *Echinococcus multilocularis*.

Epizootiology

As stated above, the cat is a potential host of this parasite, although it appears that it is not a significant host in most settings. In areas where the parasite is present and where large numbers of the normal final hosts, foxes and coyotes, are present, there should be concern that cats may play a role in serving as the final host of this parasite. The concern is that if cats assume the role of final host, this parasite that is typically present in wild animals will gain access to the owners of pets. The disease caused by the larval stage of this parasite in humans is often severe with grave consequences.

Hazards to Other Animals

The stage passed in the feces of a cat would be infective to rodents and even to dogs (Geisel et al., 1990). In these hosts, the larval stage, the alveolar hydatid cyst, would typically develop in the liver.

Hazards to Humans

Human cases of alveolar hydatid disease have been reported from almost all areas of the world where the parasite is present, including two cases within the central North American focus (Schantz et al., 1995). Human infection with the larval stage of this parasite causes clinical manifestations that are similar to those of a slowly developing carcinoma of the liver. The growing parasite destroys the liver tissue, and growth of the parasite into blood vessels allows the portions of the germinal layer to be carried by the bloodstream to other tissues where metastases can develop. The clinical diagnosis is difficult, and the disease is often mistaken for carcinoma. Alveolar hydatid disease is considered a serious disease with a grave prognosis without treatment. Treatment consists of the resection of the cystic material from the liver and prolonged administration of mebendazole or albendazole, which may be continued for the life of the patient.

REFERENCES

Crellin JR, Marchiondo AA, Anderson FL. 1980. Comparison of suitability of dogs and cats as hosts of *Echinococcus multilocularis*. AJVR 42:1980-1981.

Deblock S, Prost S, Walbaum S, Petavy AF. 1989. *Echinococcus multilocularis:* a rare cestode of the domestic cat in France. Int J Parasitol 19:687–688.

Eckert J, Müller B, Partridge AJ. 1974. The domestic cat and dog as natural definitive hosts of *Echinococcus* (*Alveococcus*) *multilocularis* in southern Federal Republic of Germany. Tropenmed Parasitol 25:334–337.

Fay FH. 1973. The ecology of *Echinococcus multilocularis* Leuckart, 1863 (Cestoda: Taeniidae) on

St. Lawrence Island, Alaska. I. Background and rationale. Ann Parasitol 48:523–542.
Geisel O, Barutzki D, Minkus G, Hermanns W, Löscher T. 1990. Hunde als Finnenträger (IntermediÑrwirt) von *Echinococcus multilocularis* (Leuckart, 1863) Vogel, 1957. Kleintierprazis 35:275–280.
Hildreth MB, Johnson MD, Kazacos KR. 1991. *Echinococcus multilocularis:* a zoonosis of increasing concern in the United States. Comp Cont Educ Pract Vet 13:727–740.
Kamiya M, Ooi HK, Oku Y, Yagi K, Ohbayashi M. 1985. Growth and development of *Echinococcus multilocularis* in experimentally infected cats. Jap J Vet Res 33:135–140.
Leiby PD, Kritsky DC. 1972. *Echinococcus multilocularis:* a possible domestic life cycle in central North America and its public health implications. J Parasitol 58:1213–1215.
Leuckart R. 1863. Die menschlichen Parasiten und die von ihnen herruhrenden Krankheiten. Vol 1. Lepzig u Heidelberg.
Morsy TA, Michael SA, El Disi AM. 1980. Cats as reservoir hosts of human parasites in Amman, Jordan. J Egypt Soc Parasitol 10:5–18.
Rausch RL. 1995. Life cycle patterns and geographic distribution of *Echinococcus* species. In *Echinococcus* and Hydatid Disease, ed RCA Thompson and AJ Lymbery, pp 89–134. Wallingford, UK: CAB International.
Rausch RL, Schiller EL. 1951. Hydatid disease (Echinococcosis) in Alaska and the importance of rodent intermediate hosts. Science 113:57–58.
Schantz PM, Chai J, Craig PS, Eckert J, Jenkins DJ, Macpherson CNL, Thakur A. 1995. Epidemiology and control of hydatid disease. In *Echinococcus* and Hydatid Disease, ed RCA Thompson and AJ Lymbery, pp 231–233. Wallingford, UK: CAB International.
Thomas LJ, Babero BB, Galicchio V, Lacey RJ. 1954. Echinococcosis on St. Lawrence Island, Alaska. Science 120:1102–1103.
Thompson RCA, Eckert J. 1983. Observations on *Echinococcus multilocularis* in the definitive host. Z Parasitenk 69:335–345.
Vogel H. 1955. Ueber den Entwicklungszyklus und die zuhöorigkeit des europaischen Alveolarechinococcus. Dtsch Med Wchschr 80:931–932.
Vogel H. 1957. über den *Echinococcus multilocularis* Süddeutschlands. 1. Das Bandwurmstadium von Stämmen menschlicher und tierischer Herkunft. Z Tropenmed Parasitol 8:405–454.
Vogel H. 1960. Tiere als naturliche Wirte des *Echinococcus multilocularis* in Europa. Z Tropenmed Parasitol 11:36–42.
Wobeser G. 1972. The occurrence of *Echinococcus multilocularis* (Leuckart, 1863) in cats near Saskatoon, Saskatchewan. Can Vet J 12:65–68.
Zeyhle E. 1982. Distribution of *Echinococcus multilocularis* in southwest Germany. Abstr 5th Int Cong Parasitol, Toronto, Canada.
Zeyhle E, Bosche D. 1982. Comparative experimental infections of cats and foxes with *Echinococcus multilocularis*. Zbl Bakteriol 277:117–118.

ACANTHOCEPHALA

The Acanthocephala is a small phylum of wormlike creatures that is very important relative to fish, aquatic reptiles, and aquatic birds. There are a few of the Acanthocephala that have developed life cycles that allow them to make good use of terrestrial hosts; for the most part, they are seen almost exclusively by individuals working in wildlife biology or medicine.

The adult worms can be less than 1 cm to more than 35 cm in length depending on the species involved. The adult worms do not have an intestinal tract, and on the anterior end of the worm, there is a protrusible proboscis that is covered with hooks. The adult worms are all parasites of the intestinal tract where they live with their proboscis embedded in the intestinal mucosa. There are separate sexes, males and females, and the females produce eggs that are characteristic in that they typically have three marked components to the shell and have a larva inside that has a lot of hooklets on one end. In the typical life cycle, there is the requirement for some type of arthropod as the first intermediate host. Depending on the species, the life cycle can also involve various paratenic vertebrate hosts. When cats become infected, they have typically done so by eating either an intermediate host or a vertebrate paratenic host.

The majority of reports of Acanthocephala in cats have come from Australia (O'Callaghan and Beveridge, 1996; Thompson et al., 1993; Shaw et al., 1983; Coman et al., 1981; Ryan, 1976; Coman 1972). Almost all these reports have dealt with cats being infected with a species of *Oncicola.* In the most recent of these reports (O'Callaghan and Beveridge, 1996), the species in the cats from the Northern Territory of Australia was identified as *Oncicola pomatostomi.* In the 188 cats that were examined in this study, this was the most common helminth recovered, being present in over 65 percent of the cats, and infected cats had anywhere from 1 to 1,000 worms. In the other studies, the prevalence of infection was lower. Cats probably acquired infections with this acanthocephalan through the ingestion of a paratenic host. The arthropod intermediate host has not been described, but birds and small mammals can probably serve as paratenic hosts.

In most cases, the genus, let alone the species, of the Acanthocephala parasite has not been identified. In Somalia, a cat was reported as being infected with a species of *Moniliformis,* which is typically found in rodents and which uses an arthropod as the intermediate host (Gadale et al., 1989). Reports from Japan (Asato et al., 1986), India (Balasubramaniam, 1972), Malaysia (Amin Babjee, 1978), and Chile (Bonilla-Zepeda, 1980) have simply reported the presence of these worms. Chandler (1925) recorded *Centrorhynchus erraticus* from a cat in Calcutta.

REFERENCES

Amin Babjee. 1978. Parasites of the domestic cat in Selangor, Malaysia. Kajian Vet 10:107–114.

Asato R, Hasegawa H, Kuniyoshi S, Higa T. 1986. Prevalence of helminthic infections in cats on Okinawa Island, Japan. Jap J Parasitol 35:209–214.

Balasubramaniam G. 1972. Report of an acanthocephalan infection in a domestic cat (*Felis domesticus*). Cheiron 1:116–117.

Bonilla-Zepeda C. 1980. Estudio de la fauna helmintologica del gato en la ciudad de Valdivia, Chile. Arch Med Vet 12:277.

Chandler AC. 1925. The helminthic parasites of cats in Calcutta and the relation of cats to human helminthic infection. Ind J Med Res 13:213.

Coman BJ. 1972. A survey of the gastro-intestinal parasites of the feral cat in Victoria. Aust Vet J 48:133–136.

Coman BJ, Jones EH, Driesen MA. 1981. Helminth parasites and arthropods of feral cats. Aust Vet J 57:324–327.

Gadale OI, Capelli G, Ali AA, Poglayen G. 1989. Intestinal helminths of cats. First reports in Somalia. Boll Sci Fac Zootech Vet Univ Naz Somala 1989:8–24.

O'Callaghan MG, Beveridge I. 1996. Gastro-intestinal parasites of feral cats in the Northern Territory. Trans Roy Soc S Aust 120:175–176.

Ryan GE. 1976. Gastro-intestinal parasites of feral cats in New South Wales. Aust Vet J 52:224–227.

Shaw J, Dunsmore H, Jakob Hoff, R. 1983. Prevalence of some gastrointestinal parasites in cats in the Perth area. Aust Vet J 60:151–152.

Thompson RCA, Meloni BP, Hopkins RM, Deplazes P, Reynoldson JA. 1993. Observations on the endo- and ectoparasites affecting dogs and cats in Aboriginal communities in the north-west of Western Australia. Aust Vet J 70:268–270.

4 THE NEMATODES

Nematodes constitute a phylum of bilaterally symmetrical tubular organisms that are present upon the earth in fairly innumerable quantities. The vast majority of nematodes are free-living, being found in soils of most of the earth's ecosystems. However, some have also developed the means of surviving within niches in other living hosts. In this relationship, nematodes have come to be recognized as important parasites of plants and animals. This chapter focuses on those that live within the feline host.

The external surface of the nematode is covered with a noncellular surface called the cuticle. Under the cuticle is a syncytium that is called the hypodermis. Under the hypodermis is a layer of muscle cells that are arranged along the long axis of the tubular worm. The muscles of nematodes are divided into four quadrants by dorsal and ventral nerve cords and two lateral cords that are composed of extensions of the hypodermis. Within the tubular nematode is a tubular digestive tract that extends from the mouth on the anterior end to the anus at the posterior of the worm. This digestive tract is composed of a muscular esophagus that connects to a simple intestine that is composed of a single layer of intestinal epithelial cells. The nervous system is centered in a nerve ring that encircles the esophagus and that extends into the ventral and dorsal nerve cords. Nematodes have a third body opening called the excretory pore, which represents the opening of the excretory system that varies in structure in different nematode groups. The excretory pore is usually located anteriorly on the ventral surface between the mouth and the base of the esophagus.

Female nematodes have a fourth body orifice, the vulval opening of the female reproductive tract. The typical female reproductive system consists of a vagina that leads into the uterus and ovary; most typically, the uterus is branched into two tubes and each tube is connected to its own tubular ovary. The portion of the uterus nearest the vulva is typically packed full of the stages that are to be ejected from the female; thus, the terminal uterus may contain eggs with single cells, eggs with several cells or larvae, or free larvae.

Males have no additional orifices, and the male reproductive tract typically consists of a single tube that opens into the rectum and that opens to the exterior through the anus. Most male nematodes have paired cuticularized structures called spicules that are inserted into the vulva of the female during copulation. Some male nematodes also possess expansions of the body on the posterior end that form a muscular bursa copulatrix that functions to grasp the female during copulation. The sperm of nematodes is ameboid and after being introduced into the female makes its way through the uterus to the oviduct to fertilize the eggs.

The entire structure of nematodes functions on the basis of a very high internal turgor pressure that is maintained in the body cavity, the pseudocoelom, in which the different tubes of the body are suspended. Thus, the esophagus functions to pull food into the body, while the muscular vulva found in some nematodes functions to keep eggs from being extruded before they reach proper maturity. In the same fashion, the digestive tract is emptied when the sphincter muscles open the anus and allow the feces to be pushed out of the body. The longitudinal muscles of the body cavity allow the nematode to flex by working against the internal pressure that is maintained. The internal pressure in nematodes can be demonstrated by a simple pinprick, which will cause the internal organs to burst out of the body through the hole made by the pin.

The life cycle of nematodes is determined in part by the external cuticle that is present. This cuticle has to be shed every time the nematode changes its external morphology. All nematodes shed their cuticle (i.e., ecdyse) and undergo morphological metamorphosis (i.e., molt) four times during their lives, and thus, there are four larval stages between the egg and the adult. There are two major groups of nematodes, the Secernentea and the Adenophorea. Typically, the stage of secernentean nematodes that infects the vertebrate final host is the larva that has undergone two molts (i.e., the third-stage larva). The stage of adenophorean nematodes that infects the vertebrate final host is typically a larva that has never molted (i.e., a first-stage larva). Typically, adult-like characters first appear in the fourth-stage larva, but the uterus typically does not have a vulva with a patent opening to the exterior until the nematode completes its final molt to the adult stage. In some secernentean nematodes, the cuticle from the earlier stage or stages is maintained by the third-stage larva as a protective sheath. In other secernentean nematodes, both molts occur within the eggshell, so the nematode that hatches from the egg is a third-stage larva.

The cat is parasitized by both secernentean and adenophorean nematodes. There are four orders of secernentean nematode parasites in the cat, the Rhabditida, the Strongylida, the Ascaridida, and the Spirurida. The cat is also parasitized by a few representatives of the adenophorean nematodes. In the Secernentea nematodes, the anus is found in a subterminal ventral position; thus, there tends to be a tail that protrudes beyond the anus in this group of nematodes. In the case of the Adenophorea, the anus is typically terminal in position, thus, there is no tail extending beyond the end of the body.

SECERNENTEA

RHABDITIDA

The Rhabditida is a group of nematodes that is currently best known for the free-living member of the group, *Caenorhabditis elegans,* which is used extensively in genetic and developmental research. The best-known parasite in this group is *Strongyloides stercoralis,* which is parasitic as an adult in humans, dogs, and occasionally cats. Members of the Rhabditida are unusual nematodes in that they tend towards atypical sexual differentiation. In *Caenorhabditis elegans,* the female, so called because of the fact that she produces eggs and has the general morphological characteristics of a female, is a true hermaphrodite in that both male and female sex cells develop within the same reproductive tract. True males also are produced as part of this life cycle. These features allow self-fertilization for the perpetuation of clonal lines, and the presence of males allows the introduction of specific genetic crosses that makes this worm of such use to geneticists. *Strongyloides* species are also atypical in that the parasitic stage is a parthenogenetic female (i.e., it produces offspring without fertilization). In the case of *Strongyloides* species, there is also the possibility of the production of free-living male and female stages that morphologically resemble *Caenorhabditis elegans* more than their elongate parasitic form.

The only members of the Rhabditida that are parasitic in cats are members of the genus *Strongyloides.* The free-living stages, larvae and adults, have morphology that is typical of this group, which includes an esophagus that is divided into three distinct portions, the corpus, the isthmus, and the bulbus; a vulva that is near midbody; and a male that does not have a bursa. The parasitic forms have atypical morphology in that the female is relatively elongate compared with the free-living form and the esophagus is very long and cylindrical, taking up from one-fourth to one-third of the total length of the digestive tract. There are two major groups within the species of *Strongyloides.* In one group, the parasitic parthenogenetic females have ovaries that coil about the digestive tract and that produce embryonated eggs that are passed in the feces. In the second group of species, the parasitic parthenogenetic females have ovaries that simply fold back on themselves, and with these species the stage passed in the feces is a first-stage larva.

Another rhabditoid nematode that has been reported from cats is *Rhabditis strongyloides.* This is typically a free-living nematode that is capable of facultative parasitism (i.e., it can live in a host when introduced under appropriate conditions).

Rhabditis strongyloides (Schneider, 1860) Schneider, 1866

There has been a single report of *Rhabditis strongyloides* (reported as *Pelodera strongyloides*) from the urine of a cat. (Kipnis and Todd, 1977). In this case the cat presented with hematuria. The bladder was manually expressed, and an analysis of the urine sediment revealed numerous red blood cells along with larvae and an adult male *Pelodera strongyloides*. Treatment of this cat consisted of chloramphenicol three times daily and a urinary acidifier twice daily. By the sixth day of treatment, urine parameters had returned to normal.

Rhabditis strongyloides is typically a free-living nematode that is found in decaying organic material. It has been observed on the hair and in lesions in the skin of dogs, cows, sheep, and horses that have been housed on dirty bedding or under conditions where they have been sick or debilitated with difficulty in rising. In the skin of mammals, the only stage found is the larva (Fig. 4.1). The males of this nematode are about a millimeter long; the females are about 1.3 to 1.5 mm long. The esophagus has the typical rhabditoid shape with a corpus, isthmus, and bulbus. The buccal space is about one-fifth the length of the esophagus and has three metastomal teeth where it joins the esophagus. The vulva of the female is located slightly posteriad to midbody, and the uterus contains eggs that are 34–39 by 55–65 μm in width and length. The life cycle is direct.

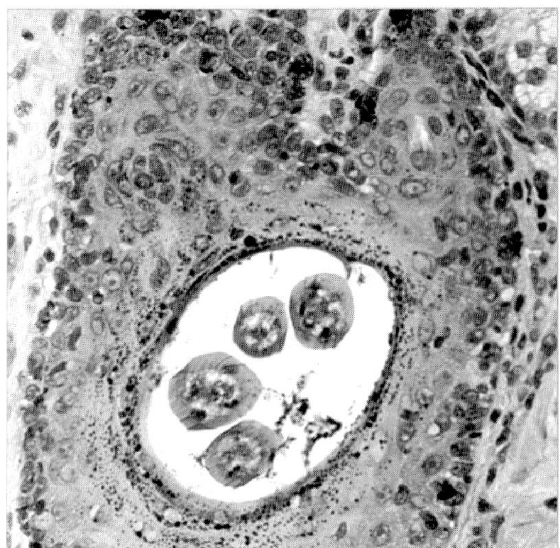

Fig. 4.1. *Rhabditis strongyloides.* A histological section through the hair follicle of a dog showing the larva of this facultative parasite.

REFERENCES

Kipnis RM, Todd KS. 1977. *Pelodera strongyloides* in the urine of a cat. Feline Pract 7:16–19.

Sudhaus VW, Schulte F. 1986. Auflösung des Artenkomplexes *Rhabditis (Pelodera) strongyloides* (Nematoda) und Beschreibung zweier nur kryptischer Arten mit Bidlung an Nagetieren. Zoologische Jahrbücher (Systematik) 113:409–428.

Sudhaus W, Schulte F. 1988. *Rhabditis (Pelodera) "strongyloides"* (Nematoda) als Verursacher von Dermatitis, mit systematischen und biologischen Bemerkungen über verwandte Arten. Zoologische Jahrbücher (Systematik) 115:187–205.

Sudhaus W, Schulte F, Hominick WM. 1987. A further sibling species of *Rhaditis (Pelodera) strongyloides* (Nematoda): *Rhabditis (P.) cutanea* n.sp. from the skin of wood mice (*Apodemus sylvaticus*). Revue de Nematologie 10:319–326.

Strongyloides Species

The genus *Strongyloides* is composed of small parasitic worms with parthenogenetic adult females that live within the mucosa of the intestinal epithelium of their hosts. The parasitic stages are characterized by the possession of a muscular esophagus that is about one-third of the length of the body; this type of esophagus is called a filariform esophagus. The parasitic females fall into two major groups, (1) those with ovaries that simply fold over at their distal ends to produce a hair-pin shape and that produce eggs that hatch before they leave the intestine and (2) those with ovaries that distally spiral around the intestine and that produce eggs that are passed in the feces (Little, 1966). For species of both types of *Strongyloides,* there are also free-living stages that do not resemble the adults in that they appear to be shorter and stockier. These free-living stages have a short esophagus that is divided into three distinct sections (i.e., the corpus, isthmus, and bulbus); this type of esophagus is called a rhabditiform esophagus. When eggs or larvae passed in the feces undergo development into free-living stages, the first-stage rhabditiform larvae that are passed in the feces or hatch from the eggs develop through four feeding larval stages to produce free-living adult males and females. The free-living adults produce eggs that hatch, and typically rhabditiform first- and second-stage larvae develop into infective filariform third-stage larvae. On rare occasions the free-living cycle may repeat itself one more time. Infective filariform larvae also can develop directly from the stages passed in the feces of the host. When the cycle involves the development of free-living stages, it is termed a heterogonic cycle. When the cycle involves the direct development of infective larvae, it is called a homogonic cycle.

Cats are hosts to three species of *Strongyloides*. *Strongyloides felis* is a species with hair-pin turns to the ovaries that is found in the small intestine of the infected cat. *Strongyloides planiceps* is a species with spiral ovaries that is also found in the small intestine of the feline host. *Strongyloides tumefaciens* is a parasite that has been recovered on a few occasions from the nodules in the mucosa of the large intestine of the feline host. *Strongyloides stercoralis,* a parasite of the small intestine of humans and dogs, will produce infections in experimentally infected cats (Sandground, 1926), but it has not been observed in naturally infected cats.

REFERENCES

Little MD. 1966. Comparative morphology of six species of *Strongyloides* (Nematoda) and redefinition of the genus. J Parasitol 52:69-84.

Sandground JH. 1926. The role of *Strongyloides stercoralis* in the causation of diarrhea. Some observations on the condition of dogs and cats experimentally infected with this parasite. Am J Trop Med 6:421–432.

Strongyloides planiceps Rogers, 1943

Etymology

Strongyl = round and *oides* = like for the genus and *planiceps* for the species name of the rusty tiger cat, *Felis planiceps,* the host from which the parasite was isolated by R.T. Leiper in 1927.

Synonyms

Strongyloides cati Rogers, 1939.

Geographic Distribution

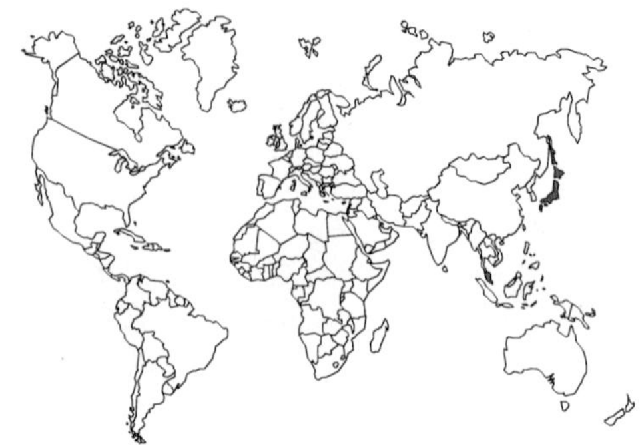

Fig. 4.2.

Strongyloides planiceps was originally described from Malaya (Rogers, 1943) and subsequently found in wild carnivores and occasionally domestic cats in Japan (Horie et al., 1981; Fukase et al., 1985). It has not been observed in the United States.

Location in Host

Strongyloides planiceps is present in the anterior portion of the small intestine.

Parasite Identification

Parasitic females are 2.4–3.3 mm long (mean, 2.8 mm); the ovaries of the female have a spiral appearance. Partially embryonated eggs measuring 58–64 by 32–40 μm (mean, 61 by 35 μm) are excreted in the feces. Infections with *Strongyloides planiceps* can be identified by finding embryonated eggs in fecal smears or fecal flotations. Fresh samples should be examined to avoid confusion with hookworm eggs. The tip of the tail of the parasitic female of *Strongyloides planiceps* abruptly narrows to a blunt end, while that of *Strongyloides felis* is longer and narrows more slowly to the tip of the tail (Horie et al., 1981).

Life Cycle

Cats become infected by oral ingestion of infective larvae or by skin penetration (Rogers, 1939). Larvae can be found in the lungs by 4 days after infection, and young parthenogenic adult females can be found in the small intestine 6 days after skin penetration. Eggs are excreted in the feces 10 to 11 days after infection.

Clinical Presentation and Pathogenesis

There has been no description of clinical signs in infected cats. It is possible that large numbers are capable of causing disease, but this is likely to require careful research in which this species is examined in cats known to be free of other helminths, particularly, *Strongyloides felis.*

Treatment

This is likely to be similar to that reported for *Strongyloides felis.* It is expected that therapeutic doses of ivermectin may also be efficacious.

Epizootiology

This parasite is probably as common in its range in dogs as it is in cats (Fukase et al., 1985). These authors report finding this parasite in 4 of 420 dogs, 4 of 105 domestic cats, 26 of 40 raccoon dogs (*Nyctereutes procyonoides viverrinus*), and two of five Japanese weasels (*Mustela sibirica itatsi*). Cats can become infected either by the oral inoculation of larvae or by skin penetration, and it would appear that where the range of cats overlaps that of wildlife reservoir hosts, cats will be at risk of infection with this parasite.

Hazards to Other Animals

Strongyloides planiceps is found in wildlife in areas of the world where it is present. It has been reported from dogs, raccoon dogs, Japanese weasels, and the rusty tiger cat in Malaysia. It appears that a red fox from Hokkaido Japan was also infected with this parasite (Fukase et al., 1985).

Hazards to Humans

There are no records of this parasite in humans.

REFERENCES

Fukase T, Chinone S, Itagaki H. 1985. *Strongyloides planiceps* (Nematoda; Strongyloididae) in some wild carnivores. Jap J Vet Sci 47:627–632.

Horie M, Noda R, Higashino J. 1981. Studies on *Strongyloides* sp. isolated from a cat and raccoon dog. Jap J Parasitol 30:215–230.

Rogers WP. 1939. A new species of *Strongyloides* from the cat. J Helminthol 17:229–238.

Rogers WP. 1943. *Strongyloides planiceps,* new name for *S. cati* Rogers. J Parasitol 29:160.

Strongyloides felis Chandler, 1925

Etymology

Strongyl = round and *oides* = like along with *felis* for the cat host.

Synonyms

None.

History

Chandler (1925a) described a new species of *Strongyloides* from cats in Calcutta. Further features of this species were described by Goodey (1926) and by Baylis (1936), but there were no additional findings presented on this worm until the 1980s when Speare and Tinsley (1986, 1987) reported that over 50 percent of cats examined in Townsville, Australia, were infected with this parasite.

Geographic Distribution

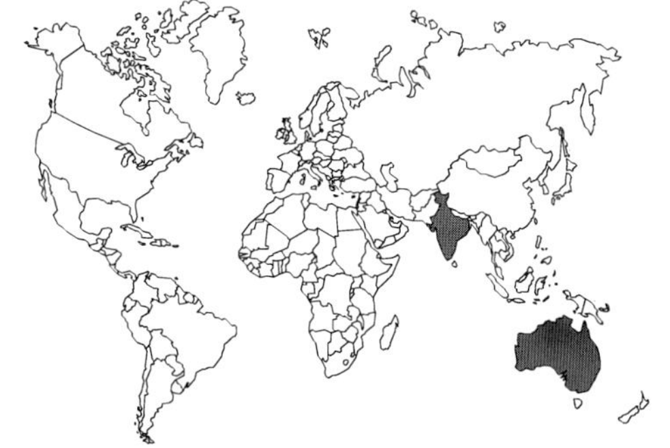

Fig. 4.3.

India and Australia.

Location in Host

The parasitic female is found in the mucosa of the anterior half of the small intestine of its host.

Parasite Identification

Strongyloides felis differs from *Strongyloides stercoralis* in that the parasitic female of *Strongyloides felis* has a narrower tail and the free-living female of *Strongyloides felis* has a postvulval constriction of the body that is lacking in the free-living female of *Strongyloides stercoralis.* The parasitic females of *Strongyloides felis* and *Strongyloides stercoralis* have ovaries that are straight, while the ovaries of the parasitic females of *Strongyloides planiceps* are spiral. Also, infections with *Strongyloides felis* and *Strongyloides stercoralis* result in larvae being passed in the feces of the infected cat, while infections with *Strongyloides planiceps* produce eggs that are found in freshly deposited feces. *Strongyloides tumefaciens* differs from the other species of *Strongyloides* present in the cat by having a longer parasitic female (5 mm long) that is found in tumors in the mucosa of the large intestine.

Diagnosis of infection is best performed using the Baermann technique. Larvae can be detected using a direct smear of feces, but because most cats shed less than 50 larvae per gram of feces, the sensitivity of this method is low. To determine whether a cat is infected with *Strongyloides felis* or *Strongyloides stercoralis,* it is necessary to perform fecal cultures that will generate the free-living adult stages.

Life Cycle

The life cycle of this parasite has been described by Spear and Tinsley (1986). The adult parthenogenetic female lives in the mucosa of the small intestine and produces eggs that hatch in the small intestine to produce first-stage rhabditiform larvae that are passed in the feces. The larvae passed in the feces will typically develop into free-living adults, males and females. At 20°C, the free-living adults will typically produce eggs that hatch to yield larvae that mature to the infective filariform third-stage larvae in about 6 days (Figs. 4.4 and 4.5). Occasionally, the larvae passed in the feces will develop directly to infective-stage larvae in about 2 days. There is only one generation of the short-lived free-living adults; most of the adults produced die within 10 days after cultures are established (Fig. 4.6). Infection of the cat is by the penetration of the skin by the infective-stage larva. After skin penetration, the infective larvae are carried to the lungs, break through the alveolar spaces, and migrate up the trachea and down the esophagus to the small intestine. The prepatent period is 11 (9 to 14) days. The fact that infections are found almost exclusively in older cats and that kittens of infected queens remain uninfected would suggest that transmammary infection with this species does not occur. Infections have been shown to persist for over 2 years in experimentally infected cats.

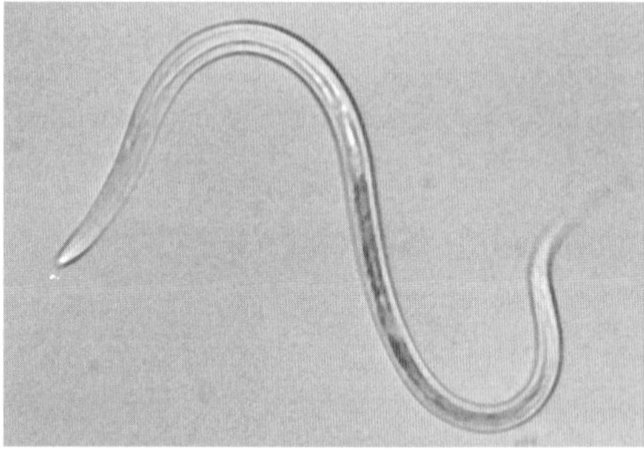

Fig. 4.4. *Strongyloides stercoralis.* Third-stage infective larva. This is the stage that penetrates the skin of its host.

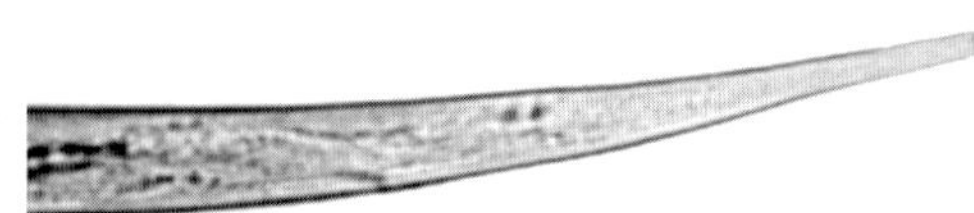

Fig. 4.5. *Strongyloides stercoralis.* Tail of third-stage infective larva. Note the forked appearance at the tip.

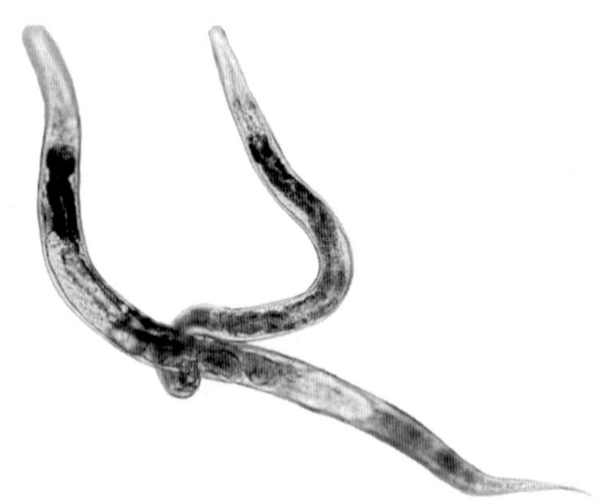

Fig. 4.6. *Strongyloides ratti.* Free-living male and female in copulation. These are the stages that sometimes develop within the environment.

Clinical Presentation and Pathogenesis

There are no pathognomonic clinical signs of infection with this parasite (Speare and Tinsley, 1986). Diarrhea is not a typical feature of infection, although some cats with naturally acquired infections had acute watery diarrhea that cleared after treatment (see below). The experimental infection of cats with 500 larvae produced no signs other than a slight unthriftiness and unkempt coats. Alertness and appetite remained normal in experimentally infected cats.

There does not appear to be an inflammatory response associated with the intestinal phase of the infection, but some worms were found to be associated with an adenomatous metaplasia of the glandular epithelium of the intestinal crypts (Speare and Tinsley, 1986). There were focal granulomas, subpleural inflammatory plaques, and a vasculitis associated with the migration of the larval stages through the lungs of experimentally infected cats.

Treatment

Thiabendazole (25 mg/kg BID for 2 days) has been found to be 100 percent efficacious in three cats. Fenbendazole (20 mg/kg SID for 3 days) caused no change in the numbers of larvae shed by two cats but caused a transient disappearance of larvae in a third cat. Oxfendazole (8 to 9 mg/kg SID for 2 days) caused only slight larval reductions. Levamisole (10 mg/kg) in combination with niclosamide (200 mg/kg) caused a temporary drop in larvae being produced in two cats. Pyrantel emboate (12.5 mg/kg) and pyrantel pamoate (25 mg/kg) both had no effect following a single treatment. Praziquantel (25 mg/kg) was also without effect (Spear and Tinsley, 1986). Ivermectin, 200 μg/kg, is probably an effective treatment.

Epizootiology

The infective stage larvae survive for a maximum of 3 weeks in the external environment and are very susceptible to dehydration. Infections are confined mainly to adult cats with cats less than 6 months of age only rarely being infected. Speare and Tinsley (1986) reported that 56 percent of 198 adult cats from Townsville and Ingham, Australia, were infected with this parasite, while only 9 percent of 63 kittens and juvenile cats were infected. Most natural infections are not heavy, with there typically being less than 50 larvae per gram of feces and less than 100 adult worms present.

Hazards to Other Animals

Unknown.

Hazards to Humans

Unknown.

Control/Prevention

Because infections are obtained by the direct penetration of the skin with larvae, it is difficult to prevent infections in cats that are allowed outside.

REFERENCES

Baylis HA. 1936. Nematoda, vol. 1 (Ascaroidea and Strongyloidea). The Fauna of British India, Including Ceylon and Burma. 808 pp.

Chandler AC. 1925a. The helminthic parasites of cats in Calcutta and the relationship of cats to human helminthic infections. Ind J Med Res 13:213–227.

Chandler AC. 1925b. The species of *Strongyloides* (Nematoda). Parasitology 17:426–433.

Goodey T. 1926. Observations on *S. fulleborni* von Linstow, 1905, with some remarks on the genus *Strongyloides*. J Helminthol 4:75–86.

Speare R, Tinsley DJ. 1986. *Strongyloides felis:* An "old" worm rediscovered in Australian cats. Aust Vet Pract 16:10–18.

Speare R, Tinsley DJ. 1987. Survey of cats for *Strongyloides felis*. Aust Vet J 64:191–192.

Strongyloides tumefaciens Price and Dikmans 1941

Etymology

Strongyl = round and *oides* = like for the genus and *tumefaciens* to reflect the tumor-like nodules induced by the parasite.

Synonyms

None.

History

Price and Dikmans first reported lesions caused by this parasite in 1929 from a cat from Louisiana. They provided a description of the lesions and worms from the original cat and an additional case from Florida in 1941 and named the parasite *Strongyloides tumefaciens.*

Geographic Distribution

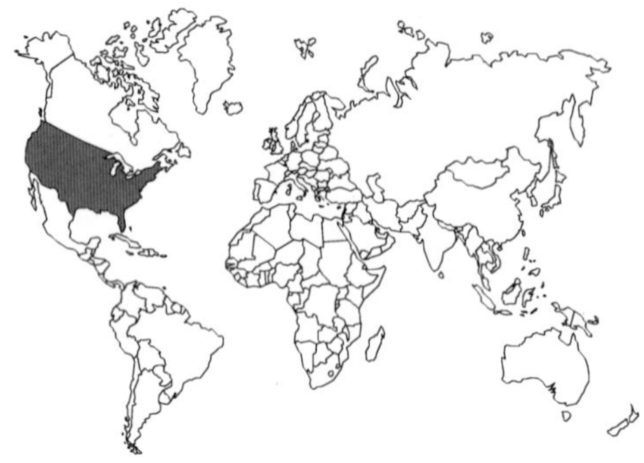

Fig. 4.7.

Strongyloides tumefaciens has been found in a small number of domestic cats from the southeastern United States in Louisiana, Florida, Texas, and Georgia (Price and Dikmans, 1941; Malone et al., 1977; Lindsay et al., 1987). It also has been observed in two wild cats, *Felis chaus,* in India (Dubey and Pande, 1964). A *Strongyloides* species, most likely *Strongyloides tumefaciens,* has been observed in three Florida bobcats, *Felis rufus,* and a Florida panther, *Felis concolor coryi* (Forrester, 1992).

Location in Host

Strongyloides tumefaciens eggs, larvae, and adults are found in grossly visible tumor-like nodules in the large intestine. Migrating larvae may be observed in various tissues during migration to the large intestine.

Parasite Identification

Parthenogenic females of *Strongyloides tumefaciens* dissected from formalin-fixed nodules are about 5 mm long (Price and Dikmans, 1941); the species of *Strongyloides* present in the small intestine of the cat tend to be around 3.5 mm or less in length. Eggs from females of *Strongyloides tumefaciens* are embryonated and measure 114 to 124 by 62 to 68 μm. Fecal cultures of larvae at room temperature will result in third-stage larvae that have a "split tail" appearance (typical for *Strongyloides* species) and a filariform esophagus (Malone et al., 1977).

Life Cycle

The life cycle is unknown. Infections are probably acquired by oral ingestion or skin penetration by third-stage larvae. Parthenogenic females are found in grossly visible tumor-like nodules in the large intestine. Eggs and larvae are also present in the nodules. Eggs hatch in the nodules, and larvae are excreted in the feces. No parasitic males exist.

Clinical Presentation and Pathogenesis

Abdominal palpation of cats with *Strongyloides tumefaciens* may reveal a firm and fibrotic colon (Malone et al., 1977). *Strongyloides tumefaciens* produces characteristic tumor-like nodules in the large intestine. Grossly white, glistening nodules present on the mucosal surface are elevated 1 to 3 mm above the mucosa and are 2 to 3 mm in diameter (Fig. 4.8). These nodules may be visualized on colonoscopy. A central depression may also be present. Microscopically, hyperplastic nodules of crypt epithelium are present in the submucosa (Fig. 4.9). A connective tissue capsule surrounds the nodules. The mucosal epithelium covering the nodules may be degenerative and infiltrated by neutrophils and lymphocytes. Parthenogenic females are present and confined to the nodules (Fig. 4.10). Eggs can be observed within the females and free in the nodules (Fig. 4.11). Rhabditiform larvae can be found in the nodules, in adjacent submucosal tissues, and free in the lumen.

Treatment

Thiabendazole is effective in treating cats with *Strongyloides tumefaciens* when administered orally at 125 mg daily for 3 days (Malone et al., 1977). The feces become normal, and larvae are eliminated by day 4 posttreatment. Ivermectin, 200 μg/kg, is probably an effective treatment.

Hazards to Other Animals

Unknown. A similar lesion containing *Strongyloides* was observed in the jejunum of a chimpanzee (Blacklock and Adler, 1922).

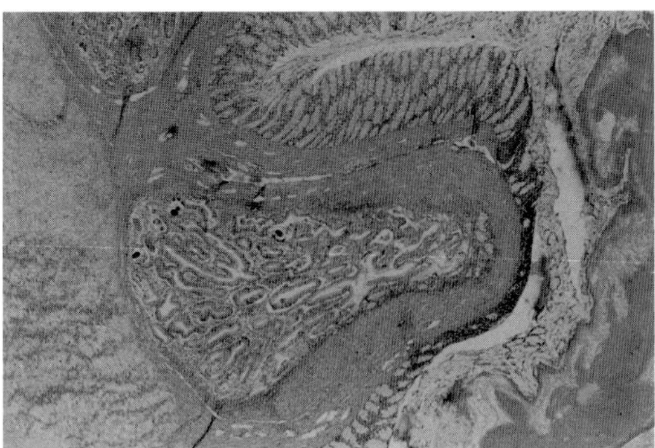

Fig. 4.8. *Strongyloides tumefaciens.* Transverse section through a nodule in the colon of a cat showing the hyperplastic mucosa and muscularis containing numerous worms.

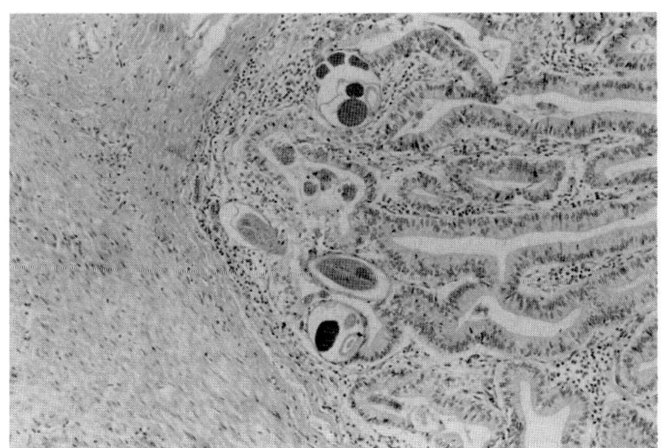

Fig. 4.9. *Stongyloides tumefaciens.* Transverse section showing several sections through the parthenogenetic female.

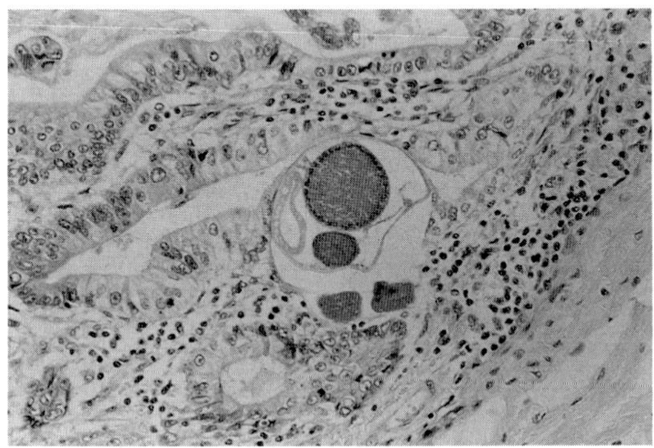

Fig. 4.10. *Strongyloides tumefaciens.* Section through a female worm at the level of the ovary.

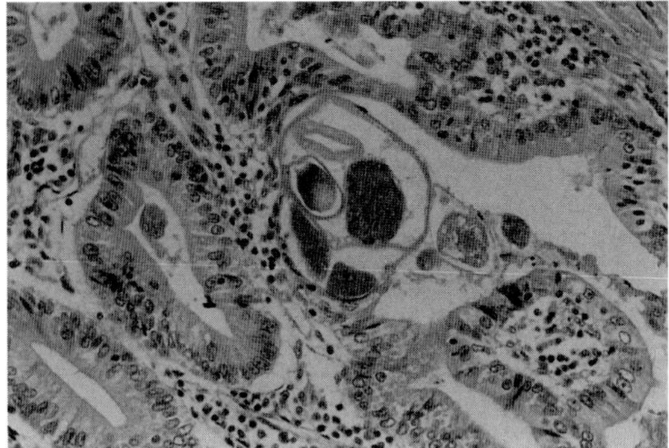

Fig. 4.11. *Strongyloides tumefaciens.* Section through the worm at the level of the uterus. Also present are laid eggs in various stages of development.

Hazards to Humans

Unknown.

REFERENCES

Blacklock B, Adler S. 1922. The pathological effects produced by *Strongyloides* in a chimpanzee. Ann Trop Med Parasitol 16:383–390.

Dubey JP, Pande BP. 1964. On helminthic lesions encountered in the alimentary canal of the Indian wild cat (*Felis chaus*). Agra Univ J Res Sci 13:169–184.

Forrester DJ. 1992. Parasites and Diseases of Wild Mammals in Florida. Gainesville: University of Florida Press, pp 174–203.

Lindsay DS, Blagburn BL, Stuart BP, Gosser HS. 1987. *Strongyloides tumefaciens* infection in a cat. Compan Anim Pract 1:12–13.

Malone JB, Butterfield AB, Williams JC, Stuart BP, Travasos H. 1977. *Strongyloides tumefaciens* in cats. J Am Vet Med Assoc 171:278–280.

Price EW, Dikmans G. 1929. Multiple adenomata of the large intestine of a cat caused by a species of *Strongyloides.* J Parasitol 16:104.

Price EW, Dikmans G. 1941. Adenomatous tumors in the large intestine of a cat caused by *Strongyloides tumefaciens,* n. sp. Proc Helminthol Soc Wash 8:41–44.

STRONGYLIDA

Cats are parasitized by all four superfamilies of nematodes that make up the order Strongylida. This order of nematodes forms a fairly cohesive group of worms whose males are characterized by the possession of a copulatory bursa. Also, all four groups typically have a muscular esophagus. The females of these groups tend to lay eggs that contain four to eight cells when they are passed in the feces, although some produce eggs that contain larvae. The longitudinal muscles that appear under the hypodermis of the worms tend to be few in number in each quadrant. The vulva may be located anywhere from midbody to just anterior to the anus.

The anterior end of these nematodes typically contains characters that can be used to assign these nematodes to one of the four superfamilies. Members of the Ancylostomatoidea (the hookworms) have a large buccal cavity that typically is armed with anteriorly placed teeth or cutting plates. Members of the Strongyloidea (the strongyles) have a large buccal cavity that is often delineated anteriorly by a set or two of fine fibrous teeth that produce the leaf crown or corona radiata of the buccal capsule. There may be large teeth present in the base of the buccal capsule of these worms. Members of the Trichostrongyloidea (trichostrongyles) tend to have very small buccal capsules that may or may not contain a single tooth called a lancet. Adult hookworms are typically parasites of the small intestine, adult strongyles are typically parasites of the large intestine, and adult trichostrongyles are typically parasites of the stomach or small intestine. The fourth superfamily, the Metastrongyloidea (the metastrongyles), is typically found associated with parasitism of the lungs or vascular system, and like the trichostrongyles, the metastrongyles tend to have a small buccal cavity. The metastrongyles also tend to have a copulatory bursa that is quite reduced, sometimes to the point of being very difficult to recognize.

The typical life history of the hookworms, strongyles, and trichostrongyles is direct (i.e., there is no intermediate host involved in the life cycle). Eggs are passed in the feces that develop and hatch in the soil to produce larvae. The larvae then develop to infective third-stage larvae, which often maintain the second-stage larval cuticle as a protective sheath. Infection with hookworms is often through the skin; infections with strongyles and trichostrongyles is typically through the ingestion of the larvae. In the case of metastrongyles, the stage passed in the feces is typically the first-stage larvae that require a molluscan intermediate host (snail or slug) for the development of the larvae to the infective third-stage larvae. In the case of the metastrongyles of carnivores, the larvae in the mollusk typically can infect a small vertebrate paratenic host where the larvae persist in the tissues until they are ingested by the carnivore. Another rare form of transmission of metastrongyles is the infection of the next host by first-stage larvae.

ANCYLOSTOMATOIDEA

The cat is host to several species of worms that are members of the Ancylostomatoidea. The disease most typically associated with hookworm infection is anemia due to blood loss in the intestine that is caused by the adult worms. These nematodes are found as adults in the small intestine and are characterized by the possession of a copulatory bursa, a large dorsally flexed buccal cavity that is armed on its anterior edge with either teeth or cutting plates, and by their length—they tend to be 1–3 cm long. Although cats are probably often infected by the penetration of the skin by the infective third-stage larvae of this worm, the larvae are also capable of utilizing small vertebrates as paratenic hosts. It is not known to what extent the hookworms of the cat utilize transmammary infection, which is a very common mode of transmission for the canine hookworm *Ancylostoma caninum.*

The two genera of worms present in the cat are *Ancylostoma* and *Uncinaria.* The genus *Ancylostoma* is characterized by the possession of large teeth on the front of the buccal capsule, while the genus *Uncinaria* is characterized by the possession of cutting plates on the front of the buccal capsule. The most common hookworm of the cat is probably *Ancylostoma tubaeforme.* In coastal areas of Africa and the Americas, another hookworm of the cat, *Ancylostoma braziliense,* is found that is a parasite that cats share with dogs. A similar worm, *Ancylostoma ceylanicum,* is found in cats, dogs, and humans in Asia. Another worm, *Ancylostoma pleuridentatum* (Alessandrini, 1905) Schwartz, 1927, is very similar to *Ancylostoma braziliense* but has only been reported from members of the Felidae other than the domestic cat. This species differs from *Ancylostoma braziliense* in that there are three small tooth-like projections on each side of the buccal capsule opposite to the large teeth present on front of the buccal capsule. *Uncinaria stenocephala* has only rarely been reported from the cat.

Ancylostoma tubaeforme (Zeder, 1800)

Etymology

Ancylo = curved and *stoma* = mouth; *tubae* = straight trumpet and *forme* = shape. The original spelling of the genus was *Agchylostoma* due to improper transliteration of the Greek root, and this was later corrected to *Ancylostoma.*

Synonyms

Strongylus tubaeforme, Ancylostoma caninum var. *longespiculum.*

History

This worm was originally described as a separate species parasitizing the cat by Zeder in 1800. However, it was later considered a variety of the dog hookworm, *Ancylostoma caninum.* It was finally given a firm position as a separate species within the genus by Burrows (1962), who compared the adults of *Ancylostoma tubaeforme* with those of *Ancylostoma caninum.*

Geographic Distribution

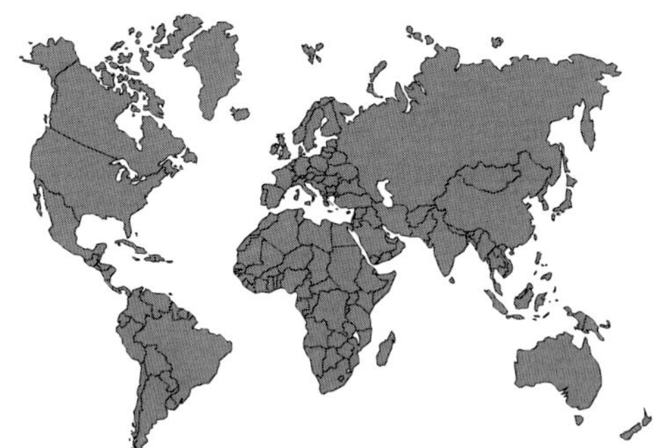

Fig. 4.12.

This worm is found throughout the world, wherever there are domestic cats (Rep, 1966).

Location in Host

The adult worms are found within the small intestine of the feline host. Most adult worms are found within the portion of the jejunum closest to the duodenum.

Parasite Identification

The adults of *Ancylostoma tubaeforme* are 7 to 12 mm long. If it is necessary to distinguish the adult specimens of hookworms found in the cat, the separations can be made on the basis of the shape of the buccal capsule. First, members of the genus *Ancylostoma* can be separated from those of *Uncinaria* by determining whether or not there are ventral teeth in the buccal capsule. Specimens of *Ancylostoma* have large teeth within the buccal capsule, while specimens of *Uncinaria* are recognized by the presence of cutting plates. Adults of *Ancylostoma tubaeforme* can be differentiated from the adults of *Ancylostoma braziliense* and *Ancylostoma ceylanicum* by the presence of three teeth on either side of the ventral midline (*Ancylostoma brazileinse* and *Ancylostoma ceylanicum* each possess two such teeth).

The eggs of the different *Ancylostoma* species found in the cat are apparently indistinguishable from each other (Fig. 4.13). The eggs of *Ancylostoma tubaeforme* have been measured to be 55–76 by 34–45 μm with means of 61 by 40 μm. The eggs of *Uncinaria* are larger than those of *Ancylostoma,* being 70 to 90 μm long by 40 to 50 μm wide. The two types of eggs are easy to distinguish in mixed infections (Ehrenford, 1953).

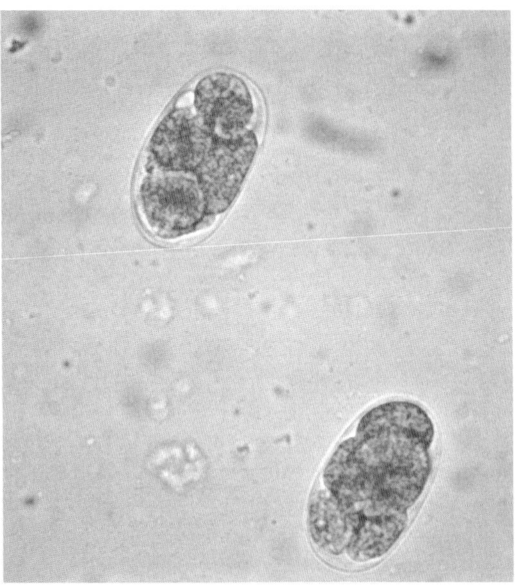

Fig. 4.13. *Ancylostoma tubaeforme.* Eggs of this hookworm as they are passed in the feces of the feline host.

Life Cycle

The life cycle of *Ancylostoma tubaeforme* has been studied in some detail (Okoshi and Murata, 1967a–d). The optimal temperature for larval development is 68°F (20°C), which is lower than the optimal temperature for developing larvae of *Ancylostoma caninum.* The infective third-stage larvae of *Ancylostoma tubaeforme* can infect cats both orally or through skin penetration.

After oral inoculation, the larvae enter the wall of the stomach and proximal small intestine where they remain for 10 to 12 days while developing to the adult stage. The adults then reenter the lumen. The prepatent period of *Ancylostoma tubaeforme* following oral administration is 18 to 28 days, which is longer that the prepatent period of the other cat hookworms. The worms have reached their maximum length about 1 month after the cat was initially infected.

After larvae penetrate the skin, they migrate through the lungs, up the trachea, and down the esophagus. The larvae then spend very little time within the wall of the gastrointestinal tract. Development of fourth-stage larvae is more rapid in larvae that have penetrated the skin, but there is no apparent growth of the larvae before they reach the intestinal tract. The prepatent period is between 19 to 25 days following skin penetration. Penetration of the skin is likely due to the secretion of proteolytic enzymes, although an early investigation failed to reveal any when the larvae of *Ancylostoma tubaeforme* were examined (Mathews, 1975).

Rodents can serve as paratenic hosts. After both oral and percutaneous infection, larvae are found concentrated in the cranial aspect of their murine host, where they have remained alive for up to 10 months (Norris, 1971). Larvae from mice have been shown to infect other mice where they are capable of again entering the tissues and persisting. There does not appear to have been any attempts to infect cats with larvae from mice.

It is assumed that there is neither transplacental nor transmammary transmission of hookworms from the queen to her kittens. This assumption is consistent with the lack of hookworm disease seen in young kittens and the small number of larvae that have been recovered from the viscera and musculature of kittens after the queen has been infected with larvae either by the oral or percutaneous route (Okoshi and Murata, 1967d). However, this question has never been carefully addressed experimentally.

The life expectancy of the adult worms has been observed to be 18 months to 2 years in experimentally infected cats (Okoshi and Murata, 1967c). Cats tend to harbor relatively few adult worms. The examination of cats in New Jersey revealed between 1 to 123 worms per cat (with a mean of 20) in 235 cats that had adult worms. There has been no examination as to the number of eggs produced by a female each day or the effects of the age of cats on the ability of worms to mature to the adult stage within the intestine.

Clinical Presentation and Pathogenesis

The main clinical signs associated with an infection of *Ancylostoma tubaeforme* are weight loss and a regenerative anemia (Onwuliri et al., 1981). When cats were given 1,000 to 2,000 infective-stage larvae, they lost weight when compared with cats receiving 0, 100, or 500 larvae. The cats that received 1,000 or 2,000 larvae died, and in these cats, hemoglobin levels fell to 4 g/dl, and packed cell volumes fell to 20 percent after the cats were infected for a month. In the cats receiving fewer larvae, the hemoglobin levels and packed cell volumes also fell, but then the levels seemed to stabilize after 6 weeks.

The hookworms cause significant blood loss from the intestinal mucosa (Fig. 4.14). Cats experimentally infected with *Ancylostoma tubaeforme* can die from the infection. Rohde (1959) gave cats infective larvae, and within 12 to 47 days after the cats were infected, 16 of them died. Examination of the intestines after death revealed that these cats harbored between 7 to 290 adult worms (mean of about 100 worms per cat). Nine Siamese cats given 2,000 larvae and six of nine Siamese cats given 1,000 infective-stage larvae died within 46 days of the initiation of the infection. These cats were found to harbor between 183 to 213 adult worms within their small intestines.

Treatment

There are several products marketed for the treatment of *Ancylostoma tubaeforme* in cats. Oral treatments with dichlorvos (11.1 mg/kg body weight), febantel, and a febantel-praziquantel

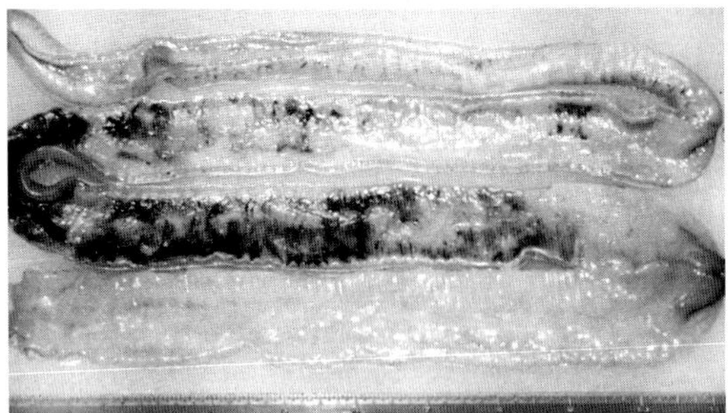

Fig. 4.14. *Ancylostoma tubaeforme.* Intestine of a cat that had been infected with approximately 100 adult hookworms. Note the amount of free blood within the intestinal lumen.

mixture (10 mg febantel/kg in cats and 15 mg febantel/kg in kittens), and n-Butyl chloride (400 mg/kg) are marketed for cats as well as disophenol sodium (10 mg/kg body weight, SQ) (Bowman, 1992). Ivermectin is now available as a chewable for cats, with an efficacy of 90.7 percent for treatment of *Ancylostoma caninum* in cats (Nolan et al., 1992). Selamectin (Revolution™) is labeled for the treatment of *Ancylostoma tubaeforme* in cats as a single topical dose.

Epizootiology

It is highly likely that cats become infected both by the ingestion of larvae (larvae penetrating the skin) or the ingestion of infected rodent paratenic hosts. Thus, there is every reason to believe that cats become infected while eating grass, by ingesting larvae while grooming, or by larvae penetrating the skin of cats when they walk on infected soils. Also, cats that hunt would have a greater likelihood of becoming infected.

Hazards to Other Animals

Mice and other rodents can become infected with the larval stages of this hookworm. It would appear that *Ancylostoma tubaeforme* does not develop to the adult stage in any hosts except felines.

Hazards to Humans

Adult *Ancylostoma tubaeforme* have not been recovered from humans. Also, it would appear that *Ancylostoma tubaeforme* is not a major cause of cutaneous larva migrans since it appears that this occurs mainly in geographical areas where *Ancylostoma braziliense* is prevalent.

Control/Prevention

If cats have access to the outside, prevention will be difficult. The marketing of a new monthly product with efficacy against this hookworm will provide control of this parasite in cats placed on this program.

REFERENCES

Bowman DD. 1992. Anthelmintics for dogs and cats effective against nematodes and helminths. Comp Cont Ed Pract Vet 14:597–599.

Burrows RB. 1962. Comparative morphology of *Ancylostoma tubaeforme* (Zeder, 1800) and *Ancylostoma caninum* (Ercolani, 1859). J Parasitol 48:715–718.

Ehrenford FA. 1953. Differentiation of the ova of *Ancylostoma caninum* and *Uncinaria stenocephala* in dogs. Am J Vet Res 14:578–580.

Mathews BE. 1975. Mechanism of skin penetration by *Ancylostoma tubaeforme* larvae. Parasitology 70:25–38.

Nolan TJ, Niamatali S, Bhopale V, Longhofer SL, Schad GA. 1992. Efficacy of a chewable formulation of ivermectin against a mixed infection of *Ancylostoma braziliense* and *Ancylostoma tubaeforme* in cats. Am J Vet Res 53: 1411–1413.

Norris DE. 1971. The migratory behavior of the infective-stage larvae of *Ancylostoma braziliense* and *Ancylostoma tubaeforme* in rodent paratenic hosts. J Parasitol 57:998–1009.

Okoshi S, Murata Y. 1967a. Experimental studies on ancylostomiasis in cats. II. Morphology of the eggs and larvae of *Ancylostoma tubaeforme* Zeder, 1800 and *Ancylostoma caninum* Ercolani, 1859. Jap J Vet Sci 29:133–140.

Okoshi S, Murata Y. 1967b. Experimental studies on ancylostomiasis in cats. III. Egg culture of *Ancylostoma tubaeforme* Zeder, 1800 and *Ancylostoma caninum* Ercolani, 1859. Jap J Vet Sci 29:174–177.

Okoshi S, Murata Y. 1967c. Experimental studies on ancylostomiasis in cats. IV. Experimental infection of *Ancylostoma tubaeforme* and *Ancylostoma caninum* in cat. Jap J Vet Sci 29:251–258.

Okoshi S, Murata Y. 1967d. Experimental studies on ancylostomiasis in cats. V. Visceral migration of larvae of *Ancylostoma tubaeforme* and *A. caninum* in cats. Jap J Vet Sci 29:315–327.

Onwuliri COE, Nwosu ABC, Anya AO. 1981. Experimental *Ancylostoma tubaeforme* infection of cats: changes in blood values and worm burden in relation to single infections of varying size. Ztsch Parasitenk 64:149–155.

Rep BH. 1966. On the polyxenia of Ancylostomidae and the validity of the characters used for their differentiation. II. Trop Geogr Med 12:271–326.

Rhode K. 1959. Vergleichende Untersuchungen über die Hakenwürmer des Hundes und der Katze un Betrachtungen über ihre Phylogenie. Ztsch Tropenmed Parasitol 10:402–426.

Zeder JGH. 1800. Erster Nachtrag sur Narugeschichte der Eingeweidewürmer, mit Zusätzen un Anmerkungen herausgegeben. Leipzig.

Ancylostoma braziliense Gomes de Faria, 1910

Etymology

Ancylo = curved + *stoma* = mouth; *braziliense* for the geographical location where the worms were first found.

Synonyms

Agchylostoma braziliense.

History

This worm was described in 1910 by Dr. Gomes de Faria from specimens recovered from the intestines of cats and dogs. It was later decided that this species was synonymous with *Ancylostoma ceylanicum,* which had been found in cats, dogs, and people in Asia (Lane, 1922; Leiper, 1913). Biocca (1951) redescribed both species and presented convincing evidence that the species were different. Similarly, Beaver (1956) discussed the fact that there had been no confirmed human infections with *Ancylostoma braziliense* in the United States where it was the only one of these two species present. More recently Rep et al. (1968) and Rep (1972) have further proven that these are separate species by performing single-sex crossover experiments in dogs. However, there was a period of about 50 years when the majority of researchers thought that these were identical forms; thus, it is difficult to examine earlier reports relative to the geographical distribution of these two parasites.

Geographic Distribution

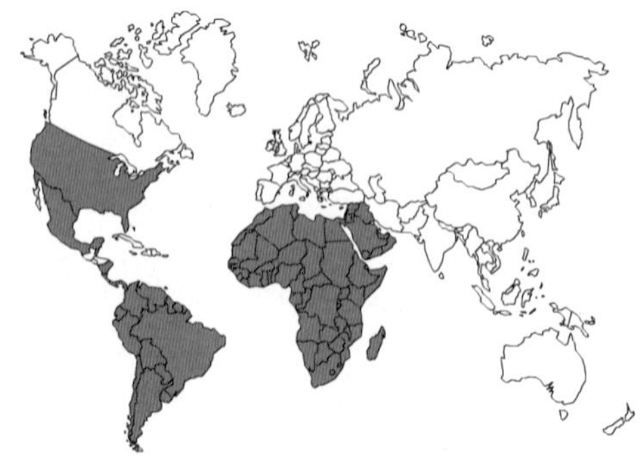

Fig. 4.15.

It would appear that *Ancylostoma braziliense* represents an American or African form of the *Ancylostoma ceylanicum* hookworm of Asia. Biocca (1951) only identified specimens of *Ancylostoma braziliense* from Africa and South America. This worm has also been reported from Central and North America. Yoshida et al. (1974) reported that it appears in Japan, and there have been additional reports of mixed infections in cats with *Ancylostoma braziliense* and *Ancylostoma ceylanicum* in Indonesia (Soeripto et al., 1978) and Malaysia (Amin-Babjee, 1978; Yoshida et al., 1973). *Ancylostoma braziliense* appears to prefer coastal areas, at least in the Americas; hence the prevalence of this parasite tends to drop as one moves inland. It is possible that *Ancylostoma braziliense* has higher requirements for sandy conditions or can withstand more readily the higher levels of salt found in coastal soils.

Location in Host

The adults are found within the anterior small intestine of the feline host. It appears that larvae are capable of persisting in the tissues of the feline host, but this has not been examined in any detail.

Parasite Identification

The adults of *Ancylostoma braziliense* are 4 to 10.5 mm long. Members of the genus *Ancylostoma* can be distinguished from those of *Uncinaria* by determining whether or not there are ventral teeth in the buccal capsule. Specimens of *Ancylostoma* have large teeth within the buccal capsule, while specimens of *Uncinaria* are recognized by the presence of cutting plates. The adults of *Ancylostoma braziliense* and *Ancylostoma ceylanicum* possess only two teeth on the ventral aspect of the buccal cavity, with the lateral tooth being large and the median tooth quite small. The adults of *Ancylostoma tubaeforme* have three teeth on each side of the buccal capsule. *Ancylostoma braziliense* can be differentiated from *Ancylostoma ceylanicum* by careful examination of the teeth within the buccal cavity. The medial teeth are smaller in *Ancylostoma braziliense* than they are in *Ancylostoma ceylanicum.* Another means of separating these two species is by careful examination of the copulatory bursa of the male. The lateral lobes of the bursa are relatively shorter in *Ancylostoma ceylanicum* than they are in *Ancylostoma braziliense,* and the branching of the externo-dorsal rays occurs more posteriad in *Ancylostoma ceylanicum* than it does in *Ancylostoma braziliense.* Finally, Yoshida (1971a) showed that if the adults are killed in hot water (149°F or 65°C) prior to fixation, about 90 percent of the females of *Ancylostoma braziliense* are noted to have a distinct 20 degree bend in the body at the level of the vulva (about two-thirds back on the body from the anterior end). This bend does not occur with *Ancylostoma ceylanicum* adults.

The eggs of the different *Ancylostoma* species found in the cat are apparently indistinguishable from each other. The eggs of *Ancylostoma braziliense* are considered by most researchers (e.g., Sarles, 1929) to be slightly smaller (55 μm × 34 μm) than those of *Ancylostoma caninum* (62 μm × 38 μm). The eggs of *Uncinaria* are considered larger than those of *Ancylostoma,* being 70 to 90 μm long by 40 to 50 μm wide. The two eggs are easy to distinguish in mixed infections (Ehrenford, 1953).

Yoshida (1971b) showed that the infective-stage larvae of *Ancylostoma braziliense* average 662 μm in length, which made them recognizably shorter than the larvae of *Ancylostoma ceylanicum,* which averaged 712 μm in length. The larvae of *Ancylostoma braziliense* are thus slightly longer than the larvae of *Ancylostoma caninum,* which average 630 μm in length (Lucker, 1942) and slightly longer than the larvae of *Ancylostoma tubaeforme* that have been reported to be 630 μm long (Okoshi and Murata, 1967). The infective-stage larvae of the *Ancylostoma* species are all longer than the larvae of *Uncinaria stenocephala,* which measure only 500 to 580 μm in length. Thus, ranking the infective-stage larvae of the four major feline hookworms, there is *Ancylostoma ceylanicum* (712 μm), *Ancylostoma braziliense* (660 μm), *Ancylostoma tubaeforme* (630 μm), and *Uncinaria stenocephala* (<600 μm).

Life Cycle

Cats can be infected by the ingestion of larvae or by the larvae penetrating the skin. When cats are infected orally with third-stage larvae, these infective larvae enter the intestinal mucosa. Within the mucosa, these larvae develop to the fourth stage. The larvae then appear in the intestinal lumen after the second day of infection. The prepatent period of the infection in cats following oral infection is 14 to 16 days. If cats are infected through the skin, the larvae migrate via the bloodstream to the lungs, migrate up the trachea, and are then swallowed. When the larvae reach the small intestine, most are still young third-stage larvae. The prepatent period following percutaneous infection can be 13 to 27 days (Dove, 1932).

Cats can also be infected by the ingestion of paratenic hosts. In mice after oral or percutaneous infection, the larvae migrate via the bloodstream to the lungs and then proceed to the area of the head of the mouse, where they persist for up to 18 months. In mice, most larvae are found within salivary glands or within the nasopharyngeal epithelium (Norris, 1973). Cats have been experimentally infected by feeding them larvae recovered from infected mice (Norris, 1971).

On the basis of a single trial, it would appear that transplacental and transmammary transmissions of *Ancylostoma braziliense* do not occur in dogs (Miller, 1971). This has not been examined in the cat.

The adults of *Ancylostoma braziliense* have been reported to live about 4 to 8 months (Sarles, 1929). A single female worm produces between 200 to 6,000 eggs per day (Sarles, 1929). As the infection matures, the number of eggs produced by a single female will decline. The infection of younger cats can be more easily obtained than the infection of older cats (Sarles, 1929).

Clinical Presentation and Pathogenesis

When *Ancylostoma braziliense* was originally described, it was noted that this hookworm was not as pathogenic as *Ancylostoma caninum* (Gomes de Faria, 1910). Very little hemorrhage occurs at the site of larval development or adult attachment. Using ^{51}chromium-labeled erythrocytes, it has been shown that the blood loss due to infections of adult worms in kittens is about 1 to 2 μl of blood/worm/day (Miller, 1966). Blood loss was first detected in cats 10 days after infection, and the experimentally infected kittens maintained hemoglobin levels, hematocrit values, and weight gains that were comparable to uninfected age-matched control kittens.

Treatment

Products approved for the treatment of *Ancylostoma braziliense* by oral administration include

(Bowman, 1992): toluene (in a dichlorophen-toluene mixture with a dose of 264.5 mg toluene per kilogram body weight), dichlorvos (11.1 mg/kg), febantel (as a febantel-proaziquantel mixture; 10 mg/kg BW febantel for adult cats and 15 mg/kg BW febantel for kittens), and n-Butyl chloride (400 mg/kg). Ivermectin as a chewable product (administered at 24 μg/kg) that is to be administered monthly is reported to reduce infections by 98.1 percent as compared with infections in untreated controls (Nolan et al., 1992). Disophenol sodium is approved at 10 mg/kg in a formulation that is to be administered subcutaneously.

Epizootiology

Ancylostoma braziliense is a parasite that is most commonly found in coastal areas with sandy soils. The development of the infective-stage larva has been shown to undergo optimal development at 27°C (Rep, 1965). There has been little examination of the effects of salinity on the development of the infective larvae of this hookworm, but one would suspect that the larvae can develop in rather high salt concentrations. It is also likely that these worms do not develop well in areas where there are freezing temperatures that occur for extended periods.

Hazards to Other Animals

Ancylostoma braziliense is a parasite that is capable of infecting dogs as well as cats. It is also highly likely that if the conditions are appropriate for the development of the larvae, they could infect and persist in the tissues as larvae in small mammals that share ground with the infected cat. There has been almost no attention given to the actual disease caused in rodent hosts.

Hazards to Humans

Ancylostoma braziliense is probably the major cause of human cases of cutaneous larva migrans. Dove (1932) clearly showed that this was the major cause of hookworm-induced cutaneous larva migrans in the United States. Cases of cutaneous larva migrans continue to be not uncommon, especially in travelers who have visited the Caribbean (Davies et al., 1993). Occasionally, cases of creeping eruption are reported from unusual temperate locations (Klose et al., 1996). In some instances, the large numbers of larvae that enter an individual will undergo the initial portion of a somatic migration and cause severe pneumonitis that might require hospitalization (Beaver et al., 1984).

Control/Prevention

Cats are infected by the ingestion of larvae when eating grass or grooming, by larvae penetrating the skin, or by the ingestion of larvae in paratenic hosts. Thus, whenever cats are in an endemic area and have access to the outside, they are probably at risk of contracting this infection. The recent availability of a monthly heartworm preventative that is also capable of treating adult hookworm infections will make it possible to protect cats from infections with this parasite.

REFERENCES

Amin-Babjee. 1978. Parasites of the domestic cat in Selangor, Malaysia. Kajian Vet 10:107–114.

Beaver PC. 1956. The record of *Ancylostoma braziliense* as an intestinal parasite of man in North America. Am J Trop Med Hyg 5:737–789.

Beaver PC, Jung RC, Cupp EW. 1984. Clinical Parasitology. 9th edition. Philadelphia, Pa: Lea and Febiger. 825 pp.

Biocca E. 1951. On *Ancylostoma braziliense* (de Faria, 1910) and its morphological differentiation from *A. ceylanicum* (Looss, 1911). J Helminthol 25:1–10.

Bowman DD. 1992. Hookworm parasites of dogs and cats. Comp Cont Educ Pract Vet 14:585–595.

Davies HD, Sakuls P, Keystone JS. 1993. Creeping eruption. A review of clinical presentation and management of 60 cases presenting to the tropical disease unit. Arch Dermatol 129:588–591.

Dove WE. 1932. Further studies of *Ancylostoma braziliense* and the etiology of creeping eruption. Am J Hyg 15:664–711.

Ehrenford FA. 1953. Differentiation of the ova of *Ancylostoma caninum* and *Uncinaria stenocephala* in dogs. Am J Vet Res 14:578–580.

Gomes de Faria J. 1910. Contribuição para a sistematic helmitolojioca braziliera. 3. *Ancylostoma braziliense* n. sp. parazito dos gatos e cãis. Mem Ist Oswaldo Cruz 2:286–293.

Klose C, Mravak S, Geb M, Bienzle U, Meyer CG. 1996. Autochthonous cutaneous larva migrans in Germany. Trop Med Int Health 1:503–504.

Lane C. 1922. *Ancylostoma braziliense*. Ann Trop Med Parasitol 16:347–352.

Leiper RT. 1913. The apparent identity of *Ancylostoma ceylanicum* (Looss, 1911) and *Ancylostoma braziliense* (Faria, 1910). J Trop Med Hyg 16:334–335.

Lucker JT. 1942. The dog *Strongyloides* with special reference to occurrence and diagnosis of infections with the parasite. Vet Med 37:128–137.

Miller TA. 1966. Blood loss during hookworm infection, determined by erythrocyte labeling with radioactive ^{51}chromium. II. Pathogenesis of *Ancylostoma braziliense* infection in dogs and cats. J Parasitol 52:856–865.

Miller TA. 1971. Vaccination against the canine hookworm diseases. Adv Parasitol 9:153–183.

Nolan TJ, Niamatali S, Bhopale V, Longhofer SL, Schad GA. 1992. Efficacy of a chewable formulation of ivermectin against a mixed infection of *Ancylostoma braziliense* and *Ancylostoma tubaeforme* in cats. Am J Vet Res 53:1411–1413.

Norris DE. 1971. The migratory behavior of the infective-stage larvae of *Ancylostoma braziliense* and *Ancylostoma tubaeforme* in rodent paratenic hosts. J Parasitol 57:998–1009.

Norris DE. 1973. Migratory behavior of infective stage larvae of *Ancylostoma* species in rodent paratenic hosts (abstr). Proc 9th Int Cong Trop Med Malaria 1:175–176.

Okoshi S, Murata Y. 1967. Experimental studies on ancylostomiasis in cats. II. Morphology of the eggs and larvae of *Ancylostoma tubaeforme* Zeder, 1800 and *Ancylostoma caninum* Ercolani, 1859. Jap J Vet Sci 29:133–140.

Rep BH. 1965. The pathogenicity of *Ancylostoma braziliense*. II. Cultivation of hookworm larvae. Trop Geogr Med 17:329–333.

Rep BH. 1972. Unfertilized hookworm eggs. Trop Geogr Med 24:363–369.

Rep BH, Vetter JC, Eijsker M. 1968. Cross-breeding experiemnts in *Ancylostoma braziliense* de Faria, 1910 and *A. ceylanicum* Looss, 1911. Trop Geogr Med 20:367–378.

Sarles MP. 1929. Quantitative studies on dog and cat hookworms, *Ancylostoma braziliense,* with special emphasis on age resistance. Am J Hyg 10:453–475.

Soeripto N, Loehoeri S, Soenarno, Baedhowi C, Soetarti, Daryono. 1978. Studies on the prevalence of hookworms in the dog's intestine and the pathology of the intestinal wall. Southeast Asian J Trop Med Publ Health 9:237–243.

Yoshida Y. 1971a. Comparative studies on *Ancylostoma braziliense* and *Ancylostoma ceylanicum.* I. The adult stage. J Parasitol 57:983–989.

Yoshida Y. 1971b. Comparative studies on *Ancylostoma braziliense* and *Ancylostoma ceylanicum.* II. The infective larval stage. J Parasitol 57:990–992.

Yoshida Y, Okamoto K, Matsuo K, Kwo EH, Retnassabapthy A. 1973. The occurrence of *Anscylostoma braziliense* (De Faria, 1910) and *Ancylostoma ceylanicum* (Looss, 1911) in Malaysia. Southeast Asian J Trop Med Publ Health 4:498–503.

Yoshida Y, Kondo K, Kurimoto H, Fukutome S, Shirasaka S. 1974. Comparative studies on *Ancylostoma braziliense* and *Ancylostoma ceylanicum.* III. Life history in the definitive host. J Parasitol 60:636–641.

Ancylostoma ceylanicum (Looss, 1911)

Etymology

Ancylo = curved and *stoma* = mouth; *ceylanicum* for the location from where the host containing these parasites was originally obtained.

Synonyms

Agchylostoma ceylanicum, Ancylostoma gilsoni.

History

Ancylostoma ceylanicum, like *Ancylostoma tubaeforme,* was originally described as a separate species parasitic in the cat and then considered for a period as a synonym of a canine parasite, in this case *Ancylostoma braziliense.* Looss (1911) described *Ancylostoma ceylanicum* based on specimens recovered from a civet cat in Ceylon. A couple of years later, three human prisoners in India were found to have hookworms that were identified as *Ancylostoma ceylanicum* by Lane (1913). However, others felt that *Ancylostoma ceylanicum* should be considered identical to *Ancylostoma braziliense* (Lane, 1922; Leiper, 1913). It was in 1951 that the redescription of Biocca established the criteria upon which this species can be separated from *Ancylostoma braziliense.* Rep et al. (1968) and Rep (1972) performed single-sex crossover experiments between males and females of *Ancylostoma ceylanicum* and *Ancylostoma braziliense* in dogs and found that fertilized eggs were produced only when both sets of worms represented the same species.

Geographic Distribution

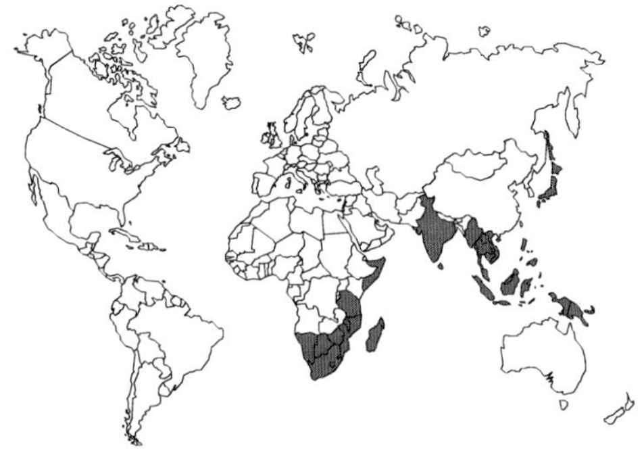

Fig. 4.16.

During the first half of the twentieth century, when *Ancylostoma ceylanicum* was considered a synonym of *Ancylostoma braziliense,* distinctions were not drawn between the two in different surveys. However, after 1951, most reports have dealt with the two species separately. *Ancylostoma ceylanicum* is a parasite capable of developing to the adult stage in humans and hamsters, while *Ancylostoma braziliense* remains restricted to feline and canine hosts. Thus, earlier surveys of humans where infections were identified as being caused by *Ancylostoma braziliense* probably represent infections with *Ancylostoma ceylanicum* (Beaver, 1956). The distribution of *Ancylostoma ceylanicum* seems to extend south from India (Chowdhury and Schad, 1972; Ray et al., 1972) down the eastern coast of Africa to Madagascar and South Africa (Baker et al., 1989; Yoshida, 1971a; Yoshida et al., 1973). The range also extends east from India into Indonesia, Singapore, Malaysia, and Thailand (Amin-Babjee, 1978; Rohde, 1962; Setasuban et al., 1976; Soeripto et al., 1978; Yoshida, 1971a; Yoshida et al., 1973). *Ancylostoma ceylanicum* has also been reported from some Pacific islands, including Taiwan and Okinawa (Yokogawa and Hsieh, 1961), Philippines (Arambulo et al., 1970), Sri Lanka (Dissanaike, 1961), British Solomon Islands (Haydon and Bearup, 1963), Fiji (Yoshida, 1971a), and Japan (Yoshida and Okamoto, 1972).

Location in Host

Adults of *Ancylostoma ceylanicum* are found within the small intestine of the cat, with the majority being found within the jejunum (Baker et al., 1989). After the oral inoculation of larvae, the worms remain within the intestinal tract; if a dog is infected by skin penetration, the worms migrate through the lungs before entering the intestinal tract. It is not known if there are any arrested stages in the tissues of cats as there would be with *Ancylostoma caninum* in the dog or to a smaller extent with *Ancylostoma tubaeforme* in the cat.

Parasite Identification

The adults of *Ancylostoma ceylanicum* are 6 to 10 mm long and appear to be slightly stouter than the adults of *Ancylostoma braziliense.* Members of the genus *Ancylostoma* can be distinguished from *Uncinaria* by determining whether or not there are ventral teeth in the buccal capsule. Specimens of *Ancylostoma* have large teeth within the buccal capsule, while specimens of *Uncinaria* are recognized by the presence of cutting plates. Like *Ancylostoma braziliense,* the adults of *Ancylostoma ceylanicum* possess only two teeth on the ventral aspect of the buccal cavity, with the lateral tooth being large and the median tooth quite small. The adults of *Ancylostoma tubaeforme* have three teeth on each side of the buccal capsule. *Ancylostoma ceylanicum* can be differentiated from *Ancylostoma braziliense* by careful examination of the teeth within the buccal cavity. The medial teeth are larger in *Ancylostoma ceylanicum* than they are in *Ancylostoma braziliense.* Another means of separating these two species is by careful examination of the copulatory bursa of the male. The lateral lobes of the bursa are relatively shorter in *Ancylostoma ceylanicum* than they are in *Ancylostoma braziliense,* and the branching of the externo-dorsal rays occurs more posteriad in *Ancylostoma ceylanicum* than it does in *Ancylostoma braziliense. Ancylostoma ceylanicum* has transverse striations in the cuticle that occur about 4 μm to 5 μm apart, while the similar striae in *Ancylostoma braziliense* are about 8 μm to 9 μm apart.

The eggs of the different *Ancylostoma* species found in the cat are apparently indistinguishable from each other. The eggs of *Ancylostoma ceylanicum* have been measured to be 60 μm by 2 μm (Arambulo, et al., 1970). The eggs of *Uncinaria* are larger than those of *Ancylostoma,* being 70 to 90 μm long by 40 to 50 μm wide. The two eggs representative of these different genera are easy to distinguish in mixed infections (Ehrenford, 1953).

Yoshida (1971b) showed that the infective-stage larvae of *Ancylostoma ceylanicum,* which measured 712 μm in length were significantly longer (712 μm) than the larvae of *Ancylostoma braziliense,* which measured 662 μm in length. Also, Yoshida demonstrated that the distance from the tip of the tail of the infective-stage larva to the end of the sheath was greater in *Ancylostoma ceylanicum* than it was in *Ancylostoma braziliense.* The larvae of *Ancylostoma ceylanicum* were similar in length to the larvae of *Ancy-*

lostoma duodenale, the human-infecting species of *Ancylostoma.* Kumar and Pritchard (1992) showed that lectins could be used to distinguish between the larvae of *Ancylostoma ceylanicum* and *Ancylostoma duodenale.*

Life Cycle

The life cycle has been examined by Yoshida (1971a, b) and Yoshida et al. (1974). Work was presented following both oral infection of puppies and after cutaneous infection. In the case of oral infection, the third-stage larvae molted in the intestinal wall 2 to 3 days after infection. The fourth-stage larvae entered the lumen, and immature adult hookworms were recovered beginning the sixth day after infection. In these puppies the prepatent period was 14 days. When puppies were infected by larvae penetrating the skin, the larvae underwent a lung migration and molted to the fourth stage in the trachea and stomach. Following skin penetration, many larvae are associated with the hair-follicle system, and most of the larvae were found in the skin 6 hours after larval application (Vetter and Leegwater-Linden, 1977). Fourth-stage larvae were recovered 3 days after infection, and adults were recovered beginning 7 days after the puppies were infected. The prepatent period was the same as in oral infection. The number of worms recovered following oral infection was 90 percent, but only 15 percent of the worms that infected via skin penetration were recovered. Yoshida (1968) reported the prepatent period in cats to be 14 to 17 days. Puppies continued to excrete eggs in their feces for 36 weeks after infection, which is when this study was terminated (Carroll and Grove, 1984).

An examination of dogs that were challenged with additional infective-stage larvae after their previous infection had been cleared by anthelmintic medication (pyrantel pamoate and bunamidine hydrochloride) indicated that there is some resistance to secondary infection (Carroll and Grove, 1985). When the dogs were reinfected a month after the clearing of the primary infection, the adult worm burdens were reduced 77 percent compared with the numbers in control dogs infected at the same time. Thus, for at least a month after the clearance of the primary infection, there appears to be some resistance to additional infection. In a second set of experiments, dogs were given a superimposed infection 4 weeks after the primary infection was induced (Carroll and Grove, 1986). Thus, dogs received 500 larvae and no challenge, 500 larvae and a challenge of 5,000 larvae, or only the 5,000 challenge larvae. In this experiment, the number of eggs produced by the dogs receiving 500 larvae remained the same throughout the trial, while the number of eggs produced by the group receiving only 5,000 larvae was much higher. The number of worms recovered from the superinfected group (the group receiving 500 and then an additional 5,000 larvae) was reduced 78 percent below that of the dogs receiving only the 5,000 challenge larvae. The dogs receiving 5,000 larvae developed anemia, while the other dogs did not.

Mice can serve as paratenic hosts, but it would seem that the percentage of larvae persisting in the mice is quite small. Fukutome (1975) found only 0.1 percent of the original inoculum present in the muscles of the infected mice. Ray and Bhopale (1972) succeeded in infecting hamsters with the adults of *Ancylostoma ceylanicum.*

Clinical Presentation and Pathogenesis

As with other hookworms, the major presentation of an infected animal is regenerative anemia. Areekul et al. (1975) examined the amount of blood loss in experimentally infected dogs using ^{51}chromium-labeled red cells. They found that blood was first detected in the feces 10 to 13 days after cutaneous and 8 to 16 days after oral infection. The mean blood loss was found to be around 0.035 ml per worm per day. When dogs were given 12,150 larvae, they developed bloody diarrhea and iron-deficient anemia (Carroll and Grove, 1984). When dogs were given 2,000 infective-stage larvae and monitored over a 36-week period, they developed normocytic anemia and eosinophilia. Dogs with severe microcytic anemia show greater autohemolysis of the blood cells when in the presence of glucose (Carroll et al., 1984). There are no appreciable clinical signs in either experimentally or naturally infected cats.

An examination of the feeding sites of *Ancylostoma ceylanicum* in dogs reveals that the heads are deeply buried in the mucosa of the wall of the small intestine (Carroll et al., 1985). Atrophy and villous ulceration surround the attachment sites. Large numbers of erythrocytes are found surrounding sites where worms have detached. Around the heads of the worms there is an infiltration of neutrophils, eosinophils, and plasma cells (Carroll et al., 1984). Erythrocytes were found extravascularly within the lamina propria, and the mucosa within the buccal capsules of the worms was in varying stages of lysis. The mucosa around the head of the worm was ulcerated, and surrounding enterocytes were small and displayed a loss of microvilli.

Treatment

There appear to be no reports of treatment of infected cats. Infections in dogs can be cleared using pyrantel pamoate and bunamidine hydrochloride (Carroll and Grove, 1985). Work in experimentally infected hamsters has indicated that the worms appear sensitive to mebendazole, but relatively refractory to thiabendazole (Misra et al., 1981); however thiabendazole can be efficacious in hamsters when used at 200 mg/kg body weight (Kamath et al., 1985). Oxfendazole (20 mg/kg body weight) has also proven highly efficacious in the hamster (Bhopale et al., 1984). Ivermectin at 100 μg/kg body weight was 100 percent efficacious in experimentally infected hamsters, and pyrantel pamoate was 100 percent efficacious when given at 100 mg/kg. Children infected with *Ancylostoma ceylanicum* have been successfully treated with mebendazole (Nontasut et al., 1987).

Epizootiology

There is very little information available on the development of the larvae of *Ancylostoma ceylanicum* from the egg to the infective-stage larva. Yoshida et al. (1974) found that larvae were more likely to develop to the adult stage after oral inoculation than after skin penetration.

Hazards to Other Animals

Dogs are routinely infected with this parasite. Thus, if dogs and cats are sharing the same pens or yards, there is a good chance that both hosts will be infected.

Hazards to Humans

Humans can serve as hosts to *Ancylostoma ceylanicum.* The larvae are capable of penetrating the skin and cause papular eruptions at the sites of larval penetration (Wijers and Smit, 1966). The prepatent period in humans is 18 to 26 days (Bearup, 1967; Yoshida, et al., 1972). Thus, in areas where this hookworm is found, it is of extra importance that cats be kept free from infection. It is also important that the staff of animal hospitals be made aware of the cross-transmission capabilities of this parasite.

Control/Prevention

Ancylostoma ceylanicum has the broadest host range of any of the hookworms infecting the cat. The worms can survive in dogs and humans, as well as in the feline host. Thus, it is important that the control of this parasite include routine examinations and treatments of cats if necessary.

REFERENCES

Amin-Babjee. 1978. Parasites of the domestic cat in Selangor, Malaysia. Kajian Vet 10:107–114.

Arambulo PV, Jueco NL, Sarmiento RV, Cada AB. 1970. The occurrence of *Ancylostoma ceylanicum* (Looss, 1911) in a native dog in the Philippines. Philipp J Vet Med 9:85–90.

Areekul S, Saenghirun C, Ukoskit K. 1975. Studies on the pathogenicity of *Ancylostoma ceylanicum:* 1. Blood loss in experimental dogs. Southeast Asian J Trop Med Publ Health 6:235–240.

Baker MK, Lange L, Verster A, Plaat S. 1989. A survey of helminths in domestic cats in the Pretoria area of Transvalal, Republic of South Africa. Part 1. The prevalence and comparison of burdens of helminths in adult and juvenile cats. J S Afr Vet Assoc 60:139–142.

Bearup AJ. 1967. *Ancylostoma braziliense* (Correspondence). Trop Geogr Med 19:161–162.

Beaver PC. 1956. The record of *Ancylostoma braziliense* as an intestinal parasite of man in North America. Am J Trop Med Hyg 5:737–789.

Behnke JM, Rose R, Garside P. 1993. Sensitivity to ivermectin and pyrantel of *Ancylostoma ceylanicum* and *Necator americanus.* Int J Parasitol 23:945–952.

Bhopale GM, Kumar A, Nayar PRG. 1984. Development of host resistance to *Ancylostoma ceylanicum* after the elimination of primary infection with oxfendazole. Hind Antibiot Bull 26:140–141.

Biocca E. 1951. On *Ancylostoma braziliense* (de Faria, 1910) and its morphological differentiation from *A. ceylanicum* (Looss, 1911). J Helminthol 25:1–10.

Carroll SM, Grove DI. 1984. Parasitological, hematologic, and immunologic responses in acute and chronic infections of dogs with *Ancylostoma ceylanicum:* a model of human hookworm infection. J Infect Dis 150:284–294.

Carroll SM, Grove DI. 1985. Resistance of dogs to reinfection with *Ancylostoma ceylanicum* following anthelmintic therapy. Trans Roy Soc Trop Med Hyg 79:519–523.

Carroll SM, Grove DI. 1986. Response of dogs to challenge with *Ancylostoma ceylanicum* during the tenure of a primary hookworm infection. Trans Roy Soc Trop Med Hyg 80:406–411.

Carroll SM, Robertson TA, Papadimitriou JM, Grove DI. 1984. Transmission electron microscopical studies of the site of attachment of *Ancylostoma ceylanicum* to the small bowel mucosa of the dog. J Helminthol 58:313–320.

Carroll SM, Robertson TA, Papadimitriou JM, Grove DI. 1985. Scanning electron microscopy of *Ancylostoma ceylanicum* and its site of attachment to the small intestinal mucosa of the dog. Ztsch Parasitenk 71:79–85.

Chowdhury AB, Schad GA. 1972. *Ancylostoma ceylanicum:* a parasite of man in Calcutta and environs. Am J Trop Med Hyg 21:300–301.

Dissanaike AS. 1961. On some helminths of dogs in Colombo and their bearing on human infections, with a description of a new trematode *Heterophysopsis yehi* sp. nov. (Heterophyidae) Ceylon J Med Sci 10:1–12.

Ehrenford FA. 1953. Differentiation of the ova of *Ancylostoma caninum* and *Uncinaria stenocephala* in dogs. Am J Vet Res 14:578–580.

Fukutome S. 1975. The migratory behaviour and development of *Ancylostoma braziliense* and *Ancylostoma ceylanicum* in the mouse. Jap J Parasitol 24:49–54.

Haydon GAM, Bearup AJ. 1963. Correspondence: *Ancylostoma braziliense* and *A. ceylanicum.* Trans Roy Soc Trop Med Hyg 57:76.

Kamath VR, Bhopale MK, Bhide MB. 1985. *Ancylostoma ceylanicum* (Looss, 1911) in golden hamsters (*Mesocricetus auratus*): immune response after application of anthelmintics. Helminthologia 22:203–210.

Kumar S, Pritchard DI. 1992. Distinction of human hookworm larvae based on lectin-binding characteristics. Parasite Immunol 14:233–237.

Lane C. 1913. *Ancylostoma ceylanicum,* a new human parasite. Ind Med Gaz 48:217–218.

Lane C. 1922. *Ancylostoma braziliense.* Ann Trop Med Parasitol 16:347–352.

Leiper RT. 1913. The apparent identity of *Agchylostoma ceylanicum* (Looss, 1911) and *Agchylostoma braziliense* (Faria, 1910). J Trop Med Hyg 16:334–335.

Looss A. 1911. The anatomy and life history of *Ancylostoma duodenale* Dub. II. The development in the free state. Rec Egypt Minist Educ 4: 163–613.

Misra A, Viusen PKS, Katiya JC. 1981. Comparative efficacy of standard antihookworm drugs against various test nematodes. J Helminthol 55:273–278.

Nontasut P, Singhasivanon V, Maipanich W, Yamput S, Visiassuk K. 1987. Comparative study of different doses of mebendazole in hookworm infection. Southeast Asian J Trop Med Publ Health 18:211–214.

Ray DK, Bhopale KK. 1972. Complete development of *Ancylostoma ceylanicum* (Looss, 1911) in golden hamsters, *Mesocricetus auratus.* Experientia 28:359–361.

Ray DK, Bhopale KK, Shrivastava VB. 1972. Incidence of *Ancylostoma ceylanicum* infection in dogs and its zoonotic potential. Ind Vet J 49:661–664.

Rep BH. 1972. Unfertilized hookworm eggs. Trop Geogr Med 24:363–369.

Rep BH, Vetter JC, Eijsker M. 1968. Cross-breeding experiments in *Ancylostoma braziliense* de Faria, 1910 and *A. ceylanicum* Looss, 1911. Trop Geogr Med 20:367–378.

Rohde K. 1962. Helminthen aus Katzen und Hunden in Malaya; Bemerkungen zu ihrer epdemiologischen Bedeutung für den Menschen. Ztsch Parasitenk 22:237–244.

Setasuban P, Vajrasthira S, Muennoo C. 1976. Prevalence and zoonotic potential of *Ancylostoma ceylanicum* in cats in Thailand. Southeast Asian J Trop Med Publ Health 7:534–539.

Soeripto N, Loehoeri S, Soenarno, Baedhowi C, Soetarti, Daryono. 1978. Studies on the prevalence of hookworms in the dog's intestine and the pathology of the intestinal wall. Southeast Asian J Trop Med Publ Health 9:237–243.

Vetter JCM, Leegwater-Linden ME. 1977. Skin penetration of infective hookworm larvae. III. Comparative studies on the path of migration of the hookworms *Ancylostoma braziliense, Ancylostoma ceylanicum,* and *Ancylostoma caninum.* Ztsch Parasitenk 53:155–158.

Wijers DJB, Smit AM. 1966. Early symptoms after infection of man with *Ancylostoma braziliense.* Trop Geogr Med 18:48–52.

Yokogawa M, Hsieh HC. 1961. A critical review of human infections of *Ancylostoma braziliense* in Taiwan, Ryukyu (Okinawa) and Japan. Jap J Parasitol 10:329–335.

Yoshida Y. 1968. Pathobiologic studies on *Ancylostoma ceylanicum* infection. 8th Int Cong Trop Med Malaria 170–171.

Yoshida Y. 1971a. Comparative studies on *Ancylostoma braziliense* and *Ancylostoma ceylanicum.* I. The adult stage. J Parasitol 57:983–989.

Yoshida Y. 1971b. Comparative studies on *Ancylostoma braziliense* and *Ancylostoma ceylanicum.* II. The infective larval stage. J Parasitol 57:990–992.

Yoshida Y, Okamoto K. 1972. On the hookworms in stray dogs in Kagoshima Prefecture, southern part of Japan, with special reference to *Ancylostoma ceylanicum.* Jap J Parasitol 21:328–332.

Yoshida Y, Okamota K, Chiu JK. 1972. Experimental infection of man with *Ancylostoma ceylanicum*. Chin J Microbiol 4:157–167.

Yoshida Y, Okamoto K, Matsuo K, Kwo EH, Retnasabapathy A. 1973. The occurrence of *Ancylostoma braziliense* (De Faria, 1910) and *Ancylostoma ceylanicum* (Looss, 1911) in Malaysia. Southeast Asian J Trop Med Publ Health 4:498–503.

Yoshida Y, Kondo K, Kurimoto H, Fukutome S, Shirasaka S. 1974. Comparative studies on *Ancylostoma braziliense* and *Ancylostoma ceylanicum*. III. Life history in the definitive host. J Parasitol 60:636–641.

Uncinaria stenocephala Railliet, 1884

Etymology

Uncin = hooked + *aria* referring to the body and *steno* = narrow + *cephala* = head.

Synonyms

Dochmoides stenocephala; Uncinaria polaris Looss, 1911*; Strongylus trigonocephala* Gurlt, 1831; *Dochmius trigonocephala* Ercolani, 1859; *Ankylostoma trigonocephala* Linstow, 1885.

History

Uncinaria stenocephala was recognized and described as a species of canine hookworm by Railliet in 1884.

Geographic Distribution

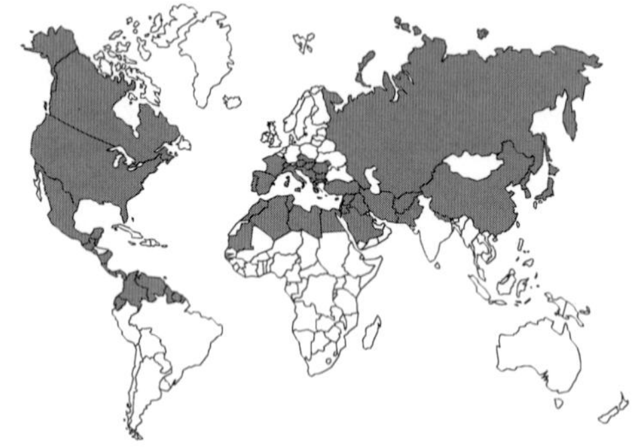

Fig. 4.17.

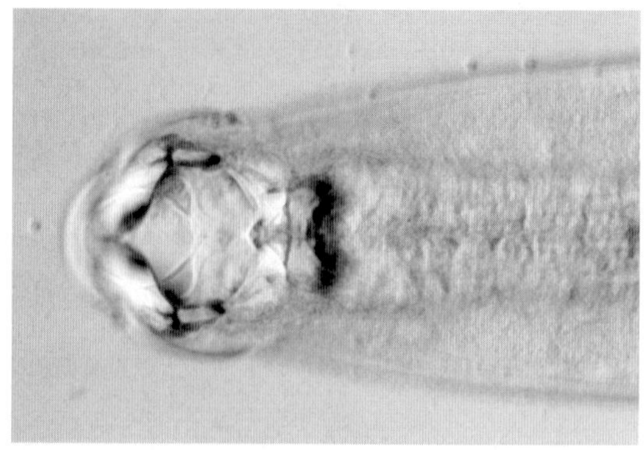

Fig. 4.18. *Uncinaria stenocephala.* Anterior end of adult worm showing the cutting plates within the buccal capsule.

Uncinaria stenocephala is considered to be a parasite that is commonly found in climates that are more temperate or cooler than those where *Ancylostoma* species are typically found. It is, therefore, confined mainly to the temperate and subarctic climates of the northern and southern hemispheres.

Reports of *Uncinaria stenocephala* in naturally infected cats are rare. Burrows (1968) reported finding *Uncinaria stenocephala* in only 1 of 2,735 cats examined in New Jersey (6 percent of dogs were infected).

Location in Host

The adults of this parasite are found in the small intestine of the feline host.

Parasite Identification

The adults of *Uncinaria stenocephala* are 3 mm to 12 mm in length. They can be distinguished from the other hookworms found in the cat by the presence of cutting plates within the buccal capsule, as opposed to the teeth that are present in species of *Ancylostoma* (Fig. 4.18). The eggs of this worm can also be differentiated from those of *Ancylostoma* by their larger sites. The eggs of *Uncinaria stenocephala* are approximately 70 to 90 μm long by 40 to 50 μm wide and are especially easy to differentiate from the eggs of *Ancylostoma* when present in mixed infections (Ehrenford, 1953) (Fig. 4.19).

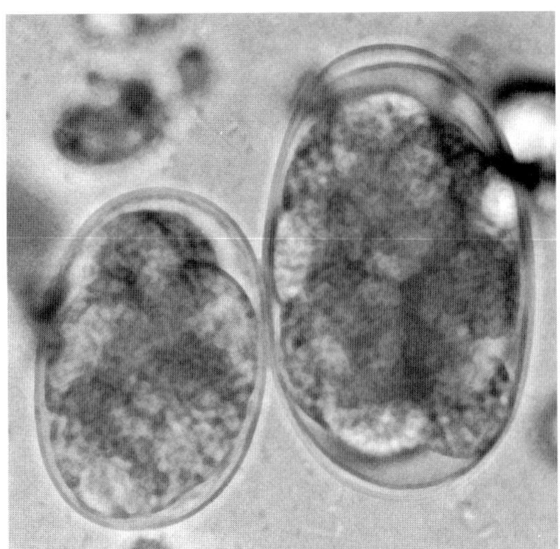

Fig. 4.19. *Uncinaria* and *Ancylostoma* eggs from the same fecal sample. The larger egg is that of *Uncinaria.*

Life Cycle

Cats are relatively refractory to infection with *Uncinaria stenocephala* (Rohde, 1959; Hurley et al., 1990). The experimental infection of six cats with larvae cultured from dog feces produced patent infections in only three of the cats. In these cats the number of eggs produced were very few, and they were present in the feces only for a very short period of time. In another study in Istanbul, cats were readily infected with larvae cultured from dog feces (Merdivenci, 1966a).

The course of infection with *Uncinaria stenocephala* has been described in experimentally infected dogs (Gibbs, 1958; Gibbs, 1961; Mihatsch, 1984). When larvae are administered to dogs orally, the larvae undergo a limited somatic migration where they enter the crypts of the gastric glands in the pyloric region of the stomach and the glands of the duodenal mucosa for the first 2 days after infection. The larvae then reenter the intestinal tract, and as the worms develop, they move in a caudal direction within the intestine. At maturity in the dog, the worms are found in the third quarter of the small intestine. The prepatent period can range from 13 to 21 days. Application of larvae to the skin results in lower infection rates. After larvae are applied to the skin, the larvae migrate to the lungs before reentering the gastrointestinal tract through the trachea and esophagus. The prepatent period following percutaneous infection is 15 to 17 days.

Transplacental and transmammary transmissions apparently do not occur with *Uncinaria stenocephala* (Mihatsch, 1984). The infection of two bitches, each with 20,000 larvae at the time of conception, failed to induce infection in the puppies produced by the pregnancies. The infection of four bitches with 20,000 larvae at the time of whelping also failed to produce infection in the nursing pups. The necropsies of these bitches 28 days after infection revealed adult *Uncinaria stenocephala* in the intestines, but no larvae were found in the organs of the body.

It has been reported that adults of *Uncinaria stenocephala* live in the dog for 4 months (Kalkofen, 1987). A source dog used for experimental infections at Cornell University was infected for approximately 1 year. Other investigators have reported that patent infections will persist for about 6 months (Dow et al., 1961). The number of eggs produced by a single female per day has been calculated to be 3,000 to 5,000 eggs per female per day (Rep and Bos, 1979) and 16,000 to 19,000 per female per day (Merdivenci, 1966b).

The larvae of *Uncinaria stenocephala* have been shown to persist within the musculature of orally or percutaneously infected mice (Feilke, 1985). Again, as with the dog, more larvae were recovered following oral infection than following percutaneous infection. It was also shown that very low numbers of larvae could be transmitted from the mothers to the mouse pups if the mothers were percutaneously infected on the day of parturition.

Clinical Presentation and Pathogenesis

Because of the rarity of infections in cats, the description of clinical signs and studies on the pathogenic effects of infection have all been described in dogs. In dogs, it would appear the *Uncinaria stenocephala* is probably the least pathogenic of the hookworm infections. Blood loss caused by *Uncinaria stenocephala* adults within the intestine has been calculated to be 0.3 μl per worm per day (Miller, 1971). This is only about 1 to 2 percent of the amount of blood lost due to the presence of a single *Ancylostoma caninum* in a dog. In beagle puppies, the oral inoculation of 1,000 larvae caused no signs of disease (Merdivenci, 1966b). The oral inoculation of infective larvae has, however, been reported to induce severe diarrhea and a 10 percent reduction in plasma protein levels (Miller, 1971). Infections of greyhounds or beagles with 87 to 1,850 adults caused protein-losing enteropathy and suboptimum growth (Walker and Jacobs, 1985). The oral inoculation of adult beagle bitches at the time of conception or whelping with 20,000 larvae caused only slight diarrhea that was on occasion accompanied with bloody mucus and a slight peripheral blood eosinophilia 2 weeks postinfection. Examination of the tissues of animals within a few days after infection have indicated that there are minimal lesions associated with the larvae that are found in the glands of the stomach and duodenum the first couple days after infection and that the appearance of the fourth-stage larvae in the ileum is marked by the appearance of petechial mucosal hemorrhages (Gibbs, 1958). There is marked inflammation around larvae that penetrate the skin, and the larvae within the lungs are found in focal areas of inflammation (Gibbs, 1958).

Treatment

Uncinaria stenocephala appears more refractory to treatment with certain compounds than the canine hookworm, *Ancylostoma caninum.* Treatment of dogs with ivermectin at a dose of 6 μg/kg was 27 percent to 51 percent and 57 percent to 90 percent effective against the adults of *Uncinaria stenocephala* and *Ancylostoma caninum,* respectively (Egerton et al., 1985). Similarly, milbemycin oxime at a dose of 0.5 mg/kg body weight was found to be 100 percent efficacious in the case of adult *Ancylostoma caninum,* but without effect on populations of adult *Uncinaria stenocephala* (Bowman et al., 1991).

Attempts have been made to prevent infections of dogs with *Uncinaria stenocephala* by vaccination with larvae (Dow et al., 1959, 1961). Dogs that had received infections with normal larvae were found to be refractive to challenge infection when they were challenged 200 days after having been given the primary infection. Dogs receiving larvae irradiated with 40 Krads of gamma irradiation developed patent infections after being inoculated with the irradiated larvae, but their infections produced much lower egg counts than dogs inoculated with normal larvae. When these dogs that had been vaccinated with irradiated larvae were challenged with normal larvae, there was a marked reduction in the number of adults that developed in these animals compared with unvaccinated controls.

Epizootiology

For *Uncinaria stenocephala,* a parasite of cooler climates, cooler temperatures proved the optimum environment for larval development. The ideal temperature for larval development is 68°F (20°C) (Gibbs and Gibbs, 1959). The maintenance of a fecal culture containing eggs of both *Ancylostoma caninum* and *Uncinaria stenocephala* at 59°F (15°C) will only produce the larvae of *Uncinaria stenocephala* after 8 days of incubation (Hill and Roberson, 1985). The eggs and larvae of *Uncinaria* can also survive temperatures of 32°F (0°C) for days to a week, while those of *Ancylostoma caninum* die within a few days (Balasingam, 1964).

On the grass exercise paddocks at two large greyhound kennels in England, most of the infective-stage larvae of *Uncinaria stenocephala* were found on the herbage of the paddock in late fall, with substantial numbers being found on the herbage throughout the winter, with a few being present in early spring (Jacobs, 1978). Also, it has been observed that dogs infected with *Uncinaria stenocephala* that have been kept in substandard housing conditions have developed cutaneous pedal lesions similar to those seen in cases of ground itch in people infected with the human hookworms, *Ancylostoma duodenale* and *Necator americanus* (Smith and Eliot, 1969)

Hazards to Other Animals

If a cat were infected with *Uncinaria stenocephala,* it could serve as a source of infection for other animals in the establishment. However, because of the rarity of this infection in cats, it is more likely that cats will be the recipients of an infection from some other infected animal.

Hazards to Humans

Adult *Uncinaria stenocephala* has not been found in humans. The larvae of this parasite have been shown to cause cutaneous larvae migrans on rare occasions. Using his own skin, Fülleborn (1927) showed that these larvae were capable of causing cutaneous larva migrans in humans.

Control/Prevention

Cats should be protected from sharing space with dogs infected with this parasite.

REFERENCES

Balasingam E. 1964. Comparative studies on the effects of temperature on free-living stages of *Placoconus lotoris, Dochmoides stenocephala,* and *Ancylostoma caninum.* Can J Zool 42:907–918.

Bowman DD, Lin DS, Johnson RC, Hepler DI. 1991. Effects of milbemycin oxime on adult *Ancylostoma caninum* and *Uncinaria stenocephala* in dogs with experimentally induced infections. Am J Vet Res 52:64–67.

Burrows RB. 1968. Internal parasites of dogs and cats from central New Jersey. Bull NJ Acad Sci 3:3–8.

Dow C, Jarrett WFH, Jennings FW, MacIntyre WIM, Mulligan W. 1959. The production of active immunity against the canine hookworm *Uncinaria stenocephala.* JAVMA 135:407–411.

Dow C, Jarrett WFH, Jennings FW, MacIntyre WIM, Mulligan W. 1961. Studies on immunity to *Uncinaria stenocephala* infection in the dog—double vaccination with irradiated larvae Am J Vet Res 22:352–354.

Egerton JR, Eary CH, Suhayada D. 1985. Dose-titration studies of ivermectin against experimental *Ancylostoma caninum* and *Uncinaria stenocephala* infections. Am J Vet Res 46:1057–1059.

Ehrenford FA. 1953. Differentiation of the ova of *Ancylostoma caninum* and *Uncinaria stenocephala* in dogs. Am J Vet Res 14:578–580.

Feilke M. 1985. Untersuchungen über die Mögligkeit pränataler und galaktogener Infektiononen mit *Uncinaria stenocephala* Railliet 1884 (Ancylostomidae) beim Hund (Beagle). Thesis, Institut für Parasitologie der Tierärtzlichen Hochschule Hannover. 65 pp.

Fülleborn F. 1927. Durch Hakenwurmlarven des Hundes (*Uncinaria stenocephala*) beim Menschen erzeugte "Creeping Eruption." Hamburgishce Universität. Abhandl Gebiet Auslandskunde. 26(D,2):121–133.

Gibbs HC. 1958. On the gross and microscopic lesions produced by the adults and larvae of *Dochmoides stenocephala* (Railliet, 1884) in the dog. Can J Comp Med Vet Sci 22:382–385.

Gibbs HC. 1961. Studies on the life cycle and developmental morphology of *Dochmoides stenocephala* (Railliet 1884) (Ancylostomidae: Nematodea) Can J Zool 39:325–348.

Gibbs HC, Gibbs KE. 1959. The effects of temperature on the development of the free-living stages of *Dochmoides stenocephala* (Railliet, 1884) (Ancylostomidae: Nematodea). Can J Zool 37:247–257.

Hill RL, Roberson EL. 1985. Temperature-induced separation of larvae of *Uncinaria stenocephala* from a mixed fecal culture containing *Ancylostoma caninum.* J Parasitol 71:390–391.

Hurley KJ, Bowman DD, Frongillo MK, French TW, Hornbuckle WE. 1990. Experimental infections with *Uncinaria stenocephala* in young dogs: treatment with nitroscanate (abstr). Proc Am Assoc Vet Parasitol no 42.

Jacobs DE. 1978. The epidemiology of hookworm infection of dogs in the UK. Vet Annu 18:220–224.

Kalkofen UP. 1987. Hookworms of dogs and cats. Vet Clin North Am [Small Anim Pract] 17:1341–1354.

Merdivenci A. 1966a. The experimental infection of cats with *Uncinaria stenocephala* [in Turkish]. Etlik Vet Bakt Enst Dergisi 3:58–66.

Merdivenci A. 1966b. The daily egg production of a female *Uncinaria stenocephala* [in Turkish]. Etlik Vet Bakt Enst Dergisi 3:72–74.

Mihatsch D. 1984. Zum verhalten de Larven von *Uncinaria stenocephala* Railliet 1884 (Ancylostomaidae) in der Maus. Thesis, Institut für Parasiotologie der Tierärtzlichen Hochschule Hannover, 1984. 46 pp.

Miller TA. 1971. Vaccination against the canine hookworm diseases. Adv Parasitol 9:153–183.

Rep BH, Bos R. 1979. Enige epidemiologische apecten van *Uncinaria stenocephala* infecties in Nederland. Tidsch Diergeneesk 104:747–758.

Rohde K. 1959. Vergleichende Untersuchungen über die Hakenwürmer des Hundes und der Katze un Betrachtungen über ihre Phylogenie. Ztsch Tropenmed Parasitol 10:402–426.

Smith BL, Eliot DC. 1969. Canine pedal dermatitis due to percutaneous *Uncinaria stenocephala* infection. NZ Vet J 17:235–239.

Walker MJ, Jacobs DE. 1985. Pathophysiology of *Uncinaria stenocephala* infection of dogs. Vet Annu 25:263–271.

STRONGYLOIDEA

The cat is host to only a single representative genus of the Strongyloidea. This genus is *Mammomonogamus,* which is an unusual representative of this group in that the adult worms tend to be parasites of the airways rather than of the large bowel as is typical of the strongyles found in horses and ruminants. These parasites have a large buccal capsule but lack the corona radiata or leaf crown that is so typical of most of the members of this superfamily. The genus *Mammomonogamus* appears to be most closely related to parasites of birds (e.g., *Syngamus, Boydinema,* and *Cyathostoma*) and to a form that is found in rodents, *Rodentogamus.*

Mammomonogamus Species

This genus is distinguished from the genera in birds by the fact that it is found in mammals and that there are longitudinal ribs on the inner walls of the buccal capsule of those found in mammals (Barus and Tenora, 1972; Lichtenfels, 1974). The genus *Mammomonogamus* is differentiated from *Rondentogamus* of palearctic rodents by the fact that the members of the rodent genus have a well-developed collar around the oral opening and operculate eggs, neither or which occur in species of *Mammomonogamus.* In most cases, human infections with *Mammomonogamus* have been ascribed to *Mammomonogamus nasicola* (e.g., Mornex et al., 1980) or *Mammomonogamus laryngeus* (e.g., Pipitgool et al., 1992; Timmons et al., 1983). Cases in cats have typically been ascribed to other species such as *Mammomonogamus ierei,* which seems to infect cats mainly in the Caribbean. A strange species parasitic in the inner ear was described from cats in China, but there have been no recent reports of this worm. As of now, the life cycle of members of this genus has not been described.

REFERENCES

Baruš V, Tenora F. 1972. Notes on the systematics and taxonomy of the nematodes belonging to the family Syngamidae Leiper, 1912. Acta Univ Agric Brno Fac Agron 20:275–286.

Lichtenfels JR. 1974. No. 7. Keys to the genera of the superfamily Strongyloidea. In CIH Keys to the Nematode Parasites of Vertebrates, ed RC Anderson, AG Chabaud, and S Wilmott, pp 1–41. Farnham Royal, Bucks, England: Commonwealth Agricultural Bureaux.

Mornex JF, Magdeleine J, De Thore J. 1980. Human syngamosis (*Mammomonogamus nasicola*) as a cause of chronic cough in Martinique. 37 recent observations. Novelle Press Medicale 9:3628.

Pipitgool V, Chaisiri K, Visetsupakarn P, Srigan V, Maleewong W. 1992. *Mammomonogamus* (*Syngamus*) *laryngeus* infection: a first case report in Thailand. Southeast Asian J Trop Med Publ Health 23:336–337.

Severo LC, Conci MA, Camargo JJP, Andre–Alves MR, Palombinin BC. 1988. Syngamosis: two new Brazilian cases and evidence of a possible pulmonary cycle. Trans Roy Soc Trop Med Hyg 82:467–468.

Timmons RF, Bowers RE, Price DL. 1983. Infection of the respiratory tract with *Mammomonogamus* (*Syngamus*) *laryngeus:* a new case in Largo, Florida, and a summary of previously reported cases. Am Rev Resp Dis 128:566–569.

Villon A, Foulon G, Ancelle R, Nguyen NQ, Martin-Bouyer G. 1983. Prevalence des parasitoses intestinales en Martinique. Bull Soc Pathol Exot 76:406–416.

Mammomonogamus auris (Faust and Tang, 1934) Ryzhikov, 1948

Etymology

Mammo (= mammal) and *monogamus* (for the finding of the worms in pairs of males and females); plus *auris* for ear.

Synonyms

Syngamus auris Faust and Tang, 1934.

History

These worms were recovered from the middle ear of 11 of 48 cats during 1932 and the spring and fall of 1933. There have been no reports of this worm being recovered since the report of Faust and Tang in 1934.

Geographic Distribution

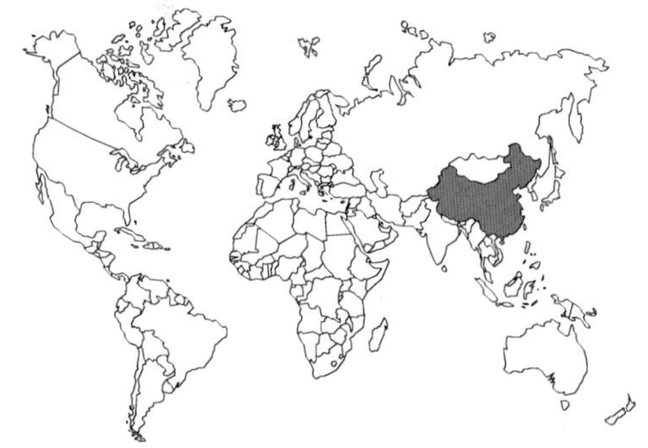

Fig. 4.20.

Foochow, Fukien Province, China.

Location in Host

Middle ear of the cat. All other species of *Mammomonogamus* appear to be located within the trachea and larynx; thus, the location within the middle ear is surprising.

Parasite Identification

The males are orange red, 3.3 to 8.1 mm long, with delicate, subequal spicules. The females are blood red, 14 to 30 mm long; the vulva is 43 percent to 46 percent behind the anterior of the worm. The adults are found consistently with the bursa of the male surrounding the vulva of the female; giving the worms a Y-shaped appearance. The eggs are 48 μm by 88 μm, with a thick, transparent sculptured shell that is in the four- to eight-celled morula stage when laid.

Life Cycle

Very little is known about the biology of these parasites. The eggs apparently pass down the eustachian tubes into the pharynx, are swallowed, and pass out in the feces.

Clinical Presentation and Pathogenesis

These parasites were not found attached to the wall of the middle ear; however, the mucosa was hemorrhagic. The tympanic membranes of the cats were not injured.

Treatment

Not known.

Epizootiology

Not known.

Hazards to Other Animals

Not known.

Hazards to Humans

Not known.

Control/Prevention

Not known.

REFERENCES

Buckley JJC. 1934. On *Syngamus ierei* sp. nov. from domestic cats with some observations on its life-cycle. J Helminthol 12:89–98.

Faust ECF, Tang CC. 1934. A new species of *Syngamus* (*S. auris*) from the middle ear of the cat in Foochow, China. Parasitology 26:455–459.

Ryzhikov KM. 1948. Phylogenetic relationships of nematodes of the family Syngamidae and an attempt to reconstruct their systematics. Dokl Acad Nauk SSSR 62:733–736.

Mammomonogamus ierei (Buckley, 1934) Ryzhikov, 1948

Etymology

Mammo (= mammal) and *monogamus* (for the finding of the worms in pairs of males and females); *ierei* for Dr. Iere.

Synonyms

Syngamus ierei Buckley, 1934.

History

This worm was first described by Buckley with specimens from domestic cats collected in Trinidad. Buckley differentiated this species from *Mammomonogamus felis,* which was reported from the tiger (Cameron, 1931), on the basis of its lack of supporting ribs in the mouth capsule. Of the two major species in ruminants, *Mammomonogamus nasicola* and *Mammomonogamus laryngeus,* only *Mammomonogamus laryngeus* is considered to have spicules (Macko et al., 1981). It has also been noted that, for *Mammomonogamus laryngeus* in Cuba, some specimens have reduced ribs in the buccal capsule. Thus, it is possible that *Mammomonogamus ierei* is a synonym of this parasite of ruminants. When humans who are from or have traveled to the Caribbean Islands, Brazil, or Southeast Asia are infected with *Mammomonogamus,* the species is typically considered to be *Mammomonogamus laryngeus.*

Geographic Distribution

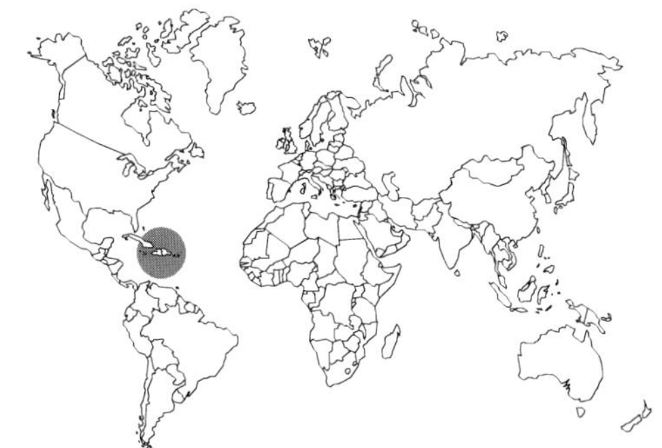

Fig. 4.21.

This worm was initially reported from the island of Trinidad where 15 of 32 cats were infected. It was found in cats from various parts of the island including Port of Spain, St. Augustine, Manzanilla, and Mayaro (Buckley, 1934). It appears that this worm is also rather common in Puerto Rico where a survey revealed that 13 of 40 cats were infected with this parasite (Cuadrado et al., 1980).

Location in Host

The worms are restricted to the nares and nasopharynx.

Parasite Identification

The females are about 20 mm long, with the maximum length reported by Buckley being 23.8 mm. The males are 5 to 6.9 mm long and rather stocky in appearance. The worms are found with the bursa of the male attached at the level of the vulva of the female. There is a large buccal capsule that has eight large teeth at its base. There are no supporting ribs extending up the sides of the capsule. The vulva of the female is located approximately one-third of the body length behind the anterior end of the worm. The esophagus is about one-tenth to one-twentieth of the total body length and is large and muscular. The male has spicules that are subequal in length: the left spicule ranges from 36 to 47 μm in length, and the right spicule ranges from 44 to 58 μm in length. Buckley distinguished *Mammomonogamus ierei* from *Mammomonogamus felis* on the basis that *Mammomonogamus ierei* had no supporting ribs in the mouth capsule, generally smaller buccal capsules, and larger spicules.

The eggs of *Mammomonogamus ierei* were illustrated by Buckley as being ovoid with a shell that is clear and marked with fine, irregular transverse striations. The eggs averaged 49.5 (48–52) μm by 92 (84–100) μm. The eggs when passed in the feces are typically in a four- to six-celled stage. Cuadrado et al. (1980) reported that the eggs of *Mammomonogamus* were typically larger than those of *Ancylostoma,* that the eggs had a thicker shell, and that the shell in a salt flotation preparation was typically found with attached debris.

Life Cycle

There has not been a complete description of the life cycle of any of the species of *Mammomonogamus.* Birds have been found to be infected by species of the related avian-infecting genera, *Cyathostoma* and *Syngamus,* through the ingestion of their embryonated eggs, free larvae, or the earthworm paratenic hosts (Anderson, 2000). Also, it appears that *Syngamus trachea* can utilize other invertebrate paratenic hosts such as snails and slugs. Attempts to infect sheep with earthworms infected with *Mammomonogamus nasicola* or with free larvae of this parasite failed to induce infections with this parasite (Euzeby et al., 1977).

Buckley (1934) examined the development of the egg. At 26° to 30°C, a first-stage larva appeared in 3 to 4 days. The second-stage larva appeared 1 to 2 days later. The third-stage larva appears about 8 days after the cultures are established. The hatched larva bears two sheaths and is about 450 μm long and 16 μm wide. The posterior end of the esophagus is between one-third to one-half of the body from the anterior end. The anus is about 40 μm from the tip of the tail, and there is a small genital primordium at midbody. Buckley fed third-stage larvae to two cats and two kittens, but none of them developed patent infections over the next 1.5 months. Interestingly, 14 days after this experiment was begun, one of the control cats began to pass eggs of *Mammomonogamus.* The fact that human cases have been reported in the United States in individuals within a week after their short trips to Jamaica, Martinique, and St. Lucia would indicate that the adults are capable of developing within a few days to 2 weeks (Nosanchuk et al., 1995; Gardiner and Schantz, 1983).

Clinical Presentation and Pathogenesis

Cuadrado et al. (1980) reported that histologically there is evidence of chronic inflammation of the nasopharynx. Humans with this infection have reported nonproductive and sometimes violent coughs (Freitas et al., 1995; Nosanchuk et al., 1995; Correa de Lara et al., 1993). No such clinical signs have been reported in cats.

Treatment

Treatment in humans has been performed with mebendazole (Correa de Lara et al., 1993; Timmons et al., 1983).

Epizootiology

Little is known about the epizootiology of this parasite; however, the confinement of the parasite to tropical areas would indicate that the cycle is not readily completed in colder climates.

Hazards to Other Animals

The life cycle is not known, and it is possible that the free larvae are capable of infecting other hosts such as ruminants that might ingest them.

Hazards to Humans

It is possible that once the infective-stage larvae have developed and hatched from the eggs, they are infective to humans upon ingestion. However, it does not appear that these larvae are capable of skin penetration based on trials by Buckley (1934).

Control/Prevention

This will not be possible until the biology of this parasite has been adequately described.

REFERENCES

Anderson RC. 2000. Nematode Parasites of Vertebrates. Their Development and Transmission. Wallingford, Oxon, UK: CABI Publishing. 650 pp.

Buckley JJC. 1934. On *Syngamus ierei* sp. nov. from domestic cats with some observations on its lifecycle. J Helminthol 12:89–98.

Cameron TWM. 1931. On some lungworms of the Malay tiger. J Helminthol 9:147–152.

Correa de Lara TA, Barbosa MA, Rodrigues de Oliveira M, Godoy I, Queluz TT. 1993. Human syngamosis. Two cases of chronic cough caused by *Mammomonogamus laryngeus.* Chest 103:264–265.

Cuadrado R, Maldonado-Moll JF, Segarra J. 1980. Gapeworm infection of domestic cats in Puerto Rico. J Am Vet Med Assoc 176:996–997.

Euzeby J, Graber M, Gevrey J, Mejia A. 1977. Recent findings concerning *Mammomonogamus* infection in America and the West Indies. Bull Acad Vet France 50:267–273.

Freitas AL, Carli G, Blankenhein MH. 1995. *Mammomonogamus* (*Syngamus*) *laryngeus* infection: a new Brazilian human case. Rev Inst Med Trop Sao Paulo 37:177–179.

Gardiner CH, Schantz PM. 1983. *Mammomonogamus* infection in a human. Report of a case. Am J Trop Med Hyg 32:995–997.

Macko JK, Birova V, Flores R. 1981. Deliberations on the problems of *Mammomonogamus* species (Nematoda, Syngamidae) in ruminants. Folia Parasitol 28:43–49.

Nosanchuk JS, Wade SE, Landolf M. 1995. Case report and description of parasite in *Mammomonogamus laryngeus* (human syngamosis) infection. J Clin Microbiol 33:998–1000.

Ryzhikov KM. 1948. Phylogenetic relationship of nematodes of the family Syngamidae and an attempt to reconstruct their systematics. Dokl Acad Nauk SSSR 62:733–736.

Timmons RF, Bowers RE, Price DL. 1983. Infection of the respiratory tract with *Mammomonogamus* (*syngamus*) *laryngeus:* a new case in Largo, Florida, and a summary of previously reported cases. Am Rev Resp Dis 128:566–569.

Mammomonogamus mcgaughei Seneviratna, 1954

This species of *Mammomonogamus* was reported from a domestic cat in Sri Lanka. A recent survey of cattle in Sri Lanka revealed that 40 percent of the cattle were infected with *Mammomonogamus laryngeus* (Aken et al., 1989). In this single report of infection in the cat, the worms were found in the frontal sinuses, nasal sinuses, and pharynx. The females were 9 to 22 mm long; the males 3 to 5.5 mm long. The males had spicules ranging from 23.5 μm to 27 μm in length. There was a large buccal capsule. The eggs in the frontal sinuses and feces measured 47–55 μm by 86–94 μm. The eggs were passed in the feces in the 6- to 12-celled stage. Nothing is known about the biology of the worms or clinical signs associated with the infection.

REFERENCES

Aken D, Bont J, Fransen J, Vercruysse J. 1989. *Mammomonogamus laryngeus* (Railliet, 1899) infections in cattle from Sri Lanka. J Helminthol 63:47–52.

Mammomonogamus dispar (Diesing, 1851) Ryzhikov, 1948

Diesing originally described this worm from a Brazilian cougar (*Felis concolor*). Power (1964) reported that he found this worm in the bronchi of 1 of 100 cats necropsied in Maracay, Venezuela. Buckley (1934) felt that Diesing's original description of 1851 was inadequate but that his figures of this species in 1857 showed that there were buccal ribs that distinguished it from *Mammomonogamus ierei.* Power (1964) described the site of infection as the bronchi. Diesing stated that the worms were in the trachea. The finding of the worms in the trachea and bronchi in these two cases is interesting because *Mammomonogamus ierei* has not been found in this location. The females are 20 to 27 mm long, and the males are 5 to 7 mm long. The vulva is located about one-fourth of the length of the body from the anterior end.

REFERENCES

Buckley JJC. 1934. On *Syngamus ierei* sp. nov. from domestic cats with some observations on its lifecycle. J Helminthol 12:89–98.

Diesing KM. 1857. Sechzehn Arten von Nematoideen. Denkscrh Akad Wiss Wien 13:1–21.
Power LA. 1964. Contribucion al conocimiento de los helmintos parasitos del gato, "*Felis* (*Felis*) *catus domesticus*," de Maracay y sus Alrededores. Rev Med Vet Parasit, Maracay 20:99-135.

Other *Mammomonogamus* Species

Linquist and Austin (1981) reported on the infection of a 2-year-old Siamese cat with an unidentified species of *Mammomonogamus.* The cat had lived most of its life in Nigeria. The cat had exhibited upper respiratory tract congestion with open mouth breathing. Upon examination the cat sneezed, and out came several small reddish brown worms. There are no other reports of *Mammomonogamus* infections in cats in Africa.

REFERENCES

Lindquist WD, Austin ER. 1981. Exotic parasitism in a Siamese cat. Feline Pract 11:9–11.

TRICHOSTRONGYLOIDEA

The trichostrongyles compose a group of bursate nematode parasites that have reduced buccal capsules and that inhabit the stomach or small intestine of all types of vertebrates. The trichostrongyles compose the superfamily of parasitic nematodes with the largest number of genera and species, but the cat is only host to two members of this genus, and both are within the same family, the Molineidae, which has representative parasites in bats, primates, rodents, lagomorphs, and ruminants. The two genera that occur in the domestic cat are *Ollulanus* and *Molineus. Ollulanus* is characterized by being ovoviviparous and having a female tail ending with several tubercles. *Molineus* contains oviparous females that have a tail terminating in a single caudal spine.

Ollulanus tricuspis Leuckart, 1865

Etymology

Ollula (diminutive of *olla; olla* = earthen pot, jar) + *anus* (anus) and *tri* (three) + *cuspis* (a point) relative to the three cusps on the tail of the adult female.

Synonyms

Ollulanus skrjabini, Ollulanus suis.

History

Leuckart (1865) found a small bursate nematode in the stomach of a domestic cat that he named *Ollulanus tricuspis.* Leuckart believed that the intermediate host was the mouse, but he was looking at the larvae of the lungworm, *Aelurostrongylus abstrusus.*

Geographic Distribution

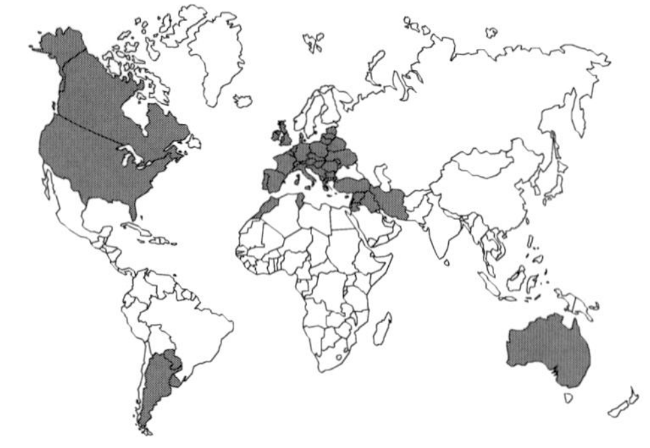

Fig. 4.22.

Hasslinger (1984) presented the geographical distribution of *Ollulanus tricuspis* in Europe and around the world. Hasslinger cited reports for Canada, the United States, Argentina, Chile, Egypt, and Australia. It also appears that this worm is much more commonly found in colony cats. Hasslinger reported that it was found in about 40 percent of cats that were allowed to roam freely in Germany; Schuster et al. (1997) reported the parasite in 12 percent of 155 cats from the eastern part of the state of Brandenburg.

Location in Host

These worms live in the mucosa of the stomach of the cat (Fig. 4.23).

Parasite Identification

The adult worms are quite small (Cameron, 1923). The anterior end of the worm usually coils around on itself. There is a relatively large, "cup-shaped" buccal capsule that contains no teeth, cutting plates, or other ancillary structures. The esophagus is about one-third to one-half the

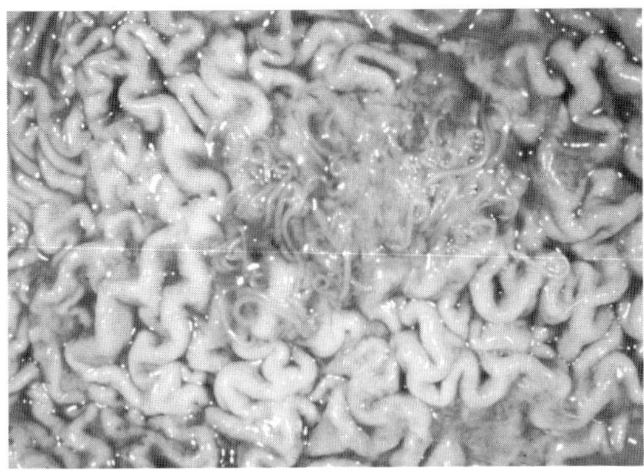

Fig. 4.23. *Ollulanus tricuspis.* Mucosal surface of a cat's stomach with a lesion containing numerous adults of this species.

length of the intestine and is slightly swollen where it joins the intestine. The male is 0.7 to 0.98 mm long by about 0.035 mm wide and has a well-developed copulatory bursa. The female is 0.8 mm to 1.0 mm long by 0.04 mm wide. The tail of the female bears three major cusps or bumps that may occasionally be accompanied by two minor ones. The vulva is in the posterior part of the body of the female, and she has only a single ovary and uterus and does not possess a muscular ovijector (Cameron, 1927). The eggs in the female are few in number and large relative to the size of the female. The egg undergoes embryonation within the female and hatches within the uterus. The first-stage larva inside the female is about 0.35 mm long, or about one-third the length of the female worm. The second- and third-stage larvae also develop within the female, who gives birth to the third-stage larva.

The antemortem diagnosis of infection is difficult. The adults and larvae of *Ollulanus tricuspis* that enter the intestine are usually dead, killed, destroyed, or digested before they are passed in the feces. Thus, it is only on rare occasions that diagnosis is made by direct fecal smears or fecal flotation methods (Hargis et al., 1983a). Hasslinger (1984) recommended two methods for antemortem diagnosis: induction of vomiting and stomach irrigation. Emesis is induced by the administration of xylazine. Hargis et al. (1983a) reported that the examination of induced vomitus is successful in making a diagnosis in about 70 percent of infected cats. Using physiologic saline, stomach irrigation is performed in anesthetized cats. The fluid collected in the irrigation is then examined after centrifugation or after larvae are collected using a Baermann apparatus.

Postmortem diagnosis of infection can be made from washings or scraping of the stomach mucosa or by peptic digestion of the stomach wall (Hasslinger, 1984). The washings of the stomach wall are centrifuged and then examined microscopically. For examination of the stomach by scraping, Hasslinger reported the examination of "rice-grain" size scrapings from each of 10 sites on the stomach wall: 2 sites on the cardiac stomach, 4 on the fundus, and 4 on the pyloric stomach. The samples were placed on a slide with a drop of saline and examined with low power (35×) microscopy. To aid in the examination, KOH was often then added to the material to aid in the dissolution of the mucosal particles removed by the scraping. A preparation of routine pepsin digestion fluid digested the stomach wall. The stomach was then opened, everted, and pinned to a cork that was suspended to an extension on the top of a funnel. The funnel was closed by attaching tubing bearing a pinch clamp. The digest was maintained at 37°C for 4 to 8 hours; then the clamp was opened, and the material collected in the bottom of the funnel was examined. This procedure worked best for fresh material containing live parasites.

Life Cycle

Transmission from cat to cat appears to be direct through the consumption of vomitus. Cameron (1927) examined the life cycle and found that there were third-stage larvae within the adult female and free within the lumen of the cat stomach. The larvae within the female were 0.4 mm long, while those in the stomach were 0.5 mm long. Fourth-stage larvae were usually found on the surface of the gastric mucosa and were around 0.65 mm long. Cameron (1927) felt that the transmission was through vomition and that there were not paratenic hosts involved in the life cycle. Wittmann (1982), like Cameron, also failed to produce infections in mice that were fed the third-stage larvae. Wittmann (1982) showed that the infection can be transmitted between cats by the feeding of the adult males and females, fourth-stage larvae, or third-stage larvae. Thus, all stages passed in the vomitus are capable of infecting another host. Also, he showed that the parasites can live in the vomitus for up to 12 days. The period required for an infection with third-stage larvae to produce the next generation of third-stage larvae appears to be from 33 to 37 days.

Internal autoinfection is believed to play a role in maintaining these infections and may lead to the clinical signs when they are observed. Wittmann (1982) showed that if cats are fed adult males and females, the number of adults present at necropsy will be greater than the number of worms fed to the cat. The large numbers of worms found in single cats, such as one reported by Collins and Charleston (1972) that harbored around 4,500 worms, are best explained by the buildup of large numbers of worms through internal autoinfection. Hasslinger and Trah (1981) found that cats harbored an average of 1,500 worms and that a single cat harbored 11,028 worms.

Clinical Presentation and Pathogenesis

Cats infected with *Ollulanus tricuspis* generally have a history of chronic vomiting (Cameron, 1932; Greve, 1981). Hänichen and Hasslinger (1977) reported on a Persian cat that died due to chronic gastritis caused by *Ollulanus tricuspis*. This cat was 3 years old and had been imported from England about a year previously. The cat lived in a household with 10 other pets. The cat became anorexic but continued to drink milk. Prior to death, the cat was dehydrated with a subnormal temperature. Linde-Sipman et al. (1992) reported on three cases of chronic infections in cats that resulted in two of the cats being euthanatized due to their wasted condition and chronic vomiting while the third cat died shortly after the appearance of blood in its vomit and feces. Necropsies revealed stomachs with signs of chronic inflammation very similar to that reported by Hänichen and Hasslinger.

The infection is capable of causing chronic gastritis in infected cats (Fig. 4.24). Cameron (1932) examined the pathogenicity of *Ollulanus tricuspis* in cats and felt that the worms caused only moderate local erosion of the gastric mucosa and increased mucous secretion. In other cases the pathologic changes are more severe, and lesions include hyperplasia of the stomach epithelium, inflammation, cellular infiltration, and sclerosis of the epithelium (Hänichen and Hasslinger, 1977). The worms are found under a layer of mucus or partially embedded head first in gastric glands (Hargis et al., 1983b). In stomachs of infected cats, there is a significant increase in mucosal fibrous tissue and mucosal lymphoid aggregates (Hargis et al., 1983b). Also, the lymphoid aggregates tend to have large germinal centers. There is also an increase in the globule leukocytes, and some cats may have over 100 globule leukocytes per high power field.

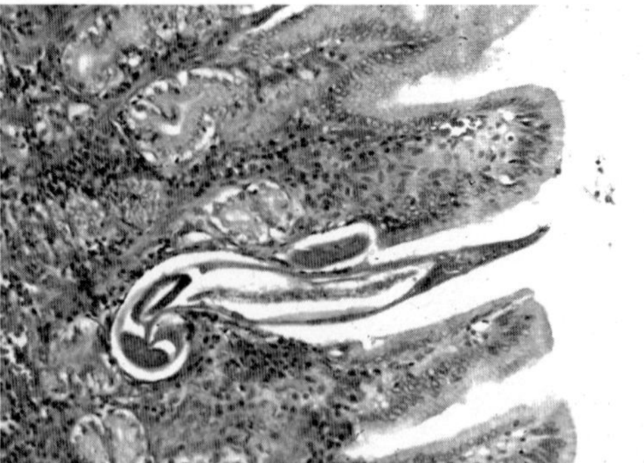

Fig. 4.24. *Ollulanus tricuspis.* Section of the stomach mucosa showing an adult worm within the mucosa.

Treatment

It has been reported that tetramisole (a 2.5 percent formulation administered at 5 mg/kg body weight) has proved efficacious and without side effects (Hasslinger, 1984).

Epizootiology

The cats most likely to be infected are feral cats and colony-reared cats (Hargis et al., 1981, 1983a). The high prevalence in colony cats is probably due to the concentration of cats in a single area, which increases the opportunities for the ingestion of another animal's vomitus containing the infective stages. As stated above, the infective stages are capable of living in vomitus for up to 12 days.

Hazards to Other Animals

Ollulanus tricuspis has been reported from other feline hosts including lions, cheetahs, and tigers

(Hasslinger, 1985). It has also been found to infect dogs (Himonas, 1968) and foxes (Hinaidy, 1976). It has also been reported from pigs on several occasions (Kotlan and von Mocsy, 1933; Stockdale and Lautenslager, 1973), but some consider the species in swine to be *Ollulanus suis,* another species within this genus (Kazello, 1972). Similarly, it is believed that the lion is host to *Ollulanus skrjabini,* a species specific to the lion (Burdelev, 1950), but others consider this a synonym of *Ollulanus tricuspis* (Hasslinger and Wittmann, 1982). Thus, it would seem that infected cats could easily serve as a source of infection for any other felines and perhaps dogs with which they are housed.

Hazards to Humans

There have been no reports of human infections with this parasite.

Control/Prevention

In catteries, it is important to watch for signs of increased vomiting, and if this does occur, cat vomitus should be checked for the presence of these worms.

REFERENCES

Burdelev TE. 1950. Novaja Nematoda—*Ollulanus skrjabini* nov. sp. iz Piscer voda I Zeludka Iva. Dokl Akad Naukj SSSR 74:163–164.

Cameron TWM. 1923. On the morphology of *Ollulanus tricuspis* Leuckart, 1865, a nematode parasite of the cat. J Helminthol 1:157–160.

Cameron TWM. 1927. Observations on the life history of *Ollulanus tricuspis* Leuck, the stomach worm of the cat. J Helminthol 5:67–80.

Cameron TWM. 1932. On the pathogenicity of the stomach and lung worms of the cat. J Helminthol 10:231–234.

Collins GH, Charleston WAG. 1972. *Ollulanus tricuspis* and *Capillaria putorii* in New Zealand cats (Correspondence). NZ Vet J 20:82.

Greve JH. 1981. A nematode causing vomiting in cats. Feline Pract 4:17–19.

Hänichen T, Hasslinger MA. 1977. Chronische Gastritis durch *Ollulanus tricuspis* (Leuckart, 1865) bei einer Katze. Berl Much Tierärztl Wschr 90:59–62.

Hargis AM, Prieur DJ, Wescott RB. 1981. A gastric nematode (*Ollulanus tricuspis*) in cats in the Pacific Northwest. J Am Vet Med Assoc 178:475–478.

Hargis AM, Haupt KH, Blanchard JL. 1983a. *Ollulanus tricuspis* found by fecal flotation in a cat with diarrhea. J Am Vet Med Assoc 182:1122–1123.

Hargis AM, Prieur DJ, Blanchard JL. 1983b. Prevalence, lesions, and differential diagnosis of *Ollulanus tricuspis* infection in cats. Vet Pathol 20:71–79.

Hasslinger MA. 1984. *Ollulanus tricuspis,* the stomach worm of the cat. Feline Pract 14:22–35.

Hasslinger MA. 1985. Der Magenwurm der Katze, *Ollulanus tricuspis* (Leuckart, 1865)—zum gegenwärtigen Stand der Kenntnis. Tierärztl Praxis 13:205–217.

Hasslinger MA, Trah M. 1981. Untersuchungen zur Verbreitung und zum Nachweis des Magenwurmes der Katze, *Ollulanus tricuspis* (Leuckart, 1865). Berl Münch tierärtzl Wschr 94:235–238.

Hasslinger MA, Wittmann FX. 1982. The tail morphology of different developmental stages of *Ollulanus tricuspis* (Leuckart, 1865) (Nematoda: Trichostrongyloidea). J Helminthol 56:351–352.

Himonas CA. 1968. The parasitic helminths of dogs in Greece and their public health importance. Epistemon Epeter, Ekdid Kteniat Scholes Aristol Panipistem. Thesis, Thessaloniki. 9:157–390.

Hinaidy HK. 1976. Ein Weiterer Beitrag sur Parasitenfauna des Rotfuchses, *Vulpses vulpes* (L.), in Osterreich. Zbl Vet Med B 23:66–73.

Kazello AB. 1972. *Ollulanus suis*—Nematoda iz Zeludka Svini. Problemy Veterinarii na Dalnem Vostoke. Blagovescensk, Chabarovskoc Kn Uzdvo 182–184.

Kotlan A, von Mocsy J. 1933. *Ollulanus tricuspis* Leuck. als Ursache Einer Chronischen Magenwurmseuche beim Schwein. Dtsch tierärtzl Wschr 41:689–692.

Leuckart R. 1865. Bericht uber die Naruwissenschaftlichen Leistungen in der Naturgeschichte der Niederen Thiere Während der Jahre 1864 und 1865. Arch Naturgesch 31:229–268.

Linde-Sipman JS, Boersema JH, Berrocal A. 1992. Drie gevallen van hypertrofische gastritis, geassocieerd met een *Ollulanus tricuspis*-infectie bij de kat. Tidschr Diergeneeskd 117:727–729.

Schuster R, Kaufmann A, Hering WS. 1997. Untersuchungen zur Endoparasitenfauna der Hauskatze in Ostbrandenburg. Berl. Münch Tierärztl Wschr 110:48–50.

Stockdale PHG, Lautenslager JP. 1973. Unusual gastric nematodes of swine in Ontario. Can Vet J 14:215–216.

Wittmann FX. 1982. *Ollulanus tricuspis* (Leuckart, 1865): Untersuchungen zur Diagnose, Morphologie, Entwicklung, Therapie Sowie zum Wirtspektrum. Thesis, Munich, 1982. 55 pp.

Molineus barbatus Chandler, 1942

Etymology

Molineus for Dr. Molin of Padua, and *barbatus* for the hair-like nature of these worms.

Synonyms

None.

History

This worm was originally described by Chandler (1942) from raccoons in east Texas. It has since been found on rare occasions in cats.

Geographic Distribution

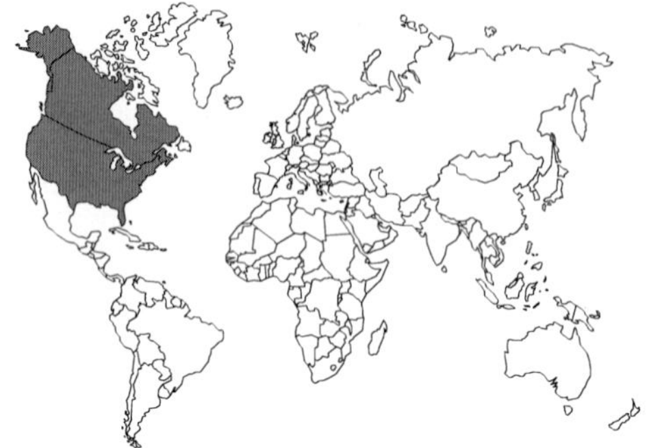

Fig. 4.25.

This parasite has been recorded as a parasite of raccoons, *Procyon lotor,* in North America. It has been found by Shoop et al. (1991) in cats from Arkansas. Out of 13 random-source cats, 7 were found to harbor worms. The cat with the most worms had 21 adults.

Location in Host

Small intestine.

Parasite Identification

The adults of this species are quite small and delicate (Chandler, 1942). The worms are red. The females are 5.5 to 6.6. mm long, and the males are 4.3 mm to 4.7 mm long. The cuticle is finely striated with 24 to 28 longitudinal ridges. The anterior end has a cephalic inflation. The bursa is well developed, the spicules are 90 µm to 100 µm long, and there is a gubernaculum present. The vulva is about 1 mm from the posterior end of the female. The eggs are elliptical, 50 to 53 µm long by 32 µm to 37 µm wide (Chandler, 1942). Gupta (1961) gave the dimensions of the eggs as 54 µm to 61 µm by 38 µm to 45 µm. Shoop et al. (1991) gave the size of the eggs as 60 µm long by 40 µm wide and similar to hookworm eggs in appearance. The eggs are passed in the morula stage. It would be interesting to perform careful observations to determine if the eggs can be readily separated. Schmidt (1965) presents a key to the different species of *Molineus* that have been described. The very small size of these worms may cause them to be overlooked at necropsy unless precautions are taken to use procedures that will recover worms as small as the feline hookworms.

Life Cycle

Gupta (1961, 1963) described the free-living stages and life cycle in experimentally infected ferrets (*Putorius putorius*). The egg is passed in the morula stage, and after around a day at 20°C, the first-stage larva hatches from the eggshell. Two molts occur over the next 4 days, producing a sheathed third-stage larva 520 µm long. When larvae were given orally to seven ferrets, eggs appeared in the feces of five of the ferrets 8 to 10 days later. When larvae were administered subcutaneously to seven ferrets, eggs appeared in the feces 13 days later. Following both forms of administration, the patent periods were very brief. Balasingam (1963) infected cats with larvae orally and subcutaneously and reported prepatent periods of 8 days and more than 30 days, respectively.

Clinical Presentation and Pathogenesis

Not described.

Treatment

Not described.

Epizootiology

These larvae are acquired most likely by the ingestion of material contaminated with infective third-stage larvae. Thus, if cats tend to eat grass or other matter in a yard shared by a raccoon, it is possible that the infection could be acquired by cats in this manner.

Hazards to Other Animals

The life cycle of this parasite is direct, and dogs and ferrets, as well as cats and raccoons, could be infected. Thus, it is possible that if a cat does become infected, other household pets sharing the environment could become infected.

Hazards to Humans

It may be possible for humans to develop transient patent infections if the larvae were to be ingested.

Control/Prevention

Prevent the contamination of areas with raccoon feces where cats may hunt or graze.

REFERENCES

Balasingam E. 1963. Experimental infection of dogs and cats with *Molineus barbatus* Chandler, 1942, with a discussion on the distribution of *Molineus* spp. Can J Zool 41:599–602.

Chandler AC. 1942. The helminths of raccoons in east Texas. J Parasitol 28:255–268.

Gupta SP. 1961. The life history of *Molineus barbatus* Chandler, 1942. Can J Zool 39:579–588.

Gupta SP. 1963. Mode of infection and biology of infective larvae of *Molineus barbatus* Chandler, 1942. Exp Parasitol 13:252–255.

Schmidt GD. 1965. *Molineus mustelae* sp. n. (Nematoda: Trichostrongylidae) from the long-tailed weasel in Montana and *M. chabaudi* nom. n, with a key to the species of *Molineus*. J Parasitol 51:164–168.

Shoop WL, Haines HW, Michael BF, Eary CH, Endris RG. 1991. *Molineus barbatus* (Trichostrongylidae) and other helminthic infections of the cat in Arkansas. J Helm Soc Wash 58:227–230.

METASTRONGYLOIDEA

Metastrongyloid nematodes are characterized by having life cycles that typically require an intermediated molluscan host for the development of the third-stage larvae that are infective to vertebrates. Cats do not appear to eat many snails and typically acquire their infections with these worms through the ingestion of paratenic hosts (e.g., small birds or rodents). The majority of metastrongyles are associated with lung tissue, although the adults are often living within associated blood vessels. There are four metastrongyles that have been reported from the domestic cat. One species, *Aelurostrongylus abstrusus*, is rather common. The other three species, *Troglostrongylus subcrenatus*, *Oslerus rostratus*, and *Gurltia paralysans*, have only rarely been reported from cats and probably represent species typically parasitic in wild felids or some other nondomestic mammal.

Aelurostrongylus abstrusus (Railliet, 1898) Cameron, 1927

Etymology

Aeluro = cat and *strongylus* = round, plus *abstrusus* = hidden from view.

Synonyms

Strongylus pusillus Mueller, 1890; *Strongylus abstrusus* Railliet, 1898; *Strongylus nanus* Braun and Luehe, 1909; *Synthetocaulus abstrusus* Railliet and Henry, 1907.

History

This worm was originally found and described by Mueller (1890) as *Strongylus pusillus*. In 1898, Railliet (1898) changed the name to *Strongylus abstrusus*. Braun and Lühe (1909) described a species from the cat that they named *Strongylus nanus*. In 1907, Railliet and Henry (1907) erected the genus *Sythetocaulus* to include this worm. Cameron (1927) erected the genus *Aelurostrongylus* and concluded that the larva passed in the feces was capable of infecting mice; this work has never been duplicated.

Geographic Distribution

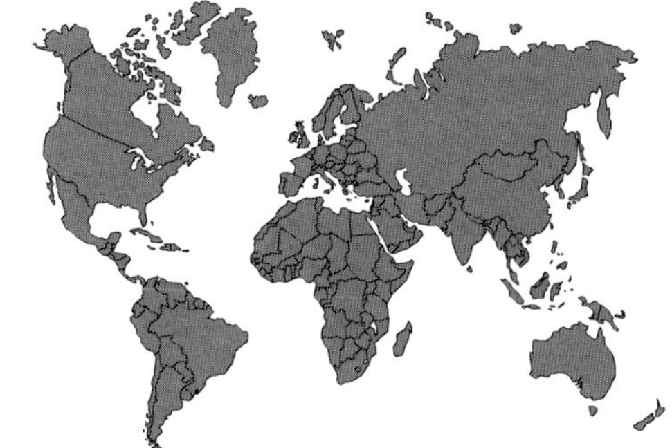

Fig. 4.26.

This is a metastrongyloid nematode parasite of the cat around the world (Ash, 1962; Center et al., 1990; Charan and Sheik-Dawood, 1984; Gathumbi et al., 1991; Martinez et al., 1990; Naylor et al., 1984; Pennisi et al., 1995; Wilson-Hanson and Prescott, 1982).

Location in Host

The adults live in the terminal respiratory bronchioles and alveolar ducts.

Parasite Identification

The adult females are 9 to 10 mm long with a vulval opening that, unlike in many nematodes, occurs near the anus. The males are smaller, being 4 to 6 mm long, and have a small bursa and relatively short and stout spicules. The worms are less than a millimeter wide and have a dark brown to black appearance when observed in fresh tissue. Due to the small worms being deeply within the terminal respiratory bronchioles and alveolar ducts, it is difficult to remove entire worms by dissection. The females lay eggs that contain single cells and that embryonate within the alveolar ducts and the surrounding alveoli. The larvae hatch from the eggs and then are carried up the ciliary escalator, swallowed, and passed in the feces. The larvae of *Aelurostrongylus abstrusus* are quite active larvae that are easy to recover in the feces using a Baermann apparatus. The larva is approximately 360–390 μm long and has a characteristic dorsal spine on the tail (Figs 4.27 to 4.29).

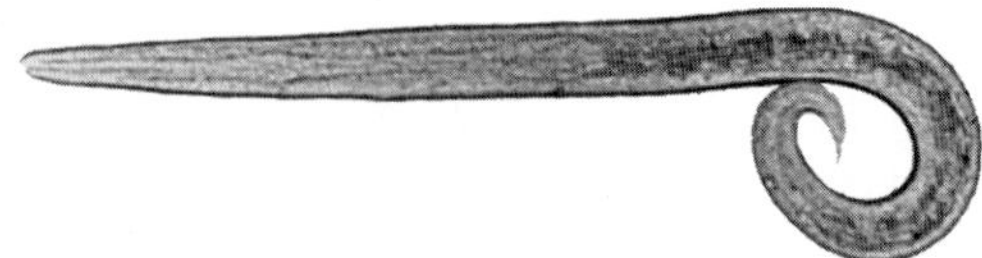

Fig. 4.27. *Aelurostrongylus abstrusus.* First-stage larva passed in the feces. The characteristic dorsal spine on the larval tail is not evident in this image.

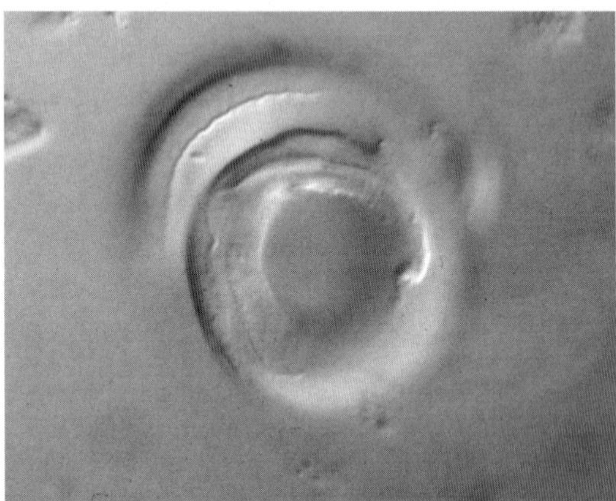

Fig. 4.28. *Aelurostrongylus abstrusus.* First-stage larva passed in the feces. This is a higher magnification (see Fig. 4.27) of the kinked tail with a dorsal spine.

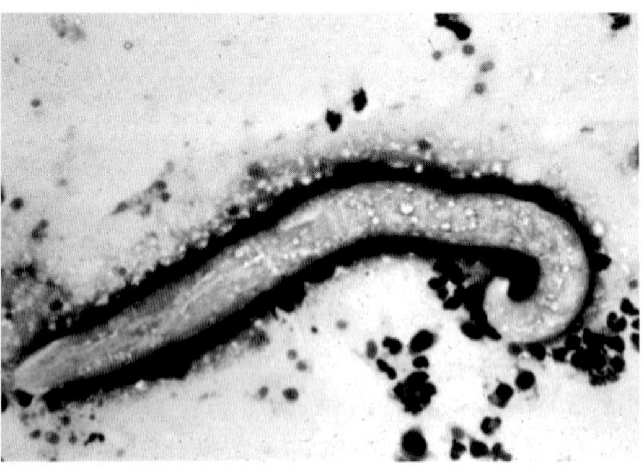

Fig. 4.29. *Aelurostrongylus abstrusus.* First-stage larva recovered in a tracheal wash from an infected cat stained with Dif-Quik.

Life Cycle

The life cycle of *Aelurostrongylus abstrusus* has been shown to involve a required snail intermediate host (Hamilton and McCaw, 1967). It has also been shown that mice that ingest the infected snails can serve as paratenic hosts (Mackerras, 1957). Hobmaier and Hobmaier (1935a) also showed that if the larvae from snails were fed to frogs, toads, snakes, lizards, ducklings, chickens, or sparrows, the larvae could later be recovered from their tissues. Thus, it seems highly possible that cats become infected typically by the ingestion of infected mice or birds. Stockdale (1970) found that the females began to lay eggs as early as 25 days postinfection; larvae have been found in the feces after 39 days of hosts' being infected with third-stage larvae (Gerichter, 1949).

Clinical Presentation and Pathogenesis

Aelurostrongylus abstrusus is known to cause severe pulmonary disease with heavy infections (Stockdale, 1970) (Figs. 4.30 to 4.32). Cats infected with 100 larvae showed early radiographic changes 2 weeks after infection (Mahaffey, 1979). The most severe disease was noted 5 to 15 weeks after infection and presented as alveolar disease. Examination of experimentally infected cats followed for up to a year after infection revealed that there was neither pulmonary hypertension nor associated right ventricular dis-

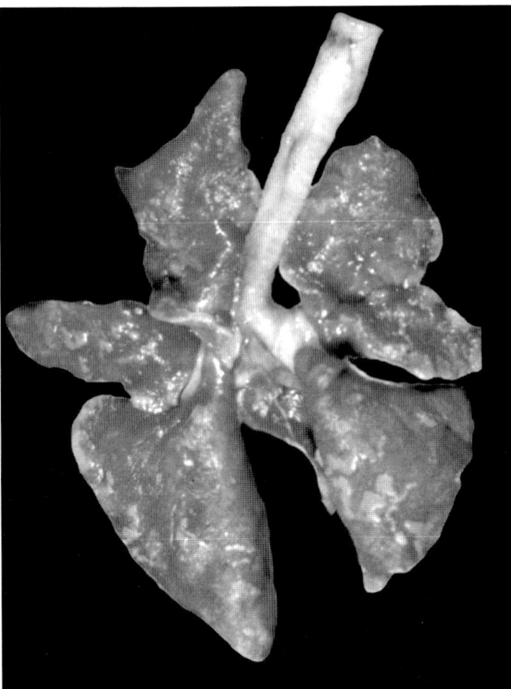

Fig. 4.30. *Aelurostrongylus abstrusus.* Lungs of an infected cat showing changes in the serosal surface.

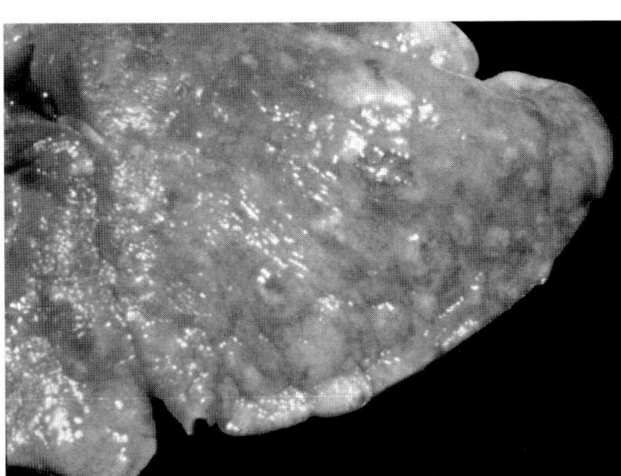

Fig. 4.31. *Aelurostrongylus abstrusus.* Higher view of lungs showing numerous areas of apparent consolidation.

ease (Rawlings et al., 1980). Pulmonary arteries in experimentally infected kittens showed disruption of the vascular endothelium and proliferation of the endothelial cells, and as early as 10 days after infection, there was disruption of the internal elastic lamina (Figs 4.33 and 4.34). Hypertrophy and hyperplasia of the medial and intimal walls of the pulmonary vessels caused complete

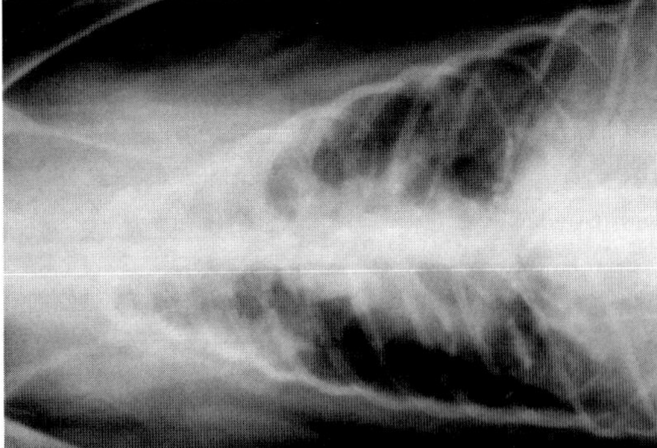

Fig. 4.32. *Aelurostrongylus abstrusus.* Radiograph of lungs of infected cat.

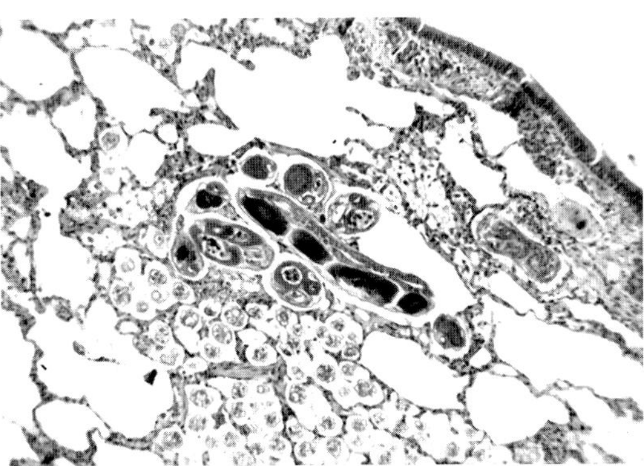

Fig. 4.33. *Aelurostrongylus abstrusus.* Histological section of lung showing sections of adult worm along with eggs within the parenchyma in various stages of development.

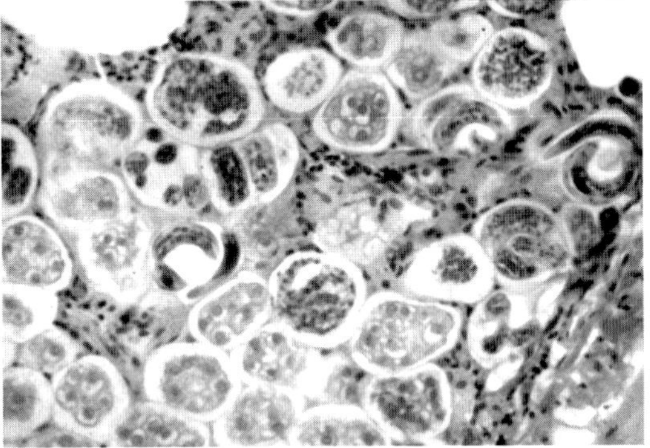

Fig. 4.34. *Aelurostrongylus abstrusus.* Transverse section through lung parenchyma showing a large number of eggs in various stages of development in the tissues as well as a few free first-stage larvae.

occlusion of many of the vessels by 24 weeks after infection (Naylor et al., 1984).

Mild infections often present with only minimal signs; however, heavy infections can cause severe bronchopneumonia with cats having rapid, open-mouthed abdominal breathing (Vig and Murray, 1986). A retrospective study of 312 cases of cats with eosinophilia revealed that 2 percent of the cases were infected with *Aelurostrongylus abstrusus,* while the majority of cases, 20.5 percent, had eosinophilia as a result of flea-bite allergy dermatitis (Center et al., 1990). Hamilton (1963) reported on one cat that was presumed to have died as a result of its lungworm infection. The 6-month-old cat developed signs of respiratory disease when 3 months old, and the disease persisted. During this 3-month period, the cat was observed to be coughing and sneezing with a muco-purulent discharge. As the disease progressed, the cat became dyspneic, anorexic, and emaciated and had hydrothorax.

Treatment

In cats infected with *Aelurostrongylus abstrusus,* treatment with fenbendazole—55 mg/kg daily for 21 days (Vig and Murray, 1986) or 20 mg/kg daily for 5 days followed by a second 5-day treatment after a 5-day hiatus—has been reported to be successful (Smith, 1980). Treatment of 15 cats experimentally infected with *Aelurostrongylus abstrusus* with fenbendazole (50 mg/kg, once daily for 3 days) stopped the shedding of larvae in the feces by 14 days after treatment, but a few days later, the larvae reappeared in small numbers in the feces of the infected cats (Roberson and Burke, 1980). Published reports on the efficacy of ivermectin has not produced conclusive results (Blagburn et al., 1987). However, there is a report of treatment with ivermectin (200 µg/kg followed by a second treatment with 400 µg/kg) clearing a cat of the *Aelurostrongylus abstrusus* infection (Kirkpatrick and Megalla, 1987).

Epizootiology

Cats probably most typically become infected by the ingestion of captured prey (e.g., small birds and rodents). Thus, to prevent infection, it is probably necessary to restrict the hunting of cats.

Hazards to Other Animals

This parasite seems restricted to cats, and the stage passed in the feces is not infectious to other avian or mammalian hosts until after a period of development in a mollusk. Thus, it is unlikely that this worm would pose a threat to other animals in a clinic.

Hazards to Humans

None.

Control/Prevention

Control would be by the prevention of hunting by cats. It is unlikely that the monthly heartworm preventatives approved for cats would have any effects on the development of this parasite in the cat.

REFERENCES

Ash LR. 1962. Helminth parasites of dogs and cats in Hawaii. J Parasitol 48:63–65.

Blagburn BL, Hendrix CM, Lindsay DS, Vaughan JL. 1987. Anthelmintic efficacy of ivermectin in naturally parasitized cats. Am J Vet Res 48:670–672.

Braun MGCC, Lühe MFL. 1909. Leitfaden zur Untersuchung der tierischen Parasiten des Menschen und der Haussäugetiere für Studierende, értze und Tierärzte. Wurtburg. 186 pp.

Cameron TWM. 1927. Observations on the life history of *Aelurostrongylus abstrusus* (Raillet) the lungworm of the cat. J Helminthol 5:55–66.

Center SA, Randolph JF, Erb HN, Reiter S. 1990. Eosinophilia in the cat: a retrospective study of 312 cases (1975–1986). J Am Anim Hosp Assoc 26:349–358.

Charan K, Sheik-Dawood MM. 1984. Lungworm infestation in a cat. Ind Vet Med J 8:245–247.

Gathumbi PK, Waruiru RM, Buoro I. 1991. A case of feline *Aelurostongylus* infection in Kenya. Bull Anim Health Prod Afr 39:361–363.

Gerichter CB. 1949. Studies on the nematodes parasitic in the lungs of Felidae in Palestine. Parasitology 39:251–262.

Hamilton JM. 1963. *Aelurostrongylus abstrusus* infestation of the cat. Vet Res 75:417–422.

Hamilton JM, McCaw AW. 1967. The role of the mouse in the life cycle of *Aelurostrongylus abstrusus.* J Helminthol 41:309–312.

Hobmaier M, Hobmaier A. 1935a. Intermediate hosts of *Aelurostrongylus abstrusus* of the cat. Proc Soc Exp Biol Med 32:1641–1647.

Hobmaier M, Hobmaier A. 1935b. Mammalian phase of the lungworm *Aelurostrongylus abstrusus* in the cat. J Am Vet Med Assoc 87:191–198.

Kirkpatrick CE, Megalla C. 1987. Use of ivermectin in treatment of *Aelurostrongylus abstrusus* and *Toxocara cati* infection in a cat. J Am Vet Med Assoc 190:1309–1310.

Mackerras MJ. 1957. Observations on the life history of the cat lungworm, *Aelurostrongylus abstrusus* (Railliet, 1898) (Nematoda: Metastrongylidae). Aust J Zool 5:188–195.
Mahaffey MB. 1979. Radiographic-pathologic findings in experimental *Aelurostrongylus abstrusus* infection in cats. J Am Vet Rad Soc 20:81.
Martinez AR, Santa-Cruz AM, Lombardero OJ. 1990. Lesiones histopatologicas en la aelurostongilosis felina. Rev Med Vet (Buenos Aires) 71:260–264.
Mueller A. 1890. Helminthologisch Mittheilungen. Deutsch Ztsche Thiermed 17:58–70.
Naylor JR, Hamilton JM, Weatherley AJ. 1984. Changes in the ultrastructure of feline pulmonary arteries following infection with the lungworm *Aelurostrongylus abstrusus*. Brit Vet J 140:181–190.
Pennisi MG, Niutta PP, Giannetto S. 1995. Longwormziekte bij katten veroozaakt door *Aelurostrongylus abstrusus*. Tijdsch v Diergeneesk 120:263–266.
Railliet A. 1898. Rectification de la nomenclature d'après les travaux recénts. Rec méd Vet Par 75:171–174.
Raillet A, Henry A. 1907. Sur les variations des strongyles de l'appareil respiratoire des mammiferes. Compt rend Soc Biol 63:751–753.
Rawlings CA, Losonsky JM, Lewis RE, Hubble JJ, Prestwood AK. 1980. Response of the feline heart to *Aelurostrongylus abstrusus*. J Am Anim Hosp Assoc 16:573–578.
Roberson EL, Burke TM. 1980. Evaluation of granulated fenbendazole (22.2%) against induced and naturally occurring helminth infections in cats. Am J Vet Res 41:1499–1502.
Smith RE. 1980. Feline lungworm infection. Vet Rec 107:256.
Stockdale PHG. 1970. The pathogenesis of the lesions elicited by *Aelurostrongylus abstrusus* during its prepatent period. Pathol Vet 7:102–115.
Vig MM, Murray PA. 1986. Successful treatment of *Aelurostrongylus abstrusus* with fenbendazole. Comp Cont Educ Pract Vet 8:214–222.
Wilson-Hanson SL, Prescott CW. 1982. A survey for parasites in cats. Aust Vet J 59:109.

Troglostrongylus subcrenatus (Railliet and Henry, 1913) Fitzsimmons, 1964

This is a metastrongyloid nematode parasite of the lungs of felids that is related to *Aelurostrongylus abstrusus* and that was originally reported from a leopard in the Congo. This nematode has been reported on a single occasion from a cat in Africa, Blantyre, Nyasaland (Fitzsimmons, 1961). The males of this species have long, slender spicules, and the vulva of the female is posterior to the middle of the body rather than near the anus as in *Aelurostrongylus*. The adults are 10 to 23 mm long—about twice the length of the adults of *Aelurostrongylus abstrusus*. The life cycle of a related parasite, *Troglostrongylus brevior*, was described by Gerichter (1948, 1949). The adults of *Troglostrongylus brevior* are found in *Felis ocreata* and *Catolynx chaus*. First-stage larvae in the feces enter a suitable mollusk, and infective larvae are present in about 8 days. The patent period for this other species was found to be 28 days in a kitten fed snails containing infective larvae.

REFERENCES

Fitzsimmons WM. 1961. *Bronchostrongylus subcrenatus* (Railliet and Henry, 1913) a new parasite recorded from the domestic cat. Vet Rec 73:101–102.
Fitzsimmons WM. 1964. On a redescription of the male of *Troglostrongylus subcrenatus* (Railliet and Henry, 1913) n. Comb., from the domestic cat and the synonymy of *Bronchostrongylus* Cameron, 1931 with *Troglostrongylus* Vevers, 1923. J Helm 38:11–20.
Gerichter CB. 1948. Observations on the life histories of lung nematodes using snails as intermediate hosts. Am J Vet Res 9:109–112.
Gerichter CB. 1949. Studies on the nematodes parasitic in the lungs of Felidae in Palestine. Parasitology 39:251–262.

Oslerus rostratus (Gerichter, 1949) Anderson, 1978

This is a metastrongyloid nematode parasite of felines that occasionally finds its way into the domestic cat. *Oslerus rostratus* is a large worm that is closely related to the canine parasite *Oslerus* (= *Filaroides*) *osleri;* some researchers consider the genus *Anafilaroides* containing the species *rostratus* to be distinct from the genus *Oslerus* (e.g., Seneviratna, 1959a). *Oslerus rostratus* has been reported from cats in the United States, Pacific Islands, Southern Europe, and the Middle East (Gerichter, 1949; Ash, 1962; Seneviratna, 1959b; Juste et al., 1992). The adult males are about 28–37 mm long, and the adult females are 48–64 mm long. The worms are typically found in the bronchial submucosa. The vulva in the female is located just anteriad to the anus. The larvae found in the feces are 335 to 412 μm long and have a tail that is similar to that of *Oslerus osleri*. The life cycle has been described by Gerichter (1949) and Klewer (1958), who found that the larvae were capable of development in slugs. Seneviratna (1959b) showed that the third-stage larvae from slugs are capable of infecting mice that serve as paratenic hosts. Similarly, he found that week-old chickens could be infected as paratenic hosts and that the larvae recovered from these chicks were capable of infecting a cat. Larvae were first observed in the cat 78 days after being given infective-stage larvae. There have been no studies on the signs of infection with this parasite or on the effectiveness of different treatments.

REFERENCES

Ash LR. 1962. Helminth parasites of dogs and cats in Hawaii. J Parasitol 48:63–65.

Gerichter CB. 1949. Studies on the nematodes parasitic in the lungs of Felidae in Palestine. Parasitology 39:251–262.

Juste RA, Garcia AL. Mecia L. 1992. Mixed infestation of a domestic cat by *Aelurostrongylus abstrusus* and *Oslerus rostratus*. Ang Parasitol 33:56–60.

Klewer HL. 1958. The incidence of helminth lung parasites of *Lynx rufus rufus* (Schabes) and the life cycle of *Anafilaroides rostratus* (Gerichter). J Parasitol 44:29.

Seneviratna P. 1959a. Studies on the family Filaroididae Schulz, 1951. J Helminthol 33:123–144.

Seneviratna P. 1959b. Studies on *Anafilaroides rostratus* Gerichter, 1949 in cats. II. The life cycle. J Helminthol 33:109–122.

Gurltia paralysans Wolffhügel, 1933

In 1933, Dr. Kurt Wolffhügel erected a new genus, *Gurltia,* and species, *paralysans,* to contain a worm causing paralysis in a cat in Chile that was named after Dr. Ernst Friedrich Gurlt. In this paper several cases of paraparesis in cats caused by this worm are described. Wolffhügel believed that the natural host of this parasite was the small wild cat, *Felis guigna.*

The worms as described by Wolffhügel had females that were 20 to 23 mm long with a maximum width of about 0.15 mm. The vulva was posterior near the anus. The males were about half as long and wide as the females and had a distinct bursa. The eggs passed by the female were about 60 μm long and about 45 μm wide. The eggs were undeveloped when laid, but eggs containing 16-celled embryos were found in the blood. Wolffhügel was unable to find any larva in the blood or feces of the feline host.

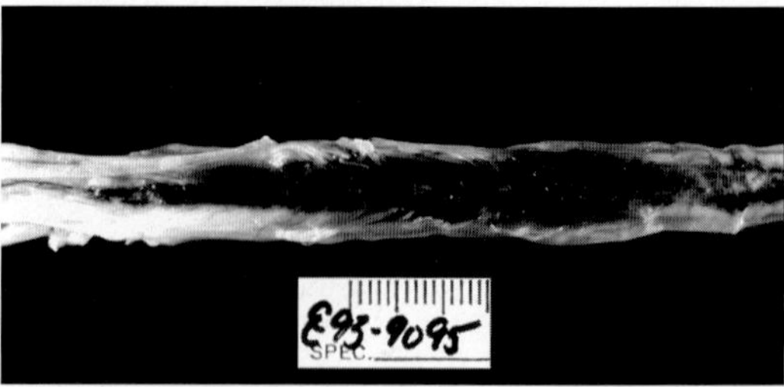

Fig. 4.35. *Gurltia paralysans.* Spinal cord of a cat that presented with signs of paralysis.

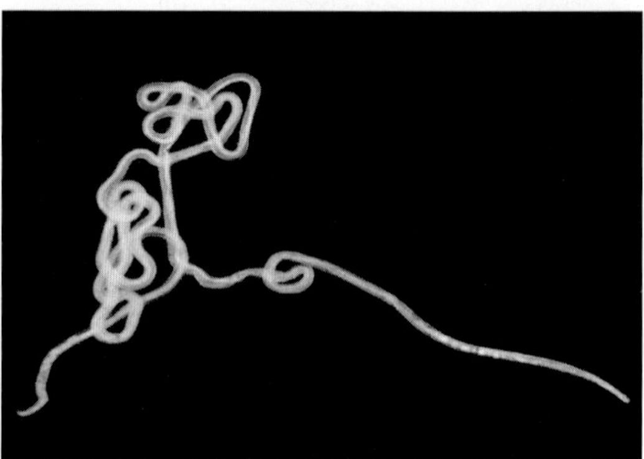

Fig. 4.36. *Gurltia paralysans.* Worm removed by Dr. M. Georgi from the lesion depicted in Fig. 4.35.

In 1993, a cat was presented to the clinic at Cornell that ultimately died with serious neurologic signs following progressive hind limb weakness leading to total fecal and urinary incontinence. At necropsy, a lesion was seen in the spinal cord with extensive hemorrhage between L3 and L6 (Fig. 4.35). The lesion contained a metastrongyle that appears to have characteristics consistent with *Gurltia paralysans* (Figs. 4.36 and 4.37). Unfortunately, the lack of a male in the material teased from the lesion made it impossible to verify the identity of the worm (Fig. 4.38).

REFERENCES

Wolffhügel K. 1933. Paraplegia cruralis parasitaria felis, causada por *Gurltia paralysans* nov. gen., n. sp. (nematodes). Rev Chilena Hist Nat 37:190–192.

Wolffhügel K. 1934. Paraplegia cruralis parasitaria durch *Gurltia paralysans* nov. gen. nov. sp (Nematoda). Ztsch Infektionskr Haustiere 48:28–47.

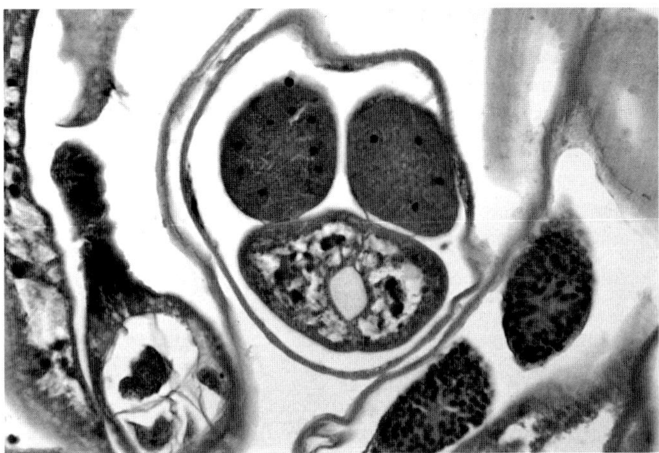

Fig. 4.37. *Gurltia paralysans.* Section through lesion depicted in Fig. 4.35 showing mature adult female worm.

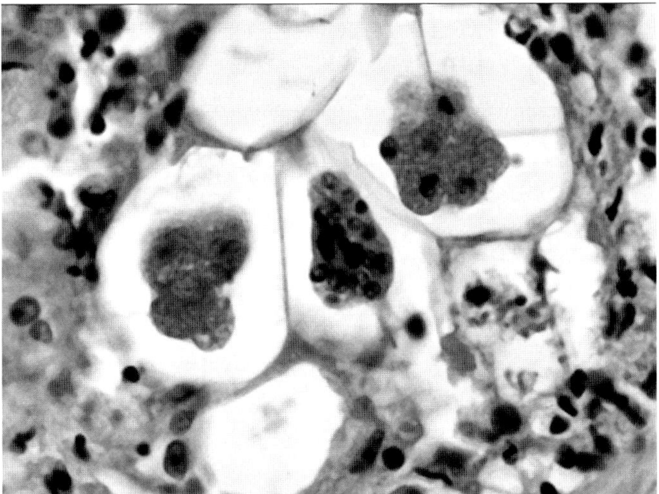

Fig. 4.38. *Gurltia paralysans.* Section through lesion in spinal cord depicted in Fig. 4.35 showing eggs in various stages of embryonation.

ASCARIDIDA

The Ascaridida is an order of nematodes that includes *Toxocara cati,* which is one of the most common parasites of the cat around the world. The ascarids are characterized by being cream-colored, robust, and relatively long as nematodes go, being 1 to more than 10 cm in length. Other characteristics of this group include (1) the presence of three large fleshy lips on the anterior end of the adult worms and (2) the eggshells produced by the species found in terrestrial hosts that typically are thick shelled and very resistant to environmental extremes. The adults of these nematodes are typically found in the small intestine, and it is there that adults of the two most common species in the cat, *Toxocara cati* and *Toxascaris leonina,* are found. Both of these species are capable of infecting cats through paratenic hosts, such as mice, where the larvae are found in the musculature. Unfortunately, the dog roundworm, *Toxocara canis,* is also capable of persisting in paratenic hosts, and on rare occasions this host can be the cat. One other ascarid parasite of the cat, *Lagochilascaris,* is a strange worm that is a rare parasite of extraintestinal sites in humans. In the cat, this worm has been found in the stomach as well as in fistulated abscesses in various locations, usually with tracts that drain into the gastrointestinal tract so that eggs are passed in the feces.

Toxocara cati (Schrank, 1788) Brumpt, 1927

Etymology

Toxo = arrow + *cara* = head, and *cati* for the domestic cat.

Synonyms

Ascaris cati Schrank, 1788; *Fusaria mystax* Zeder, 1800; *Ascaris felis* Gmelin, 1790; *Belascaris mystax* (Zeder, 1800) Leiper, 1907; *Belascaris cati* (Schrank, 1788) Brumpt, 1922; *Toxocara mystax* (Zeder, 1800) Stiles and Brown, 1924.

History

A detailed history of the name *Toxocara cati* is presented by Sprent (1956). Goeze (1782) illustrated a worm from the cat that had large cervical alae. Schrank (1788) gave this worm the name *Ascaris cati.* Zeder (1800) introduced the specific name *mystax* for this parasite. The name *cati* designated by Schrank, who referred to the figure of Goeze, therefore has priority. The genus *Toxocara* was established by Stiles and Hassall (1905), and *Lumbricus canis,* the dog ascarid, identified by Werner (1782) was considered the type species. Leiper (1907) created the genus *Belascaris* with *Ascaris mystax* of Zeder (1800) as the type species, and Leiper differentiated the genus *Belascaris* from other ascarids by the ventriculus located at the base of the esophagus. Stiles and Brown (1924) confirmed that the genus *Toxocara* had priority over *Belascaris,* and they created the name *Toxocara mystax* for the *Toxocara* species of the cat. However, the name designated by Schrank has priority over that of Zeder, and therefore, the common *Toxocara* of the cat is *Toxocara cati* (Schrank, 1788) Brumpt, 1927.

Geographic Distribution

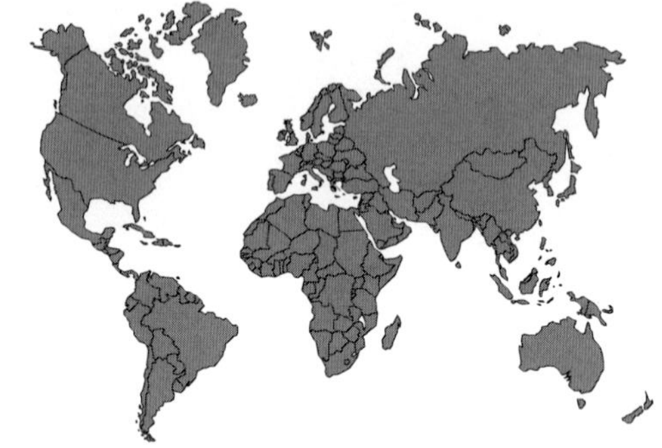

Fig. 4.39.

Toxocara cati is a cosmopolitan parasite of the domestic cat and probably one of the most commonly encountered parasites. Some prevalences that have been recorded in different countries include Germany, 45 percent of 155 cats (Schuster et al., 1997); France, 31 percent of 129 cats (Petithory et al., 1996); Tasmania, 89 percent of 39 cats (Milstein and Goldsmid, 1997); Taipei, 42 percent of 95 cats (Fei and Mo, 1997); Japan, 18.2 percent of 1,064 cats (Oikawa et al., 1991); Somalia, 28 percent of 50 cats (Gadale et al., 1988–89); South Africa, 11 percent of 1,502 cats (Baker et al., 1989). Interestingly, a survey of 188 feral cats from the Northern Territory of Australia revealed that only 1 percent of the cats were infected with *Toxocara cati* (O'Callaghan and Beveridge, 1996). In a careful study of the parasites occurring in litters of kittens in Germany, *Toxocara cati* infections were found in 54 litters of the 70 litters of free-ranging farm cats that were examined (Beelitz et al., 1992). On the other hand, of 30 litters of house cats, where both the mothers and kittens had received anthelmintic treatment between weeks 2 and 12 after delivery, only 1 litter had an infection with *Toxocara cati.* As with many other helminth infections, juvenile cats are more likely to maintain patent infections,

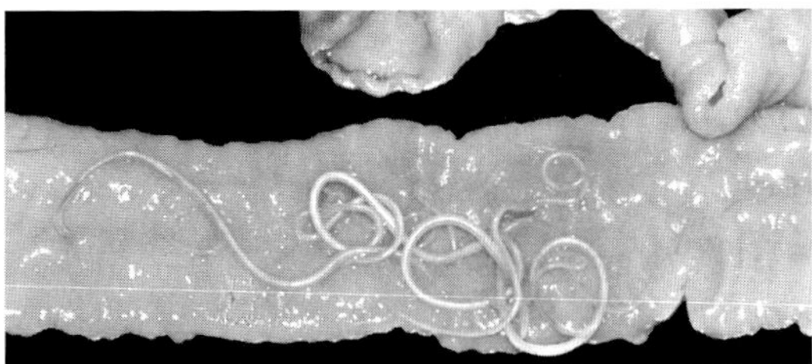

Fig. 4.40. ***Toxocara cati.*** Adult worms on the mucosa of the small intestine of a naturally infected cat.

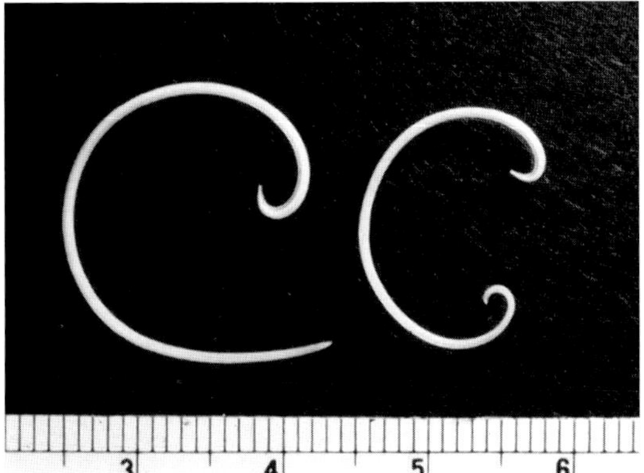

Fig. 4.41. *Toxocara cati.* Adult female and male worms, formalin fixed. Notice that the female tail is straight while both the head and the tail of the male are curled.

as shown in the survey performed in South Africa where the overall prevalence of infection with *Toxocara cati* was 11 percent but the prevalence in juvenile cats was 41 percent.

Location in Host

Adults are found in the small intestine.

Parasite Identification

The adult worms are brownish yellow or cream colored to pinkish and have a length of up to 10 cm (Figs. 4.40 and 4.41). Warren (1971) reported males as 3 to 7 cm long and females as 4 to 10 cm long. The adults have distinct cervical alae that are short and wide, giving the anterior end the distinct appearance of an arrow. The esophagus is about 2 percent to 6 percent of the total body length and terminates in a glandular ventriculus that is about 0.3 to 0.5 mm long. The vulva of the female occurs about 25 percent to 40 percent of the body length behind the anterior end. The spicules of the males range from 1.7 to 1.9 mm in length. The egg measures 65 μm by 77 μm and has the pitted eggshell typical of the eggs of this genus of ascaridoid (Fig. 4.42). The pits on the eggs of *Toxocara cati* are smaller than the pits observed on the eggs of *Toxocara canis*.

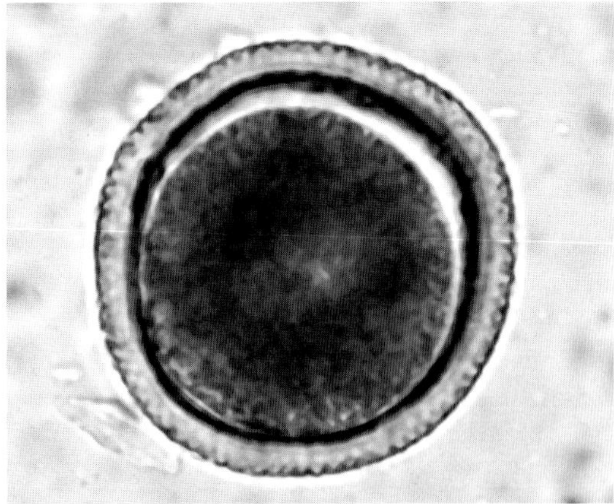

Fig. 4.42. *Toxocara cati.* Egg passed in the feces of an infected cat. The egg has the thick shell and dimpled surface.

Life Cycle

The adult worms live in the small intestine, and the female produces eggs that are passed in the feces of the cat. The egg is typically passed containing a single cell, and after a period of time in the environment, two molts occur within the eggshell to produce the infective third-stage larva. There has been considerable debate about the number of molts occurring within the eggshell of the ascaridoid parasites, but the majority of evidence seems to be that for certain genera, anyway, the infective stage is the third-stage larva.

Sprent (1956) described the details of the development of *Toxocara cati* in the feline host following oral infection with eggs and with mice that had been orally infected with eggs. After having infected kittens with 10,000 embryonated eggs, Sprent found that the larvae were found to migrate away from the alimentary tract before commencing development. By 3 days after infection, larvae were found in the liver and lungs, and there were also larvae present in the stomach wall. Five days after infection, there were larvae in the lungs, tracheal washings, and stomach wall (Figs. 4.43 and 4.44). After the tenth day of infection, many larvae were in the lungs and stomach wall, and a number of larvae began to be recovered from the muscle tissues of the cat. The larvae that made the liver-lung migration and returned to the stomach wall via the trachea then underwent considerable growth. When kittens were fed mice that had been infected with 10,000 infective eggs of *Toxocara cati,* almost all larvae were found to complete their development without undergoing a liver-lung migration, and larvae were only rarely recovered from the muscle tissues of the infected cats. The larva that escaped from the eggshell measured 0.31 mm to 0.42 mm in length. Within the stomach wall of the cat, the larvae grew from 0.4 mm to about 1.3 mm in total length. The molt from third-stage to fourth-stage larvae occurred when the larvae measured 0.999 to 1.235 mm in length, and during this molt there was a marked reorganization of the mouth with the development of the lips characteristic of ascaridoid nematode. The fourth-stage larvae were found in the stomach contents, intestinal wall, and intestinal contents. In egg-infected cats, fourth-stage larvae were first observed at 19 days after infection, whereas, in mouse-infected cats, fourth-stage larvae were first observed at 10 days after infection. When the fourth-stage larvae reached a length of about 1.5 mm, it was possible to readily distinguish males from females on the morphology of the genital rudiment, and as growth progressed, the spicules of the males became evident, and the tails of the males were broader than the tails of the female larvae. The molt from the fourth to the fifth larval or young adult stage occurred within the intestinal lumen when the larvae were 4.3 to 6.5 mm in length. The fourth-stage larvae could be distinguished from the young adults of similar length by the much thinner cuticular annulations on the adults. The smallest female observed by Sprent to have eggs in its uterus was 5.5 mm long. Eggs were first observed in the feces beginning 56 days after the infection of the cats. Dr. Stoye (personal correspondence with Dr. J.C. Parsons) reported that in four older cats that were each experimentally infected with 500 embryonated eggs, the observed prepatent period was 38, 39, 39, and 40 days.

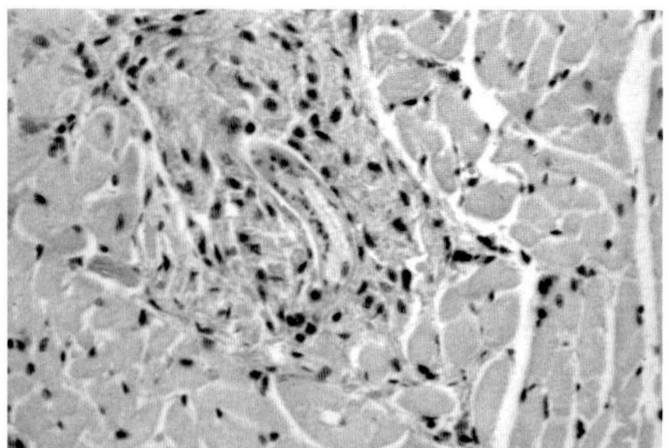

Fig. 4.43. *Toxocara cati.* This histologic section is through a larva that was discovered as an incidental finding in a cat at necropsy.

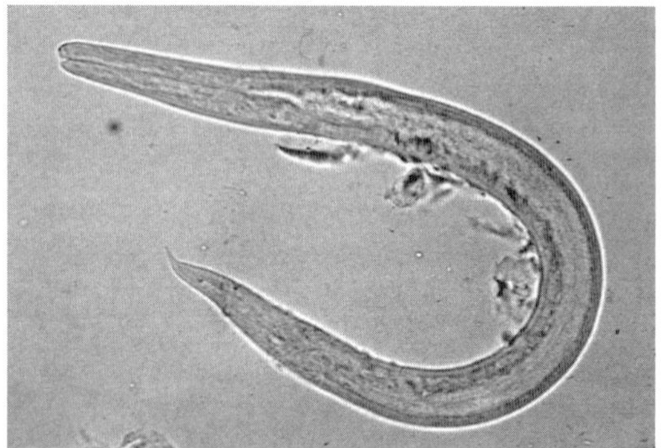

Fig. 4.44. *Toxocara cati.* Larva teased by Dr. M. Georgi from the heart tissue of the cat described in Fig. 4.43.

Sprent (1956) looked for the possibility of transplacental transmission from the queen to the developing kittens. During the last 4 weeks of gestation, a pregnant queen was given three inocula of 10,000 embryonated eggs. Larvae were not recovered from the tissues of the kittens examined 3 or 4 days after birth.

Swerczek et al. (1971) showed that transmammary transmission commonly occurs with *Toxocara cati.* The examination at birth of 78 kittens from 20 queens that were naturally infected with *Toxocara cati* and 14 kittens from 7 queens that were experimentally infected with 300 to 2,000 eggs of *Toxocara cati* per day from day 2 to 56 prepartum revealed no larvae in the organs of the kittens when they were examined. When 12 kittens were examined 15 to 22 days after natural delivery from 5 queens that had been orally infected with 2,000 eggs of *Toxocara cati* for 1 to 10 days prepartum, a total of 7,959 larvae were recovered, with most of the larvae being recovered from the gastrointestinal tract. Larvae were not found in the 5 littermates (one from each litter) that had not been allowed to nurse. These authors also found larvae in the mammary glands and milk of these 5 queens. The authors went on to show that 19 kittens that were derived by caesarean section from 6 queens and raised colostrum-free to maturity remained free of infections with *Toxocara cati.*

Paratenic hosts are probably routinely involved in the life cycle of *Toxocara cati.* The larvae are capable of persisting in the tissues of cockroaches (Sprent, 1956), earthworms (Okoshi and Usui, 1968), mice (Schön and Stoye, 1986), chickens (Okoshi and Usui, 1968; Sprent, 1956), dogs (Sprent, 1956), and lambs (Sprent, 1956). Beaver et al. (1952) showed that both *Toxocara cati* and *Toxocara canis* produced lesions in white mice that were similar to those observed in human cases of visceral larva migrans (Fig. 4.45). Fülleborn (1921), Höeppli et al. (1949), and Sprent (1952) showed that the larvae undergo a liver-lung migration in the mouse before they settle down in the musculature or brain. Sprent (1956) reported that the larvae of *Toxocara cati* are found mainly in the somatic musculature. Nichols (1956) described the morphology of the larva of *Toxocara cati* and differentiated it from the larva of *Toxocara canis;* he found the major difference in the two worms is the diameter of the body, which is narrower in *Toxocara cati* (*Toxocara cati* larvae have a width that is never greater than 18 μm, while the larvae of *Toxocara canis* are typically 18 μm wide or wider.)

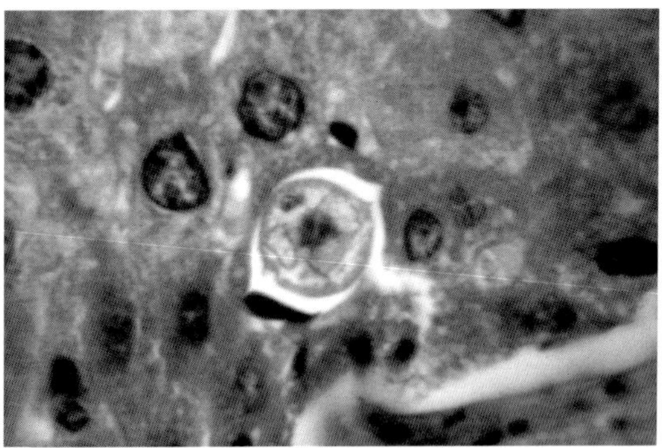

Fig. 4.45. *Toxocara cati.* Section through the liver of a mouse that has been experimentally infected with *Toxocara cati* by the feeding of eggs containing infective larvae. Note the large lateral cords characteristic of these larvae in tissue sections.

Clinical Presentation and Pathogenesis

Kittens infected with *Toxocara cati* often show no clinical signs due to the infection. However, it is generally considered that kittens are capable of displaying signs similar to puppies with moderate worm burdens (i.e., a pot-bellied appearance and a general failure to thrive). On occasion it may be possible to palpate thickened intestines.

Aoki et al. (1990) reported on a 7-year-old domestic male cat that had anorexia, vomiting, and an enlarged abdomen. A laparotomy revealed an adult *Toxocara cati* in the abdominal cavity and a gastric ulcer that had perforated the stomach wall. The next day, acute perforations of the stomach again occurred, and during a second surgery, the two new gastric perforations were repaired, and four adult *Toxocara cati* were removed from the abdominal cavity. Unfortunately, the cat died during recovery from the second emergency surgery. It is difficult to determine whether the ascarids were the cause of the gastric perforation or were simply migrating into lesions from some other underlying cause.

Swerczek (1969) and Swerczek et al. (1970), in studies on the comparative development of medial hypertrophy of the pulmonary arteries in cats with various helminth infections, described the hematological changes in experimentally infected cats. Swerczek reported that eosinophils may increase to up to 35 percent of the total leukocytes. Also, he found that anemia was typically not associated with the infection. Swerczek concluded that "*T. cati* migration produces severe lesions and is probably the most common cause of MHPA [medial hypertrophy of the pulmonary vessels] in cats." This was observed in cats that had received doses of eggs over a period of several weeks; cats that received a single inoculum had less severe lesions that were similar to those of cats receiving weekly inocula. After a single inoculum, the lungs of cats would appear to have slight lesions 10 weeks after infection and would appear normal 14 weeks after infection. The histopathological lesions of MHPA can be quite remarkable, with media of the arteries becoming very enlarged. A potential cause of the observed hypertrophy of the media of the vessels is allergy with histamine release (Weatherly and Hamilton, 1984) or pulmonary hypertension (Mecham et al. 1987).

Treatment

Treatment of gastrointestinal infections with *Toxocara cati* is relatively straightforward. Approved compounds include piperazine, pyrantel, dichlorvos, febantel formulated with praziquantel, and pyrantel formulated with praziquantel. Ridley et al. (1991) reported on the use of pyrantel pamoate for the treatment of *Toxocara cati* in kittens experimentally infected by feeding the tissues of infected mice; at 20 mg of base per kilogram body weight, this compound was 100 percent effective in removing the worms from these kittens. Febantel formulated with praziquantel has been shown to be 100 percent effective in removing *Toxocara cati* from cats (Corwin et al., 1984). Ivermectin (200 µg/kg body weight) has been found to remove adult *Toxocara cati* from infected cats (Kirkpatrick and Megella, 1987). Milbemycin oxime (500 µg/kg body weight) is also effective against the adults of *Toxocara cati.* Selamectin (Revolution™) is labeled for the treatment of *Toxocara cati* in a single topical dose.

There has been no work published on the pharmacologic prevention of the transmammary transmission of larvae. It would seem, based on work with the transplacentally migrating larvae of *Toxocara canis* in dogs, that it might be possible to prevent transmammary transmission by the targeted administration of fenbendazole or ivermectin at just prior to or just at the time of delivery. However, it does not appear that any method has been tested for this purpose.

Epizootiology

Cats can be infected by one of three routes: by the ingestion of infective eggs, by the ingestion of a mouse containing larvae, or by the transmammary infection of kittens. Dubinski et al. (1995) showed that small mammals were probably a major means by which the infection is maintained in cats that are allowed to hunt in Slovakia. Webster and MacDonald (1995) examined a total of 510 brown rats from 11 rural farms in the United Kingdom, and they found that 15 percent of the rats were infected with the larvae of *Toxocara cati.* Sprent (1956) infected chickens and recovered 10 larvae from only one of the four chicks that were given 5,000 eggs. Okoshi and Usui (1968) successfully infected a number of chickens by feeding them the eggs of *Toxocara cati* and verified that the eggs were present in the tissues of the chickens for at least 3 months after infection. However, there has been very little effort to determine the role of birds in the transmission of *Toxocara cati* between cats. Sprent did recover larvae from earthworms that were fed embryonated eggs. Takahashi et al. (1990) showed that cockroaches that ingest the eggs of *Toxocara canis* were capable of excreting the eggs in their feces over a 2-day period and that these eggs were still infectious; they went on to postulate that such insects can serve as vectors as they carry the eggs from fecal-contaminated areas to foodstuffs. It is unclear how often cats are infected by the ingestion of infective eggs. Uga et al. (1996) examined the defecation habits of cats around three sandlots in public parks in Nishinomiya City, Japan, through the use of video recordings. Around 4 to 24 cats visited each of the sandlots. Cats were observed to defecate in the three sandlots a total of 961 times in about 4.5 months while dogs were only observed to defecate in these areas 11 times. One of the three sandlots was highly contaminated with the eggs of *Toxocara,* and 8 of the 12 cats that visited this site were observed to be infected with *Toxocara cati.* However, although cats are routinely visiting such sites, there is no information on whether they are becoming infected from these types of sources. In a survey of 181 cats for *Toxocara* in Dublin (O'Lorcain, 1994), no cats less than 4 weeks old were found to be infected; the highest prevalence of infection was found in cats between 12 and 24 weeks of age, and there was no apparent difference in the prevalence of infection between male and female cats. The work of Beelitz et al. (1992) would suggest that, as expected, the levels of transmission are greatest between free-ranging cats and lowest when cats receive adequate veterinary care.

Hazards to Other Animals

Toxocara cati will infect small mammals, but there is little information on the effects on these hosts. The experimental infection of mice with the eggs of *Toxocara cati*, unlike those of *Toxocara canis*, seldom results in ocular lesions in the infected mice (Olson and Petteway, 1971). Prociv (1986) showed that in guinea pigs the larvae of *Toxocara cati* tend to remain in the musculature rather than moving into the nervous system as do the larvae of *Toxocara canis*.

Roneus (1963, 1966) presented rather convincing evidence that the larvae of *Toxocara cati* were capable of being a cause of "white-spot" disease in the liver of pigs. He showed that following infections with *Toxocara cati, Toxocara canis, Parascaris equorum*, or *Ascaris suum*, white spots appear on the surface and deep in the livers of infected pigs between a few days and up to 2 months after infection. Thus, although the disease induced in swine may not be great, there is the potential for economic loss due to this parasite if pigs are infected.

Hazards to Humans

There have been reports of humans who have passed the adult stage of *Toxocara cati*. To quote from Dr. Paul C. Beaver (Beaver et al., 1984), "Intestinal infections with adult-stage *T. canis* and *T. cati* have been reported in humans, but such records are generally unreliable. In the few cases in which an adult worm was unquestionably passed from the anus or mouth of a child, circumstances have suggested that the worm had been ingested as a mature or, more likely, an immature adult, having been taken from the feces or vomitus of an infected dog or cat (von Reyn et al., 1978)." More recently, however, Eberhard and Alfano (1998) described four cases of children in the United States who were infected with adult *Toxocara cati*. Again, it was highly possible that the children had acquired their infections by ingesting adult worms.

It is believed that most cases of human larval toxocariasis (visceral larva migrans) are due to the larvae of *Toxocara canis*. In histological sections, the larvae of *Toxocara cati* are slightly smaller, having a diameter of 15 to 16 μm, than the larvae of *Toxocara canis*, which have a diameter of 18 μm or greater. Thus, when biopsies are performed, it is often possible to identify the larvae that are observed as the larvae of *Toxocara canis*. There have been two cases where the larvae of *Toxocara cati* have been identified in the tissues of humans. Karpinski et al. (1956) reported on two cases of human larval toxocariasis, and in a 2-year-old boy from Philadelphia, they found small larvae in a liver biopsy that they thought were *Toxocara cati* due to their small size and the boy being in contact with an infected kitten and without any known canine contact. In a second case, Schoenfeld et al. (1964) found numerous larvae that were identified as *Toxocara cati* in the brain tissue of a 5-year-old girl who died after entering a hospital in Israel, comatose with fever and convulsions. Nagakura et al. (1990) reported on a serological procedure for differentiating *Toxocara canis* and *Toxocara cati* in a gel diffusion method and examined sera from 17 cases of suspected toxocariasis. Virginia et al. (1991) examined the sera of 54 children from Recife City, Brazil, who had signs of tropical eosinophilia syndrome. They found 21 sera that were positive for antibodies to *Toxocara*, and after further analysis of sera from 6 of these children, they identified 1 that they thought was due to *Toxocara cati*.

Control/Prevention

The control of *Toxocara cati* in the cat still depends on the diagnosis of infection and treatment of cats shedding eggs. The monthly preventative approved for cats, ivermectin at 24 μg/kg, does not significantly reduce the number of adult *Toxocara cati*; Blagburn et al. (1987) showed that a dose of 300 μg/kg of ivermectin administered subcutaneously was required for the removal of adult *Toxocara cati*. Thus, at this time, it is necessary to prevent cats from obtaining infections by the ingestion of infective eggs or mammalian paratenic hosts.

Transmammary transmission should be presumed to occur, and kittens should be considered as infected.

REFERENCES

Aoki S, Yamagami T, Saeki H, Washizu M. 1990. Perforated gastric ulcer caused by *Toxocara cati* in a cat. J Jap Vet Med Assoc 43:207–210.

Baker MK, Langge L, Verster A, Van der Plaat S. 1989. A survey of helminths in domestic cats in the Pretoria area of Transvaal, Republic of South Africa. Part 1. The prevalence and comparison of burdens of helminths in adult and juvenile cats. JSAVA 60:139–142.

Beaver PC, Snyder CH, Carrera GM, Dent JH, Lafferty JW. 1952. Chronic eosinophilia due to visceral larva migrans. Pediatrics 9:7–19.

Beaver PC, Jung RC, Cupp EW. 1984. Clinical Parasitology. 9th edition. Philadelphia, Pa: Lea and Febiger. 825 pp.

Beelitz P, Gobel E, Gothe R. 1992. Species spectrum and incidence of endoparasites of cat litters and their mothers under different maintenance conditions in southern Germany. Tierarztliche Praxis 20:297–300.

Blagburn BL, Hendrix CM, Lindsay DS, Vaughan JL. 1987. Anthelmintic efficacy of ivermectin in naturally parasitized cats. Am J Vet Res 48:670–672.

Brumpt. 1922. Precis de Parasitologie. 3rd Edition. Paris. 1216 pp.

Corwin RM, Pratt SE, McCurdy HD. 1984. Anthelmintic effect of febantel/praziquantel paste in dogs and cats. Am J Vet Res 45:154–155.

Dubinski P, Havasiova-Reiterova K, Petko B, Hovorka I. 1995. Role of small mammals in the epidemiology of toxocariasis. Parasitology 110:187–193.

Eberhard ML, Alfano E. 1998. Adult *Toxocara cati* infections in U.S. children: report of four cases. Am J Trop Med Hyg 59:404–406.

Fei CY, Mo KM. 1997. Survey for endoparasitic zoonoses in stray dogs and cats in Taipei City. J Chin Soc Vet Sci 23:26–33.

Fülleborn F. 1921. Ascarisinfecktion durch Verzsehren eingekapselter Larven und über gelungene intrauterine Ascarisinfektion. Arch Schiff Tropenhyg 25:367–375.

Gadale OI, Capelli G, Ali AA, Poglayen G. 1988–89. Intestinal helminths of cats. First reports in Somalia. Boletinol Scientifico della Facolta di Zootecnia e Veterinaria, Universita Nazionale Somala, Somalia, pp 813–824.

Gmelin JF. 1790. Caroli a Linne. Systema Naturae, vol 1. Editio decima tertia. J Fred Gmelin, pt. 6 (Vermes), pp 3021–3910.

Goeze JAE. 1782. Versuch einer naturgeschichte der eingeweidewürmer thierischer köroer. Xi + 471 pp, 44 (35) pls, Blankenburg.

Höeppli R, Feng C, Li F. 1949. Histological reactions in the liver of mice due to larvae of different ascaris species. Peking Nat Hist Bull 2:119–132.

Karpinski FE, Evcerts-Suarez EA, Sawitz WG. 1956. Larval granulomatosis (visceral larva migrans). AMAJ Dis Child 92:34–40.

Kirkpatrick CE, Megella BA. 1987. Use of ivermectin in treatment of *Aelurostrongylus abstrusus* and *Toxocara cati* infections in a cat. JAVMA 190: 1309–1310.

Leiper RT. 1907. Two new genera of nematodes occasionally parasitic in man. Br Med J 1:1296–1298.

Mecham RP, Whitehouse LA, Wrenn DS, Parks WC, Griffin GL, Senior RM, Crouch EC, Stenmark KR, Voelkel NF. 1987. Smooth muscle-mediated connective tissue remodeling in pulmonary hypertension. Science 237:423–426.

Milstein TC, Goldsmid JM. 1997. Parasites of feral cats from southern Tasmania and their potential significance. Aust Vet J 75:218–219.

Nagakura K, Kanno S, Tachibana H, Kaneda Y, Ohkido M, Kondo K, Inoue H. 1990. Serologic differentiation between *Toxocara canis* and *Toxocara cati*. J Infect Dis 162:1418–1419.

Nichols RL. 1956. The etiology of visceral larva migrans. I. Diagnostic morphology of infective second-stage *Toxocara* larvae. J Parasitol 42:349–391.

O'Callaghan MG, Beveridge I. 1996. Gastro-intestinal parasites of feral cats in the Northern Territory. Trans Roy Soc South Austral Incorp 120:175–176.

Oikawa H, Mikazuki K, Kanda M, Nakabayashi T. 1991. Prevalence of intestinal parasites with faecal examination in stray cats collected in the western area of Japan from 1983 to 1990. Jap J Parasitol 40:407–409.

Okoshi S, Usui M. 1968. Experimental studies on *Toxascaris leonina*. VI. Experimental infection of mice, chickens, and earthworms with *Toxascaris leonina, Toxocara canis,* and *Toxocara cati*. Jap J Vet Sci 30:151–166.

O'Lorcain P. 1994. Epidemiology of *Toxocara* spp. In stray dogs and cats in Dublin, Ireland. J Helminthol 68:331–336.

Olson LJ, Petteway MB. 1971. Ocular nematodiasis: results with *Toxocara cati* infected mice. J Parasitol 57:1365–1366.

Petithory JC, Vandemeulebroucke E, Jousserand P, Bisognani AC. 1996. Prevalence of *Toxocara cati* in cats in France. Bull Soc Fran Para 14:79–84.

Prociv P. 1986. *Toxocara pteropodis, T. canis,* and *T. cati* infections in guinea pigs. Trop Biomed 3:97–106.

Ridley RK, Terhune KS, Granstrom DE. 1991. The efficacy of pyrantel pamoate against ascarids and hookworms in cats. Vet Res Comm 15:37–44.

Roneus O. 1963. Parasitic liver lesions in swine experimentally produced by visceral larva migrans of *Toxocara cati*. Acta Vet Scand 4:170–196.

Roneus. 1966. Studies on the aetiology and pathogenesis of white spots in the liver of pigs. Acta Vet Scand 7:1–139.

Schoenfeld AE, Ghitnic E, Rosen N. 1964. Granulomatous encephalitis due to *Toxocara* larvae (visceral larva migrans). Harefuah 66:337–339.

Schön J, Stoye M. 1986. Pränatale und galaktogene infektionen mit *Toxocara mystax* Zeder 1800 (Anisakidae) bei der maus. J Vet Med 33:397–412.

Schrank F. 1788. Verzeichnisse der bisher hindläglich bekannten engeweiderwürmer nebst einer abhandlung über ihnre anverwandtschaften. 116 pp.

Schuster R, Kaufmann A, Hering S. 1997. Investigations on the endoparasite fauna of the domestic cat in eastern Brandenburg, Germany. Berliner und munchener Tierarztliche Wochenschrift 110: 48–50.

Sprent JFA. 1952. On the migratory behavior of the larvae of various *Ascaris* species in white mice. J Inf Dis 92:114–117.

Sprent JFA. 1956. The life history and development of *Toxocara cati* (Schrank 1788) in the domestic cat. Parasitology 46:54–77.

Stiles CW, Brown G. 1924. Nomenclature of the nematode genera *Belascaris* 1907, and *Toxascaris* 1907, and *Toxocara* 1905. J Parasitol 11:92–93.

Stiles CW, Hassall A. 1905. The determination of generic types, and a list of round-worm genera, with their original and type species. Bull no 79, Bur Anim Ind USDA, pp 1–150.

Swerczek TW. 1969. Medial hyperplasia of the pulmonary arteries of cats. University Microfilms International, Ann Arbor, Mich. 199 pp.
Swerczek TW, Nielsen SW, Helmboldt CF. 1970. Ascariasis causing pulmonary arterial hyperplasia in cats. Res Vet Sci 11:103–105.
Swerczek TW, Nielsen SW, Helmboldt CF. 1971. Transmammary passage of *Toxocara cati* in the cat. Am J Vet Res 32:89–92.
Takahashi J, Uga S, Matsumura T. 1990. Cockroach as a possible transmitter of *Toxocara canis*. Jap J Parasitol 39:551–556.
Uga S, Minami T, Nagata K. 1996. Defecation habits of cats and dogs and contamination by *Toxocara* eggs in public park sandpits. Am J Trop Med Hyg 54:122–126.
Virginia P, Nagakura K, Ferreira O, Tateno S. 1991. Serologic evidence of toxocariasis in northeast Brazil. Jap J Med Sci Biol 44:1–6.
von Reyn CF, Roberts TM, Owen R, Beaver PC. 1978. Infection of an infant with an adult *Toxocara cati* (Nematoda). J Pediatr 93:247–249.
Warren G. 1971. Studies on the morphology and taxonomy of the genera *Toxocara* Stiles, 1905 and *Neoascaris* Travasso, 1927. Zool Anz 185:393–442.
Weatherly AJ, Hamilton JM. 1984. Possible role of histamine in the genesis of pulmonary arterial in cats infected with *Toxocara cati*. Vet Rec 114:347–349.
Webster JP, MacDonald DW. 1995. Parasites of wild brown rats (*Rattus norvegicus*) on UK farms. Parasitology 111:247–255.
Werner PCF. 1782. Vermium intestinalium brevis expositionis continuatio. 28 pp. Leipzig.
Zeder JHG. 1800. Erster nachtrag zur naturgeschichte der eingeweiderwürmer, mit Zufässen und Anmerkungen herausgegeben. 320 pp.

Toxocara canis

In 1988, Parsons et al. described a case of disseminated granulomatous disease in a cat that was caused by the larvae of the dog roundworm, *Toxocara canis* (Fig. 4.46). The larvae were identified on the basis of morphology, being greater in diameter than the 17 µm of the larvae of *Toxocara cati* when they appear in tissues. This cat had been housed for 19 days in the research facilities of the School of Veterinary Medicine in Madison, Wisconsin, and had been considered normal except for being noted as pyrexic throughout the 19-day period. At necropsy, the cat was found to have well-delineated, raised, gray-to-white nodules that were up to 4 mm in diameter within the cortical parenchyma of the kidneys and within the epicardium and myocardium of both ventricles (Fig. 4.47). Lesions were also noted on the liver, lungs, spleen, diaphragm, and intestinal serosa. Upon histologic examination, the nodules were found to be large eosinophilic granulomas that contained larvae of *Toxocara canis*. In the lungs, medial hypertrophy of the pulmonary vessels was noted along with severe eosinophilic endarteritis (Fig. 4.48). Similar lesions have been noted in cats experimentally infected with *Toxocara canis* (Bhowmick, 1964; Parsons et al., 1989; Swerczek, 1969). In experimentally infected cats, peak eosinophil counts occurred at 25 to 39 days after infection, and challenge infections prolonged the period of increased eosinophilia. In some cats, eosinophils were noted to be up to 50 percent of the circulating white blood cells.

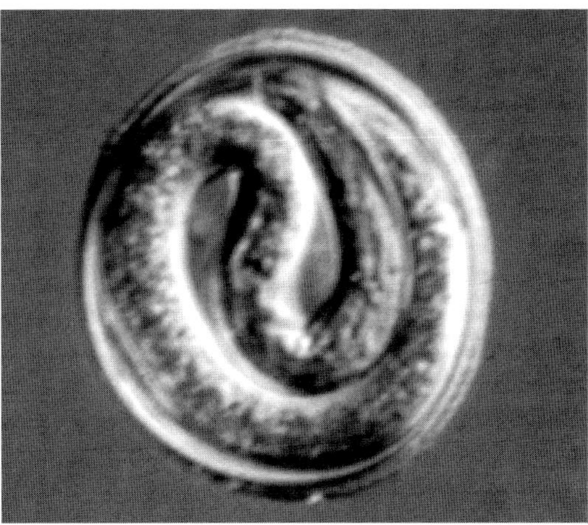

Fig. 4.46. *Toxocara canis.* Embryonated egg containing a third-stage infective larva.

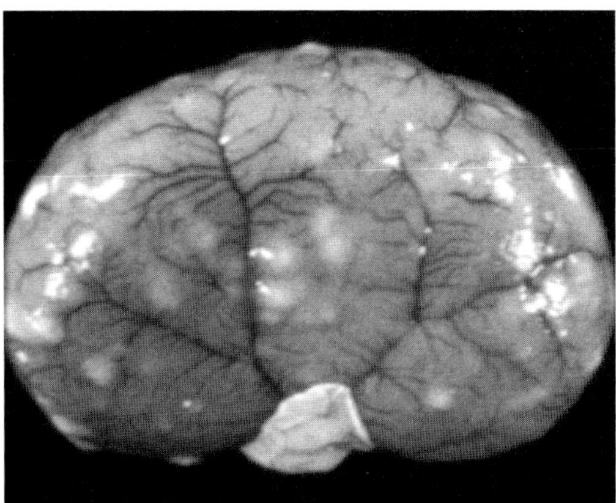

Fig. 4.47. *Toxocara canis.* Kidney of an infected cat showing the large eosinophilic granulomas that develop around the larvae of the canine species in this host.

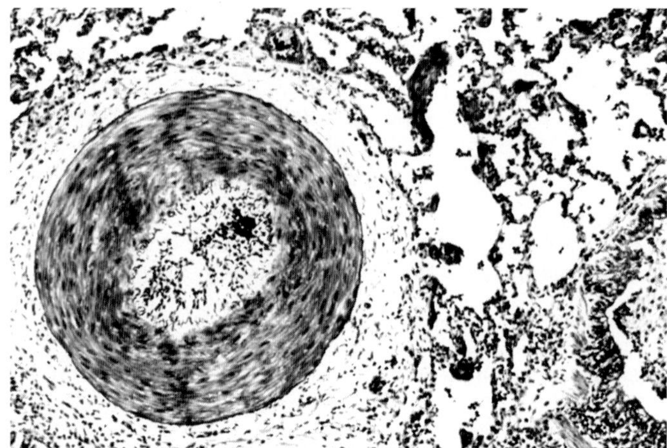

Fig. 4.48. *Toxocara canis.* Medial hypertrophy of the pulmonary vessels of a specific-pathogen-free cat necropsied 39 days after being experimentally infected with this canine ascarid. Note the highly thickened medial layer of the pulmonary vessel.

Lee et al. (1993) reported that the necropsy of 55 cats around Kuala Lumpur, Malaysia, revealed that 15 of these cats were infected with adults of the genus *Toxocara.* They stated that 12 of the cats were infected with *Toxocara cati,* 3 were infected with *Toxocara canis,* and 3 had mixed infections of *Toxocara cati* and *Toxocara canis.*

REFERENCES

Bhowmick DK. 1964. Deiträge zu dem problem der wanderweg der askaridenlarven (*Ascaris lumbricoiudes* Linné 1758 und Toxocara canis Wener 1782) im experimentellen und natüralichen Wirt. Zeitschrift für Parasitenkunde 24:121–168.

Lee CC, Cheng NY, Bohari Y. 1993. *Toxocara canis* from domestic cats in Kuala Lumpur. Trop Biomed 10:79–80.

Parsons JC, Bowman DD, Grieve RB. 1988. Disseminated granulomatous disease in a cat caused by larvae of *Toxocara canis.* J Comp Pathol 99:343–346.

Parsons JC, Bowman DD, Grieve RB. 1989. Pathological and haematological responses of cats experimentally infected with *Toxocara canis* larvae. Int J Parasitol 19:479–488.

Swerczek TW. 1969. Medial hyperplasia of the pulmonary arteries of cats. University Microfilms International, Ann Arbor, Mich. 199 pp.

Toxascaris leonina (von Linstow, 1902) Leiper, 1907

Etymology

Tox = arrow + *Ascaris,* along with *leonina* referring to the lion.

History

Sprent (1959) summarized the history and taxonomy of this species. In brief, von Linstow (1902) redescribed one of the ascaridoid parasites of the lion as *Ascaris leonina.* In 1809, Rudolphi had described the ascaridoid of the lion as *Ascaris leptoptera* and presented a description of a worm with narrow cervical alae. Unfortunately, in 1819, Rudolphi described some additional worms from the lion as *Ascaris leptoptera,* but these worms were probably *Toxocara cati.* Thus, Sprent suggested that the name *leptoptera* be suppressed. The genus name *Toxascaris* was created by Leiper (1907) to contain the arrow-headed ascaridoids with smooth eggs, and *Ascaris leonina* von Linstow, 1902, was designated at the type species.

Geographic Distribution

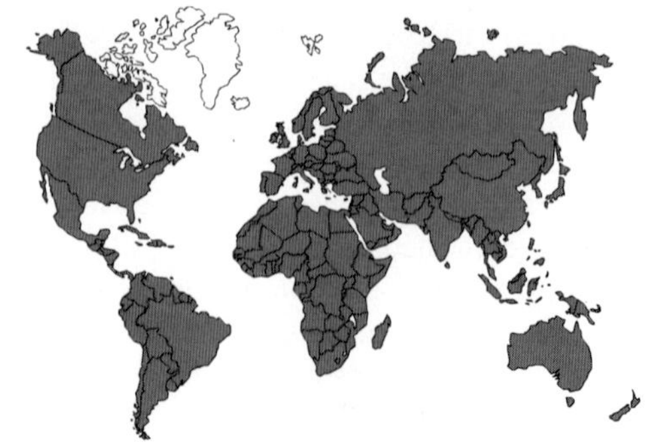

Fig. 4.49.

Sprent and Barrett (1964) summarized much of the work on the prevalence of *Toxascaris leonina* in cats up to that time. It had been reported in 1 percent to 5 percent of cats from North America, 2 percent to 20.5 percent of cats in Europe, and 11 percent of cats in Ceylon. In 1996, 82 percent of farm cats in Oxfordshire in the United Kingdom were reported to be shedding eggs of this parasite (Yamaguchi et al., 1996); Nichol (1981) found only 1.1 percent of 92 feral cats in London to be infected with *Toxascaris leonina.* In Scotland (McColm and Hutchison, 1980), 3 of 72 stray cats were found to harbor infections with *Toxascaris leonina.* In Belgium (Vanparijs et al., 1991) 60 percent of 30 stray cats had fecal samples containing the eggs of *Toxascaris leonina.* The necropsy of 567 stray cats in Moscow revealed *Toxascaris leonina* in only 1.1 percent of the animals (Vereta, 1986). In Australia, fecal examination of 376 cats revealed eggs of *Toxascaris leonina* in 3.7 percent of the cats (Moore and O'Callaghan, 1985). Okoshi and Usui reported that *Toxascaris leonina* had been previously reported from cats in Taiwan and Sakhalin but had not been reported or probably seen in Japan until the early 1960s (Okoshi and Usui, 1967). In their paper, they described five cases of feline toxascariasis, in which all cases were from imported cats (the sources were Hawaii or California) or from cats that had been housed with these imported cats. It was their belief that *Toxascaris leonina* infection in cats did not occur previously in cats in that country.

Location in Host

The adult worms are found in the small intestine of the cat. Dubey (1969) confirmed earlier findings of larvae in the musculature of infected mice beginning 7 days after infection where they appear after a lung migration. The larvae remained in the musculature where they encysted and were found in the muscles for up to 60 days after infection (Okoshi and Usui, 1968) and probably persisted in the muscles of the carcass for much longer periods.

Parasite Identification

The adults of *Toxascaris leonina* are cream colored to pinkish worms (Fig. 4.50). The females are around 6 to 15 cm in length, and the males are around 5 cm long (Okoshi and Usui, 1967). The cervical alae of *Toxascaris leonina* adults are longer and considerably narrower than those of *Toxocara cati,* and the head of *Toxascaris leonina* resembles a spear, while the head of *Toxocara cati* resembles an arrowhead (Sprent and Barrett, 1964). There is no ventriculus at the base of the esophagus of *Toxascaris leonina* (Sprent, 1968). The vulva of the female *Toxascaris leonina* is about one-third of the length of the body behind the anterior end of the worm (Okoshi and Usui, 1967). The males of *Toxascaris leonina* have tails that gradually taper to a point. The eggs of *Toxascaris leonina* have a smooth shell, are ellipsoid, and have dimensions of about 70 μm by 80 μm (Fig. 4.51); Warren (1971) reported ex utero eggs as having dimension of 54 by 74 μm. The eggs of *Toxascaris leonina* typically appear lighter colored or clearer and more translucent than the eggs of *Toxocara cati.*

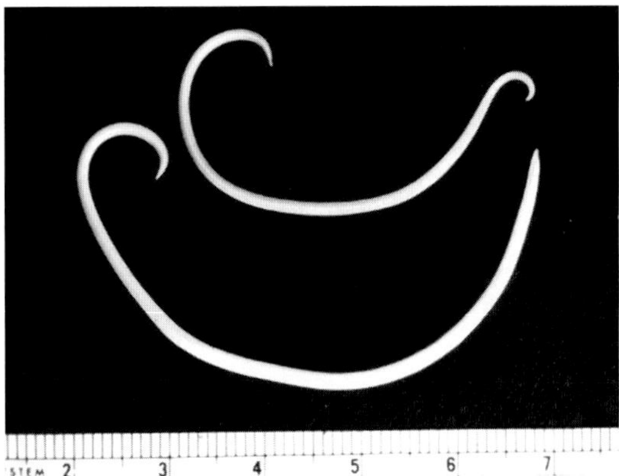

Fig. 4.50. *Toxascaris leonina.* Adult male and female fixed in 10 percent formalin. Note that the male tail curls in the opposite direction as the head.

Life Cycle

The adult male and female worms live in the small intestine, and the female produces eggs that are passed in the feces. Wright (1935) found that the eggs of *Toxascaris leonine,* unlike those of *Toxocara canis,* were capable of developing to the infective stage at 37°C. Okoshi and Usui (1967) reported that around 95 percent of eggs contained infective-stage larvae after 4 days of culture at 25°C. They reported that at 17° to 22°C it took 6 days for 99 percent of the eggs to reach the

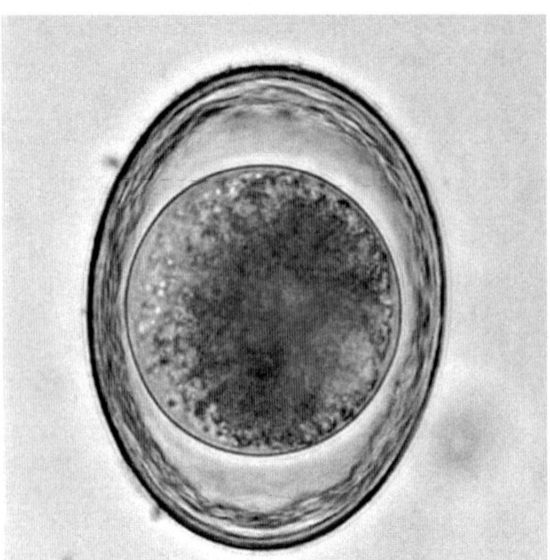

Fig. 4.51. *Toxascaris leonina.* Egg passed in feces. Notice the thick shell that has a smooth exterior.

infective stage; at 30°C it took 5 days, and confirming the work of Wright, they found that 97 percent of the eggs reached the infective stage when held at 37°C. (Also, as reported by Wright for *Toxocara canis,* the eggs of *Toxocara canis* and *Toxocara cati* failed to develop at 37°C.) When the eggs of *Toxascaris leonina* were held at 40°C, they were incapable of completing their development, and even after being returned to 25°C after 24 hours at 40°C were incapable of developing. For the purpose of this discussion, it is considered that the infective-stage larva is a third-stage larva. The tail of the infective-stage larva bears a small knob reminiscent of the small terminal projection present on the tail of the third-stage larva of *Lagochilascaris* species (see below).

Sprent (1959) and Okoshi and Usui (1968) examined the development of *Toxascaris leonina* in cats infected by the feeding of embryonated eggs. After ingestion of the eggs, Sprent found that the larvae entered the wall of the small intestine. Within the intestinal wall the larvae grew to a length of 0.5 to 0.6 mm. Then either within the wall or after returning to the intestinal lumen, the larvae molted to the fourth stage. The fourth-stage larvae grew to lengths around 6 mm, which was when the molt to the adult stage occurred. Adults appeared as early as 28 days after infection, but eggs did not appear in the feces until 74 days after infection. Okoshi and Usui found that adults were first present sometime between day 22 to day 48 after infection, and in their infections, the prepatent period was 62 to 63 days. Both Sprent and Okoshi and Usui were unable to infect cats with eggs recovered from naturally infected dogs, but Petrov and Borovkova (1959) had been successful in infecting cats and dogs with eggs recovered from foxes.

Sprent (1959) also showed that cats could be infected with the larvae present in experimentally infected mice. Infections with larvae in mice proved to be less successful than with eggs. Cats were capable of supporting larvae of both canine and feline isolates when murine tissues containing these larvae were ingested. Okoshi and Usui (1968) were also capable of recovering developing larvae of the canine isolates when the source of infection was infected murine tissue.

Sprent noted that a characteristic feature of infections with *Toxascaris leonina* in the cat was the persistence of small fourth-stage larvae in the intestinal wall and lumen of the cats for weeks to months after infection. These persistent fourth-stage larvae followed infections with either eggs from feces or larvae from mice.

Toxascaris leonina is capable of persisting in the tissues of paratenic hosts. Wright (1935) found that when eggs were fed to mice, rats, guinea pigs, and dogs, larvae could be recovered from the intestinal wall and lumen 10 days after infection and that these larvae grew to a length of around 0.7 mm. Matoff (1949) studied the migration of *Toxascaris leonina* in experimentally infected mice and found that although many of the larvae became encysted in the wall, some larvae also underwent either a hepato-pulmonary or a lympho-pulmonary migration and that these larvae later appeared in an encysted state in the musculature of the head and carcass. In 1965, Matoff and Komandarev reported on additional studies where they found considerable larvae in the abdominal cavities of mice after infection but with the majority in the wall of the intestine 10 days after infection. Okoshi and Usui (1968) fed the eggs of *Toxascaris leonina* to mice, chickens, and earthworms. In mice, they found that the larvae were mainly in the intestine up to 7 days after infection and that the number then decreased gradually and that the larvae disappeared from this organ by the fifteenth day after infection. They found small numbers of larvae in the liver and lungs between the sixth and the thirteenth day after infection, with larvae then being found in the carcass (39.6 percent of the inoculum was recovered from the carcass on the twelfth day after infection). Living larvae were recovered from the carcass 3 months after inoculation. The larvae in the mice grew to about 0.87 mm in total length. In chickens, they found that the majority of larvae stayed in the intestinal wall, although a very few were recovered from the lungs, liver, carcass, and brain. In earthworms, no larvae were recovered, although larvae of *Toxocara canis* and *Toxocara cati* were recovered from similar earthworms infected using the same methods. When larvae from mice were harvested from the carcasses 20 to 60 days after infection and orally inoculated into additional mice, larvae were again recovered from the carcasses of these mice. Larvae harvested from the carcass of one of the second group of mice 10 days after infection were infective to other mice. Thus, these authors showed that the infection could be perpetuated in mice by the repeated passage of the larvae. Dubey (1969) found larvae in the musculature of mice beginning 10 days after infection. The lungs of the mice killed 6 to 10 days after infection were found to have numerous hemorrhages and to contain larvae. Dubey however found few larvae in the liver and increasing numbers of larvae in the mesenteric lymph glands and concluded that the larvae underwent a migration to the lungs via the thoracic lymphatic duct. Prokopic and Figallova (1982) examined the migration of larvae in white mice for up to 135 days after infection. They found that although some larvae could be found in the intestinal wall during the entire observation period, the majority of larvae were present beginning 10 days after infection in the intercostal muscles and the muscles of the legs. They found larvae in the lungs as early as 4 days after infection. Karbach and Stoye (1982) found that mouse pups were not infected transplacentally if the mothers were infected while pregnant. When mothers were infected with 1,000 larvae, the largest number of larvae was recovered from the pups if the mother was infected at parturition. However, infection of pups occurred when mothers were infected 20, 40, 80, or even 160 days prior to parturition. Bowman (1987) described the morphology of the larvae of *Toxascaris leonina* recovered from murine tissues 32 days after infection.

Clinical Presentation and Pathogenesis

There appear to be few clinical signs associated with *Toxascaris leonina* infections in cats. For puppies, Okoshi and Usui (1967) described the clinical signs of digestive disturbance, allotriophagia, and unthriftiness, but they saw no such signs in adult dogs. These same authors reported no such signs for the experimentally infected cats. Fei et al. (1986) reported a fatal case of toxascariasis accompanied by bloody diarrhea in a kitten in Taiwan.

Treatment

The treatment of cats for adults of *Toxascaris leonina* is relatively straightforward. Approved compounds include toluene, dichlorvos, pyrantel, piperazine, and febantel. Mebendazole at 30 mg per kilogram body weight for 2 days is efficacious (Cardini et al., 1997). A single dose of nitroscanate at 50 mg per kilogram body weight was 100 percent effective in removing the adults of *Toxascaris leonina* from dogs (Boray et al., 1979).

Epizootiology

Cats can become infected by ingesting either the eggs or rodents that contain the larvae of *Toxascaris leonina*. The common occurrence of *Toxascaris leonina* in felids in zoological gardens would suggest that the egg is a very common source of infection. The ability of the egg to embryonate at a wide range of temperatures and to become infective as rapidly as 4 days after being passed in the feces would suggest that infective eggs can rapidly build up in the environment. Although the eggs will not develop if held at 40°C, Okoshi and Usui (1968) showed that if eggs were exposed to −15°C for up to 40 days and then returned to 25°C, almost all would complete the development to the infective stage. Thus, freezing temperatures had very little effect on their ability to later develop.

Surveys of soil samples in cities have revealed the presence of the eggs of *Toxascaris leonina*. Pfeiffer (1983) reported eggs present in 4 of 334 soil samples collected from public gardens and children's playgrounds in Vienna, Austria. Veteta and Mamykova (1984) found eggs in 5 of 311 soils collected in preschool institutions in Moscow. Rapic et al. (1983) reported eggs of *Toxascaris leonina* in 10 of 100 urban soil samples collected in Zagreb, Yugoslavia. Bettini and Canestri-Trotti (1978) reported the presence of these eggs in 10 of 204 samples collected in Bologna, Italy. The most common egg in almost all these surveys was the egg of *Toxocara* species, but there was no attempt to distinguish between the eggs of *Toxocara canis* and *Toxocara cati*.

Hazards to Other Animals

Toxascaris leonina is commonly found in canids and felids. This parasite very commonly infects large cats in zoos (Abdel-Rasoul and Fowler, 1979, 1980) and can be a common problem also in foxes. Sprent (1959) gave a host list that includes the arctic fox, jackal, dingo, dog, coyote, wolf, arctic wolf, cape hunting dog, raccoon dog, gray fox, American red fox, Indian fox, cheetah, lynx, bobcat, puma, ocelot, serval, snow leopard, jaguar, tiger, lion, leopard, and other species. As in the cat host, usually there is little disease associated with the infections in other animals. Fenbendazole has been approved for use in the treatment of helminth infections in many zoo animals and would be a very good candidate for treating infections with this parasite.

Hazards to Humans

The biology of this parasite in mice is such that it would be expected that humans would acquire infections with the larvae of this parasite by ingesting eggs in contaminated soil or on contaminated foodstuffs; however, except for the report of Beaver and Bowman (see below), there have been no reports of larval toxascarisis in humans. There are, however, two rather strange accounts of human parasitism with adult *Toxascaris leonina*. When Leiper (1907) described the genus *Toxascaris*, he included humans in the host list. Grinberg (1961) reported on a 39-year-old male patient who complained of having chronic osteomyositis for the last 15 years. He presented with an abscessed area on the right shin with five tracts and a dark brown scab covering an inflamed area. Squeezing the area produced two worms. The patient had also brought 20 more worms with him to the clinic and stated that he had extracted another 50 worms 5 years previously. The worms were 6 to 7 cm long, whitish pink, with 3 lips. The female had a rounded tail, and the male had awl-shaped spicules. The females contained smooth-shelled eggs. Based on the morphology of the 20 worms supplied by the patient and the two extracted in the clinic, a diagnosis of *Toxascaris leonina* was made.

Beaver and Bowman (1984) described a larva from the eye of a child in East Africa that was about twice the size of *Toxascaris* larvae observed in tissues. However, no species of the other similar ascaridoid genus, *Baylisascaris*, are known to occur in Africa, and it was considered that it was possible that this larva represented a case of infection with a larva of some *Toxascaris* species.

Control/Prevention

Due to the rapid development of the eggs of *Toxascaris leonine*, control in catteries requires excellent cleanliness. Abdel-Rasoul and Fowler (1980) reported finding viable eggs on the floors of cages and in the drinking water of a number of large felids in zoos in California. It also appears that older animals can be reinfected with this parasite; thus, regular deworming of cats is a must for good control to be obtained. Because domestic cats can probably also acquire their infections from hunting, if cats do go outside, it would be expected that they could be infected from either soil or the ingestion of infected rodents. Thus, regular examination of the feces of such cats for parasites would be a prudent approach to control. The amount of ivermectin in Heartgard for cats (a maximum dose of 24 μg per kilogram body weight) is probably not sufficient for 100 percent control of the infections with this parasite.

REFERENCES

Abdel-Rasoul K, Fowler M. 1979. Epidemiology of ascarid infection in captive carnivores, pp 105–106a. Philadelphia, Pa: Am Assoc Zoo Vet.

Abdel-Rasoul K, Fowler M. 1980. An epidemiologic approach to the control of ascariasis in zoo carnivores, pp 273–277. Berlin: Akademie Verlag.

Beaver PC, Bowman DD. 1984. Ascaradoid larva (Nematoda) in the eye of a child in Uganda. Am J Trop Med Hyg 33:1272–1274.
Bowman DD. 1987. Diagnostic morphology of four larval ascaridoid nematodes that may cause visceral larva migrans: *Toxascaris leonina, Baylisascaris procyonis, Lagochilascaris sprenti,* and *Hezametra leidyi.* J Parasitol 73(6):1198–1215.
Bettini P, Canestri-Trotti G. 1978. Parasitic contamination by dog and cat faeces in soil and sand-boxes in public gardens and schools in Bologna. Parassitologia 20 (1/3):211–215.
Boray PA, Strong MB, Allison JR, von Oreilli M, Sarasin G, Gfeller W. 1979. Nitroscanate: a new broad spectrum anthelmintic against nematodes of cats and dogs. Austral Vet J 55(2):45–53.
Cardini G, Grassotti G, Papini R, Valle VC. 1997. Anthelmintic activity and tolerance of a new micronized mebenzole pharmaceutical formulation (Lendue) for treating intestinal helminthoses in dogs and cats. Veterinaria (Cremona) 11:125–131.
Dubey JP. 1969. Migration and development of *Toxascaris leonina* larvae in mice. Trop Geogr Med 21:214–218.
Fei ACY, Jeng CR, Lai RY. 1986. *Toxascaris leonina* infection in a kitten. J Chinese Soc Vet Sci 12(1): 61–63.
Grinberg AI. 1961. Rare cases of *Toxascaris leonina* and *Toxocara mystax* in man. Med Parasitol 30:626.
Karbach G, Stoye M. 1982. Zum vorkommen pränataler und galaktogener infektionen mit *Toxascaris leonina.* Vet Med 29:219–230.
Leiper RT. 1907. Two new genera of nematodes occasionally parasitic in man. Br Med J 1:1296–1298.
Matoff K. 1949. Experimentelle Untersuchungen über die wanderung von *Toxocara canis, Toxascaris leonina* und *Neoascaris vitulorum* (Bulgarisch). God Vet Med 25:593–659.
Matoff K, Komandarev S. 1965. Comparative studies on the migration of the larvae of *Toxascaris leonina* and *Toxascaris transfuga.* Parasitenkunde 25:538–555.
McColm AA, Hutchison WM. 1980. The prevalence of intestinal helminths in stray cats in central Scotland. J Helminth 54(4):255–257.
Moore EO, O'Callaghan MG. 1985. Helminths of dogs and cats determined by faecal examinations in Adelaide, South Australia. Aust Vet J 62:198–199.
Nichol S. 1981. Prevalence of intestinal parasites in feral cats in some urban areas of England. Vet Parasitol 9(2):107–110.
Okoshi S, Usui M. 1967. Experimental studies on *Toxascaris leonina.* I. Incidence of *T. leonina* among dogs and cats in Japan. Jap J Vet Sci 29:185–194.
Okoshi S, Usui M. 1968. Experimental studies on *Toxascaris leonina,* IV. Development of eggs of three ascarids, *T. leonina, Toxocara canis* and *Toxocara cati,* in dogs and cats. Jap J Vet Sci 30:29–38.
Parsons JC, Bowman DD, Gillette DM, Grieve RB. 1988. Disseminated granulomatous disease in a cat caused by larvae of *Toxocara canis.* J Comp Pathol 99:343–346.
Petrov AM, Borovkova AM. 1959. Tr. Vseoyuz. Inst Gelminthol 7:53–59.
Pfeiffer H. 1983. The contamination of public gardens and sand pits in Vienna with permanent stages of human pathogenic parasites of dogs and cats. Mitteilungen, Osterreichischen Gesellschaft fur Tropenmedizin und Parasitologie 5:83–87.
Prokopic J, Figallova V. 1982. Migration of some roundworm species in experimentally infected white mice. Folia Parasitologica 29:309–313.
Rapic D, Dzakula N, Stojcevic D. 1983. Contamination of public places in Zagreb with ova of *Toxocara* and other helminths. Veterinarski Arhiv 53:233–238.
Rudolphi CA. 1809. Entozoorum sive vermium intestinalium historia naturalis. Amstelaedami. 457 pp.
Sprent JFA. 1959. The life history and development of *Toxascaris leonina* (von Linstow 1902) in the dog and cat. Parasitology 49:330–371.
Sprent JFA, Barrett MG. 1964. Large roundworms of dogs and cats: differentiation of *Toxocara canis* and *Toxascaris leonina.* Aust Vet J 40:166–171.
Sprent JFA. 1968. Notes on *Ascaris* and *Toxacaris,* with a definition of *Baylisascaris* gen.nov. Parasitology 58:185–198.
Vanparijs O, Hermans, van der Flaes L. 1991. Helminth and protozoan parasites in dogs and cats in Belgium. Vet Parasitol 38:67–73.
Vereta LE. 1986. Helminths of cats in Moscow and epizootic aspects of some helminthiases. Byulleten' Vsesoyuznogo Instituta Gel'mintologii im. K.I Skryabina 42:20–26.
Veteta LE, and Mamykova OI. 1984. Contamination of the soil with Toxocara eggs in pre-school institutions of Moscow, and its sources. Med Parazytol Parazit Bolezn 3:19–22.
von Linstow OFB. 1902. Beobachtungen an neuen und bekannten Nemathelminthen. Arch Mikr Anat 60:217–232.
Warren EG. 1971. A new species of *Toxascaris* from hyenas. J Parasitol 62:171–178.
Wright WH. 1935. Observations on the life history of *Toxascaris leonina* (Nematoda: Ascaridae). Proc Helm Soc Wash 2:56.
Yamaguchi N, MacDonald DW, Passanisi WC, Harbour DA, Hopper CD. 1996. Parasite prevalence in free-ranging farm cats, *Felis silvestris catus.* Epidemiol Infect 116:217–223.

Lagochilascaris minor Leiper, 1909

Etymology

Lago (hare) + *Chil* (lip) + *Ascaris,* along with *minor* (due to being larger than the previously described *Lagochilascaris minor*).

History

In 1909, Leiper described a new genus and species of ascaridoid nematode based on worms collected from subcutaneous lesions from the necks of two human patients in Trinidad. Sprent (1971) reviewed the genus and reviewed the 11 cases that had been reported from humans in Trinidad, Surinam, Tobago, Costa Rica, and Brazil. In these cases worms had been recovered from subcutaneous tissues of the neck, from the mastoid process, from tonsils, and passed from the nose. In 1991, it was reported that there had been a total of 62 cases from around the world and that 46 of these cases were from Brazil (Costa and Weingrill, 1991). Since that time additional cases have been reported from Surinam (Oostburg, 1992), Brazil (Aguilar-Nascimento et al., 1993; Bento et al., 1993), Bolivia (Ollé-Goig, 1996), and Mexico (Vargas-Ocampo and Alvarado-Aleman, 1997). *Lagochilascaris minor* infection has been associated with fatal encephalopathy (Rosemberg et al., 1986; Orihuela et al., 1987). Volcán et al. (1992) performed experimental infections that incriminated the cat as a potential final host of this nematode.

Geographic Distribution

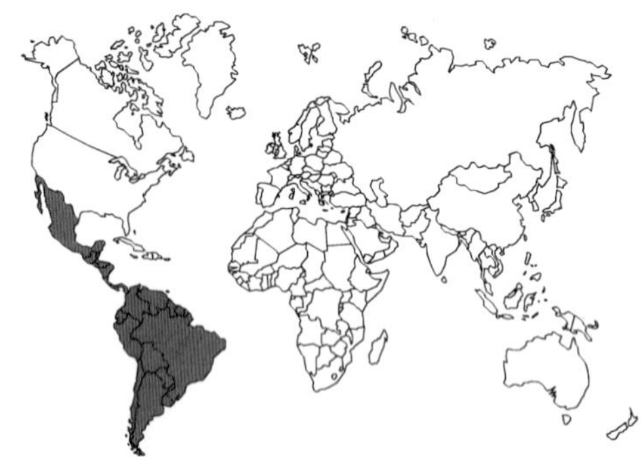

Fig. 4.52.

All reports of natural infections have been in humans. Sprent (1971) summarized 11 cases from Trinidad, Tobago, Surinam, Costa Rica, and Brazil. More recent cases have included Brazil (Bento et al., 1993); Bolivia (Ollé-Goig, 1996); Mexico (Vargas-Ocampo et al., 1997); Surinam (Oostburg, 1992); Colombia (Botero and Little, 1984); and Venezuela (Orihuela et al., 1987). Two female worms recovered from the larynx of a bush dog (*Speothos venaticus*) in Venezuela appeared to be *Lagochilascaris minor* (Volcán et al., 1991). A species of *Lagochilascaris* was also found in the larynx of an ocelot (*Felis pardalis mearnsi*) in Costa Rica (Brenes and Frenkel, 1972).

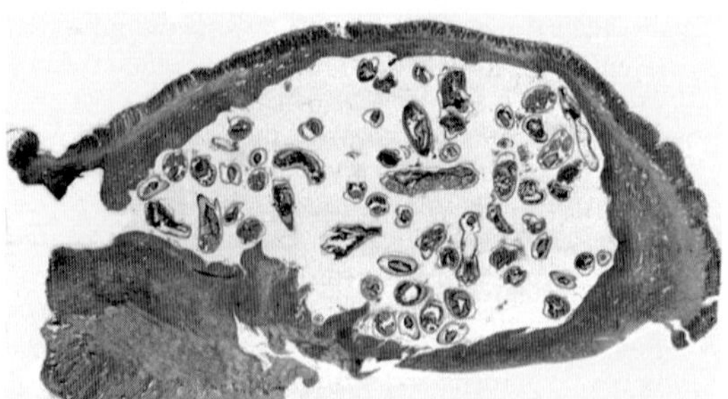

Fig. 4.53. *Lagochilascaris sprenti.* Section through the wall of the stomach of an opossum, *Didelphis virginiana,* showing the adult worms living in the typical submucosal excavation.

Location in Host

In humans, the worms have been recovered from subcutaneous abscesses in the neck, the inner ear, the mastoid process, the tonsil, and the parenchyma of the brain. In the cats that have been experimentally infected, worms have been recovered from the lungs, cervical region, larynx, pharynx, rhinopharynx, and sacs at the base of the tongue. Eggs are passed in the feces of these experimentally infected cats. In the North American opossum, *Didelphis virginiana,* the related species *Lagochilascscaris sprenti* is found in excavations under the mucosa of the stomach (Fig. 4.53)

Parasite Identification

Adults of *Lagochilascaris* tend to be rather small worms, with the total length of the males being around 17 to 20 mm and the length of the females being around 18 to 21 mm. The worms are cream colored. The vulva of the female is located at or slightly behind midbody. The lips are a distinguishing feature in that the dorsal lip and each of the subventral lips have a deep central cleft in the anterior border that gives them the typical "harelip" appearance. The anterior end of the worm is constricted between the base of the lips and the body of the worm, and there is an inflation of cuticle on the anterior of the worm behind this indentation that has been termed a collar. Extending anteriad from the collar are prolongations called interlabia, which protrude forward between the three lips. The eggs of *Lagochilascaris* are the feature that can most easily be used to distinguish *Lagochilascaris major* from *Lagochilascaris minor.* Although the eggs are similar in size (around 60 μm in diameter) and in general appearance (having a thickened brown shell), the eggs of *Lagochilascaris minor* have approximately 15 to 25 pits around the circumference, while those of *Lagochilascaris major* have approximately 33 to 45 pits around the circumference. It appears that the collar is more apparent on the anterior end of *Lagochilascaris minor* and that the lips of *Lagochilascaris minor* tend to be the same width or narrower than the collar while those of *Lagochilascaris major* appear wider than the collar.

Life Cycle

Volcán et al. (1992) and Campos et al. (1992) showed that the cat could be infected by being fed mice that had been infected for 40 days; both sets of researchers also reported that cats were not infected when simply fed eggs containing infective-stage larvae (Fig. 4.54). In the work of Volcán et al. (1992) eggs first appeared in the feces beginning 17 days after infection, and 9 of the 10 cats fed mice were positive by 40 days after infection. Campos et al. (1992) found that 9 to 20 days after cats were fed mice, adult worms were present within the esophagus, pharynx, trachea, and cervical lymph nodes. Also, in one cat that had been infected for 43 days, the lesions in the lungs and cervical region contained adults, eggs containing developing larvae, and hatched third-stage larvae in various stages of development, and Campos et al. postulated that the autoinfective cycle that is characteristic of human lesions may occur in the cat (Figs. 4.55 to 4.58).

Campos and Freire-Filha (1992) found that some of the larvae given to mice in infective eggs were capable of developing to adults within cysts in the muscles. Similar growth of larvae to adults in cysts in the muscle of mice was reported for the related species *Lagochilascaris sprenti* when eggs of this parasite of the opossum (*Didelphis virginiana*) were fed to mice. The morphology of the larva of *Lagochilascaris sprenti* that is typically found in the muscle of mice was described by Bowman (1987). The fact that *Lagochilascaris sprenti* is typically found in the stomach wall of the opossum may indicate that the final host of *Lagochilascaris minor* has actually yet to be found.

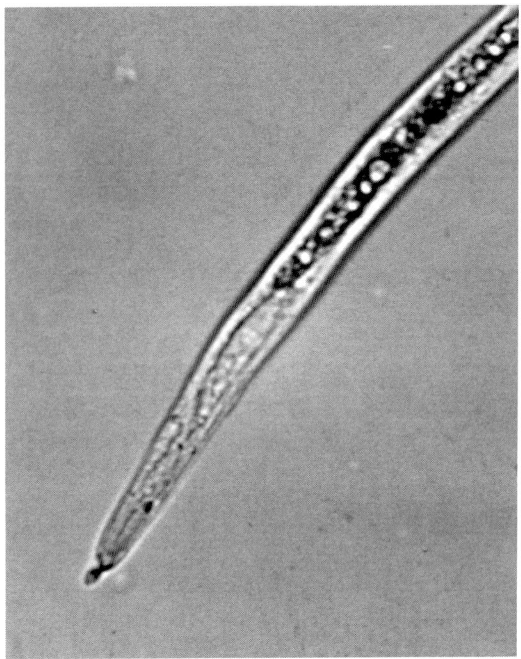

Fig. 4.54. *Lagochilascaris sprenti.* Infective third-stage larva expressed from an embryonated egg. Note the pedunculated knob at the end of the tail.

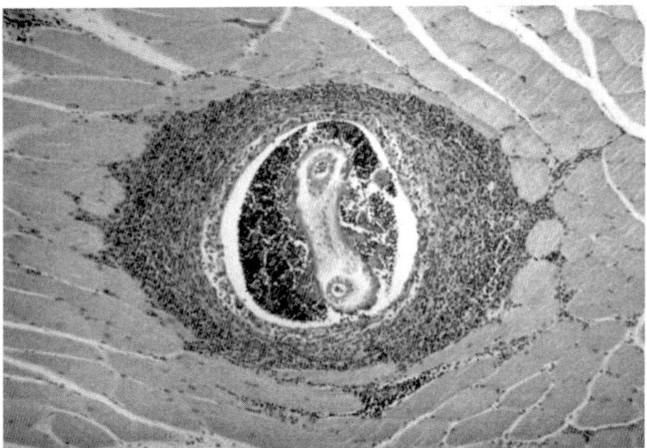

Fig. 4.55. *Lagochilascaris sprenti.* Section through the muscle tissue of an experimentally infected mouse showing the larva within an eosinophilic granuloma.

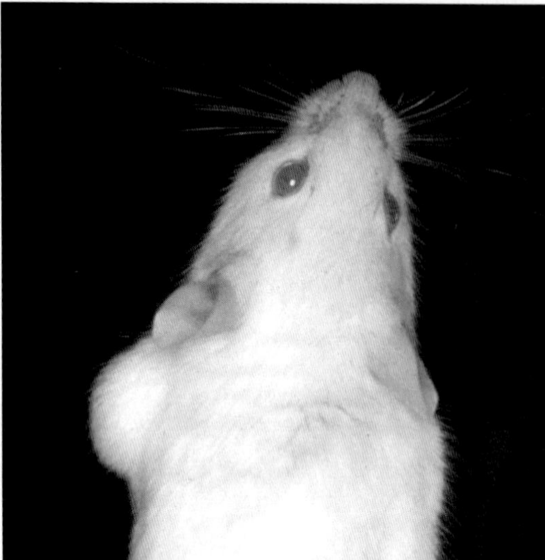

Fig. 4.56. *Lagochilascaris sprenti.* Large cyst that developed on the leg of a mouse experimentally infected with this worm.

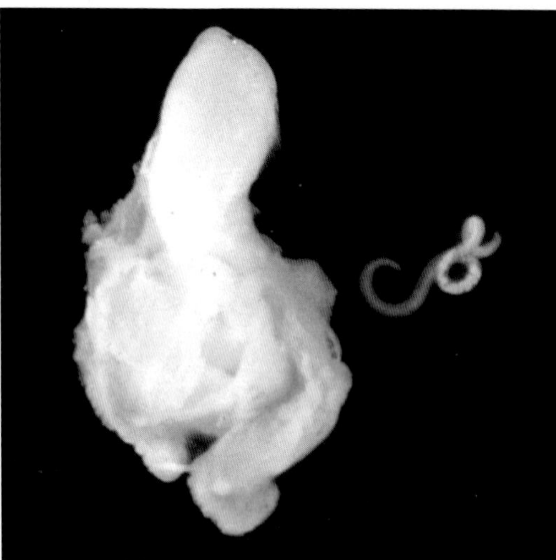

Fig. 4.57. *Lagochilascaris sprenti.* When the lesion from the leg in Fig. 4.56 was opened, it was found to contain an adult nematode.

Clinical Presentation and Pathogenesis

Cats show some signs of infection beginning 9 days after being fed experimentally infected mice (i.e., slightly decreased motor activity, weak vocalizations, and frequent sneezing) (Volcán et al., 1992). One of 10 experimentally infected cats developed a fistula in the posterior wall of the pharynx. A second cat developed destructive lesions at the base of the tongue with sacks that had inflamed walls and that contained mucus, eggs, and adult worms.

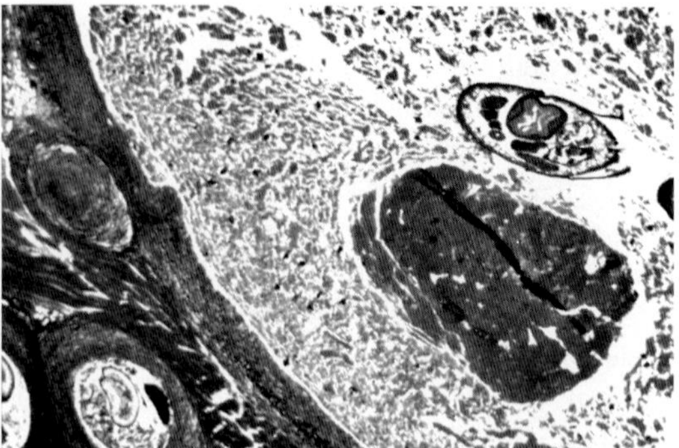

Fig. 4.58. *Lagochilascaris sprenti.* Section through a large cyst in an experimentally infected mouse showing the presence of both a large cyst containing an adult female and two sections through smaller cysts containing larvae.

Treatment

Infections of humans with *Lagochilascaris minor* have proven refractory to treatment with anthelmintics. In humans the lesions may persist, and living worms may be removed from the lesions for periods of several years. Treatment with high doses of diethylcarbamazine has apparently worked (de Leão et al., 1978) but has also been unsuccessful (Draper, 1963). Worms were recovered from one lesion for up to 10 years after the first diethylcarbamazine treatment (Sprent, 1971). Thiabendazole has worked in some cases (Oostburg, 1971) but has failed in other cases (Oostburg and Verma, 1968; Mondragon et al., 1973). Levamisole has apparently also worked on occasion (Santos, 1990) and failed on other occasions (Aguilar-Nascimento et al., 1993). Ivermectin has apparently successfully treated one human case of infection (Bento et al., 1993).

Epizootiology

The cat is probably not the normal final host of either *Lagochilascaris minor* or *Lagochilascaris major.* Interestingly, cats have not been reported as naturally infected with *Lagochilascaris minor,* but infections in cats have been described as due to *Lagochilascaris major.* The difference in pits on the circumference of the egg is a fairly easily discernable taxonomic character, suggesting that most diagnoses have been correct. Cats are probably acquiring their infections with these nematodes by the ingestion of intermediate hosts.

Hazards to Other Animals

Mice and agoutis (*Dasyprocta leporina*) have been experimentally infected by the feeding of *Lagochilascaris minor* eggs. In some mice, the larvae develop into adults in abscesses within the musculature (Campos and Freire-Filha, 1992); similar growth of adults of *Lagochilascaris sprenti* in the muscles of mice has also been described (Smith et al., 1983). The eggs passed in the feces require days to become infectious and, thus, pose no threat when passed in the feces.

Hazards to Humans

Humans are considered the host most at risk for infections with *Lagochilascaris minor.* At this time, it is unclear how humans are becoming infected. They may be obtaining their infections by the ingestion of some improperly cooked meat and mimicking a final host in a manner similar to the cat when fed the larvae of an infected mouse. On the other hand, humans developing lesions may be serving as some form of intermediate host, and like the mouse that ingests eggs that develop to the adult stage in abscesses, humans may have acquired their infections by the ingestion of eggs containing infective-stage larvae.

Control/Prevention

This infection will be prevented by preventing cats from hunting.

REFERENCES

Aguilar-Nascimento JE, Silva GM, Tadano T, Valadares-Filho M, Akiyama AMP, Castelo A. 1993. Infection of the soft tissue of the neck due to *Lagochilascaris minor.* Trans Roy Soc Trop Med Hyg 87:198.

Bento R-F, Mazza C, Motti EF, Chan YT, Guimaraes JRR, Miniti A. 1993. Human lagochilascariasis treated successfully with ivermectin: a case report. Revista do Instituto de Medicina Tropical de Sao Paulo 35:373–375.

Botero D, Little MD. 1984. Two cases of human *Lagochilascaris* infection in Colombia. Am J Trop Med Hyg 33:381–386.

Bowman DD. 1987. Diagnostic morphology of four larval ascaridoid nematodes that may cause visceral larva migrans: *Toxascaris leonine, Baylisascaris procyonis, Lagochilascaris sprenti,* and *Hexametra leidyi.* J Parasitol 73:1198–1215.

Brenes MRR, Frenkel J. 1972. Discovery of *Lagochilascaris* sp. in the larynx of a Costa Rican ocelot (*Felis pardalis mearnsi*). J Parasitol 58:978.

Campos DMB, Freire-Filha LG. 1992. Consideraçoes sobre o desenvolvimento de *Lagochilascaris minor* Leiper, 1909 em camundongos isogênicos da linhagem C57B1/6. Rev Pat Trop 21:219–233.

Campos DMB, Freire-Filha LG, Vieira MA, Paçôm JM, Moacir AM. 1992. Experimental life cycle of *Lagochilascaris minor* Leiper, 1909. Rev Inst Med Trop São Paulo 34:277–287.

Costa VR, Weingrill EC. 1991. Lagoquilascaríase. Report of the 12 Congress of the Brazilian Society of Parasitology, Encarte 13:5.

de Leão RN, Leao-Filho J, Brago-Dias L, Calheiros LB. 1978. Human infection with *Lagochilascaris minor* Leiper, 1909. A case history from Para State. Rev Inst Med Trop de Sao Paulo 20:300–306.

Draper JW. 1963. Infection with *Lagochilascaris minor.* Br Med J 1:931–932.

Leiper RT. 1909. A new nematode worm from Trinidad: *Lagochilascaris minor* sp. n. Proc Zool Soc Lond 4:35–36.

Mondragon H, Cano MR, Botero DR. 1973. Primer caso de infecciíon humana por *Lagochilascaris minor* en Colombia. Antioquia medica 23:463–464.

Ollé-Goig JE. 1996. First case of *Lagochilascaris minor* infection in Bolivia. Trop Med Int Heal 1:851–853.

Oostburg BFJ. 1971. Thiabendazole therapy of *Lagochilascaris minor* infection in Surinam, a report case. Am J Trop Med Hyg 20:580–583.

Oostburg BFJ. 1992. The sixth case of *lagochilascariasis minor* in Surinam. Trop Geogr Med 44:154–159

Oostburg BFJ, Verma AAO. 1968. *Lagochilascaris minor* infection in Surnam, a report case. Am J Trop Med Hyg 17:548–550.

Orihuela R, Botto C, Delgado O, Ortiz A, Suarez JA, Arguello C. 1987. Human *Lagochilascaris* infection in Venezuela. Description of a fatal case. Inst Med Trop, Venezuela 20:217–221.

Rosemberg S, Lopes MBS, Masuda Z, Campos R, Vieira Bressan MCR. 1986. Fatal encephalopathy due to *Lagochilascaris minor* infection. Am J Trop Med Hyg 35:575–578.

Santos VM. 1990. Relato de caso de infecçao humana por *Lagochilascaris minor.* An Bras Dermatol 65:189–192.

Smith JL, Bowman DD, Little MD. 1983. Life cycle and development of *Lagochilascaris sprenti* (Nematoda: Ascarididae) from opossums (Marsupialia: Didelphidae) in Louisiana. J Parasitol 69:736–745.

Sprent JFA. 1971. Speciation and development in the genus *Lagochilascaris.* Parasitology 62:71–112.

Vargas-Ocampo F, Alvarado-Aleman J. 1997. Infestation from *Lagochilascaris minor* in Mexico. Int J Dermatol 36:37–58.

Volcán GS, Medrano CE, Quiñones D. 1991. Infeccion natural de *Speothos venaticus* (Carnivora: Canidae) por estadios adultos de *Lagochilascaris* sp. Rev Inst Med Trop São Paulo 33:451–458.

Volcán GS, Medrano CE, Payares G. 1992. Experimental heteroxenous cycle of *Lagochilascaris minor* Leiper, 1909 (Nematoda:Ascarididae) in white mice and in cats. Mem Inst Oswald Cruz, Rio de Janeiro 87:525–532.

Lagochilascaris major Leiper, 1910

Etymology

Lago (hare) + *Chil* (lip) + *Ascaris,* along with *major* (due to being larger than the previously described *Lagochilascaris minor*).

History

Leiper (1910) originally described this worm from a lion from the area of Kilimanjaro. Durette (1963) presented the next description from a lion in the Congo. Clapham (1945) reported on specimens of *Lagochilascaris* found in an unknown host from West Africa, probably a harrier hawk in the genus *Lagochilascaris,* and it is assumed that this was a spurious finding based on the bird having ingested adult worms. In 1971, Sprent determined that specimens of *Lagochilascaris* recovered from the esophagus, stomach, and trachea of a cat in Argentina by Led et al. (1968) were *Lagochilascaris major* on the basis of the morphology of the lips and the number of pits around the circumference of the eggshell. In 1990, Armato et al. published a report of two cases of *Lagochilascaris major* in domestic cats from Petropólis, Brazil, and discussed an earlier unpublished case from a cat that occurred in São Paulo, Brazil.

Geographic Distribution

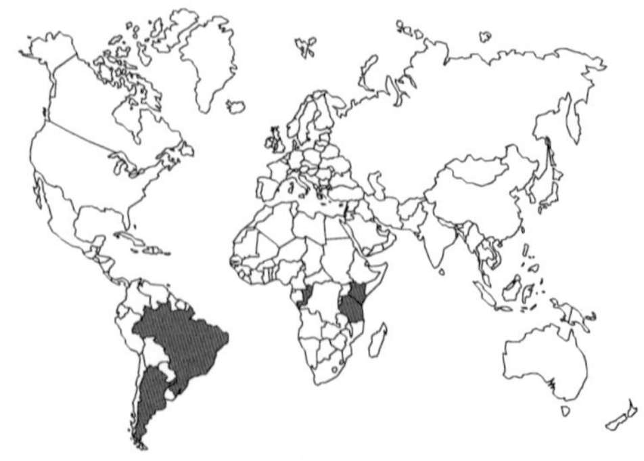

Fig. 4.59.

Described from domestic cats in Argentina and Brazil and from lions in Africa.

Location in Host

In Argentina, the worms have been described from the stomach, esophagus, and trachea (Led et al., 1968). Romero and Led (1985) also described from Argentina a fistulated abscess in the masseter muscle of a cat. In Brazil, the worms in the two cases described by Armato et al. (1990) were recovered from a fistulated abscess at the level of the first pharyngeal ring of each of the two cats. Dell'Porto and Schumaker (1988) described a case of a fistulated abscess in the neck of a cat that contained 35 adult *Lagochilascaris major.*

Parasite Identification

Adults of *Lagochilascaris* tend to be rather small worms with the total length of the males being around 17 to 20 mm and the length of the females being around 18 to 21 mm. The worms are cream colored. The vulva of the female is located at or slightly behind midbody. The lips are a distinguishing feature in that the dorsal lip and each of the subventral lips have a deep central cleft in the anterior border that gives them the typical "hare-lip" appearance. The anterior end of the worm is constricted between the base of the lips and the body of the worm, and there is an inflation of cuticle on the anterior of the worm behind this indentation that has been termed a collar. Extending anteriad from the collar are prolongations called interlabia that protrude forward between the three lips. The eggs of *Lagochilascaris* are the feature that can most easily be used to distinguish *Lagochilascaris major* from *Lagochilascaris minor.* Although the eggs are similar in size (around 60 μm in diameter) and in general appearance (having a thickened brown shell), the eggs of *Lagochilascaris major* have approximately 33 to 45 pits around the circumference, while those of *Lagochilascaris minor* have approximately 15 to 25 pits around the circumference. In the case of Romero and Led (1985) the eggs from the cat were described as having 29 to 31 pits around the circumference of the eggshell. In the case of Dell'Porto and Schumaker (1988), the eggs were described as having 21 to 31 pits around the circumference of the eggshell. It also appears that the collar is more apparent on the anterior end of *Lagochilascaris minor* and that the lips of *Lagochilascaris major* appear to be wider than the collar while those of *Lagochilascaris minor* tend to be the same width or narrower than the collar.

Life Cycle

The life cycle of *Lagochilascaris major* has not been described. It is assumed, based on work done with *Lagochilascaris sprenti* by Smith et al. (1983) and by work done with *Lagochilascaris minor* by Volcán et al. (1992), that there is a mammalian intermediate host that has mature larvae in its muscle tissues. The feline host would then become infected by the ingestion of the intermediate host. The embryonated eggs of *Lagochilascaris major* were fed to a cat and to an opossum (*Didelphis azarae*), but neither adult worms nor larvae were recovered from these animals at necropsy (Romero and Led, 1985).

Clinical Presentation and Pathogenesis

The case described by Led et al. (1968) was a mixed-breed, 8-month-old female cat that had not eaten for 3 days and that presented with buccal paralysis. This cat died 4 days after the first signs appeared. In the first presentation of the case of Romero and Led (1985), a total of 6 adult worms were recovered from the abscess. Twenty-six days after the initial presentation, an examination of the abscess revealed another adult male and female worm. Seventy-two days after the first presentation, the abscess was found to contain 24 adult worms. In the case of Dell'Porto and Schumaker (1988), the cat was found to have a fistulated abscess on the neck, and following lavage with physiological saline, a total of 50 male and 65 female worms were recovered. The clinical signs associated with the two cases described by Armato et al. (1990) were weakness, coughing, and an inability to swallow. The cats both had an abscess on the right side at the level of the first pharyngeal ring. The abscess in one cat contained 45 adult nematodes; the abscess in the other cat contained 31 adult nematodes.

Treatment

Romero and Led (1985) treated the cat with oral membendazole for 7 days, and no worms were observed over the next 7 months. However, this treatment was applied after the abscess had been washed on several occasions.

Epizootiology

Cats are probably being infected by the ingestion of some small rodent intermediate host.

Hazards to Other Animals

The eggs are not embryonated when passed, and thus, with routine removal of cat feces, other animals should be protected from infection. However, rodents probably can become infected with this parasite.

Hazards to Humans

Lagochilascaris major has not been reported from humans. *Lagochilascaris minor* has been.

Control/Prevention

Because the means by which cats obtain their infection is not clear at this time, it is difficult to determine the best mode of control or prevention. Cats may be acquiring their infection by the ingestion of rodent intermediate hosts, or they may be becoming infected by the ingestion of infective eggs.

REFERENCES

Armato JFR, Grisi L, Neto MP. 1990. Two cases of fistulated abscesses caused by *Lagochilascaris major* in the domestic cat. Mem Inst Oswald Cruz, Rio de Janeiro 85:471–473.

Clapham PA. 1945. Some helminths from West Africa. J Helminthol 21:90–92.

Dell'Porto A, Schumaker TTS. 1988. Ocorrencia de *Lagochilascaris major* Leiper, 1910 em gato (*Felis catus domesticus* L.) no estado de São Paulo, Brasil. Rev Fac Med Vet Zootec 25:173–180.

Durette MC. 1963. Remarques sur les anomalies du genre *Lagochilascaris*. Bull Soc Pathol Exot 56:129–133.

Led JE, Colombo E, Baraboglia E. 1968. Primera comprobacion en Argentina de parasitismo en gato (*Felis catus domesticus*) por nematode del genero *Lagochilascaris*, Leiper 1909. Gaceta Vet, Buenos Aires 30:407–410.

Leiper RT. 1910. Nematodes. Wissenschaftliche ergebnisse der schwedischen zoologischen expedition nach dem Kilimandjaro, dem meru und den umgebenden massaisteppen Deutsch- Ostafrikas 1905–1906 unter letung von Prof. Dr. Yngve Sjöstedt. Hrsq. mit unterstützung von der Konigl. Schwedischen Akademie der Wissenschaften, Stockholm. Vermes 3, 22:23–26.

Romero JR, Led JE. 1985. Neuevo caso de *Lagochilascaris major* (Leiper 1910) en la República Argentina, parasitando al gato (*Felis catus domesticus*). Zbl Vet Med B 32:575–582.

Smith JL, Bowman DD, Little MD. 1983. Life cycle and development of *Lagochilascaris sprenti* (Nematoda: Ascarididae) from opossums (Marsupialia: Didelphidae) in Louisiana. J Parasitol 69:736–745.
Sprent JFA. 1971. A note on *Lagochilascaris* from the cat in Argentina. Parasitology 63:45–48.
Volcán GS, Medrano CE, Payares G. 1992. Experimental heteroxenous cycle of *Lagochilascaris minor* Leiper, 1909 (Nematoda:Ascarididae) in white mice and in cats. Mem Inst Oswald Cruz, Rio de Janeiro 87:525–532.

SPIRURIDA

The Spirurida is an order of nematodes of which many different families occur in cats. The bodies of spirurids tend to be white, although some of them can be red or yellowish, as in the case of the gnathostomes. All spirurid parasites of the cat probably utilize some form of arthropod as an intermediate host. In some cases the cat is infected by the ingestion of the arthropod (e.g., in the case of *Dracunculus*), while in other cases, the cat probably ingests a vertebrate intermediate host (e.g., *Gnathostoma*). The filarioids (e.g., *Brugia* or *Dirofilaria*) infect the cat by the bite of the mosquito intermediate host.

Most of the spirurid parasites of the cat are rather rare or often unreported. Many are more commonly found in tropical developing nations and, thus, have received little study as they relate to disease within the domestic cat. It is expected that this will change to some degree in the next few decades.

DRACUNCULOIDEA

The Dracunculoidea is a group of spirurid nematodes that live within the tissues of their vertebrate hosts. The adults tend to be rather long and are associated with hosts that have contact with fresh water. Intermediate hosts include various crustaceans such as copepods, although some parasites in fish use ectoparasitic branchiuran crustacea as hosts. The reports from cats are few and consist solely of a very few reports of infection with *Dracunculus*.

Dracunculus Species

The species of *Dracunculus* (*Draco* = snake or serpent) that has been reported from cats has often been identified as *Dracunculus medinensis* (Linnaeus, 1758) Gallandat, 1773. This worm was known to the ancients of Medina in Arabia as being the cause of lesions in the feet and ankles of humans. One of the earliest cases recorded from the domestic cat is that of Sonsino (1889). Due to great strides in providing clean water and mass chemotherapy programs, the distribution of human infections with *Dracunculus medinensis* is rapidly shrinking, bordering on extinction. Due to humans being the major host for this parasite, the areas of the world where infections in cats might be expected are also rapidly diminishing. Left around the world are only a few sites in northern Africa, the Near East, and parts of India and Pakistan.

The females of these species are large white worms that are typically seen protruding from a blister on the leg or foot of the host. Identification is readily made by putting a drop of the exudate on a glass slide with a little water and seeing the 600 μm long larvae with their long tails swimming about. For purposes of determining whether a cat is infected with *Dracunculus medinensis* or *Dracunculus insignis,* the easiest means of identification will be by the geographic range of the parasite. *Dracunculus medinensis* is found in the Old World, and *Dracunculus insignis* is found only in the Americas (Fig. 4.60). Of course, if the cat has traveled and hunted during its excursions,

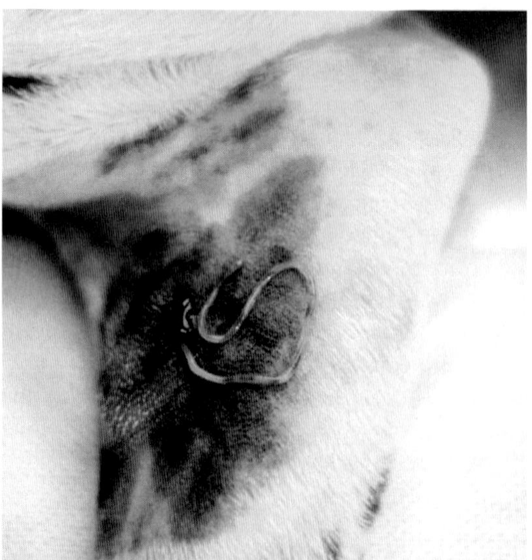

Fig. 4.60. *Dracunculus insignis* emerging from the leg of a naturally infected dog. (Photo courtesy of Dr. Susan L. Giovengo)

it will be very difficult to determine the identity of the worm causing the infection. Also, around the world, there are probably still-to-be-described species of *Dracunculus* of wild animals that may also find their way into domestic cats; thus, on many occasions it will be impossible to assign a specific name to a specimen recovered from a cat.

The female nematode lives under the skin and gains access to the outside through a blister in the skin. The typical site of the blister is on the legs. From the blister, the female slowly protrudes and releases first-stage larvae from her degenerating body into the environment. If released into water, the first-stage larvae move actively and are eaten by copepods. Within the copepod, the larva develops to a third-stage larva, which is infective to the final host. The final host becomes infected by drinking water containing infected copepods. Once ingested, the larvae penetrate the intestinal mucosa and make their way to the thoracic and abdominal muscles. By 43 days after infection, they have made their way to the subcutaneous tissues and sometime soon thereafter undergo the final molt to the adult stage. The males only reach a size of 1 to 3 cm, but the females reach lengths of up to 80 cm. The males seem to die within 6 months after infection, but the females move to the extremities between 8 to 10 months after infection. After moving to the extremities, the females induce the blister from which the larvae are released. Thus, the entire cycle takes about 1 year to reach completion.

Using a species that commonly occurs in North America in the raccoon, *Dracunculus insignis* (Leidy, 1858) Chandler, 1942, Crichton and Beverly-Burton (1977) and Eberhard and Brandt (1995) have shown that this species is capable of using tadpoles as paratenic hosts. After the tadpoles are infected, it is possible to ultimately recover infective larvae from the adult frogs that develop. The larvae recovered from the adult frogs were shown capable of infecting ferrets. Thus, with this species and potentially other members of this genus, it is possible that cats might be infected by the ingestion of a paratenic host.

There have been almost no cases of *Dracunculus* described from naturally infected cats. Muller (1968) described cases in experimentally infected cats and found a single adult female emerging from the leg of one of seven cats that had been infected 365 days previously, but no larvae were recovered from this worm. Young stages were found in three cats upon dissection. Chun-Siun (1966) reported on a case of dracunculosis in a cat in Kazakhstan. A second report of *Dracunculus* from cats in Kazakhstan was made by Genis in 1972. Fu et al. (1999) described a case in a cat from Yanzhou, China.

Ivermectin has been very successful in the treatment of human cases of dracontiasis, and it is likely to prove just as efficacious in cats.

REFERENCES

Chun-Siun F. 1966. Med Parazit Parazitar Bolezni 35:374–375 [Russian].

Crichton VFJ, Beverly-Burton M. 1977. Observations on the seasonal prevalence, pathology and transmission of *Dracunculus insignis* (Nematoda: Dracunculoidea) in the raccoon (*Procyon lotor* [L.]) in Ontario. J Wildl Dis 13:273–280.

Eberhard ML, Brandt FH. 1995. The role of tadpoles and frogs as paratenic hosts in the life cycle of *Dracunculus insignis* (Nematoda: Dracunculoidea). J Parasitol 81:792–793.

Fu A, Tao JP, Wang ZX, Jiang BL, Liu YX, Qiu HH. 1999. Observations on the morphology of *Dracunculus medinensis* from a cat in China. Chin J Zoonoses 15:35–38.

Genis DE. 1972. New cases of *Dracunculus medinensis* infection in domestic animals (cats and dogs) in Kazakhstan. Med Parazit Parazitar Bolezni 50:365.

Muller RL. 1968. Experimental dracontiasis in animals. Parasitology 58:7p–8p.

Sonsino P. 1889. Studie e notizie elmintologiche. Atti Soc Tosc Sc Nat Proc Verb 6/7:273–285.

GNATHOSTOMATOIDEA

The Gnathostomatoidea is a group of spirurid nematodes that like *Dracunculus* have a first intermediate host that is a small copepod crustacean. Unlike *Dracunculus,* the genera in this superfamily tend to routinely use paratenic hosts for the purpose of completing their life cycle. The fact that the list of potential paratenic hosts is rather large, as well as the fact that the final hosts in the wild include various carnivores, means that cats are very capable of entering the chain of events that ultimately leads to their infection. The adults of these worms are robust forms that are several centimeters long and that have spine-covered heads that are often embedded within the mucosa of the stomach, which is the organ in which they are usually found. Thus, infections in cats can often produce gastritis.

Gnathostoma spinigerum Owen, 1836

Etymology

Gnathos = jaw and *stoma* = mouth, along with *spinigerum* representing the rings of spines on the anterior end of the parasite.

Synonyms

Cheiracanthus robustus Diesing, 1838; *Cheiracanthus socialis* Leidy, 1859; *Filaria radula* Schneider, 1866; *Cheiracanthus siamensis* Levinson, 1889; *Gnathostoma paronai* Porta, 1908; *Gnathostoma spinigerum* Mitter, 1912.

History

This worm was described by Owen (1836) from the stomach of a tiger in the London Zoo. It was first reported as a parasite of the domestic cat by Gedoelst (1911). Chandler (1925) reported finding *Gnathostoma spinigerum* in 10 percent to 30 percent of cats in India. It has since been reported from cats and other felines.

Geographic Distribution

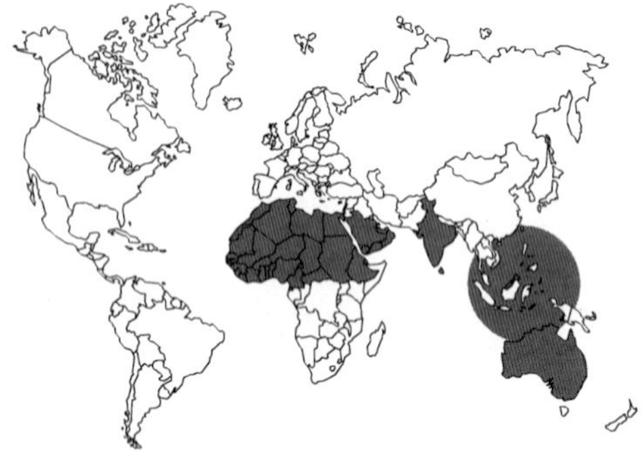

Fig. 4.61.

This parasite has been encountered mainly in Asia, including reports from India (Sur and Biswas, 1988), Laos (Scholtz and Ditrich, 1990), Malaysia (Rohde, 1962), Japan (Miyazaki, 1960), and Thailand (Daengsvang, 1980a). The parasite has been found on several occasions in cats in Australia (Barton and McEwan, 1993; Beveridge et al., 1978; Trueman and Ferris, 1977). This worm has also been found in the Philippines (Refuerzo and Garcia, 1938) and has been reported from cats in Egypt (Arafa et al., 1978). A cat experimentally infected with fish containing larvae developed a patent infection with worms that were identified as *Gnathostoma spinigerum* (Wenceslao-Ollague et al., 1988).

Location in Host

The adult worms live in the stomach. The anterior end of the worm is embedded into the mucosa of the stomach, and there may be a large cyst up to 2.5 cm in diameter that contains worms and a canal leading to the stomach lumen.

Parasite Identification

The adult worms are large, stout, and characterized by having a large inflation or head bulb on the anterior end. The head bulb and the anterior of the body are covered with spines. Adult females are 1 to 3 cm long, and the adult males are about 1 to 2.5 cm long. The vulva of the female is one-third to one-half of the body length from the posterior of the worm. The eggs are 60 to 70 μm long and 35 to 40 μm wide, contain a several-celled embryo or morula stage when passed in the feces, have a rather thick brownish shell that is thickened on one end by a clear inflation that resembles the plug in the egg of a *Trichuris* species

Life Cycle

In the life cycle of *Gnathostoma spinigerum* and the other species of *Gnathostoma,* two different intermediate hosts are required for larval development to be completed. When the eggs passed in the feces enter fresh water, they undergo development and ultimately produce a sheathed second-stage larva. At 25°C to 31°C, the second-stage larva will hatch spontaneously from the egg about 9 days after development has begun. The first intermediate host is a small freshwater crustacean, a cyclopoid copepod (Prommas and Daengsvang, 1933). The genera of copepods involved include *Cyclops, Eucyclops, Mesocyclops,* and *Thermocyclops.* After the free-swimming larva is ingested by the copepod, it sheds its sheath, penetrates the intestinal wall, and enters the body cavity of the crustacean. It takes about a week at 29°C to 31°C for the larva to then develop to the third stage within the copepod; this third-stage larva is about 0.5 mm long and has a head bulb with spines similar to the head bulb present on the adult worms.

This larva is not infective to the final host but requires passage through a second intermediate host. The larvae of *Gnathostoma spinigerum* then enter the fish that ingest the copepod hosts (Prommas and Daengsvang, 1936, 1937). The larvae first undergo a migration through the liver of the fish, and after about 1 week, they become encapsulated within the muscles and grow to lengths of 3 to 4 mm. Any one of a wide variety of animals other than fish (e.g., frogs, toads, snakes, chickens, rodents, and primates) can serve as the second intermediate host after ingesting an infected copepod and will have larvae present in muscles and other viscera (Daengsvang et al., 1966). Paratenic hosts are an important part of the life cycle, and it has been found that the advanced third-stage larvae from one host can be transferred by feeding to a second host (Daengsvang, 1971). Cats and dogs become infected by eating fish or paratenic hosts that contain third-stage larvae. The larvae penetrate the stomach and enter the liver. From the liver, the larvae, while growing, migrate about in the muscles and connective tissue before they return to the stomach where they mature in the tumors in the stomach wall (Ueki, 1957). The prepatent period after the ingestion of the third-stage larvae is somewhere between 100 to 225 days (Prommas and Daengsvang, 1937; Miyazaki, 1960).

Although it may not be important in the regular biology of this parasite, Daengsvang et al. (1970) also showed that the advanced third-stage larvae recovered from the snake-headed fish, *Ophiocephalus striatus,* are capable of infecting cats by skin penetration if the free larvae are placed on the skin. The penetration of the skin took about 5 minutes to over an hour. Once the larvae penetrated the skin, they moved into the nearby muscle tissue and were later found in the liver, diaphragm, abdominal tissues, and chest wall. Ultimately, 2 to 7.5 months later, eggs were found in the feces of cats infected by the percutaneous application of these larvae.

Clinical Presentation and Pathogenesis

Trueman and Ferris (1977) described clinical signs in three cats that were found to have gnathostomiasis. One cat died after an illness of 3 weeks, one stray cat was emaciated, and another stray cat was apparently normal. All three cats were necropsied, and it was found that the cat that died had expired due to a perforated stomach wall. The emaciated cat had a small serosal perforation on a gastric lesion, and the cat that appeared normal had a well-developed gastric lesion but no perforation of the wall. Histological examination of the lesions revealed a marked proliferation of fibrous tissues, foci of inflammatory cells, necrotic tracts, and a submucosal cavity in which the adult worms were found.

Treatment

Daengsvang et al. (1971) found that disophenol (2,6-diiodo-4-nitrophenol), "Ancylol" or "DNP," was effective in removing adult *Gnathostoma spinigerum* from the stomachs of infected cats. All adult worms in the gastric tumors were killed by around 3 days after the subcutaneous administration of the drug. These authors found that larvae present in the liver, diaphragm, and skeletal muscle were not killed at the dosage level tested. To examine the potential for eliminating the larval stages, Daengsvang (1980b) infected 10 cats with 50 to 99 third-stage larvae that were recovered from mice. Eight of the cats were then treated, and two cats served as untreated controls. Each cat received 12 doses of the compound at 10-day intervals. Two cats received 0.05 ml per pound, two cats received 0.04 ml per pound, two cats received 0.03 ml per pound, and two cats received 0.02 ml per pound. Necropsies were performed 19 to 24 days after the last dose. There were no worms found in the cats receiving the highest dose, one cat given 0.04 ml per pound had two larvae, and one cat given 0.03 ml per pound had one larva. Both cats treated with 0.02 ml per pound had worms: one had an immature adult and nine larvae, and the other cat had six larvae. The two control cats were necropsied 180 days after infection and had eight immature adults and eight larvae.

Epizootiology

Cats acquire their infections with *Gnathostoma spinigerum* by the ingestion of infected prey. The initial larval stage requires development in freshwater copepods; thus, the parasite is present around freshwater. In this situation it will be very difficult to prevent cats from hunting for prey that might be infected due to the wide range of hosts that are potentially infected.

Hazards to Other Animals

The eggs passed in the feces of cats are not infectious unless first ingested by copepods. Thus, with proper disposal of feces, this parasite should not pose a threat to other animals. However, an infected cat on the premises where a pond is present may produce water that contains infected copepods capable of infecting other animals.

Hazards to Humans

There have been a number of human cases of gnathostomiasis. They occur from the ingestion of raw or undercooked fish or other animals containing the larval stages. On occasion, infections have proven fatal (Chitanondh and Rosen, 1967). In humans, the larvae migrate through the stomach wall, and this is followed with epigastric pain and possibly peritonitis. The larvae migrate through the liver and peritoneum. Very typically in humans there is a cutaneous involvement where the larvae migrate about under the skin. On occasion the larvae also may enter the nervous system, causing life-threatening illness.

Control/Prevention

Control is achieved by preventing cats from hunting in areas where the parasite is found. The wide range of intermediate and paratenic hosts makes it more difficult to prevent infection in cats.

REFERENCES

Arafa MS, Nasr NT, Khalifa R, Mahdi AH, Mahmoud WS, Khalil MS. 1978. Cats as reservoir hosts of *Toxocara* and other parasites potentially transmissible to man in Egypt. Acta Parasitol Polonica 25:383–392.

Barton MA, McEwan DR. 1993. Spirurid nematodes in dogs and cats from central Australia. Aust Vet J 70:270.

Beveridge I, President PJA, Arundel JH. 1978. *Gnathostoma spinigerum* infection in a feral cat from New South Wales. Aust Vet J 54:46.

Chandler, AC. 1925. The helminthic parasites of cats in Calcutta and the relationship of cats to human helminthic infections. Ind J Med Res 13:213–227.

Chitanondh H, Rosen L. 1967. Fatal eosinophilic encephalomyelitis caused by the nematode *Gnathostoma spinigerum*. Am J Trop Med Hyg 16:638–645.

Daengsvang S. 1971. Infectivity of *Gnathostoma spinigerum* larvae in primates. J Parasitol 57:476–478.

Daengsvang S. 1980a. A monograph on the genus *Gnathostoma* and gnathostomiasis in Thailand. 87 pp.

Daengsvang S. 1980b. Chemotherapy of feline *Gnathostoma spinigerum* migrating stage with multiple subcutaneous doses of Ancylol. Southeast Asian J Trop Med Publ Health 11:359–362.

Daengsvang S, Thienprasitthi P, Chomcherngpat P. 1966. Further investigations on natural and experimental hosts of larvae of *Gnathostoma spinigerum* in Thailand. Am J Trop Med Hyg 15:727–729.

Daengsvang S, Sermwatsri B, Youngyi P, Guname D. 1970. Penetration of the skin by *Gnathostoma spinigerum* larvae. Ann Trop Med Parasitol 64:399–402.

Daengsvang S, Sermwatsri B, Youngyi P, Guname D. 1971. A preliminary study of chemotherapy of *Gnathostoma spinigerum* infections in cats with Ancylol, disophenol (2,6-diido-4-nitrophenol). Southeast Asian J Trop Med Publ Health 2:359–361.

Gedoelst L. 1911. Synopsis de parasitologie de l'homme et des animaux domestiques. 332 pp. Lierre et Bruxelles.

Heydon GM. 1929. Creeping eruption or larva migrans in North Queensland and a note on the worm *Gnathostoma spinigerum* (Owen). Med J Aust 1:583–591.

Miyazaki I. 1960. On the genus *Gnathostoma* and human gnathostomiasis, with special reference to Japan. Exp Parasitol 9:338–370.

Owen R. 1836. Anatomical descriptions of two species of Entozoa from the stomach of a tiger (*Felis tigress* Linn), one of which forms a new genus of Nematoidea, *Gnathostoma.* Proc Zool Soc London 47:123–126.

Prommas C, Daengsvang S. 1933. Preliminary report of a study on the life cycle of *Gnathostoma spinigerum.* J Parasitol 19:287–292.

Prommas C, Daengsvang S. 1936. Further report of a study on the life cycle of *Gnathostoma spinigerum.* J Parasitol 22:180–186.

Prommas C, Daengsvang S. 1937. Feeding experiments on cats with *Gnathostoma spinigerum* larvae obtained from the second intermediate host. J Parasitol 23:115–116.

Refuerzo PG, Garcia EY. 1938. The crustacean intermediate hosts of *Gnathostoma spinigerum* in the Philippines and its pre- and intercrustacian development. Philipp J Anim Indust 5:351–362.

Rohde K. 1962. Helminthen aus Katzen un Hunden in Malaya; Bemerkungen zu ihrer epideiologischen Bedeutung für den Menschen. Ztsch Parasitenk 22:237–244.

Scholtz T, Ditrich O. 1990. Scanning electron microscopy of the cuticular armature of the nematode *Gnathostoma spinigerum* Owen, 1836 from cats in Laos. J Helminthol 64:255–262.

Sur SK, Biswas G. 1988. Cat—a source of human parasitic infection. Ind J Publ Health 32:211.

Trueman KF, Ferris PBC. 1977. Gnathostomiasis in three cats. Aust Vet J 53:498–499.

Ueki T. 1957. Experimental studies on the third-stage larva of *Gnathostoma spinigerum.* Egaku Kenkyu Fukuoka 27:1162–1196.

Wenceslao-Ollague L, Eduardo-Gomez L, Manuel Briones I. 1988. Infeccion experimental de un gato domestico adulto con el tercer estado larvaio de *Gnathostoma spinigerum* procedente de un pez de agua dulce. Medicina Cutanea Ibero-Latino-Americana 16:295–297.

Gnathostoma procyonis and Other *Gnathostoma* Species

Gnathostoma procyonis was described from raccoons in Texas by Chandler (1942); the life cycle was described by Ash (1962a, b). As part of his studies, Ash (1962b) experimentally infected seven kittens with larvae from naturally infected snakes. Only a single larva was recovered from the diaphragm of a kitten necropsied 6 days after infection. Two adult cats were examined 3 and 4 months after infection, and no worms were found in these cats. It thus appears that this species does not infect cats.

Kirkpatrick et al. (1987) described a case of gastric gnathostomiasis in a cat from Pennsylvania. This was a 10-year-old domestic cat that had a brief history of listlessness and inappetence accompanied by bouts of diarrhea. An abdominal mass was revealed by palpation and radiography, and an exploratory laparotomy revealed that there was a mass about 3 cm in diameter on the stomach wall. The mass was found to contain a single 1 cm long female gnathostome. The worm was a young adult, and the eggs within the uterus were misshapen and possibly unfertilized. These authors hypothesized that the worm was a species that would typically be found in some wild mammal in North America.

REFERENCES

Ash LR. 1962a. Development of *Gnathostoma procyonis* Chandler, 1942, in the first and second intermediate hosts. J Parasitol 48:298–305.

Ash LR. 1962b. Migration and development of *Gnathostoma procyonis* Chandler, 1942, in mammalian hosts. J Parasitol 48:306–313.

Chandler AC. 1942. The helminths of raccoons in east Texas. J Parasitol 28:255–268.

Kirkpatrick CE, Lok JB, Goldschmidt MK, Mellman SL. 1987. Gastric gnathostomiasis in a cat. J Am Vet Med Assoc 190:1437-1439.

PHYSALOPTEROIDEA

There are three genera of physalopteroid spirurid nematodes, *Physaloptera, Turgida,* and *Abbreviata,* that have been recovered from the domestic cat. These nematodes are usually found in the stomachs of their vertebrate hosts, where they are attached to the mucosa by the means of large pseudolabia. The adults tend to be white to pinkish and are 3–5 cm in length. The vertebrate hosts include amphibia, reptiles, birds, and mammals, but those nematodes found in the cat are typically species that are true cat parasites or that are typically found in other mammalian hosts. The typical intermediate host of these worms is an insect, often something that feeds on feces like a cockroach or a beetle. It appears that the larvae are capable of persisting in paratenic hosts, and it seems that as more work is done on this group, cats will be found to be commonly infected by this route. The genera in the cat can be differentiated by the appearance of the head and the number of uterine branches. *Turgida* has seven or more uterine branches, while *Physaloptera* and *Abbreviata* have only two. *Physaloptera* species have a collarette behind the pseudolabia, which is not obvious in members of the genus *Abbreviata.*

Physaloptera praeputialis von Linstow, 1889

Etymology

Physalis = bubble and *ptero* = wing, along with *praeputialis* to describe the cuticular projection of the cuticle over the posterior end of the body.

History

This parasite was originally described by Linstow (1889) from a domestic cat in Brazil. Since that time, it has been the most commonly described species of *Physaloptera* reported from domestic cats, and it appears to utilize the cat as its major or sole definitive host.

Geographic Distribution

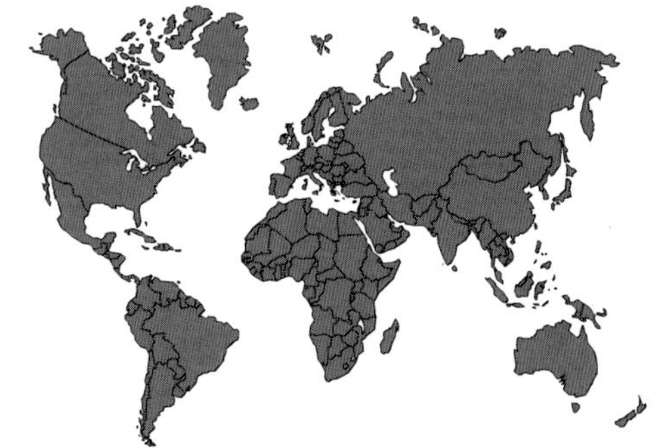

Fig. 4.62.

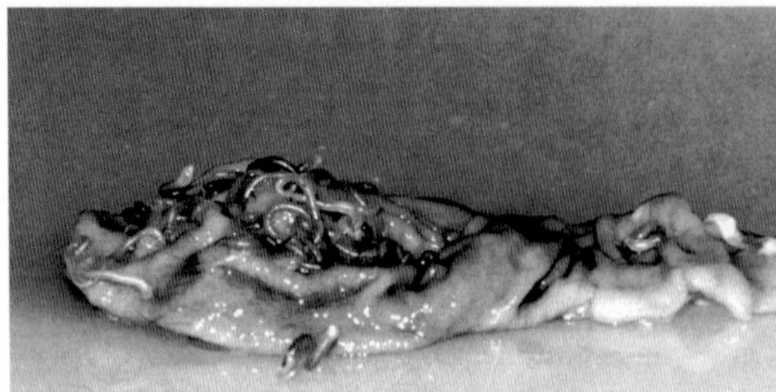

Fig. 4.63. *Physaloptera praeputialis.* Adult worms in situ in the stomach of a cat at necropsy.

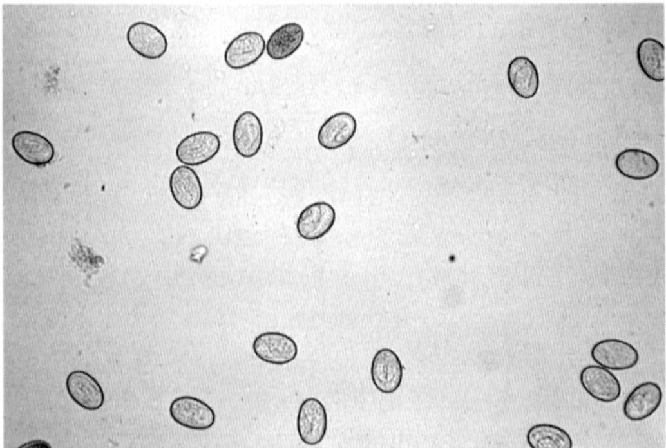

Fig. 4.64. *Physaloptera praeputialis.* Eggs of this worm in a fecal flotation.

Physaloptera praeputialis has been reported from cats around the world. In the Americas it has been reported from the United States (Gufstafson, 1995; Levine, 1968) and the Bahamas (Clarkson and Owen, 1959), Mexico (Zarate-Ramos et al., 1991), Venezuela (Power, 1964), Argentina (Santa-Cruz and Lombardero, 1987), and Brazil (Campos et al., 1974; Ogassawara et al., 1986). From Southeast Asia and the South Pacific, this species has been reported from cats in Hawaii (Ash, 1962), the Philippines (Tongson and San-Pablo, 1979), Japan (Hayasaki et al., 1982), Malaysia (Retnasabapathy and San, 1970), and Australia (Barton and McEwan, 1993). From Asia and the Middle East, this parasite has been reported from cats in Iraq (Daoud et al., 1988), Iran (Mirzayans, 1972), Turkey (Burgu et al., 1985), Turkmenia in the former USSR (Velikanov and Sharpillo, 1984), and India (Gill, 1972). From Europe, the only report is from Greece (Haralampides, 1978). From Africa, the only report is from South Africa (Baker et al., 1989).

Location in Host

Within the cat, the adults and larvae of *Physaloptera praeputialis* are found in the stomach, usually with their anterior end attached to the mucosa (Fig. 4.63).

Parasite Identification

Physaloptera praeputialis is a pink worm that is characterized by having a cuticular sheath that covers the posterior end of the body of both sexes and that appears prepuce-like. The males are 1 cm to 4.5 cm in length; the females are 1.5 to 6 cm long. The vulva is slightly anterior to mid-body. The eggs are 45 to 58 μm long and 30 to 42 μm wide. The egg has a thick, clear shell and contains a fully formed larva when passed in the feces (Figs. 4.64 and 4.65). The eggs are very clear and are relatively easy to miss when examining a fecal specimen, especially following sugar flotations.

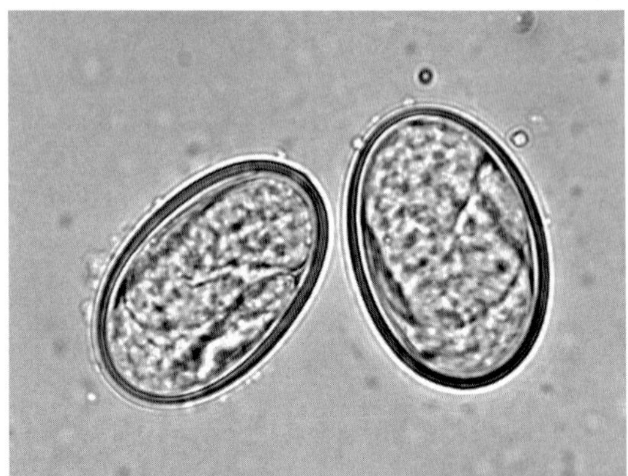

Fig. 4.65. *Physaloptera praeputialis.* Higher-power view of eggs showing the larvae, which are already developed at the time that the eggs are passed in the feces.

The species of *Physaloptera* described from cats fall into two groups, those with and those without preputial-like sheaths that cover the posterior of the body. *Physaloptera praeputialis, Physaloptera pseudopraeputialis,* and *Physaloptera brevispiculum* (not actually reported from the domestic cat) represent those species that have preputial-like sheaths. *Physaloptera rara* and *Physaloptera pacitae* represent the species without preputial-like sheaths. Only *Physaloptera praeputialis* and *Physaloptera rara* have been commonly reported from the domestic cat.

Life Cycle

Petri and Ameel (1950) were the first to show that an arthropod was a required part of the life cycle of *Physaloptera praeputialis*. These authors succeeded in infecting German cockroaches (*Blatella germanica*), camel crickets (*Ceutiphilus* species), and field crickets with eggs from cat feces. Zago Filho (1957, 1962) examined development in experimentally infected crickets (*Acheta assimilis*) and showed that third-stage infective larvae were present by 23 days after infection in the body cavities of crickets held at 22°C to 24°C. In cats given these larvae, the third molt occurred 45 days after infection, and the fourth molt occurred 95 days after infection. The prepatent period was 131–156 days. Cats fed larvae from naturally infected lizards (*Varanus griseus*) and the long-eared hedgehog (*Hemiechinus aratus*) from Turkmenia in the former USSR were found to develop patent infections 60 days after being fed the third-stage larvae from these paratenic hosts (Velikanov and Sharpillo, 1984). Thus, it would appear that cats are more likely to be infected by the ingestion of paratenic hosts than by the ingestion of arthropod intermediate host.

Clinical Presentation and Pathogenesis

Vomiting, with vomitus containing one or more worms, is not an atypical presentation of infection with *Physaloptera praeputialis*. Gufstafson (1995) described two cats that had intermittent vomiting of several months' duration. The adult worms were detected in the vomitus. Clinical signs included melena with anemia and eosinophilia. Zarate-Ramos et al. (1991) reported that 6 of 32 cats in Monterrey, Mexico, were infected with this parasite, and though the necropsies revealed moderate catarrhal gastritis and multiple pseudogranulomas, none of the six infected cats had been noted to have signs of gastritis before being euthanatized.

Treatment

Ivermectin (200 µg/kg body weight) was shown by Gufstafson (1995) to remove the clinical signs of *Physaloptera praeputialis* infection. Smith (1979) found that 2 of 44 cats that were infected with a *Physaloptera* species prior to treatment expelled their worms within 24 hours after treatment with levamisole solution injected subcutaneously at a dosage of 8 mg/kg body weight. With the levamisole, about 5 percent of the treated cats had side effects of vomiting and salivation for 1 to 2 hours after treatment.

Epizootiology

Velikanov and Sharpillo (1984) found seven species of reptiles and three species of mammals naturally infected with the larvae of *Physaloptera praeputialis*. Thus, it would appear that the paratenic hosts probably play an essential role in the infection of cats.

Hazards to Other Animals

The eggs of *Physaloptera praeputialis* passed in the feces are infective only to arthropods. The fact that German cockroaches can serve as the intermediate host would suggest that catteries with less than perfect sanitation could serve to spread the infection between animals. Thus, with sanitation that includes arthropod control, this parasite should not pose a problem.

Hazards to Humans

Humans have on rare occasions been infected with *Physaloptera,* but the infections are obtained by the ingestion of the intermediate and paratenic hosts, and an infected cat in a household would thus present only a very minimal risk to its owners.

Control/Prevention

Control requires that cats be prevented from hunting. The monthly preventatives given to cats for heartworm prevention are likely to have no effect on the larvae of this parasite if they are ingested by hunting cats.

REFERENCES

Ash LR. 1962. Helminth parasites of dogs and cats in Hawaii. J Parasitol 48:63–65.

Baker MK, Lange L, Erster A, Plaat S van der. 1989. A survey of helminths in domestic cats in the Pretoria area of Transvaal, Republic of South Africa. Part 1. The prevalence and comparison of burdens of helminths in adult and juvenile cats. J S Afr Vet Assoc 60:139–142.

Barton MA, McEwan DR. 1993. Spirurid nematodes in dogs and cats from central Australia. Aust Vet J 70:270.

Burgu A, Tinar R, Doganay A, Toparlak M. 1985. Ankara'da sokak kedilerinin ekto-ve endoparazitleri uzerinde bir arastirma [Turkish]. Vet Fak Dergisi, Ankara Univ 32:288–300.

Campos DMB, Garibaldi IM, Carneiro JR. 1974. Prevalencia de helmintos em gatos (*Felis catus domesticus*) de Goiania. Rev Patologia Trop 3:355–359.
Clarkson MJ, Owen LN. 1959. The parasites of domestic animals in the Bahama islands. Ann Trop Med Parasitol 53:341–346.
Daoud IS, Al-Tae ARA, Salman YJ. 1988. Prevalence of gastro-intestinal helminths in cats from Iraq. J Biol Sci Res 19:363–368.
Gill HS. 1972. Incidence of gastro-intestinal helminths in cat (*Felis catus*) in Delhi. J Commun Dis 4:109–111.
Gufstafson BW. 1995. Ivermectin in the treatment of *Physaloptera praeputialis* in two cats. J Am Anim Hosp Assoc 31:416–418.
Haralampides ST. 1978. Contribution to the study of cat's parasites and their public health importance. Hellenike Kteniatrike 21:117–119.
Hayasaki M, Ohishi I, Munakata A. 1982. Incidence of stomach worm, *Physaloptera praeputialis* von Linstow, 1889, in two cats and a dog in Tokyo, Japan. Jap J Parasitol 31:499–506.
Levine ND. 1968. Nematode Parasites of Domestic Animals and Man. Minneapolis, Minn: Burgess Publishing Company. 600 pp.
Linstow OFB. 1889. Helminthologisches. Arch Naturg, Berlin 54, 1:235–246, plate 16.
Mirzayans A. 1972. The incidence of gastro-intestinal helminths of domestic cats in Tehran area of Iran [Persian with English summary]. J Vet Fac Univ Tehran 28:29–35.
Ogassawara S, Benassi S, Larsson CE, Leme PTZ, Hagiwara MK. 1986. Prevalencia de infeccoes helminticas em gatos na cidade de Sao Paulo. Rev Fac Med Vet Zootec Univ Sao Paulo 23:145–149.
Petri LH, Ameel DJ. 1950. Studies on the life cycle of *Physaloptera rara* Hall and Wigdor, 1918 and *Physaloptera praeputialis* Linstow, 1889. J Parasitol 36(suppl):40.
Power LA. 1964. Contribucion al conocimiento de los helmintos parasitos del gato, "*Felis* (*Felis*) *catus domesticus*", de Maracay y sus Alrededores. Rev Med Vet Parasitol, Maracay 20:99–135.
Retnasabapathy A, San KT. 1970. Incidence of stomach worm *Physaloptera praeputialis* in local cats. Malaysian Vet J 5:14–16.
Santa-Cruz AM, Lombardero OJ. 1987. Resultados parasitologicos de 50 necropsia de gatos de la ciudad de Corrientes. Vet Argent 4:735–739.
Smith JP. 1979. Efficacy of levamisole as an anthelmintic in domestic cats. Feline Pract 9:14, 16, 18.
Tongson MS, San-Pablo FG. 1979. A study on the prevalence of gastro-intestinal worms of cats in Metropolitan Manila. Philipp J Vet Med 18:1–15.
Velikanov VP, Sharpillo VP. 1984. Experimental identification of *Physaloptera praeputialis* and *Pterygodermatites cahirensis* larvae (Nematoda, Spirurata) from paratenic hosts [in Russian]. Vestnik Zoologii 6:25–29.
Zago Filho H. 1957. Contribuição para o conhecimento de hospedeiros intermediarios e definitivos da *Physaloptera praeputialis* Linstow, 1889 (Nematoda, Spiruroidea). Rev Brasil Biol 17:513–520.
Zago Filho H. 1962. Contribuição para o conhecimento do ciclo evolutivo da *Physaloptera praeputialis* von Linstow, 1889 (Nematoda: Spiruroidea). Arquivos de Zoologia do Estado de Sao Paulo (Years 1958–1962) 11, 59–98.
Zarate-Ramos JJ, Craig TM, Avalos-Ramirez R, Guzman-Garcia MA, Davalos-Aranda G, Ramirez-Romero R. 1991. Gastritis verminosa por *Physaloptera praeputialis* en el gato. Vet Mex 22:185–190.

Physaloptera pseudopraeputialis Yutuc, 1953

These worms were recovered from the stomachs of 28 of 78 necropsied cats. The cats were from Manila, Quezon City, and Santa Cruz in the Philippines. These cats were part of an efficacy trial for cesticidal products, and no clinical signs of the infections were noted in any of the animals. The maximum number of worms recovered from a single cat was 32. Typically, the white to whitish pink worms were recovered attached firmly to the mucosa of the stomach by their anterior ends. There were no lesions associated with the sites of attachment. In both the males and females the posterior of the body is covered by a preputial-like sheath. The males were 21 to 34 mm long; the right spicules were 0.60 to 0.70 mm long, and the left spicules were 0.85 to 1.20 mm long. The females were 27 to 44 mm long with an esophagus that was 4.4 to 6.4 mm long. The vulva was located about 10 to 19 mm behind the anterior end. The eggs were 50 μm to 60 μm long, were ovoid, and had a thick shell. The eggs were larvated when laid. In none of the fecal samples from the 28 positive cats were eggs identified, although there is no indication given of the method used for fecal analysis. It was felt that this species differed from *Physaloptera praeputialis* based on the arrangement of the papillae on the male tail and the appearance of the teeth on the anterior end.

Tacal and Corpuz (1962) described a case where 55 worms were found in the stomach of a cat that was known to be infected with *Physaloptera* and that gradually became emaciated, depressed, and anorectic. The cat died, and the necropsy revealed frothy exudate in the bronchi and a left lung that was edematous and congested. The apical lobe of the right lung was collapsed. Three adult *Physaloptera pseudopraeputialis* were recovered from the larynx, and 55 of these worms were recovered from the stomach of this cat. It was suggested that the worms in the larynx either made their way there as larvae or that they were regurgitated and subsequently inhaled.

REFERENCES

Tacal JV, Corpuz ZV. 1962. Abnormal location of the stomach worm, *Physaloptera pseudopraeputialis,* in a cat. JAVMA 140:799–800.

Yutuc LM. 1953. *Physaloptera pseudopraeputialis* n. sp.—a stomach worm of the cat (Nematoda: Physalopterinae). Philipp J Sci 82:221–226.

Yutuc LM, Cosio HF. 1953. The incidence and frequency distribution of parasitic worms in naturally infected cats. Tharpar Commem Vol, pp 305–308.

Physaloptera brevispiculum von Linstow, 1906

This worm has been described on a single occasion from specimens collected from a rusty-spotted cat (*Felis rubiginosa*) in Kandy, Ceylon (von Linstow, 1906). These worms were about a centimeter long, and the male had spicules that were equal and about 0.8 mm long.

REFERENCES

von Linstow O. 1906. Helminthes from the collection of the Colombo Museum. Spolia Zeylanica 3:163–188.

Physaloptera rara Hall and Wigdor, 1918

Etymology

Physalis = bubble and *ptero* = wing, along with *rara* = *rarus* (thin).

Synonyms

Physaloptera felidis Ackert, 1936.

History

Physaloptera rara was originally described by Hall and Wigdor (1918) from the dog. This worm is now considered mainly a parasite of the coyote (*Canis latrans*) that has developed a domestic cycle in the cat, dog, and other wildlife species. Ackert (1936) found a parasite in the cat that he described as *Physaloptera felidis,* but the descriptions of *Physaloptera felidis* and *Physaloptera rara* are very similar, and it would warrant additional work on the biology and taxonomy of these species to verify that they are actually distinct.

Geographic Distribution

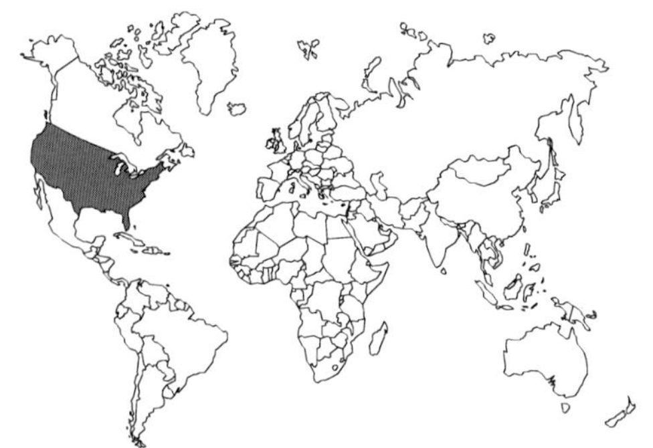

Fig. 4.66.

Hitchcock (1953) reported that she found *Physaloptera rara* in kittens in Michigan. Baughn and Bliznick (1954) found it in cats in New York. Ackert (1936) recovered his specimens from cats in Kansas. Ackert and Furumoto (1949) also found it in cats in Kansas. Shoop et al. (1991) reported *Physaloptera rara* from cats in Arkansas. Marchiondo and Sawyer (1978) recovered specimens from cats in Utah.

Location in Host

The adult worms are found in the stomach and very anterior portion of the duodenum of the cat.

Parasite Identification

Physaloptera rara differs from *Physaloptera praeputialis* in that there is no sheath over the posterior portion of the body of the male or female. The males are 2.5 to 3 cm long; the females are 3 to 6 cm in length. These worms tend to be white. The male has caudal alae and pedunculate papillae on its tail. The vulva of the female is anterior to the middle of the body. The eggs are thick shelled, ellipsoid, 42 μm to 53 μm long, and 29 μm to 35 μm wide and contain a larva when passed in the feces. Like the eggs of *Physaloptera praeputialis,* the eggs of *Physaloptera rara* are quite clear and difficult to see, especially in sugar flotations.

Life Cycle

Petri (1950) showed that the German cockroach, *Blatella germanica,* and grain beetles, *Tribolium confusum,* could serve as intermediate hosts of

Physaloptera rara. Petri and Ameel (1950) added ground beetles, *Harpalus* species, and crickets, *Acheta assimilis,* to the list of intermediate hosts. Olsen (1980) added grasshoppers, *Melanoplus femurrubrum,* to the list of intermediate hosts. Widmer (1967) found larvae attached to the mucosa of the stomachs of rattlesnakes in Colorado, and he used these larvae to experimentally infect cats (Widmer, 1970). Olsen (1980) used larvae from rattlesnakes to infect cats and found the prepatent period to be 75 to 79 days. Olsen also showed that mice and frogs could serve as paratenic hosts, with the larvae persisting attached to the mucosa of the gastrointestinal tract. Using larvae recovered from frog feces 21 days after infection, a cat developed a patent infection 156 days after infection.

Clinical Presentation and Pathogenesis

Reports of clinical signs due to this parasite are rare. Santen et al. (1993) reported on signs including vomiting and diarrhea in a 7-month-old cat that was infected with *Physaloptera rara* and *Toxocara cati.*

Treatment

The only description of treatment in the cat is that of Santen et al. (1993), who treated an infected cat with pyrantel pamoate (5 mg/kg body weight pyrantel pamoate). Examination of the feces of the cat 6 weeks after treatment revealed the continued presence of eggs of *Physaloptera rara* and *Toxocara cati.* The cat was then treated with two oral doses of pyrantel pamoate (5 mg/kg body weight) 3 weeks apart. Repeat fecal examinations revealed no additional eggs in the feces of this cat.

Epizootiology

Cats apparently can become infected with *Physaloptera rara* by the ingestion of the arthropod intermediate host or through the ingestion of paratenic hosts. The failure of Olsen (1980) to infect chickens with larvae suggests that birds may not be important as paratenic hosts of this parasite. The fact that German cockroaches could serve as intermediate hosts could mean that this parasite could become a problem in catteries with less than adequate cleanliness.

Hazards to Other Animals

The larvated eggs passed in the feces are not infectious unless ingested by arthropod intermediate hosts.

Hazards to Humans

Humans have been reported infected with *Physaloptera* species, but it is unclear which species have been involved in these infections (Nicolaides et al., 1977). Infections are probably acquired by the accidental ingestion of arthropod hosts or by the ingestion of uncooked paratenic hosts.

Control/Prevention

Control would involve preventing cats from hunting paratenic hosts or preying on the arthropod intermediate hosts.

REFERENCES

Ackert JE. 1936. *Physaloptera felidis* n. sp., a nematode of the cat. Trans Am Microsc Soc 55:250–254.

Ackert JE, Furumoto HH. 1949. Helminths of cats in eastern Kansas. Trans Kans Acad Sci 52:449–453.

Baughn CO, Bliznick A. 1954. The incidence of certain helminth parasites of the cat. J Parasitol 40 (suppl):19.

Hall MC, Wigdor M. 1918. A *Physaloptera* from the dog, with a note on the nematode parasites of the dog in North America. J Am Vet Med Assoc 53:6:733–744.

Hitchcock DJ. 1953. Incidence of gastrointestinal parasites in some Michigan kittens. North Am Vet 34:428–429.

Marchiondo AA, Sawyer TW. 1978. Scanning electron microscopy of the head region of *Physaloptera felidis* Ackert, 1936. Proc Helm Soc Wash 45:258–260.

Nicolaides NJ, Musgrave J, McGuckin D, Moorhouse DE. 1977. Nematode larvae (Spirurida: Physalopteridae) causing infarction of the bowel in an infant. Pathology 9:129–135.

Olsen JL. 1980. Life history of *Physaloptera rara* Hall and Wigdor, 1918 (Nematoda: Physalopteroidea) of canids and felids in definitive, intermediate, and paratenic hosts. Rev Iberica Parasitol 40:489–525.

Petri LH. 1950. Life cycle of *Physaloptera rara* Hall and Wigdor, 1918 (Nematoda: Spiruroidea) with the cockroach, *Blatella germanica* serving as intermediate host. Trans Kans Acad Sci 53:331–337.

Petri LH, Ameel DJ. 1950. Studies on the life cycle of *Physaloptera rara* Hall and Wigdor, 1918 and *Physaloptera praeputialis* Linstow, 1889. J Parasitol 36(suppl):40.

Power LA. 1971. Helminths of cats from the Midwest with a report of *Ancylostoma caninum* in this host. J Parasitol 57:610.

Santen DR, Chastain CB, Schmidt DA. 1993. Efficacy of pyrantel pamoate against *Physaloptera* in a cat. J Am Anim Hosp Assoc 29:53–55.
Shoop WL, Haines HW, Michael BF, Eary CH, Endris RG. 1991. *Molineus barbatus* (Trichostrongylidae) and other helminthic infections of the cat in Arkansas. J Helm Soc Wash 58:227–230.
Widmer EA. 1967. Helminth parasites of the prairie rattlesnake, *Crotalus viridis* Rafinesque, 1818, in Weld County, Colorado. J Parasitol 53:362–363.
Widmer EA. 1970. Development of third-stage *Physaloptera* larvae from *Crotalus viridis* Rafinesque, 1818 in cats with notes on pathology of the larvae in the reptile (Nematoda, Spiruroidea). J Wildl Dis 6:89–93.

Physaloptera pacitae Tubangi, 1925

This species was described (Tubangui, 1925) on the basis of specimens collected from worms encysted in the stomach wall of a cat in Los Baños, Laguna, Luzon, Philippines. It seems that there have been no additional reports of infections of cats with this worm. The male is 19 to 22 mm long, and the female is 23 to 25 mm long. There is no preputial sheath on the tail of the male or female specimen. The spicules of the male are dissimilar, with the right spicule being the shorter: the right spicule is 0.61 mm long; the left spicule 0.91 mm long. The vulva of the female is located at the posterior end of the body on the ventral surface. The eggs were thick shelled, 48 μm to 50 μm long, and ovoid with a width of about 30 μm. The eggs were not shown to contain larvae, although it is expected that they would when passed in the feces.

REFERENCES

Tubangui MA. 1925. Metazoan parasites of Philippine domesticated animals. Philipp J Sci 28:11–37, plates 1–3.

Abbreviata gemina (von Linstow, 1899)

Abbreviata gemina was originally described from the stomach and small intestine of a domestic cat in Egypt under the name of *Physaloptera gemina* by von Linstow. Other potential synonyms are *Physaloptera caucasica* Linstow, 1902, and *Abbreviata mordens* (Leiper, 1908). Specimens of *Abbreviata* are very similar to members of the genus *Physaloptera* but tend to lack the cuticular collarette characteristic of that genus. The males of this species tend to be 1 cm long; the females 2 cm long. The eggs are thick shelled, ellipsoidal, larvated when passed, and 52 μm by 32 μm in length and width. The life cycle of a related species found in primates (*Abbreviata caucasica*) involves German cockroaches, *Blatella germanica,* and grasshoppers, *Schistocerca gregaria,* as intermediate hosts (Poinar and Quentin, 1972). There have been no reports on clinical presentation or treatment of these infections in cats. Because the life cycle can probably utilize cockroaches, infections could theoretically become a problem in unclean catteries.

REFERENCES

Gedoelst L. 1911. Synopsis de parasitologie de l'homme et des animaux domestiques. Lierre et Bruxelles. 332 pp.
Linstow OFB. 1899. Nematoden aus der Berliner zoologischen Sammlung. Mitt Zool Samml Mus Naturk Berl 1:3–28, plates 1–6.
Morgan BB. 1945. The nematode genus *Abbreviata* (Travasos, 1920) Schulz, 1927. Am Midl Nat 34:485–490.
Poinar GO, Quentin JC. 1972. The development of *Abbreviata caucasica* (von Linstow) (Spirurida: Physalopteridae) in an intermediate host. J Parasitol 58:23–28.
Travassos L. 1920. Contribuites para o conhecimento da fauna helmintolojica brazileira. X. Sobre es especies do genero *Turgida.* Mem Inst Oswaldo Cruz 12:73–77.

Turgida turgida (Rudolphi, 1819) Travassos, 1920

Turgida turgida is a common parasite of the stomachs of opossums, *Didelphis virginiana* and *Didelphis paraguayensis,* in North and South America. The life cycle is similar to that of various *Physaloptera* species with which it is closely related. The adults differ from those of *Physaloptera* species in that the female has typically seven or more uterine branches whereas typically only two uterine branches are present in the species of *Physaloptera* found in cats. Alicata (1937) showed that the German cockroach, *Blatella germanica,* could serve as the first intermediate host of this parasite. Gray and Anderson (1982a, 1982b) used the field cricket, *Acheta pennsylvanicus,* as the intermediate host of this parasite. Alicata gave larvae to one cat and later found larvae in washings of the stomach of the cat at necropsy. On the other hand, Zago Filho (1958) and Gray and Anderson (1982b) were unable to infect cats with third-stage larvae that were infective to opossums.

REFERENCES

Alicata JE. 1937. Larval development of the spirurid nematode *Physaloptera turgida* in the cockroach, *Blatella germanica.* Papers on Helminthology Published in Commemoration of the 30th Year Jubileum KI Skrjabin and 15th Anniversary All-Union Institute of Helminthology, pp 11–14.

Gray JB, Anderson RC. 1982a. Observations on *Turgida turgida* (Rudolphi, 1819) (Nematoda: Physalopteroidea) in the American opossum (*Didelphis virginiana*). J Wildl Dis 18:279–285.

Gray JB, Anderson RC. 1982b. Development of *Turgida turgida* (Rudolphi, 1819) (Nematoda: Physalopteroidea) in the American opossum (*Didelphis virginiana*). Can J Zool 60:1265–1274.

Zago Filho H. 1958. Contribuição para o conhecimento de hospedeiros intermediarios e definitivos da *Turgida turgida* (Rud., 1819) Travassos, 1920 (Nematoda, Spiruroidea). Rev Brasil Biol 18:41–46.

RICTULARIOIDEA

This group of spirurid nematodes consists of a single genus, *Pterygodermatites,* that has been recovered from cats. The adults of these worms live in the small intestine and utilize insect intermediate hosts. The larvae can also survive in paratenic hosts, and it appears that cats likely become infected by the ingestion of infected lizards or frogs. Other species are found in rodents and occasionally primates. All members of this superfamily possess a sclerotized buccal capsule and rows of lateroventral spines that are distinctive.

Pterygodermatites cahirensis (Jägerskiöld, 1909) Barus, Petavy, Deblock, and Tenora, 1996

Etymology

Pterygo = wing, and *dermatites* refers to the lateroventral cuticular spines or wings, and *cahirensis* refers to the original description being from cats in Cairo, Egypt.

Synonyms

Rictularia cahirensis Jägerskiöld, 1909.

History

This worm was originally described by Jägerskiöld in 1904 in an abstract describing specimens collected from a cat in Egypt, but the name was considered a *nomen nudum* until it was republished in a paper in 1909. For a period of time, it was considered to be a synonym of *Rictularia affinis* Jägerskiöld, 1909, and has also appeared under the name of *Pterygodermatites affinis.* In 1996, Barus et al. reexamined *affinis* and several other species within the genus *Pterygodermatites* and determined that *cahirensis* was a valid species occurring mainly in felids.

Geographic Distribution

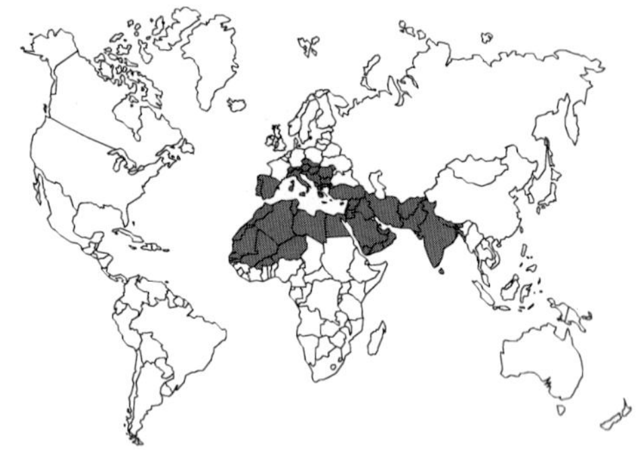

Fig. 4.67.

This worm has been reported from cats in North Africa and the Middle East (Abdul Salam and Baker, 1990; Dalimi and Mobedi, 1992; Daoud et al., 1988; Jägerskiöld, 1909; Quentin et al., 1976; Witenberg, 1928). The worm has also been reported from cats in India (Arya, 1979, 1980; Gupta and Pande, 1970, 1977; Srivastava, 1940).

Location in Host

Small intestine.

Parasite Identification

These are white worms. The females are 8.75 to 13.5 mm long, and the males are 3.7 to 4.8 mm long. (Jägerskiöld, 1909). The number of lateroventral spines on the male is 96, and the number of cuticular ornamentations on the lateroventral flanges of the female is 126 to 135. The ovoid egg contains a larva, is thick shelled, and is about 30 μm by 40 μm. The distinctive feature of the worm is the lateral appearance of the sclerotized buccal capsule, which can be used to distinguish this species from that of *Pterygodermatites affinis* of the fox.

Life Cycle

The first intermediate host of *Pterygodermatites cahirensis* is an arthropod, and Quentin et al. (1976) found larvae in the insect *Tachyderma hispida* in Algeria. When these larvae were fed to a young cat, eggs appeared in the feces 38 days later. Witenberg (1928) and Gupta and Pande (1970) found larvae encapsulated in the wall of the intestine and in abdominal mesenteries of lizards. Gupta and Pande (1970), using larvae recovered from these lizards, successfully infected a cat experimentally. Later, Gupta and Pande (1977), using larvae recovered from a naturally infected frog, *Rana tigrina,* infected puppies and found a prepatent period of 25 to 40 days.

Clinical Presentation and Pathogenesis

There have been no descriptions of signs associated with infections of cats with this parasite.

Treatment

There have been no attempts at treating infected cats.

Epizootiology

The life cycle requires an arthropod intermediate host and amphibian and reptilian paratenic hosts. Thus, cats become infected by the ingestion of these hosts.

Hazards to Other Animals

None.

Hazards to Humans

None.

Control/Prevention

Prevention of hunting by cats with a predisposition to prey on lizards and arthropods.

REFERENCES

Abdul Salam J, Baker K. 1990. Prevalence of intestinal helminths in stray cats in Kuwait. Pak Vet J 10:17–21.

Arya SN. 1979. Redescription of *Rictularia cahirensis* Jägerskiöld, 1904 from the cat (*Felis domesticus*) from Jodhpur, India. Parasitol Hung 12:87–89.

Arya SN. 1980. First record of male of *Rictularia cahirensis* Jägerskiöld, 1904 (Nematoda: Rictularioidea) from a cat, *Felis domesticus* in India. Ind J Parasitol 4:35–36.

Barus V, Petavy AF, Deblock S, Tenora F. 1996. On *Pterygodermatities* (*Multipectines*) *affinis* and other species of *Multipectines* (Nematoda, Rictulariidae). Helminthologia 33:93–100.

Dalimi A, Mobedi I. 1992. Helminth parasites of carnivores in northern Iran. Ann Trop Med Parasitol 86:395–397.

Daoud IS, Al Tae ARA, Salman YJ. 1988. Prevalence of gastro-intestinal helminths in cats from Iraq. J Biol Sci Res 19:363–368.

Gibbs HC. 1957. The taxonomic status of *Rictularia affinis* Jägerskiöld, 1909, *Rictularia cahirensis* Jägerskiöld, 1909, and *Rictularia splendida* Hall, 1913. Can J Zool 35:405–410.

Gupta VP, Pande BP. 1970. *Hemidactylus flaviviridis*, a paratenic host of *Rictularia cahirensis*. Curr Sci 23:535–536.

Gupta VP, Pande BP. 1977. Development of re-encapsulated larva of *Rictularia cahirensis* in experimental pups. Ind J Parasitol 1:177–180.

Jägerskiöld LAKE. 1909. Nematoden aus Aegypten und dem Sudan (eigesammelt von der schwedischen zoologischen Expedition). Results Swedish Zoological Expedition Egypt and White Nile 1901 (Jägerskiöld). Pt. 3, 66 pp, 4 plates.

Miquel J, Cassanova JC, Tenora F, Felieu C, Torres J. 1995. A scanning electron microscope study of some Rictulariidae (Nematoda) parasites of Iberian mammals. Helminthologia 32:3–14.

Quentin JC, Seureau C, Vernet R. 1976. Cycle biologique du nematode rictulaire *Pterygodermatites* (*Multipectines*) *affinis* (Jägerskiöld, 1904). Ann Parasitol Hum Comp 51:51–64.

Srivastava HD. 1940. An unrecorded spirurid worm, *Rictularia cahirensis* Jagerskiold, 1904, from the intestine of an Indian cat. Ind J Vet Sci Anim Husb 10:113–114.

Tiner JD. 1948. Observations on the *Rictularia* (Nematoda: Thelaziidae) of North America. Trans Am Microsc Soc 67:192–200.

Witenberg GG. 1928. Reptilien als Zchwischenwirte parasitischer Würmer von Katze und Hund. Tierärztl Rundschau 34:603.

THELAZIOIDEA

This is a group of nematodes that contains eye worms of mammals and birds (*Thelazia* and *Oxyspirura*). Two of these eye worms, *Thelazia californiensis* and *Thelazia callipaeda,* have been reported from the eyes of cats. The Thelazioidea also contains a group of morphologically related nematodes, the Pneumospiruridae, found in the lungs of mammalian hosts. Cats are infected by two species of the Pneumospiruridae, *Vogeloides massinoi* and *Vogeloides ramanujacharii.* Species of *Thelazia* use flies as their intermediate hosts. It is expected that members of the Pneumospiruridae also use arthropod intermediate hosts.

Thelazia californiensis Price, 1930

Etymology

Thelazia for Dr. Thelaz; *californiensis* for the location from where the specimens were collected.

Synonyms

None.

History

Allerton (1929) reported on a *Thelazia* species from the eye of a dog collected in the area of Los Angeles, California. The worms in this report were identified by Dr. Ackert as *Thelazia callipaeda.* In 1930, Price recognized the worm as a new species and gave it the name *Thelazia californiensis.* Most reports have been made from dogs.

Geographic Distribution

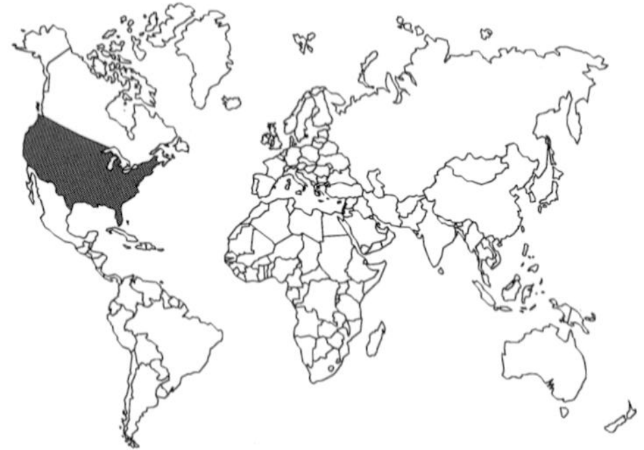

Fig. 4.68.

Parmelee et al. (1956) presented the geographical distribution of this parasite in California. Douglas (1939) reported that the cat could serve as a host of this parasite. Cases from humans in Utah have also been reported (Doezie et al., 1996).

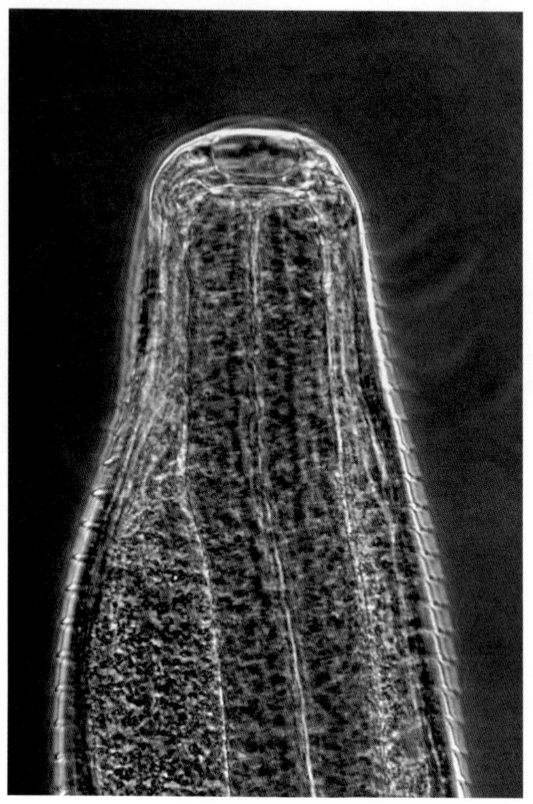

Fig. 4.69. *Thelazia* species. View of the anterior end showing the anterior of the esophagus, the striations in the cuticle, and the anteriorly projecting uterus.

Location in Host

These worms are parasites of the orbits of the eye, being found on the conjunctiva and under the lids and nictitating membrane.

Parasite Identification

These are white to cream colored worms. The males are 12 to 13 mm long with dissimilar spicules, the longer being 1.5 to 1.7 mm long and the shorter being 0.15 to 0.19 mm long. The females are 15 to 17 mm long. The vulva of the female is located behind the esophageal intestinal junction and is 0.8 to 1 mm from the anterior end (Fig. 4.69). The eggs in the uterus measure 52 μm by 29 μm. The species differs from *Thelazia callipaeda* in that, in the latter, the vulva is located anterior to the junction of the esophagus and intestine.

Life Cycle

Burnett et al. (1957) reported on the life cycle of *Thelazia californiensis.* Sheathed larvae from worms were fed to various species of flies, and developmental stages of the worm were recovered from species of the muscoid fly, *Fannia canicularis.* These authors also collected similar larval forms from *Fannia benjamini* collected near San Bernadino, California and felt that they represented natural infections of the flies with this parasite. When the fly feeds on fluids around the eye, the larvae that have migrated to the mouth parts are deposited, and they enter the eye to begin development in their vertebrate host. Weinmann et al. (1974) showed that the vector of *Thelazia californiensis* is actually a new species of *Fannia.* This fly was described as *Fannia thelaziae* by Turner (1976).

Clinical Presentation and Pathogenesis

None reported.

Treatment

Treatment would most typically be by the application of local anesthetic and the careful removal of the worms from the eye.

Epizootiology

There is very little information on the prevalence of this parasite and no information as to whether it is transmitted seasonally.

Hazards to Other Animals

Other known hosts include the dog, coyote, bear, jackrabbit, and silver fox (Burnett and Wagner, 1958). These animals are infected from larvae deposited by flies, so there is no direct transmission between cats and other animals without flies being present.

Hazards to Humans

There have been a number of published cases of human infection with this worm. Cases in humans have come from the Sierra Nevada and Siskiou Mountains, the Mojave Desert, and the Rocky Mountains in Utah. Lee and Parmlee (1958) reported on six human cases, including summarizing the three earlier cases reported by Kofoid and Williams (1935), Hosford et al. (1942), and Freidman (1951). Knierim and Jack (1975) reported on a case in a pathology resident who recalled contact with a small fly or gnat while riding on a motorcycle. Kirschner et al. (1990) reported a case from a woman who reported symptoms beginning 2 weeks after getting a small fly in the eye while hiking in the Sierra Nevada foothills. Doezie et al. (1996) reported on two cases from the eyes of patients in the Rocky Mountains of Utah.

Control/Prevention

Control would be by preventing the flies from feeding around the eyes of cats. There is no information as to whether monthly ivermectin for cats would prevent infections with this worm; however, because of the external site of development, it is likely that this would not be effective.

REFERENCES

Allerton FR. 1929. Worm parasites on conjunctiva in dog. North Am Vet 10:56.

Burnett HS, Wagner ED. 1958. Two new definitive hosts for the eye worm, *Thelazia californiensis* Price, 1930. J Parasitol 44:502.

Burnett HS, Parmelee WE, Lee RD, Wagner ED. 1957. Observations on the life cycle of *Thelazia californiensis* Price, 1930. J Parasitol 43:433.

Doezie AM, Kucius RW, Aldeen W, Hale D, Sith DR, Mamalis N. 1996. *Thelazia californiensis* conjunctival infestation. Ophthal Surg Lasers 27:716–719.

Douglas JR. 1939. The domestic cat, a new host for *Thelazia californiensis* Price, 1930 (Nematoda: Thelaziidae). Proc Helm Soc Wash 6:104.

Freidman M. 1951. Thelaziasis der Conjunctiva, ein Nachtrat. Ophthalmologica 122:252–254.

Hosford GN, Stewart MA, Sugarman EI. 1942. Eye worm (*Thelazia californiensis*) infection in man. Arch Ophthalmol 27:1165–1170.

Kirschner BI, Dunn JP, Ostler HB. 1990. Conjunctivitis caused by *Thelazia californiensis.* Am J Ophthalmol 110:573–574.

Knierim R, Jack MK. 1975. Conjunctivitis due to *Thelazia californiensis.* Arch Ophthalmol 93:522–523.

Kofoid CA, Williams OL. 1935. The nematode *Thelazia californiensis* as a parasite of the eye of man in California. Arch Ophthalmol 13:176–180.

Kofoid CA, Williams OL, Veale NC. 1937. *Thelazia californiensis,* a nematode eye worm of dog and man, with a review of the *Thelazia*s of domestic animals. Univ Calif Publ Zool 41:225–234.

Lee RD, Parmlee WE. 1958. Thelaziasis in man. Am J Trop Med Hyg 7:427–428.

Parmelee WE, Lee RD, Wagner ED, Burnett HS. 1956. A survey of *Thelazia californienesis,* a mammalian eye worm, with new locality records. JAVMA 129: 325–327.

Price EW. 1930. A new nematode parasitic in the eyes of dogs in the United States. J Parasitol 17: 112–113.

Turner WJ. 1976. *Fannia thelaziae,* a new species of eye-frequenting fly of the *benjamini* group from California and description of *F. conspicua* female (Diptera: Muscidae). Pan-Pacific Entomol 52:234–241.

Weinmann CJ, Anderson JR, Rubtzoff P, Connolly G, Longhurst WM. 1974. Eyeworms and face flies in California. Cal Agric 28:4–5.

Thelazia callipaeda Railliet and Henry, 1910

Etymology

Thelazia for Dr. Thelaz and *calli* = beautiful + *paeda* = child, referring to the beautiful larvae within the female worm.

Synonyms

None.

History

This worm was described by Railliet and Henry (1910) for specimens collected from the nictitating membrane of a dog in Pawal Pindi, Punjab, India.

Geographic Distribution

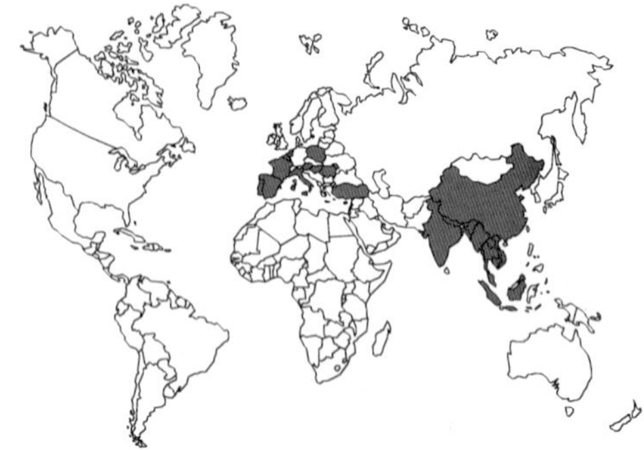

Fig. 4.70.

Europe, China, India, and Southeast Asia. Di Sacco et al. (1995) described an infection with *Thelazia callipaeda* in the eye of a cat in Italy. Morishige et al. (1992) found *Thelazia callipaeda* in 5 of 11,581 cats in Japan; the cats were examined by the inversion of the eyelid. Shi et al. (1988) reported on two of four cats and 37 of 39 dogs infected in Guang Hua of Hubei Province, China; there were also 37 human cases diagnosed during the same 5-year period, 1970 to 1975.

Location in Host

These worms are parasites of the orbits of the eye, being found on the conjunctiva and under the lids and nictitating membrane.

Parasite Identification

These are white- to cream-colored worms. The males are 9 to 12 mm long with dissimilar spicules, the left being 1.3 to 2.3 mm long and the right being 0.12 to 0.16 mm long. The females are 10 to 18 mm long. The vulva of the female is located anterior to the esophageal intestinal junction and is 0.5 to 0.7 mm from the anterior end. This species differs from *Thelazia californiensis* in that, in the latter, the vulva is located posterior to the junction of the esophagus and intestine.

Life Cycle

Kozlov (1962 and 1963; Wang et al. 1990; Wang and Yang, 1993) reported on the life cycle of this worm. Sheathed larvae were fed to flies of the *Drosophila* family, *Amiota* (= *Phortica*) *variegata,* where within about 3 weeks they had become infective third-stage larvae. The larvae present in the flies had genital systems that were much more highly advanced than is typical of third-stage larvae, the testes were already quite extended, and both branches of the uterus in the female were readily apparent. When larvae were placed in the eyes of dogs, Kozlov found adult males and females present by 3 weeks after infection, and a few days later, the uterus of the female contained larvated eggs. By 55 days after infection, motile larvae were present in the vagina of the female.

Clinical Presentation and Pathogenesis

The cat described by Di Sacco et al. (1995) was a castrated 10-year-old male. The cat presented with blepharospasm and epiphora of the left eye. There was a monolateral keratoconjunctivitis with corneal opacities noted on the nasal quadrant of the eye starting at the limbus. The worms were noted on ocular examination and removed. A total of four worms, three females and a male, were recovered. The worms were about 8 to 12 mm long.

Treatment

Treatment would most typically be by the application of local anesthetic and the careful removal of the worms from the eye.

Epizootiology

Kozlov (1962) reported that adult worms were found in the eyes of dogs throughout the year. It thus appears possible that there may be various populations of worms infecting the eye throughout the year in areas where the prevalence is high.

Hazards to Other Animals

Other known hosts include canids and rabbits. There would not be direct transmission from cats to other hosts, but because the intermediate host is a gnat, it seems highly possible that gnats could set up a cycle in the vicinity of a cattery and pose as a threat to the health of the animals.

Hazards to Humans

Infections of humans with this species of eye worm have been more commonly reported than infections in the United States with *Thelazia californiensis*. Human infections have been reported from throughout southeastern Asia. Examples of human cases from various countries include China (Lu, 1996; Hsü, 1933); Thailand (Bhaibulaya et al., 1970); Japan (Arizono et al., 1976); Indonesia (Kosin et al., 1989); and Korea (Hong et al., 1985).

Control/Prevention

Control would be by preventing the flies from feeding around the eyes of cats. There is no information as to whether monthly ivermectin for cats would prevent infections with this worm; however, because of the external site of development, it is likely that this would not be effective.

REFERENCES

Arizono N, Yopshida Y, Kondo K, Kuimoto H, Oda K, Shiota T, Shimada Y, Ogino K. 1976. *Thelazia callipaeda* from man and dogs in Kyoto and its scanning electron microscopy [in Japanese]. Jap J Parasitol 25:402–408.

Bhaibulaya M, Prasetsilpa S, Vajrasthira S. 1970. *Thelazia callipaeda* Railliet and Henry, 1910, in a man and dog in Thailand. Am J Trop Med Hyg 19:476–479.

Di Sacco B, Ciocca A, Sirtori G. 1995. *Thelazia callipaeda* (Railliet and Henry, 1910) nel sacco congiuntivale di un gatto di Milano. Veterinaria 9:81–84.

Hong ST, Lee SH, Kim SI. 1985. A human case of *Thelazia callipaeda* infection with reference to its internal structures. Kor J Parasitol 26:137–140.

Hsü HF. 1933. On *Thelazia callipaeda* Railliet and Henry, 1910, infection in man and dog. Arch Schiffs Tropenhyg 37:363–369.

Kosin E, Kosman ML, Depary AA. 1989. First case of human thelaziasis in Indonesia. Southeast Asian J Trop Med Publ Health 20:233–236.

Kozlov DP. 1962. The life cycle of the nematode, *Thelazia callipaeda*, parasitic in the eye of man and carnivores [in Russian]. Doklady Akademii Nauk SSSR 142:732–733.

Kozlov DP. 1963. Biology of *Thelazia callipaeda* Railliet and Henry, 1910 [in Russian]. Trudi Gelmintologisscheskoi Laboratorii 13:330–346.

Lu YF. 1996. An infant with *Thelazia callipaeda* infection [in Chinese]. Chin J Parasitol Parasi Dis 14:138.

Morishige K, Saito T, Maeda S, Tongu Y. 1992. Infection rate of *Thelazia callipaeda* in dogs and cats in Bingo District and Okayama City. Jap J Parasitol 41:431–433.

Shi YE, Han JJ, Yang WY, Wei DX. 1988. *Thelazia callipaeda* (Nematoda: Spirurida): transmission by flies from dogs to children in Hubei, China. Trans Roy Soc Trop Med Hyg 82:627.

Railliet A, Henry ACL. 1910. Nouvelles observations sur les thélazies nématodes parasites de l'oiel. Compt Rend Soc Biol, Paris 68:783–785.

Wang ZX, Yang ZX. 1993. Studies on the development of *Thelazia callipaeda* larva in the intermediate host *Amiota variegata* in China. Chin J Zool 28:4–8.

Wang ZX, Yang ZX, Du JS. 1990. The discovery of *Amiota variegata* as an intermediate host of *Thelazia callipaeda* in China. Chin J Zool 25:55.

Vogeloides massinoi (Davtjan, 1933) Dougherty, 1952

In 1933, Davtjan reported on worms recovered from the small bronchioles and lungs of 30 percent of some 100 cats that were examined in Armenia. The worms were white. The males were 8 to 14 mm long, and the females 26 to 40 mm long. The worms had six well-developed lips surrounding the mouth. The esophagus was clearly divided into an anterior muscular and a posterior glandular portion. The male had a pointed tail, spicules that were similar and about 200 μm long, and a gubernaculum. The vulva of the female was located near the anus. The eggs were thick shelled and ovoid with a length of 38 to 58 μm and a width of 25 to 34 μm. The mature eggs contained larvae. In 1952, Dougherty transferred the species described by Davtjan to a new genus, *Vogeloides.* There appears to be no other reports of this species from cats.

In 1977, Pence and Stone described the pathology associated with *Vogeloides felis* in the bobcat, *Felis rufus,* in west Texas. They found that the severity of the pathology observed depended on the intensity of infection with these worms. There was a patchy interstitial pneumonia with edema of the alveolar sept observed immediately adjacent to infected bronchioles. In bobcats with more than 100 worms, the lesions expanded to involve most of the lungs. The parenchymal changes were tentatively attributed to an interstitial pneumonia resulting from a blockage of the terminal air passages by the nematodes.

REFERENCES

Davtjan EA. 1933. Ein neuer Nematode aud den Lungen der Hauskatze. *Osleroides massino,* nov. sp. Deutsch Tierärztl Wchschr 41:372–374.

Dougherty EC. 1952. A note on the genus *Metathelazia* Skinker, 1931 (Nematoda: Metastrongylidae). Proc Helm Soc Wash 19:55–63.

Pence DB, Stone JE. 1977. Lungworms (Nematoda: Pneumospiruridae) from west Texas carnivores. J Parasitol 63:979–991.

Vogeloides ramanujacharii Alwar, Lalitha, and Seneviratnaa, 1958

This species was described based on a collection of worms from the lungs of 12 of 50 cats that were examined in Madras, India. Each cat was found infected with only one to four worms, except from two cats that each harbored about a dozen adult worms. The worms were white and thread-like. The males were about 7 to 15 mm long, and the females 13 to 30 mm long. The esophagus was divided into a distinct slender anterior muscular portion and a longer posteriad glandular portion. The excretory pore was posterior to the nerve ring and anteriad to the junction of the muscular and glandular portions of the esophagus. The spicules were similar and measured about 150 μm to 190 μm in length; a gubernaculum was present. The vulva of the female was located just anterior to the anus; the posterior portion of the uterus contained thick shelled, embryonated, ovoid eggs that measured 40 μm to 45 μm long by 25 μm to 35 μm in width.

REFERENCES

Alwar VS, Lalitha CM, Seneviratna P. 1958. *Vogeloides ramanujacharii* n. sp., a new lungworm from the domestic cat (*Felis catus* Linne), in India. Ind Vet J 35:1–5.

SPIRUROIDEA

The Spiruroidea is represented in cats by a number of species that parasitize the stomach of the feline host. Typically, these worms produce small, thick-shelled eggs that are infectious to some arthropod hosts. The larvae that live in the arthropod are capable of utilizing various vertebrate paratenic hosts that will transmit the worms to the feline final host.

Spirura rytipleurites (Deslongchamps, 1824) Railliet, 1916

Etymology

Spirura from the name of the group (round), *ryti* = wrinkled cuticle, and *pleurites* for the location of the cysts in the pleural cavity of the intermediate host.

Synonyms

Filaria gastrophila of Müller, 1894; *Spirura gastrophila* of Marotel, 1912.

History

These worms were originally described by Deslongchamp (1824) from larvae recovered from the body cavity of the oriental cockroach (*Periplaneta orientalis*). Müller (1894) was probably the first to illustrate the adult forms of this species. In 1954, Chabaud divided the species into two subspecies. *Spirura rytipleurites rytipleurites* is considered a parasite of the cat and accidentally sometimes the rat; the intermediate host of this subspecies is the cockroach. The other subspecies, *Spirura rytipleurites seurati,* is considered a parasite of the mongoose *(Herpestes),* fox *(Vulpes),* hedgehog *(Eiinaceus),* and striped polecat *(Zorilla),* and the intermediate hosts are considered to be beetles rather than cockroaches.

Geographic Distribution

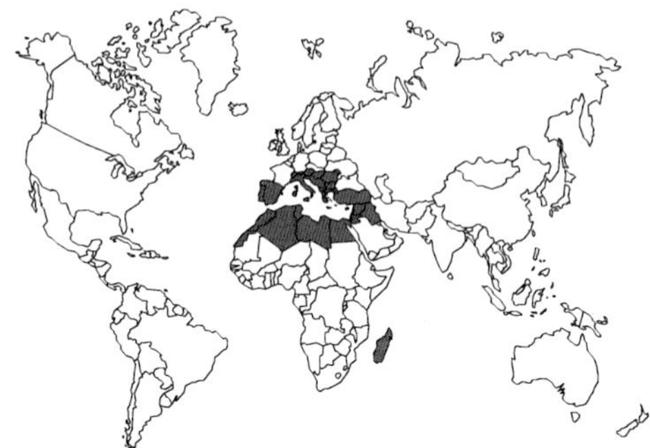

Fig. 4.71.

These worms are common in North Africa and probably into parts of southern Europe as evidenced by their appearance in hedgehogs in Sicily (Gianetto and Trotti, 1995). Marotel (1912) reported on infections in cats, one from Lyon and one from Madagascar. Sonsino (1896) reported on worms recovered from a cat in Egypt.

Location in Host

The adults live in the wall of the esophagus and stomach.

Parasite Identification

The adults of this genus are recognized by the presence of one or two ventral cuticular bosses (inflations) in the cervical region. The eggs are ovoid; each has a smooth, thick shell and contains a first-stage larva with a cephalic hook when passed in the feces.

Life Cycle

Stefanski (1934b) showed that the larvae were capable of developing in cockroaches that become infected when they ingest the eggs. The larvae grow within capsules in the abdominal cavities of the cockroaches where they become quite long, over 1 cm in length. The third-stage larvae within the abdominal cavity of the insects have well-developed reproductive systems. Cats become infected through the ingestion of infected cockroaches. Stefanski fed 17 larvae to a cat and recovered 11 adult worms.

Clinical Presentation and Pathogenesis

Not described.

Treatment

Not described.

Epizootiology

Chabaud (1954) stated that the larvae of *Spirura rytipleurites* are in extraordinary abundance in North Africa, being present within the body cavities of some 30 percent of the "Moricas, Pimelies, and Blaps" dissected around Casablanca. The larvae are also commonly found in various vertebrates (e.g., species of skinks, *Chalcides,* and frogs, *Bufo*). It would appear that cats are becoming infected by eating either the arthropods or the small vertebrate paratenic hosts.

Hazards to Other Animals

It appears that it would be unlikely that other hosts would be seriously affected; however, the development of the spiny hedgehog as a pet and the potential of oriental cockroaches serving as intermediate hosts could lead to the development of large number of parasites causing disease under confinement situations.

Hazards to Humans

None.

Control/Prevention

As with many of the parasites, it is important to keep cats from hunting. At the same time, the large numbers of oriental cockroaches that can be present in houses would mean that infections could be very hard to control in many parts of the world.

REFERENCES

Chabaud AG. 1954. Le cycle évolutive des spirurides et de nématodes ayant une biologie comparable. Valeur systématique des caractères biologiques. Ann Parasitol Hum Comp 29:42–88, 206–249, 358–425.

Deslongchamp EE. 1824. Spiroptère. Spiroptera. Encycl. Méthodique, Paris, vol 2, p 697.
Galeb O. 1878. Observations sur les migrations du *Filaria rytipleurites,* parasite des blatteset des rats. Compt Rend Hebd Séances Acad Sc, Paris 88:75–77.
Gianetto S, Trotti GC. 1995. Light and scanning electron microscopy of *Spirura rytipleurites seurati* Chabaud, 1954 (Nematoda: Spiruridae) from *Erinaceus europaeus* in Sicily. J Helminthol 69:305–311.
Marotel G. 1912. Nouveau Spiroptère stomacal du chat. Rec méd vét 86:827–828.
Müller A. 1894. Helminthologische Beobachtungen an bekannten und unbekannten Entozoen. Arch Naturgesch 60:113.
Sonsino P. 1896. Forme nuove, o poco conosciute, in parte indeterminate, di entozoi raccolti, o osservati in Eggito. Centr Bak Parasit, Abt. 1 20:437–449.
Stefanski M. 1934a. *Spirura rytipleurites* (Deslonchamps, 1824) parasite peu connu du chat. Wiadom Wet 13:177–180.
Stefanski M. 1934b. Sur le dévelopment et les caratères spécifiques de *Spirura rytipleurites.* Ann Parasitol 12:203–217.

Cyathospirura seurati Gibbs, 1957

Etymology

Cyatho = cup shaped + *spirura* = speiroieides (spiral) and *seurati* after Dr. Seurat.

Synonyms

Cyathospirura dasyuridis Mawson, 1968.

History

Gibbs (1957) first described this from a fennec fox in Egypt. Mawson (1968) described a new species, *Cyathospirura dasyuridis,* from dasyurid marsupials (*Dasyurops maculatus* and *Dasyurus quoll*) of Australia and Tasmania. In 1993, Hasegawa et al., after comparing specimens of *Cyathospirura* collected from rodents in Okinawa, placed *Cyathospirura dasyuridis* in synonymy with *Cyathospirura seurati.* Seurat (1913) described a new species, *Habronema chevreuxi,* from a cat, *Felis ocreata,* from Algeria that was red and found free within the stomach. The worm was transferred to the genus *Cyathospirura* by Baylis (1934). It has since been reported from Tunisia, Central Africa, and North America (Pence et al., 1978). Chabaud (1959) confirmed the separate identity of *Cyathospirura chevrauxi,* but the distinguishing characters were mainly the host and the different geographical locations. In light of the work by Hasegawa et al. (1993), this may need to be reconsidered.

Geographic Distribution

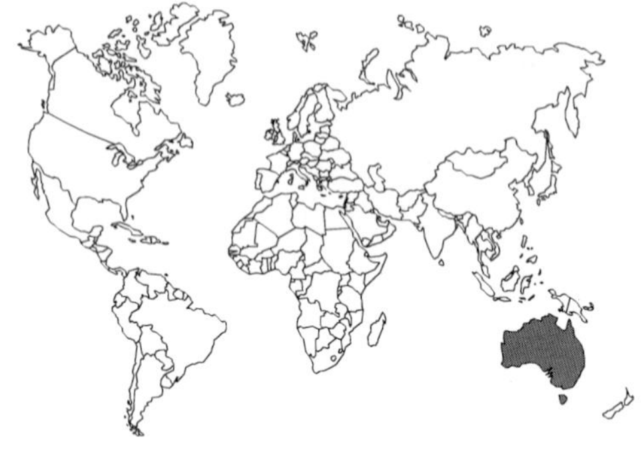

Fig. 4.72.

It has been reported from cats in Australia and Tasmania (Coman, 1972; Coman et al., 1981), Gregory and Munday (1976). It has also been reported from the fennec fox in Egypt (Gibbs, 1957) and from foxes in Australia (Coman, 1973). It has been described from *Rattus rattus* in southern Europe, North Africa, and Japan (Quentin and Werthem, 1975; Hasegawa et al., 1993).

Location in Host

The worms are found in the stomach of their host, as noted originally by Seurat (1913) and later by Coman et al. (1981). In cats in Australia, *Cyathospirura seurati* was typically found free in the lumen, while *Cylicospirura felineus* was found in tumors in the mucosa. Pence et al. (1978) noticed in bobcats that *Cyathospirura chevrauxi* was typically free in the lumen while the *Cylicospirura felineus* that was present caused tumors in the mucosa.

Parasite Identification

The red worms of *Cyathospirura seurati* are found free in the lumen of the stomach (although sometimes in the tumors formed by *Cylicospirura felineus* if also present). The worms are about 6 to

12 mm long. The worms in the genus *Cyathospirura* differ from those of *Cylicospirura* and *Spirocerca* in that the buccal cavity has one dorsal and one ventral lobe and contains eight teeth. The vulva is located near midbody. The eggs are small, clear, thick shelled and contain coiled embryos. The eggs are 33 to 35 μm long and 18 to 20 μm wide.

Life Cycle

Gupta and Opande (1981) reported on the experimental infection of dogs with spirurid larvae recovered from wall lizards, *Hemidactylus flaviviridis.* Worms were recovered from the dogs 16 to 24 days after infection. These worms were described as a new species, *Cyathospirura chabaudi,* that was considered morphologically similar to *Cyathospirura seurati.*

Clinical Presentation and Pathogenesis

There have been no descriptions of the pathologic manifestations of this parasite. Pence et al. (1978) felt that *Cyathospirura chevreuxi* was mainly a lumen dweller. Gupta and Opande (1981) found that *Cyathospirura chabaudi* in experimentally infected puppies was found deep in the mucosa and submucosa.

Treatment

None has been reported.

Epizootiology

Very little is known about the intermediate hosts of this group of worms. It would be suspected that the first intermediate host would be an arthropod. It is suspected that paratenic hosts are involved in the life cycle and that cats would become infected by either eating lizards or some other such host.

Hazards to Other Animals

There would be no direct infection of animals housed with infected cats.

Hazards to Humans

None would be likely.

Control/Prevention

Cats should be prevented from hunting.

REFERENCES

Baylis HA. 1934. On a collection of cestodes and nematodes from small mammals in Taganyika Territory. Ann Mag Nat Hist 10:338–353.

Chabaud AG. 1959. Sur la systematique des nematodes proches de *Spirocerca lupi* (Rud., 1809). Parassitologia 1:129–135.

Coman BJ. 1972. A survey of the gastro-intestinal parasites of the feral cat in Victoria. Aust Vet J 48:133–136.

Coman BJ. 1973. Helminth parasites of the fox (*Vulpes vulpes*) in Victoria. Aust Vet J 49:378–384.

Coman BJ, Jones EH, Driesen MA. 1981. Helminth parasites and arthropods of feral cats. Aust Vet J 57:324–327.

Gibbs HC. 1957. Helminth parasites of reptiles, birds and mammals in Egypt. III. *Cyathospirura seurati* sp. nov. from *Fennecus zerda.* Can J Zool 35:201–205.

Gregory GC, Munday BL. 1976. Internal parasites of feral cats from the Tasmanian Midlands and King Island. Aust Vet J 52:317–320.

Gupta VP, Opande BP. 1981. *Cyathospirura chabaudi* n. sp. from pups infected with re-encapsulated larvae from a paratenic host. Ind J Anim Sci 51: 526–534.

Hasegawa H, Arai S, Shiraishi S. 1993. Nematodes collected from rodents on Uotsuri Island, Okinawa, Japan. J Helminthol Soc Wash 60:39–47.

Mawson PM. 1968. Two species of Nematoda (Spirurida: Spiruridae) from Australian dasyurids. Parasitology 58:75–78.

Pence DB, Samoil HP, Stone JE. 1978. Spirocercid stomach worms (Nematoda: Spirocercidae) from wild felids in North America. Can J Zool 56: 1032–1042.

Quentin JC, Werthem G. 1975. Helminths d'oiseaux et de Mammifères d'Israâl. V. Spirurides nouveauz ou peu connus. Ann Parasitol 50:63–85.

Ryan GE. 1976. Gastro-intestinal parasites of feral cats in New South Wales. Aust Vet J 52:224–227.

Seurat LG. 1913. Sur deux spiroptères du chat ganté (*Felis ocreata* Gmel.). Compt Rend Soc Biol, Paris 74:676–679.

Cylicospirura felineus (Chandler, 1925) Sandground, 1932

Etymology

Cylico = cycle and *spirura* = spiral, along with *felineus* for cat.

Synonyms

Spirocerca felineus Chandler, 1925.

History

This worm was first described as *Spirocerca felineus* by Chandler in 1925 based on specimens he recovered from purulent cysts in the stomach wall of about 5 of 250 cats that he examined in Calcutta, India. In 1932, Sandground redescribed the species using specimens recovered from a Bengal tiger, and he transferred *felineus* to the genus *Cylicospirura.*

Geographic Distribution

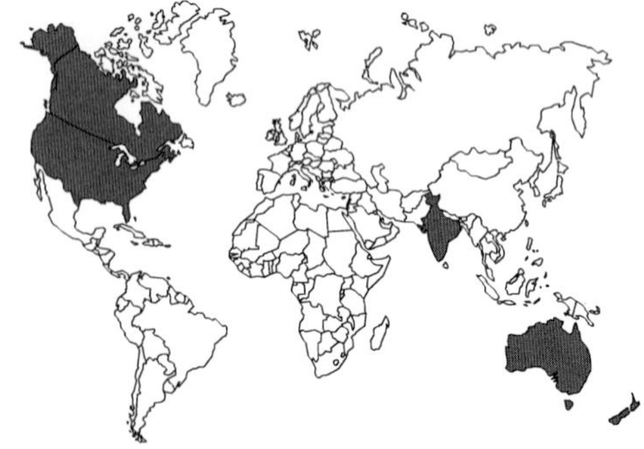

Fig. 4.73.

Cylicospirura felineus has been described from cats in India (Chandler, 1925) and from cats in Australia and surrounding regions. Gill (1972) found this worm in the stomachs of 3 of 88 cats from New Delhi, India. Pavlov and Howell (1977) reported 4 percent of 100 cats in Canberra were infected with *Cylicospirura felineus.* Coman et al. (1981) reported that around 27 percent of 327 cats in Victoria and western New South Wales were infected with *Cylicospirura felineus, Cyathospirura dasyuridis,* or both parasites. Gregory and Munday (1976) reported that 57 percent of 86 cats from the Tasmanian midlands were infected with *Cylicospirura felineus, Cyathospirura dasyuridis,* or both parasites and that 9 of 21 cats from King Island were infected with *Cylicospirura felineus.* Interestingly, Pence et al. (1978) examined parasites from Texas bobcats and Canadian lynx from Alberta, Canada, and found that these hosts were infected with *Cylicospirura felineus.*

Location in Host

Chandler described the worms as being present in purulent cysts in the stomach wall. Gregory and Munday (1976) reported that nodules in the stomach wall contained the two species of spiruroid nematodes in about equal numbers. The *Cylicospirura felineus* nematodes were typically held firmly by the fibrous tissue of the nodule, while the *Cyathospirura dasyuridis* were free within the stomach or within the nodules. Coman et al. (1981) reported that *Cylicospirura felineus* nematodes usually were found within nodules in the pyloric region. Pence et al. (1978) stated that the stomachs of bobcats often contained mixed infections of *Cylicospirura felineus* and *Cyathospirura chevreuxi.* In the bobcats, the *Cylicospirura felineus* always appeared associated with enlarged granulomas in the pyloric stomach, while *Cyathospirura chevreuxi* appeared to be a lumen dweller that sometimes secondarily invaded the lesions produced by *Cylicospirura felineus.*

Parasite Identification

These are bright or blood red worms that reach a length of 30 mm (females) and 22 mm (males). The left spicule of the male is about 2 mm long; the right spicule is about 0.5 mm long. The buccal cavity is well developed and contains six longitudinal supporting ribs that end anteriorly in trifid projections. In the case of *Cylicospirura subaequalis,* the longitudinal ribs of the buccal cavity end in bifid knobs, and in the case of *Cylicospirura advena,* the projections end in a single knob.

The vulva is located anterior to the esophageal intestinal junction. The egg is thick shelled and contains a well-developed larva. The eggs are 29 μm to 38 μm long and 13 μm to 22 μm wide.

Life Cycle

There has been no work on the life cycle of this genus of parasites. It is likely that the intermediate host is some form of beetle and that cats become infected by eating the beetle or some vertebrate paratenic host.

Clinical Presentation and Pathogenesis

There have been no reports on the clinical signs observed in infected cats. Chandler (1925) noted that the worms were in purulent cysts in the stomach wall. Gregory and Munday (1976) found that the lesions in cats in Tasmania were fibrous and nonpurulent.

Pence et al. (1978) described the lesions observed in bobcats and lynx in some detail. The cystic granulomas in the stomach wall measured from a few millimeters in size to 3 cm. Each cyst contained from 1 to 45 worms. Usually, each cyst had a small orifice from which the posterior ends of worms extended. All granulomas of 1.5 cm diameter or greater were located in the pyloric region of the stomach. The tumors were most abundant on the side of greater curvature and only rarely seen on the side of lesser curvature. Small lesions in the fundus were observed that were filled with a firm yellowish necrotic material indicative of caseous necrosis, but these lesions never contained worms. The mucosal surface of the larger lesions was normal except for the orifice from which the worms protruded. Usually, the muscularis externa and the serosal surface were normal, and the granulomas were hardly discernable from the serosal aspect. However, in two cases, pedunculate nodular lesions, about 1 cm in diameter, protruded from the serosal wall of the pyloric region. These pedunculate lesions contained worms.

Treatment

There has been no attempt to treat infections with this parasite.

Epizootiology

It would appear that cats in Australia may be the natural host of this parasite, but it is also possible that dingoes, dogs, or foxes may also be serving as hosts in the wild. The fact that the cat was relatively recently introduced into Australia and Tasmania would indicate that either the cat is an accidental host or that the parasite was introduced with the cat and found adequate intermediate hosts for the successful completion of the life cycle. Interestingly, there has only been one other report from India (Gill, 1972), although a different species of *Cylicospirura, Cylicospirura subaequalis,* has been reported from India.

Hazards to Other Animals

There would be no direct transmission to other animals. It is very unclear what the impact, if any, this feline parasite might have on the indigenous animals in Australia.

Hazards to Humans

There are no known infections of humans.

Control/Prevention

Control would involve preventing cats from hunting.

REFERENCES

Chandler AC. 1925. The helminthic parasites of cats in Calcutta and the relation of cats to human helminthic infections. Ind J Med Res 13:213–228, plates 2 and 3.

Coman BJ, Jones EH, Driessen MA. 1981. Helminth parasites and arthropods of feral cats. Aust Vet J 57:324–327.

Gill HS. 1972. Incidence of gastro-intestinal helminths in cat (*Felis catus*) in Delhi. J Comm Dis 4:109–111.

Gregory GG, Munday BL. 1976. Internal parasites of feral cats from the Tasmanian Midlands and King Island. Aust Vet J 52:317–320.

Pavlov PM, Howell MJ. 1977. Helminth parasites of Canberra cats. Aust Vet J 53:599–600.

Pence DB, Samoil HP, Stone JE. 1978. Spirocercid stomach worms (Nematoda: Spirocercidae) from wild felids in North America. Can J Zool 56:1032–1042.

Sandground JH. 1932. Report on the nematode parasites collected by the Kelley-Roosevelts expedition to Indo-China with descriptions of several new species. Part 1. Parasites of Birds. Part 2. Parasites of Mammals. Z Parasitenk 5:542–583.

Cylicospirura subaequalis (Molin, 1860) Vevers, 1922

Etymology

Cylico = cycle and *spirura* = spiral, along with *subaequalis,* which refers to the spicules of different lengths.

Synonyms

Spiroptera subaequalis Molin, 1860.

History

In 1860, Molin described *Spiroptera subaequalis* from specimens collected from cats in South America and Algeria. In 1913, Seurat described specimens from cats in Algeria. In 1922, Vevers created the genus *Cylicospirura* to include specimens recovered from animals in the London Zoo.

Geographic Distribution

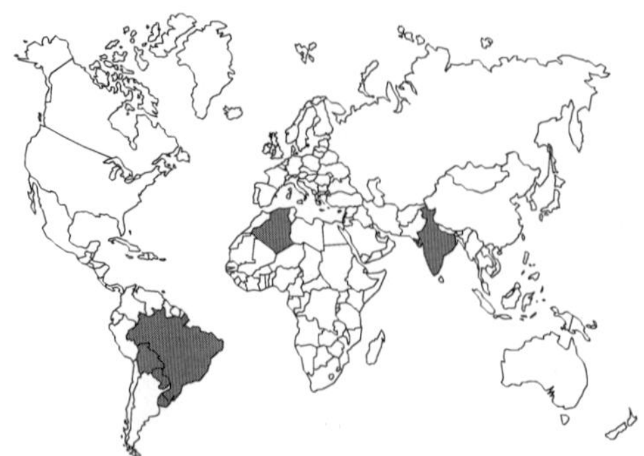

Fig. 4.74.

Reports of this species in cats have come from India (Mudaliar and Alwar, 1947; Alwar and Lalitha, 1958; Abdul Rahman et al., 1971; Pillai et al., 1981; and Silimban et al., 1996). Molin (1860) had originally described this parasite from cats in South America and Algeria. Seurat (1913) reported on the recovery of this worm from tumors in the stomach of *Felis ocreata* in Algeria and from *Felis concolor* and *Felis mellivora* from Brazil. In 1988, Waid and Pence redescribed *Cylicospirura subaequalis* from the American cougar (*Felis concolor*).

Location in Host

The adults of *Cylicospirura subaequalis* are found in cysts or tumors located in the wall of the fundus of the stomach. Waid and Pence (1988) found that in mountain lions the worms and nodules were mainly in the duodenum near the pyloric sphincter.

Parasite Identification

These are reddish brown worms. The female is 22 mm long, and the male is 20 mm long. The esophagus is about 20 percent of the total body length, and the vulva is located slightly anterior to the esophageal-intestinal junction. The spicules in the male are unequal, with the left spicule being about 2.5 mm long and the right spicule being about 0.5 mm long. The feature that differentiates *Cylicospirura subaequalis* from the other species of *Cylicospirura* is the shape of the anterior ends of the longitudinal ribs of the buccal capsule when viewed *en face* (Clark, 1981). These ribs in the case of *Cylicospirura subaequalis* are bifid at their anteriormost projection. Females of *Cylicospirura subaequalis* can be differentiated from females of *Cylicospirura felineus* by the position of the vulva relative to the esophago-intestinal junction. In *Cylicospirura subaequalis,* the vulva is located posterior to this junction; in *Cylicospirura felineus,* it is anteriad to this junction (Waid and Pence, 1988).

Life Cycle

The life has not been described for any member of this genus. Based on affinities to morphologically related forms, it is postulated that the intermediate host would be an arthropod, probably a beetle. There is also a possibility that vertebrate paratenic hosts are involved in the life cycle.

Clinical Presentation and Pathogenesis

There have been no reports actually detailing the clinical signs associated with infections with this parasite. The lesions would suggest clinical signs, but they have not yet been described.

Abdul Rahman et al. (1971) described the histopathology associated with a 4 cm nodule from the stomach of a cat in Bangalore, India. A single reddish brown worm was seen grossly protruding from the lesion, and dissection revealed a second worm within the nodule. Histopathology revealed that the nodule represented chronic inflammatory proliferation of connective tissue with suppuration around the contained worms. The lesions in the duodenum of the lions described by Waid and Pence (1988) were typically 1.5 to 2.5 cm in diameter, each with a central opening on the serosal surface. The nodules contained a necrotic cavity surrounded by fibrous encapsulation. The necrotic cavities contained debris, partially calcified remains of nematodes, and intact immature and adult nematodes.

Treatment

Not reported.

Epizootiology

This parasite is probably found in various wild felids and occasionally makes its way into the domestic cat. In North America, the potential wild hosts include mainly the lynx, bobcat, and puma, and it is unclear to what extent these populations overlap with the majority of domestic cats in the United Stated.

Hazards to Other Animals

Due to the requirement for an intermediate host, it is unlikely that these parasites would be directly transmitted from one cat to another or directly to other animals it may be living with while infected.

Hazards to Humans

There have not been reports of human infections with this parasite.

Control/Prevention

Cats that hunt are likely to be those that become infected.

REFERENCES

Abdul Rahman S, Hegde KS, Mohiyudeen S, Seshjadri SJ, Rahamathulla PM, Rajasekharan D. 1971. Study of *Cylicospirura subaequalis* (Molin, 1860) and the histopathology of the nodule in the stomach of the cat. Ind Vet J 48:683–687.

Alwar VS, Lalitha CM. 1958. Parasites of domestic cats (*Felis catus*) in Madras. Ind Vet J 35:292–295.

Bhalerao GD. 1935. Helminth parasites of domesticated animals in India. Sci Mong 6, Imper Counc Agric Res, Delhi, India.

Clark WC. 1981. *Cylicospirura advena* n. sp. (Nematoda: Spirocercidae) a stomach parasite from a cat in New Zealand, with observations on related species. Syst Parasitol 3:185–191.

Molin R. 1860. Una mongragia del genere *Spiroptera*. Sitzungsb K Akad Wissensch Wien, Math Naturw CL 38(28):7–38, 1 plate.

Mudaliar SV, Alwar VS. 1947. A check list of parasites (class Nematoda) in the Department of Parasitology, Madras Veterinary College Laboratory. Ind Vet J 24:77–94.

Pillai KM, Pythal C, Sundara RK. 1981. A note on the occurrence of *Cylicospirura subaequalis* (Molin, 1860) (Spiruridae: Nematoda) in a jungle kitten (*Felis chaus*) in Kerala. Kerrala J Vet Sci 12:155–156.

Rickard LG, Foreyt WJ. 1992. Gastrointestinal parasites of cougars (*Felis concolor*) in Washington and the first report of *Ollulanus tricuspis* in a sylvatic felid from North America. J Wildl Dis 28:130–133.

Seurat LG. 1913. Sur deux spiroptères du chat ganté (*Felis ocreata* Gmel.). Compt Rend Soc Biol, Paris 74:676–679.

Silamban S, Ramachandran KM, Devi TL, Pillai KM. 1996. Histopathology of *Cylicospirura subaequalis* induced nodule (Molin, 1860) in the stomach of a cat. J Vet Anim Sci 27:68–69.

Waid DD, Pence DB. 1988. Helminths of mountain lions (*Felis concolor*) from southwestern Texas, with a redescription of *Cylicospirura subaequalis* (Molin, 1860) Vevers, 1922. Can J Zool 66:2110–2117.

Vevers GM. 1922. On the parasitic nematoda collected from mammalian hosts which died in the gardens of the Zoological Society of London during the years 1919–1921; with a description of three new genera and three new species. Proc Zool Soc London (1922) part 4:901–919.

Cylicospirura heydoni (Baylis, 1927) Mawson, 1968

This species was originally described from a opossum, (*Dasyurus* species) collected in Cairns, north Queensland, Australia (Baylis, 1927). In 1968, the worms were redescribed by Mawson using specimens from *Dasyurus quoll* from Tasmania and *Dasyurops maculatus* from New South Wales. In 1997, Milstein and Goldsmid reported finding *Cylicospirura heydoni* in 4 of 39 cats collected in southern Tasmania. The six anteriorly directed ribs in the buccal cavity of *Cylicospirura heydoni* are each tipped with a single pointed denticle.

REFERENCES

Baylis HA. 1927. Some new parasitic nematodes from Australia. Ann Mag Nat Hist, Ser 9, 20:115–120.

Mawson PM. 1968. Two species of Nematoda (Spirurida: Spiruridae) from Australian dasyurids. Parasitology 58:75–78.

Milstein TC, Goldsmid JM. 1997. Parasites of feral cats from southern Tasmania and their potential significance. Aust Vet J 75:218–219.

Cylicospirura advena Clark, 1981

Cylicospirura advena nematodes were found in a single introduced feral cat in New Zealand. The feral cat was found to have in its stomach wall about six firm tumor-like balls, each about 1 cm in diameter. There was a fissure on the inner wall of each tumor, and nematodes were found to inhabit each tumor. The nematodes were described as a new species, *advena,* of *Cylicospirura,* where it was understood that the specific name *advena,* meaning stranger or foreigner, was an allusion to the probability that this worm was most likely of exotic origin.

The adults of these worms were about 5.5 mm long. The buccal capsule contained six heavily sclerotized ribs that terminated anteriorly in blunt knobs. Clark (1981) described the *en face* view of these ribs and used this character to distinguish the various species of *Cylicospirura*. The vulva was posterior to the base of the esophagus. The eggs were embryonated and 34 to 36 μm long and 22 to 24 μm wide.

REFERENCES

Clark WC. 1981. *Cylicospirura advena* n. sp. (Nematoda: Spirocercidae) a stomach parasite from a cat in New Zealand, with observations on related species. Syst Parasitol 3:185–191.

Spirocerca lupi (Rudolphi, 1809) Railliet and Henry, 1911

Spirocerca lupi is basically a parasite of dogs and other canids, although lesions or signs of lesions have been reported in nondomestic felids (Kikuchi et al., 1976; Murray, 1968; Pence and Stone, 1978). Infections in the domestic cat have been rare to nonexistent. Experimentally, it has been possible to cause lesions in cats although they have not been described under other circumstances.

Faust (1928) described the life cycle of *Spirocerca lupi,* showing that it was capable of utilizing beetle intermediate hosts and various vertebrate paratenic hosts. The life cycle of *Spirocerca lupi* as it relates to the canine host has been described in detail by Bailey (1965). Bailey exposed adult dung beetles of the genus *Geotrupes* to large numbers of eggs of *Spirocerca lupi.* Development to the third larval stage occurred in these intermediate hosts. These larvae were found within cysts in the body of the beetle. Some of the cysts contained two or more larvae, while one contained 25 larvae. The cysts possessed a brown sclerotized wall that conformed to the shape of the coiled larvae. When ingested by a variety of transport hosts, the larvae either continued a migration similar to that in the definitive host or localized in the wall of some portion of the digestive tract. When the infective third larval stages from either the intermediate or transport host were ingested by the canine host, the larvae excysted in the stomach and began a meandering migration. The larvae continued their migration in the wall of the gastric artery and aorta to the area between the aortic arch and diaphragm. In the canine definitive host, most of the developing larvae traveled through the wall of the aorta and invaded the wall of the esophagus where they induced the formation of a reactive granuloma. This granuloma may vary greatly in size and shape depending on the number of worms present and the pressure of the surrounding tissues. Cavernous tracts often formed around the adult worms; through these apertures, eggs passed to the lumen of the esophagus and hence to the external environment via the gut. This parasite does demonstrate a wanderlust activity; it has been reported in many unusual locations, including the kidney, wall of the urinary bladder, subcutaneous abscess, interdigital cyst, trachea, mediastinum, and lung.

Chhabra and Singh (1972) reported on the experimental infection of cats with *Spirocerca lupi.* Two adult cats given larvae did not develop any signs of infection or lesions. Three kittens that were given 50 to 100 larvae all died within 40 days of the infection. In all three kittens, the lesions that were observed were in the aorta. These authors reported that the majority of larvae were juveniles and that most of the larvae detected were degenerating. Faust (1928) reported that cats served as a model for tracing the routes of migration during early infection and that the primary lesions in the aortic wall of the cat are much less intense than they are in the dog. Faust felt that in the cat the infections were usually aborted before the worms reached maturity.

One reported case of *Spirocerca* in a domestic cat was a single, mature, infertile female; therefore no eggs were observed (Mense et al., 1992). This worm was in the stomach wall of a 7-year-old spayed domestic shorthair cat living in Florida. The cat had chronic postprandial vomiting that persisted for several weeks. On examination, no eggs were detected in the feces, and the cat began a course of antibiotics. Three weeks later, the cat returned to the hospital, radiographs appeared normal, and the cat was started on an oral petroleum-based laxative. Two weeks later, the cat was still vomiting, and a laparotomy was performed that revealed a 1.5 to 2 cm nodule in the wall of the pylorus. The nodule was removed and submitted for histological examination. The larva in section was considered to be a larva of *Spirocerca* based on the morphology of the observed sections through the worm. The sections were compared with those of *Gnathostoma* and *Physaloptera,* but comparisons were not made with *Cylicospirura felineus.* It would be of interest to determine if this cat was perhaps infected with *Cylicospirura felineus,* which is present in the United States in bobcats.

REFERENCES

Bailey WS. 1965. Parasites and cancer: sarcoma associated with *Spirocerca lupi.* Ann NY Acad Sci 108:890–923.

Chhabra RC, Singh KS. 1972. On *Spirocerci lupi* infection in some paratenic hosts infected experimentally. Ind J Anim Sci 42:297–304.

Faust EC. 1928. The life cycle of *Spirocerca sanguinolenta*—a natural nematode parasite of the dog. Science 68:407–409.

Kikuchi S, Ori M, Saito K, Hayashi S. 1976. Scanning electron microscopy of *Spirocerca lupi* obtained from the lower esophagus and cardiac opening of a marbled cat. Jap J Parasitol 25(suppl 1):13.

Mense MG, Gardiner CH, Moeller RB, Partridge HL, Wilson S. 1992. Chronic emesis caused by a nematode-induced gastric nodule in a cat. JAVMA 201:597–598.

Murray M. 1968. Incidence and pathology of *Spirocerca lupi* in Kenya. J Comp Pathol 78:401–405.

Pence DB, Stone JE. 1978. Visceral lesions in wild carnivores naturally infected with *Spirocerca lupi.* Vet Pathol 15:322–331.

Mastophorus muris (Gmelin, 1790) Chitwood, 1938

In 1924, Cram described a new species of worm, *Protospirura gracilis,* from the cat based on a single nematode that was recovered from the stomach of a cat that had been fed larval nematodes recovered from a dung beetle. The worm was about 2 cm long, with an esophagus that was about 10 percent of the body length. The mouth had three large pseudolabia, with each divided into three lobes. The central pseudolabial lobe appeared to have seven teeth. Even at the time of collection, Cram was concerned that the worm may have come from one of the rats that were fed to the cats in the colony.

Chitwood (1938) felt that the genus *Protospirura* could be separated from that of *Mastophorus* based on certain characteristics including the number of teeth and the location of the vulva. Wertheim (1962) felt that there was no good reason for the separation of the genera and placed them all in *Mastophorus.*

REFERENCES

Chitwood BG. 1938. The status of *Protospirura* vs *Mastophorus* with a consideration of the species of these genera. Libro Jub Travassos 115–118.

Cram EB. 1924. A new nematode *Protospirura gracilis,* from the cat. JAVMA 65:355–357.

Miyata J. 1939. Study of the life cycle of *Protospirura muris* (Gmelin) of rats and particularly of its intermediate hosts (in Japanese). Volumen Jubilare Pro Professore Sadao Yoshida 1:101–136.

Quentin JC. 1970. Morphogénèse larvaire du spiruride *Mastophorus muris* (Gmelin, 1790). Ann Parasitol Hum Comp 45:839–855.

Wertheim GA. 1962. A study of *Mastophorus muris* (Gmelin, 1790) (Nematoda: Spiruridae). Trans Am Miocro Soc 81:274–279.

FILARIOIDEA

The Filarioidea is a superfamily within the order Spirurida. All the species parasitic in the cat are representatives of the Onchocercidae and have microfilariae that occur dispersed in various tissues of the host, typically the blood or subcutaneous tissues. Cats are hosts to quite a few of these pathogens, but very few of those appear to be strictly parasitic in the domestic cat. In fact, most of the species found in the cat are considered to be parasites of other hosts that can infect the cat. Unfortunately, some of the nematodes can cause serious disease in the cat, and the disease in the cat caused by some of the forms that occur primarily in tropical developing countries has not really been examined for its effects on the health of the cat. Experimentally infected cats have been used to model some of the pathology observed in humans, but there has been very little done to examine the effects on any naturally infected cats living where the infections are common.

Cats are hosts to species of *Brugia* and species of *Dirofilaria. Brugia* represents relatively small worms with adults that live in the lymphatic tissue of their final hosts. The microfilariae that are produced are found in the blood, and transmission is by mosquitoes. The members of this genus are mainly found in Asia, although there are species in the raccoon in the United States that might be capable of infecting cats. *Dirofilaria* is best known in North America for the species, *Dirofilaria immitis,* which causes canine heartworm disease. This worm will also cause disease in cats. In Europe and Asia, cats also become infected on rare occasions with *Dirofilaria repens,* which is a subcutaneous-dwelling member of this genus. This long worm, up to 17 cm in length, occurs in the subcutaneous tissues, and microfilariae are found in the blood. In North America, bobcats are infected with *Dirofilaria striata,* a similar subcutaneous species, but we know very little about how often this parasite actually infects domestic cats.

The basic filarioid nematode is a hair-like structure with relatively simple features. The females produce microfilariae that circulate in the peripheral blood. The microfilariae are infective to a blood-feeding arthropod, and in the case of those parasitic in cats, all the arthropod vectors are mosquitoes. In the mosquito, the larva undergoes some essential development before it is ready to infect its next host when the mosquito takes another blood meal. Once inoculated into the cat, the larva matures over a period of several months to the adult stage, and then the cycle is repeated.

Brugia pahangi (Buckley and Edeson, 1956) Buckley, 1960

Etymology

Brugia for Dr. Brug and *pahangi* for Pahang, Malaysia, where the worm was discovered.

History

This worm was originally described as *Wuchereria pahangi* from cats and dogs in Malaysia (Buckley and Edeson, 1956) and then subsequently transferred to the genus *Brugia* by Buckley (1960).

Geographic Distribution

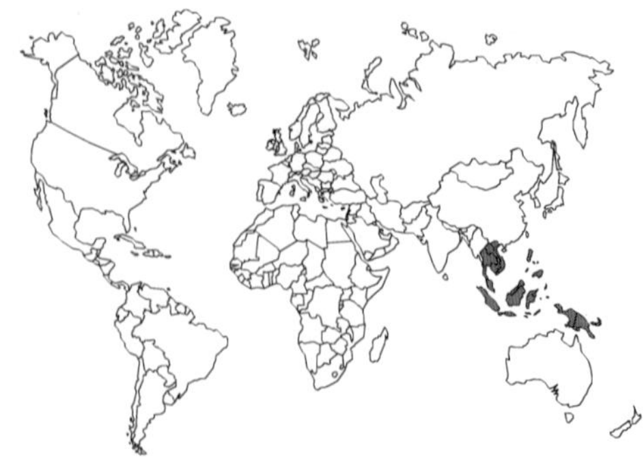

Fig. 4.75.

Brugia pahangi has been reported from cats in Malaysia; Mak et al. (1980) reported that about 11 percent of cats sampled in peninsular Malaysia were infected. In Thailand, Chungpivat and Sucharit (1993) reported that about 25 percent of blood samples from 83 cats living in Buddhist temples were found to be infected with *Brugia pahangi* in the area of Lat Krabang. About 61 of 325 cats (18.8 percent) in South Kalimantan, Indonesia, were found to have circulating microfilariae of *Brugia pahangi* (Palmieri et al., 1985).

Location in Host

The adult worms are found in the lymphatic vessels, as also are the larval stages (Schacher, 1962a). However, immature and adult worms can sometimes be recovered from subcutaneous tissues and the carcasses of infected cats.

Parasite Identification

The adult males of *Brugia pahangi* are 17.4 to 20 mm long; the adult females of *Brugia pahangi* are 38 to 63 mm long (Schacher, 1962a). The adults of *Brugia pahangi* are most easily recognized by the male spicules: those of *Brugia pahangi* are the shortest of the *Brugia* species in cats, those of *Brugia patei* are intermediate in length, and those of *Brugia malayi* are the longest. The left spicule of *Brugia pahangi* is 200 μm to 215 μm long; the right spicule is 75 μm to 90 μm long. There is probably no good way to distinguish the females of these *Brugia* species.

The microfilaria of *Brugia pahangi* is 280 μm (274 μm to 288 μm) long when collected in 2 percent formalin as in the Knott's technique, and 189 μm (186 μm to 200 μm) long when examined in a thick blood film (Schacher, 1962b).

Diagnosis of infection is made by finding the microfilariae in the blood using a Knott's technique or by direct smear (Fig. 4.76). The numbers of circulating microfilariae per milliliter of blood can often be greater than 10,000 microfilariae per milliliter; Denham et al. (1972) found that there were around 2 to 10 microfilariae per microliter of blood in experimentally infected cats. It is difficult to distinguish the microfilaria of *Brugia pahangi* from that of *Brugia malayi.* The distinction between the two species is made by the examination of the innenkorper of Giemsa-stained microfilariae, the innenkorper in the microfilaria of *Bru-*

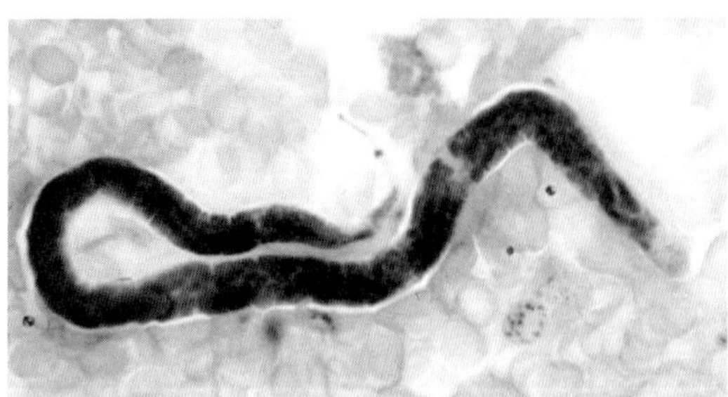

Fig. 4.76. *Brugia pahangi.* Microfilaria from experimentally infected rat. Giemsa stain. (Specimen courtesy Dr. Robin Bell)

gia pahangi is longer than that in *Brugia malayi* (Sivanandam and Mak, 1975). Also, when the microfilariae are stained using the acid phosphatase histochemical method, the microfilariae of *Brugia pahangi* tend to be red throughout their length, while those of *Brugia malayi* are red mainly at the excretory and anal pores (Redington et al., 1975). An antigen detection ELISA and counter-immunoelectrophoresis have been used to detect infections of *Brugia pahangi* in cats (Au et al., 1981; Kumar et al., 1991), but these tests are not commercially available.

Life Cycle

After a cat is inoculated with infective third-stage larvae from mosquitoes, the molt from the third to fourth stage occurs about 8 or 9 days later (Schacher, 1962a). The molt from fourth-stage larvae to adults occurs about 23 days after infection in the case of male worms and about 27 days after inoculation in the case of female worms. Microfilariae appear in the blood about 60 days after infection (Edeson et al., 1960; Schacher, 1962a). The females do not reach maximal length until about 120 days after infection; the males reach maximal length about 60 days after infection. The mean prepatent period in cats is 69 days, but it may take up to 96 days before a patent infection develops (Denham, 1974). Ewert and Singh (1969) found that experimentally infected cats first became microfilaremic about 10 weeks after infection. Microfilarial counts were around 3 or 4 microfilariae per microliter of blood. Adults worms are capable of living in some cats over 2 years.

Different cats respond to infections in different manners. Based on observations made after experimental infection, Denham et al. (1992) divided cats that had been inoculated with third-stage larvae on repeated occasions into five groups. One group represented about 70 percent of the infected cats, and these cats developed high levels of circulating microfilariae that persisted for over 2 years. Cats in this group often had large numbers of worms present in their tissues at necropsy. In group two cats, the adult worms died after about a year of infection, and in the presence of repeated inoculations of larvae, the cats became refractory to reinfection. In group three cats, the microfilariae disappeared from the blood after about a year of infection, but serum antigen levels remained high with adults being present at necropsy. In group four cats, there was only a transient presence of microfilariae in the blood, and adult worms were not recovered at necropsy. Cats in group five were refractory to infection initially and never developed circulating microfilariae or adult worms.

Microfilariae that are transfused in whole blood to naive cats are capable of being detected in the circulation for up to 136 days after injection (Pondurai et al., 1975). Kittens born to two queens with circulating microfilariae were found to be negative for microfilariae, although microfilariae were found in the lungs of one kitten killed 2 days after birth (Kimmig, 1979). The microfilariae in a transplacentally infected kitten will not grow to adults because they have not passed through a mosquito, and it also appears likely that there is little chance of kittens presenting with microfilariae acquired from the queen.

The vectors of *Brugia pahangi* are mosquitoes of the genus *Mansonia, Anopheles,* and *Armigeres* (Edeson et al., 1960). It has been shown that although this worm is not present in the United States, species of *Anopheles* and *Psorphora* found in Louisiana are capable of transmitting the infection experimentally (Schacher, 1962b). Infective larvae are found in the mouth parts of mosquitoes about 9 to 11 days after the ingestion of blood containing microfilariae.

Clinical Presentation and Pathogenesis

The clinical presentation and pathogenesis of infection in cats have been examined almost exclusively for the purpose of using cats as models of human infection. Thus, there has been very little if any work done on possible disease being seen in naturally infected cats in endemic areas. Rogers and Denham (1974) and Rogers et al. (1975) reported on the changes in the lymphatics of cats infected with 100 to 200 infective larvae in the dorsum of one hind foot and then killed from 2 days to 5 years after infection. By 14 to 15 days after infection, some of the larvae were in the lymphatic sinus, while others had migrated to the afferent lymphatic just below the popliteal node. At this stage the lymphatics were slightly dilated, and the valves were slightly thickened. By 6 weeks after infection, the varicosity of the lymphatics had increased enormously, and pockets of worms extended from the popliteal node to the tarsal joint. By 16 weeks after infection, the lymphatics showed extensive and chronic inflammation and fibrosis, and sometimes, there was obvious thrombolymphangitis. Cats that had been infected for 4 to 5 years typically improved and showed less lymphatic disorganization than cats infected for a year or so. In cats that were repeatedly infected over long periods of time (100 larvae and then rechallenged with 50 larvae at 10-day intervals for various periods), the pathological manifestations were variable. Sometimes the popliteal nodes were enormously enlarged, and other times, the nodes were scarcely palpable. In these studies of repeated inoculation, secondary inguinal lymph node systems and new lymphatics developed and ran alongside the nonfunctional lymphatic. Also, many new or enlarged skin lymphatics were observed.

A small percentage of humans infected with the related worm *Brugia malayi* will develop marked fibrosis of various lymphatic tissues and fibrosis and apparent swelling of associated limbs or tissues; this condition is known as elephantiasis. This tends to occur in only a small percentage of infected individuals (Partono et al., 1977). Although there have been several studies where cats have been examined for microfilariae of *Brugia pahangi,* there have been no reports of elephantiasis occurring naturally in cats. Rogers and Denham (1974) noted that of the cats receiving repeated infections for 3 to 5 years, the limbs of a few cats seemed to simulate cases of human elephantiasis with edema and skin thickening.

Treatment

Although cats have been a major experimental model for studying infections with lymphatic filariid parasites, there has been very little work on the direct treatment of cats infected with *Brugia pahangi.* Edeson and Laing (1959) treated experimentally infected cats with diethylcarbamazine. The activity of the drug on the microfilariae in these cats was unlike that in humans where there is a rapid die-off after treatment. In the cats, the microfilariae often remained at pretreatment levels. The microfilariae remained infectious to mosquitoes and from mosquitoes infectious to other cats. At the same time, the adult worms in the cats appeared to die following treatments ranging from 10 to 100 milligrams per day from several days to a week. Work in humans infected with *Brugia malayi* has shown that the oral administration of either diethylcarbamazine at 6 mg/kg or ivermectin at 20 to 200 μg/kg will markedly reduce the number of circulating microfilariae for 3 to 6 months in many cases (Ottesen et al., 1997). It is not known what effects either treatment has on the adults in the tissues. In the case of elephantiasis in humans, treatment is currently usually through surgical intervention.

Epizootiology

Brugia pahangi is a parasite of cats that has also been reported from dogs (Mak et al., 1980). The biology of the parasite is such that there is either no periodicity associated with the appearance of microfilariae in the blood or they are present at all times and in somewhat increased numbers either at night or during the day (Chungpivat and Sucharit, 1990; Sucharit, 1973).

Hazards to Other Animals

Infection could be transmitted from cats to dogs, but this would require the animals living together and the infection being passed to the dog through a mosquito vector. Denham and McGreevy (1977) cited the various hosts of *Brugia pahangi* and noted that it is in only a few primates, the dusky leaf monkey and the slow loris, but appears in several other animals, mainly carnivores (e.g., various civet cats, the panther, the pangolin, the moon rat, and the giant squirrel).

Hazards to Humans

Although humans have been experimentally infected with *Brugia pahangi* (Edeson et al., 1960), it would appear that there have been no natural human infections with this parasite reported (Abdullah et al., 1993). The diagnosis of infection in humans is complicated because the parasite overlaps the range of *Brugia malayi,* which has an almost indistinguishable microfilaria that is present in the same areas often in a subperiodic form.

Control/Prevention

More recent work using the related worm *Brugia malayi* (see below) would suggest that diethylcarbamazine is more likely to be a successful preventative than ivermectin.

REFERENCES

Abdullah WO, Oothuman P, Yunu H. 1993. Detection of circulating antigens and parasite specific antibodies in filariasis. Southeast Asian J Trop Med Publ Health 24:31–36.

Au ACS, Denham DA, Steward MW, Draper CC, Ismail MM, Rao CK, Mak JW. 1981. Detection of circulating antigens and immune complexes in feline and human lymphatic filariasis. Southeast Asian J Trop Med Publ Health 12:492–498.

Buckley JJC. 1960. On *Brugia* gen. nov. for *Wuchereria* spp. of the "malayi" group, i.e., *W. malayi* (Brug, 1927), *W. pahangi* Buckley and Edeson, 1956, *W. patei* Buckley, Nelson, and Heisch, 1958. Ann Trop Med Parasitol 54:75–77.

Buckley JJC, Edeson JFB. 1956. On the adult morphology of *Wuchereria* sp (*malayi?*) from a monkey (*Macaca iris*) and from cats in Malaya, and on *Wuchereria pahangi* n. sp. from a dog and a cat. J Helminthol 30:1–20.

Chungpivat S, Sucharit S. 1990. Microfilarial periodicity of *Brugia pahangi* in naturally infected cats in Bangkok. Thai J Vet Med 20:239–245.

Chungpivat S, Sucharit S. 1993. Microfilariae in cats in Bangkok. Thai J Vet Med 23:76–87.

Denham DA. 1974. Studies with *Brugia pahangi.* 6. The susceptibility of male and female cats to infection. J Parasitol 60:642.

Denham DA, McGreevy PB. 1977. Brugian filariasis: epidemiology and experimental studies. Adv Parasitol 15:243–309.

Denham DA, Rogers R. 1975. Structural and functional studies on the lymphatics of cats infected with *Brugia pahangi.* Trans Roy Soc Trop Med Hyg 69:173–176.

Denham DA, Ponnudurai T, Nelson GS, Rogers R, Guy F. 1972. Studies with *Brugia pahangi* I. Parasitological observations on primary infections of cats (*Felis catus*). Int J Parasitol 2:239–247.

Denham DA, Medeiros F, Baldwin C, Kumar H, Midwinter ICT, Birch DW, Smail A. 1992. Repeated infection of cats with *Brugia pahangi:* parasitological observations. Parasitology 104:415–420.

Edeson JFB, Laing ABG. 1959. Studies on filariasis in Malaya: the effects of diethylcarbamazine on *Brugia malayi* and *B. pahangi* in domestic cats. Ann Trop Med Parasitol 53:394–399.

Edeson JFB, Wharton RH, Laing ABG. 1960. A preliminary account of the transmission, maintenance and laboratory vectors of *Brugia pahangi.* Trans Roy Soc Trop Med Hyg 54:439–449.

Ewert A, Singh M. 1969. Microfilarial levels in cats infected with *Brugia pahangi* by two alternative routes. Trans Roy Soc Trop Med Hyg 63:603–607.

Gooneratne BWM. 1973. A chronological lymphographic study of cats experimentally infected with *Brugia filariasis* from 5 days to 5 years. Lymphology 6:127–149.

Gooneratne BWM, Nelsonn GS, Denham DA, Rurzr H, Monson E. 1971. Lymphographic changes in cats with filariasis. Trans Roy Soc Trop Med Hyg 65:195–198.

Kimmig P. 1979. Diaplacentare übertragung von Mikrofilarien der Art *Brugia pahangi* bei der Katze. Z Parasitenk 58:181–186.

Kumar H, Baldwin C, Birch DW, Kenham DA, Medeiros FD, Midwinter ITC, Smail A. 1991. Circulating filarial antigen in cats infected with *Brugia pahangi* is indicative of the presence of adult worms. Parasit Immunol 13:405–412.

Mak JW, Yen PKF, Lim KC, Ramiah N. 1980. Zoonotic implications of cats and dogs in filarial transmission in Peninsular Malaysia. Trop Geogr Med 32:259–264.

Ottesen EA, Duke BO, Karam M, Behbehani K. 1997. Strategies and tools for the control/elimination of lymphatic filariasis. Bull World Health Organ 75:491–503.

Palmieri JR, Masbar S, Purnomo Marwoto HA, Tirtokusumo S, Darwis F. 1985. The domestic cat as a host for brugian filariasis in South Kalimantan (Borneo), Indonesia. J Helminthol 59:277–281.

Partono F, Oemijati SH, Joesoef A, Clarke MD, Durfee PT, Irving GS, Taylor J, Cross JH. 1977. *Brugia malayi* in seven villages in South Kalimatan, Indonesia. Southeast Asian J Trop Med Publ Health 8:400–407.

Pondurai T, Denham DA, Rogers R. 1975. Studies on *Brugia pahangi* 9. The longevity of microfilariae transfused from cat to cat. J Helminthol 49:25–30.

Ponnampalam JT. 1972. Histological changes produced in cats by the microfilariae of *Brugia pahangi.* Southeast Asian J Trop Med Publ Health 3:511–517.

Redington BC, Montgomery CA, Jervis HR, Hockmeyer WT. 1975. Histochemical differentiation of the microfilariae of *Brugia pahangi* and subperiodic *Brugia malayi.* Ann Trop Med Parasitol 69:489–492.

Rogers R, Denham DA. 1974. Studies with *Brugia pahangi.* 7. Changes in lymphatics of injected cats. J Helminthol 48:213–219.

Rogers R, Denham DA. 1975. Studies with *Brugia pahangi:* 11. Measurements of lymph flow in infected cats. Southeast Asian J Trop Med Publ Health 6:199–205.
Rogers R, Denham DA, Nelson GS, Guy F, Ponnudurai T. 1975. Studies with *Brugia pahangi.* III. Histological changes in the affected lymph nodes of infected cats. Ann Trop Med Parasitol 69:77–84.
Sakamoto M. 1980. Changes in the lymphatic system of cats experimentally infected with *Brugia.* Trop Med 22:223–236.
Schacher JF. 1962a. Developmental stages of *Brugia pahangi* in the final host. J Parasitol 48:693–706.
Schacher JF. 1962b. Morphology of the microfilaria of *Brugia pahangi* and of the larval stages in the mosquito. J Parasitol 48:679–692.
Schacher JF, Sahyoun PF. 1967. A chronological study of the histopathology of filaria disease in cats and dogs caused by *Brugia pahangi* (Buckley and Edeson, 1956). Trans Roy Soc Trop Med Hyg 61:234–243.
Sivanandam S, Mak JW. 1975. Some problems associated with the processing and staining of blood film for filaria diagnosis. J Med Health Lab Tech Malaysia 2:4–6.
Sucharit S. 1973. *Brugia pahangi* in small laboratory animals: the microfilarial periodicity. Southeast Asian J Trop Med Publ Health 4:492–497.
Sucharit S, Harinasuta C, Viraboonchai S, Smithanonda S. 1975. The differentiation of *Brugia malayi, B. pahngi, B. tupaiae* and *Wuchereria bancrofti.* Southeast Asian J Trop Med Publ Health 6:549–554.
Suswillo RR, Denham DA, McGreevy P. 1982. The number and distribution of *Brugia pahangi* in cats at different times after a primary infection. Acta Trop 39:151–156.

Brugia patei (Buckley, Nelson, and Heisch, 1958) Buckley, 1960

In 1958, Buckley et al. described a new species of *Brugia* collected from dogs, cats, and civet cats on the Pate Island of Kenya, Africa. In 1960, Buckley created the new genus *Brugia* to contain this and two other similar worms. Buckley, in 1958, had brought the worms to London in female mosquitoes, *Mansonia africana* and *Mansonia uniformis,* and infections were then maintained in experimentally infected cats (Laurence and Pester, 1967). Laurence and Simpson (1968) did show that the spines on the anterior end of this species were smaller than those on either *Brugia pahangi* or *Brugia malayi.* Interest in this parasite relative to its presence in Africa has been virtually nonexistent because the parasite has never been reported from man or his food-producing animals. The fact that the prevalence rate in cats was 56 percent at the time of the original description (14 positive cats out of 25 examined) would indicate that this was not a case of incidental or recently imported parasitism.

The spicules of this species are intermediate in length between the species of *Brugia malayi* (the longest) and *Brugia pahangi* (the shortest). The left spicule of the male is 270 μm long, and the right spicule is 116 μm long. There is probably no good way to distinguish the females. According to the original description, the microfilaria is very similar to that of *Brugia malayi,* differing only in having a slightly shorter cephalic space.

REFERENCES

Buckley JJC. 1960. On *Brugia* gen. nov. for *Wuchereria* spp. of the "malayi" group, i.e., *W. malayi* (Brug, 1927), *W. pahangi* Buckley and Edeson, 1956, *W. patei* Buckley, Nelson, and Heisch, 1958. Ann Trop Med Parasitol 54:75–77.
Buckley JJC, GS Nelson, RB Heisch. 1958. On *Wuchereria patei* n.sp. from the lymphatics of cats, dogs and genet cats on Pate Island, Kenya. J Helm 32:73–80.
Laurence BR, Pester FRN. 1967. Adaptation of a filarial worm, *Brugia patei,* to a new mosquito host, *Aedes togoi.* J Helm 42:309–330.
Laurence BR, Simpson MG. 1968. Cephalic and pharyngeal structures in microfilariae revealed by staining. J Helm 42:309–330.

Brugia malayi (Brug, 1927) Buckley, 1960

Etymology

Brugia for Dr. Brug and *malayi* for the area in which the parasite was initially isolated.

Synonyms

Filaria malayi Brug, 1927; *Microfilaria malayi* (Brug, 1927) Faust, 1929; *Filaria bancrofti* Cobbold, 1877; *Wuchereria malayi* (Brug, 1927) Rao and Maplesonte, 1940.

History

Brugia malayi was first described as *Filaria malayi* by Dr. S. L. Brug on the basis of the morphology of microfilariae that were found in people in Indonesia by a Dr. A. Lichtenstein (Brug, 1927). Dr. Lichtenstein had noted that unlike the human parasite *Wuchereria bancrofti* in Indonesia, the microfilariae of this parasite did not increase in the peripheral circulation nocturnally and were not infective to culicine mosquitoes (Lichtenstein, 1927). Rao and Maplestone (1940) were the first to describe the adults of this species. Buckley (1960) erected a new genus, *Brugia,* on the basis of specimens of *Brugia malayi* from monkeys, *Brugia pahangi* from cats, dogs, and monkeys in Malaysia, and *Brugia patei* from cats and dogs in East Africa.

Geographic Distribution

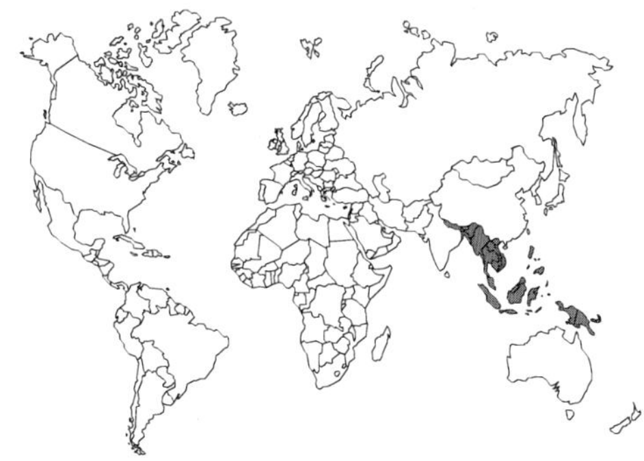

Fig. 4.77.

The location of *Brugia malayi* in Asia is illustrated by Denham and McGreevy (1977), but this illustration is based mainly on reports in people. Basically this region includes India, Sri Lanka, Sumatra, Java, Borneo, Malaysia, the Philippines, southern Thailand and northern Vietnam, South Korea, and coastal China. Cats only become infected with *Brugia malayi* in areas where this species is present in a subperiodic form (i.e., microfilariae are present in the blood throughout all hours of the day). This subperiodic form is present in Malaysia, Thailand, Vietnam, Borneo, Java, and the Philippines. In these areas, several studies have identified circulating microfilariae in cats. Chang et al. (1992) found 10.5 percent of 191 domestic cats positive for *Brugia malayi* in 12 Malay villages in Sarawak, Malaysia, and Mak et al. (1980) found infected cats in Peninsular Malaysia. Dondero and Menon (1972) found two of nine cats in Perak, Malaysia, with circulating microfilariae. Palmieri et al. (1985) in South Kalamantan, Indonesia, found 4 of 325 cats positive; Partono et al. (1977) found 13 of 51 cats positive. Phatana et al. (1987) found a cat positive for *Brugia malayi* in southern Thailand.

Location in Host

The adult worms are found in the lymphatic vessels, as also are larval stages (Ahmed, 1966). Ewert (1971) showed that if infective-stage larvae were inoculated into the foot of the cat, the worms developed within the popliteal lymph node of that same leg. Only very rarely were worms recovered from other sites.

Parasite Identification

The adult males of *Brugia malayi* are 13 to 23 mm long; the adult females are 43 to 55 mm long (Buckley and Edeson, 1956). The adults of *Brugia malayi* are most easily recognized by the male spicules: those of *Brugia malayi* are the longest, those of *Brugia patei* are intermediate in length, and the spicules of *Brugia pahangi* are the shortest of the *Brugia* species in cats. The left spicule of *Brugia malayi* is 390 μm; the right spicule is 125 μm long. There is probably no good way to distinguish the females of these *Brugia* species.

Diagnosis of infection is made by finding the microfilariae in the blood using a Knott's technique or by direct smear (Figs. 4.78 and 4.79). The microfilaria of *Brugia malayi* is 177 μm to 230 μm long when examined in a thick blood film. In humans, the microfilaria of the subperiodic strain differs from that of the periodic form in that the microfilaria of the subperiodic form tends to lose its sheath in the process of dying on slides. The number of circulating microfilariae per milliliter of blood appears to remain lower than that of the microfilariae of cats infected with *Brugia pahangi.* Burren (1972) found in experimentally infected cats that there was around a maximum of <1 to only 3 microfilariae per microliter of blood. It is difficult to distinguish the microfilaria of *Brugia malayi* from that of *Brugia pahangi.* The distinction between the two species is made by the examination of the innenkorper of Giemsa-stained microfilariae: the innenkorper in the microfilaria of *Brugia malayi* is shorter than that in *Brugia pahangi* (Sivanandam and Fredericks, 1966). Also, when the microfilariae are stained using the acid phosphatase histochemical method, the microfilariae of *Brugia malayi* are

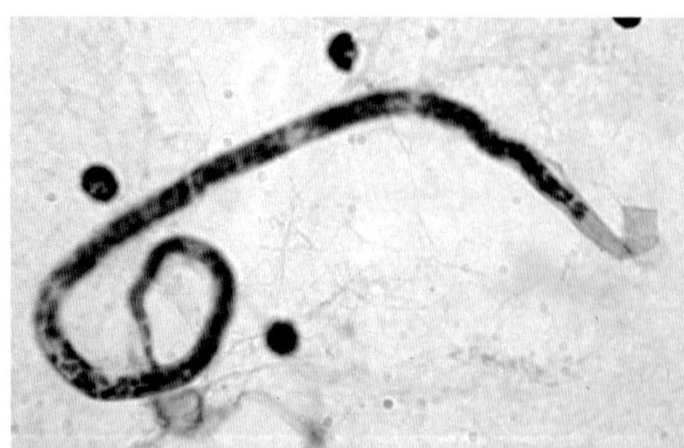

Fig. 4.78. *Brugia malayi.* Microfilaria from human. Hematoxylin stain.

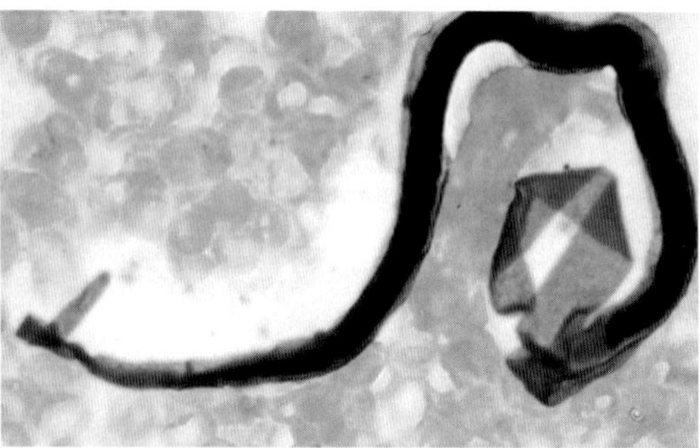

Fig. 4.79. *Brugia malayi.* Microfilaria from human. Giemsa stain.

red mainly at the excretory and anal pores, while those of *Brugia pahangi* tend to be red throughout their length (Redington et al., 1975). An antigen detection ELISA and counter-immunoelectrophoresis have been used to detect infections of *Brugia pahangi* in cats (Au et al., 1981; Kumar et al., 1991), but these tests are not commercially available. Prasomsitti et al. (1983) used an indirect fluorescence technique to examine antibody levels in cats infected with *Brugia malayi, Brugia pahangi,* and *Dirofilaria repens.*

Life Cycle

Ewert (1971) examined the development of *Brugia malayi* in experimentally infected cats. If larvae were inoculated into the hind leg, the majority of adult worms were recovered from lymph nodes associated with that same leg. In one cat, examined 16 weeks after infection, worms were recovered from soakings of the skin of the leg, and a single female worm was recovered from soakings of the scrotum and testes. Ewert (1976) found no difference in the susceptibility of male and female cats to infection; also, out of 59 female and 41 male cats that were experimentally infected, microfilariae appeared in the blood of about 90 percent of all these cats (92 percent of the females and 88 percent of the males).

In cats infected with third-stage infective larvae from mosquitoes, the prepatent period ranged from 80 to 96 days (Edeson and Buckley, 1959; Edeson and Wharton, 1957; Wharton et al., 1958). The inoculated third-stage larvae reached the regional lymph glands and vessels within 16 hours, and typically, as also shown by Ewert (1971), the site of adult development was typically related to the site of inoculation. The molt from third stage to fourth stage occurred about 10 days after the cats were infected, and the molt to the adult stage took place 35 to 40 days after infection. Ewert and Bosworth (1975) described the results of experimentally exposing cats to a second inoculation at various times after the primary inoculation. The first infection did not consistently result in lowered numbers of developing worms in the same leg, but the worms that did develop were typically farther from the inoculation site on the foot. Also, the primary infection had no apparent effect on the early migration and development of worms when the second infection was in the other hind leg.

The development in mosquitoes was described by Feng (1936). The first molt took place 4 days after the mosquito fed on the infected blood, and the second molt took place 2 days after the first molt. The infective larvae were 1.3 mm long.

Clinical Presentation and Pathogenesis

There have been no reports detailing the clinical presentation of naturally acquired *Brugia malayi* infection in cats. Ewert et al. (1972) examined the lymphographic changes in young cats that had been experimentally infected in the hind feet. After infection, lymphatic vessels in the infected limb become occluded by developing worms, and collateral lymphatics develop to maintain drainage. Eventually, infested lymphatic vessels become obliterated (Folse et al., 1981). In affected limbs, the collagen content increases

(Dresden and Ewert, 1984), and in experimentally infected cats, thrombi within the lymph vessels slowly turn into fibrous tissue that occludes the flow of lymph (Fader and Ewert, 1986). Dependent limb edema develops in cats with experimental infections that can be grossly visible (Folse and Ewert, 1988).

In an attempt to explain why some humans infected with *Brugia malayi* develop elephantiasis while the majority of those infected do not, work was performed to examine the effects of secondary bacterial infections on the course of infection of *Brugia malayi* in cats. When cats infected in one hind leg were challenged with streptococci in both hind legs, serious complications developed only in the previously worm-infected leg (Bosworth and Ewert, 1975). When similar conditions were extended to over a year, an elephantoid condition developed in the legs of five of six cats that had been repeatedly exposed to *Brugia malayi* and streptococcus (Ewert et al., 1980).

Treatment

In human infections with *Brugia malayi,* treatment has been aimed at giving both diethylcarbamazine (DEC) and ivermectin at levels that are low enough to prevent the circulation of microfilariae for a year without the induction of major side effects amongst infected individuals. In other cases, DEC has been added to salt in endemic areas (Panicker et al., 1997). There have been no reported attempts to either treat or control infections in naturally infected cats.

Ewert and Emerson (1979) reported on the effects of DEC on fourth-stage and adult *Brugia malayi* in experimentally infected cats. When the cats were treated 20 days after infection with 100 mg/kg of DEC, no worms were present in the treated cats. When the cats were treated with 50, 25, or 10 mg/kg of DEC at 20 days after infection, worms were present in all cats at necropsy, although less than in the control groups. Treatment with 1 mg/kg had no effect on the number of worms developing. When the cats were treated 8 weeks after infection, two of the five treated cats harbored one or two adult worms, while the mean number of worms present in the control cats was 23 adults. The results of treatment at 1, 10, 25, and 50 mg/kg were similar to those reported for larvae (Hillman et al., 1983).

Epizootiology

Relative to the cat, the most important aspect of the epizootiology of this disease is that cats are only infected naturally in those areas of the world where people are infected with the subperiodic form of the disease. Thus, throughout most of the range of this parasite, cats are not reservoirs of the infection. The cat can be experimentally infected with the nocturnally periodic form of the parasite, and in the experimentally infected cat, the periodic form becomes subperiodic (Denham and McGreevy, 1977; Laing, 1961). This means that cats entering an area where the nocturnal form of the disease is prevalent may be at some risk of becoming infected.

Hazards to Other Animals

Various primates and species of wild felids are considered to be susceptible to infection with *Brugia malayi.* Thus, if cats are held in places where they may be bitten by mosquitoes, the parasite could be transmitted from an infected cat to one of these other hosts.

Hazards to Humans

Brugia malayi is a significant enough human pathogen to warrant separate sections in most human parasitology texts. It is very much unclear what role the cat plays in the infection of people with *Brugia malayi.* It is assumed that cats serve as reservoirs in Malaysia and nearby countries, but it is truly not clear whether the cats or the human beings are the actual reservoirs of the observed infections.

Control/Prevention

Oral ivermectin administered to four leaf monkeys, *Prebytis cristata,* at doses of 200 μg/kg to 300 μg/kg at the same time as the subcutaneous inoculation of infective larvae failed to prevent the development of patent infections in these animals (Mak et al., 1987). On the other hand, diethylcarbamazine appears to be highly effective in preventing the infection of cats with this parasite (Ewert and Emerson, 1975). In cats that were experimentally infected with 50 larvae, the treatment of the cats the first week after infection with 10 mg of diethylcarbamazine per kilogram body weight caused only 1 of 22 cats to have any detectable living larvae at necropsy 2 weeks after infection. When cats were administered 5 mg diethylcarbamazine per kilogram body weight, a single living larva was recovered from each of two of the five treated cats. It would thus seem warranted to begin cats on daily diethylcarbamazine at 6 mg per kilogram body weight (e.g., Filaribits) before taking them into a country where this parasite is endemic.

REFERENCES

Ahmed SS. 1966. Location of developing and adult worms of *Brugia* sp. in naturally and experimentally infected animals. J Trop Med Hyg 69:291–293.

Au ACS, Denham DA, Steward MW, Draper CC, Ismail MM, Rao CK, Mak JW. 1981. Detection of circulating antigens and immune complexes in feline and human filariasis. Southeast Asian J Trop Med Publ Health 12:492–498.

Bosworth W, Ewert A. 1975. The effect of streptococcus on the persistence of *Brugia malayi* and on the production of elephantiasis in cats. Int J Parasitol 5:583–589.

Brug SL. 1927. Ein niewe Filaria-soort (*Filaria malyi*), parasiteerende bij den mensch (voorloopige mededeeling). Geneesk Tidjschr Nerderl-Indie 66:-414–416.

Buckley JJC. 1960. On *Brugia* gen. nov. for *Wuchereria* spp. of the "malayi" group, i.e., *W. malayi* (Brug, 1927), *W. pahangi* Buckley and Edeson, 1956, *W. patei* Buckley, Nelson, and Heisch, 1958. Ann Trop Med Parasitol 54:75–77.

Buckley JJC, Edeson JFB. 1956. On the adult morphology of *Wuchereria* sp. (*malayi?*) from a monkey (*Macaca irus*) and from cats in Malaya, and on *Wuchereria pahangi* n. sp. from a dog and a cat. J Helm 30:1–20.

Burren CH. 1972. The behaviour of *Brugia malayi* microfilariae in experimentally infected domestic cats. Ann Trop Med Parasitol 66:235–242.

Chang MS, Ho BC, Hardin S, Dorasisingam P. 1992. Filariasis in Kota Samarahan District Sarawak, East-Malaysia. Trop Biomed 9:39–46.

Denham DA, McGreevy PB. 1977. Brugian filariasis: epidemiological and experimental studies. Adv Parasitol 15:243–309.

Dondero TJ, Menon VVV. 1972. Clinical epidemiology of filariasis due to *Brugia malayi* on a rubber estate in West Malaysia. Southeast Asian J Trop Med Publ Health 3:355–365.

Dresden MH, Ewert A. 1984. Collagen metabolism in experimental filariasis. J Parasitol 70:208–212.

Edeson JFB. 1959. Studies on filariasis in Malaya: the periodicity of the microfilariae of *Brugia malayi* and *B. pahangi* in animals. Ann Trop Med Parasitol 53:381–387.

Edeson JFB, Buckley JJC. 1959. Studies on filariasis in Malaya: on the migration and rate of growth of *Wuchereria malayi* in experimentally infected cats. Ann Trop Med Parasitol 53:113–119.

Edeson JFB, Wharton RH. 1957. The transmission of *Wuchereria malayi* from man to the domestic cat. Trans Roy Soc Trop Med Hyg 51:366–370.

Edeson JFB, Wharton RH. 1958. The experimental transmission of *Wuchereria malayi* from man to various animals in Malaya. Trans Roy Soc Trop Med Hyg 52:25–45.

Edeson JFB, Wilson T. 1964. The epidemiology of filariasis due to *Wuchereria bancrofti* and *Brugia malayi*. Ann Rev Entomol 9:245–268.

Ewert A. 1971. Distribution of developing and mature *Brugia malayi* in cats at various times after a single inoculation. J Parasitol 57:1039–1042.

Ewert A. 1976. The comparative susceptibility of male and female and of mature and immature cats to infection with subperiodic *Brugia malayi*. Rev Biol Trop 24:262–266.

Ewert A, Bosworth W. 1975. Distribution and development of *Brugia malayi* in reinfected cats. J Parasitol 61:610–614.

Ewert A, El Bihari S. 1971. Rapid recovery of *Brugia malayi* following experimental infection of cats. Trans Roy Soc Trop Med Hyg 65:364–368.

Ewert A, Emerson GA. 1975. Effects of diethylcarbamazine on third stage *Brugia malayi* larvae in cats. Am J Trop Med Hyg 24:71–73.

Ewert A, Emerson GA. 1979. Effects of diethylcarbamazine citrate on fourth stage and adult *Brugia malayi* in cats. Am J Trop Med Hyg 28:496–499.

Ewert A, Balderach R, Elbiharia S. 1972. Lymphographic changes in regional lymphatics of cats infected with *Brugia malayi*. Am J Trop Med Hyg 21:407–414.

Ewert A, Reitmeyer JC, Folse D. 1980. Chronic infection of cats with *Brugia malayi* and streptococcus. Southeast Asian J Trop Med Publ Health 11:32–39.

Fader RC, Ewert A. 1986. Evolution of lymph thrombi in experimental *Brugia malayi* infections: a scanning electron microscopic study. Lymphology 19:146–152.

Feng LC. 1936. The development of *Microfilaria malayi* in *A. hyrcanus* var. *sinensis* Wied. Chin Med J (Suppl) 1:345–367.

Folse DS, Ewert A. 1988. Edema resulting from experimental filariasis. Lymphology 21:244–247.

Folse DS, Ewert A, Reitmeyer JC. 1981. Light and electron microscopic studies of lymph vessels from cats infected with *Brugia malayi*. Southeast Asian J Trop Med Publ Health 12:174–184.

Hillman GR, Westerfield L, Ewert A, Wang YX. 1983. Serum levels of a filaricide, diethylcarbamazine citrate, in cats following different routes of administration. Southeast Asian J Trop Med Publ Health 14:171–175.

Kumar V, Kerckhoven I, Pandey VS. 1991. Animal hosts in experimental lymphatic filariasis research. Ann Soc Belge Med Trop 71:173–186.

Laing ABG. 1961. Influence of the animal host on the microfilarial periodicity of *Brugia malayi*. Trans Roy Soc Trop Med Hyg 55:558.

Lichtenstein A. 1927. Filaria-oderzoek te Bireven. Geneesk Tijdschr Nederl-Indie 67:742–749.

Mak JW, Yen PKF, Lim KC, Ramiah N. 1980. Zoonotic implications of cats and dogs in filarial transmission in Peninsular Malaysia. Trop Geogr Med 32:259–264.

Mak JW, Lam PLW, Noor Rain A, Suresh K. 1987. Chemoprophylactic studies with ivermectin against subperiodic *Brugia malayi* infection in the leaf monkey, *Presbytis cristata.* J Helminthol 61:311–314.

Ottesen EA, Duke BO, Karam M, Behbehani K. 1997. Strategies and tools for the control/elimination of lymphatic filariasis. Bull World Health Organ 75:491–503.

Palmieri JR, Masbar S, Purnomo Marwoto HA, Tirtokusumo S, Darwis F. 1985. The domestic cat as a host for brugian filariasis in South Kalimantan (Borneo), Indonesia. J Helminthol 59:277–281.

Panicker KN, Arunachalam N, Kumar MNP, Prathibha J, Sabesan S. 1997. Efficacy of diethylcarbamazine-medicated salt for microfilaraemia of *Brugia malayi.* Natl Med J India 10:275–276.

Partono F, Oemijati S, Hudojo, Joesoef A, Clarke MD, Durfee PT, Irving GS, Taylor J, Cross JH. 1977. *Brugia malayi* in seven villages in south Kalimantan, Indonesia. Southeast Asian J Trop Med Publ Health 8:400–407.

Phantana S, Shutidamrong C, Chusattayanend W. 1987. *Brugia malayi* in a cat from southern Thailand. Trans Roy Soc Trop Med Hyg 81:173–174.

Prasomsitti P, Mak JW, Sucharit P, Liew LM. 1983. Detection of antibodies in cats infected with filarial parasites by the indirect immunofluorescence technique. Southeast Asian J Trop Med and Publ Health 14:353–356.

Rao SS, Maplestone PA. 1940. The adult of *Microfilaria malayi* Brug, 1927. Ind Med Gaz 75:159–160.

Redington BC, Montgomery CA, Jervis HR, Hockmeyer WT. 1975. Histochemical differentiation of the microfilariae of *Brugia pahangi* and sub-periodic *Brugia malayi.* Ann Trop Med Parasitol 69:489–492.

Sakamoto M. 1980. Changes in the lymphatic system of cats experimentally infected with *Brugia.* Trop Med 22:223–236.

Sivanandam S, Fredericks HJ. 1966. The "Innenkörper" in differentiation between the microfilariae of *Brugia pahangi* and *B. malayi* (sub-periodic form). Med J Malaya 20:3387–3388.

Sucharis S, Sitthai W, Surathin K. 1992. Natural infection of *Brugia malayi* in a child outside endemic area, Thailand. Mosq Borne Dis Bull 9:128–130.

Wharton RH, JFB Edeson, ABG Laing. 1958. Laboratory transmission of *Wuchereria malayi* by mosquito bites. Trans Roy Soc Trop Med Hyg 52:288.

Brugia beaveri Ash and Little, 1964

This worm was originally described from the lymph nodes, skin, and carcass of the raccoon (*Procyon lotor*) in Louisiana (Ash and Little, 1964). It was later shown that cats could be infected with it experimentally (Harbut and Orihel, 1995). Natural infections in cats in the United States with *Brugia* species are expected to include this species. Orihel and Eberhard (1998) summarized the human infections with zoonotic *Brugia* species in lymph tissue that have been observed and noted that there have been some 30 cases of human infection in the United States. The agent is probably *Brugia beaveri* of the raccoon, although *Brugia lepori* of the rabbit or some other undescribed species may be responsible.

REFERENCES

Ash LR, Little MD. 1964. *Brugia beaveri* sp. n. (Nematoda: Filarioidea) from the raccoon (*Procyon lotor*) in Louisiana. J Parasitol 50:119–123.

Orihel TC, Eberhard ML. 1998. Zoonotic filariasis. Clin Microbiol Rev 11:366–381.

Harbut CL, Orihel TC. 1995. *Brugia beaveri:* microscopic morphology in host tissues and observations on its life history. J Parasitol 81:239–243.

Dirofilaria immitis (Leidy, 1856) Railliet and Henry, 1911

Etymology

Diro = dread + *filaria* = thread along with *immitis* = cruel.

Synonyms

Filaria sanguinis Cobbold, 1869; *Dirofilaria louisianensis* Faust, Thomas, and Jones, 1941.

History

Heartworm has long been known as a disease of the canine host. Otto (1974) reviewed the history of cases that have been reported in cats from 1921 onward and listed 12 cases from cats in the United States; he suggested that the relatively common occurrence of the worm in cats mitigated against its being considered an abnormal host for this parasite. In recent years, it has become more and more obvious that if the prevalence in dogs in an area is fairly high, there is a good chance that some percentage of cats will also be infected. The cat may be relatively commonly infected with this parasite, but the inability of the cat to support large numbers of worms or patent infections would argue that in the biology of this parasite the dog and other canids are the hosts of true importance for maintaining infectious foci around the world.

Geographic Distribution

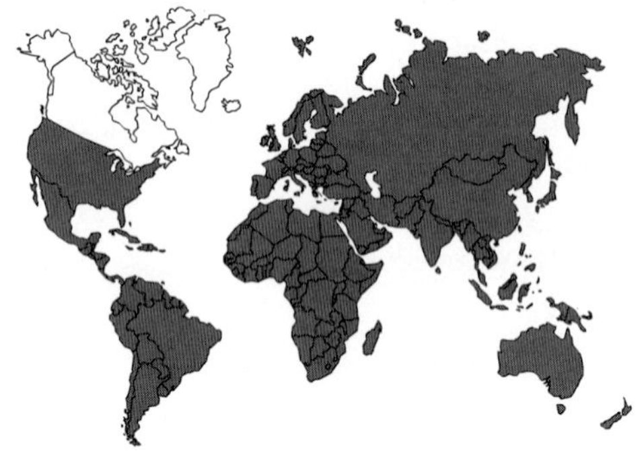

Fig. 4.80.

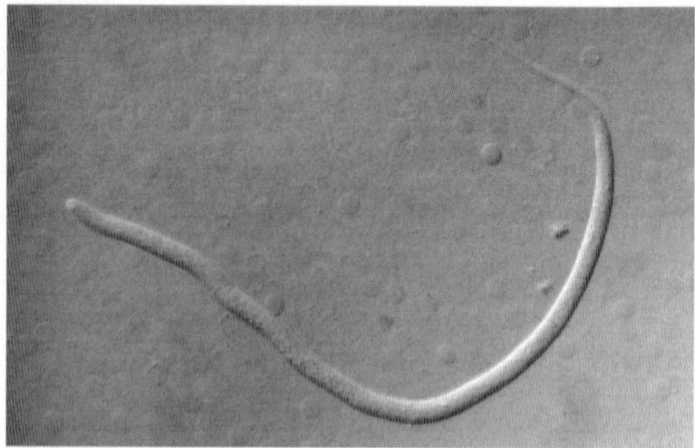

Fig. 4.81. *Dirofilaria immitis.* Microfilaria from dog blood as viewed with differential interference contrast in a Knott's preparation. Note that the width of the microfilaria at midbody is wider than a red blood cell ghost. Cats usually have very few circulating microfilariae.

Otto (1974) cited cases in cats from the United States, including Hawaii, along with cases in Brazil, the Philippines, Tahiti, New Guinea, Indonesia, China, and Japan. Since the time of this report, additional cases have been described from the United States and around the world, including Italy (Venco et al., 1999), Australia (Kendall et al., 1991), Taiwan (Fei and Mo, 1997), India (Patnaik, 1989), Japan (Roncalli et al., 1998), and Brazil (Labarthe et al., 1998).

Location in Host

In the cat the worms have usually been recovered from the right ventrical and pulmonary artery. In cats there is also a tendency for the worms to appear in ectopic sites. There have been several cases reported where heartworms have been recovered from the brains of cats at necropsy (Ader 1979; Cusick et al., 1976; Donahoe and Holzinger, 1974; Fukushima et al., 1984; Lindquist and Winters, 1981).

Parasite Identification

The adult worms are relatively easy to identify due to their size and location in the host. The long white worms are very easily recognized when removed from the cat either surgically or at necropsy. Unfortunately, relative to diagnosis, cats tend not to have circulating microfilariae (Fig. 4.81); thus, it is difficult to verify infections by examination of the blood. However, recently developed antigen detection kits make it possible to detect infections in cats as long as there are female worms present (Atkins, 1999). The antigen, which circulates in the blood of the host, is a uterine antigen produced by female worms; thus, if only male worms are present, there will be no circulating antigen.

Life Cycle

The life cycle in the cat fairly well mimics that which occurs in the dog; however, cats tend not to support anywhere near the same number of worms and are significantly refractory to infection (Zanotti and Kaplan, 1989). Cats experimentally infected with *Dirofilaria immitis* third-stage larvae (Figs. 4.82 and 4.83) appear to develop detectable levels of circulating antigen slightly later than would be expected in dogs (Mansour et al., 1995). Cats typically support only one to three adult worms, although under various experimental conditions, cats can harbor greater worm burdens (Stewart et al., 1992).

Clinical Presentation and Pathogenesis

Cats with a more typical presentation of heartworm infection will present with signs of respiratory or gastrointestinal disease. Such signs will

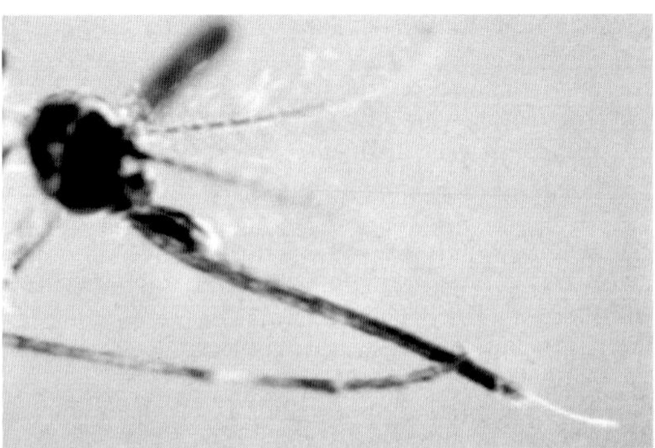

Fig. 4.82. *Dirofilaria immitis.* Infective third-stage larva emerging from the proboscis of a mosquito.

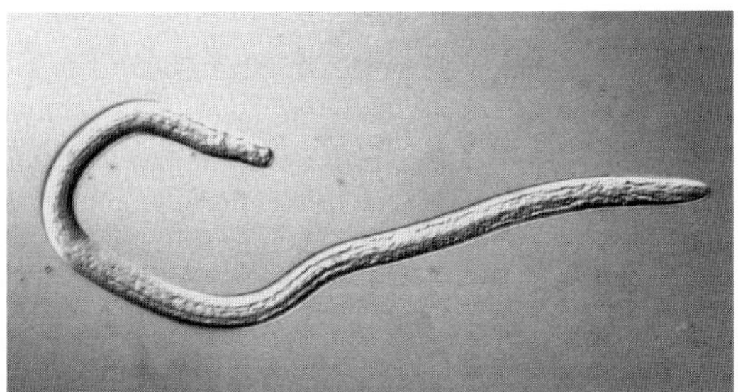

Fig. 4.83. *Dirofilaria immitis.* It can be seen that this infective third-stage larva has a fully formed intestinal tract.

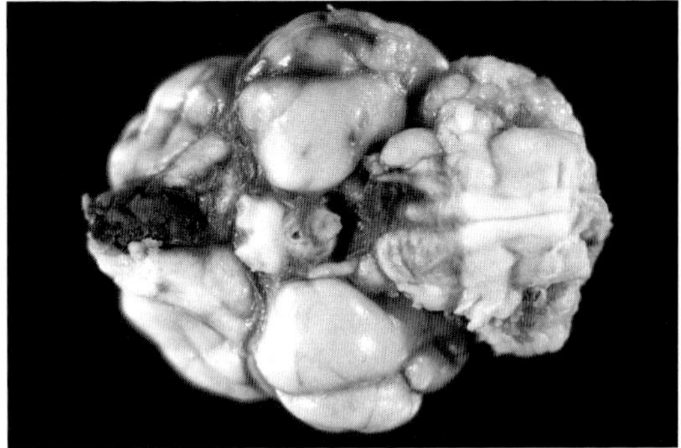

Fig. 4.84. *Dirofilaria immitis.* Damage to the brain of a cat by the ectopic migration of an adult worm.

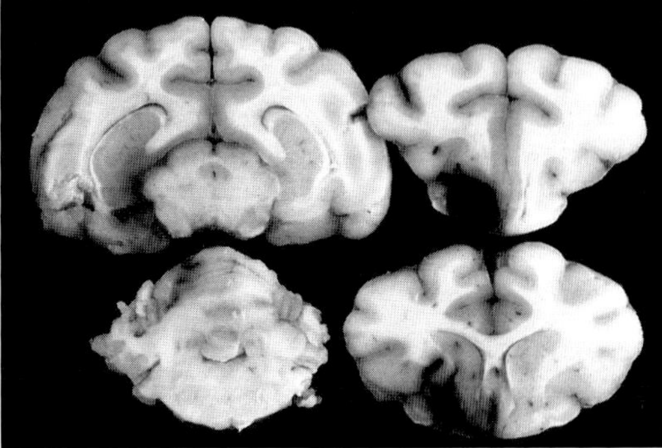

Fig. 4.85. *Dirofilaria immitis.* Extent of damage of the lesion shown in Fig. 4.84.

include dyspnea, coughing, systolic murmur, vomiting, anorexia, dysphagia, diarrhea, or syncope (Malik et al., 1998). These would be the signs expected in those animals with a chronic infection. In cats with acute onset disease, signs will be associated with the worms in either the cardiovascular system or ectopic sites. When associated with the cardiovascular system, signs may be associated with pulmonary artery obstruction, pneumothorax, or chylothorax (Birchard and Bilbrey, 1990; Smith et al., 1998). When worms enter ectopic locations such as the skin (Dillon et al., 1987) or the brain (Figs. 4.84 and 4.85), the signs associated with the infection will be related to the organ system damaged by the migrating worms. Radiography and echocardiography are both useful tools in the diagnosis of feline heartworm disease (Venco et al., 1998).

Treatment

Currently the recommendation is typically that cats be treated with symptomatic therapy because adulticide therapy using thiacetarsamid or melasormine are considered to put the cat at risk for sudden death (Atkins, 1999; Malik et al., 1998). Surgical removal of heartworms from the right atrium of cats by using catheter-bearing basket-type retrieval forceps is also successful, especially when the worms are visualized during removal with ultrasonography (Borgarelli et al., 1997).

Epizootiology

The epizootiology of feline heartworm disease seems to mimic that of dogs. It may be that other species of mosquitoes different from those typically biting dogs are more important in the transmission of the infection to cats (Borgarelli et al., 1997); however, more work needs to be done in this area.

Hazards to Other Animals

The heartworms in a cat would only be infectious to another host through transmission by the mosquito intermediate host. The fact that cats seldom are microfilaremic would suggest that they play very little role in serving as reservoirs for this infection.

Hazards to Humans

Infections in humans do occasionally occur due to canine heartworm, but people have to get bitten by a heartworm-infected mosquito to become infected. The fact that the worms in cats are poor producers of microfilariae would indicate that the infection of cats provides little risk to owners.

Control/Prevention

Prevention of heartworm infection in cats can now be easily introduced by the monthly administration of several products, ivermectin and selamectin, that are capable of preventing this infection in cats.

REFERENCES

Ader P. 1979. Heartworm (*Dirofilaria immitis*) in the brain of a cat—review and case report. Calif Vet, Nov, pp 23–25.

Atkins C. 1999. The diagnosis of feline heartworm infection. JAAHA 35:185–187.

Birchard SJ, Bilbrey SA. 1990. Chylothorax associated with dirofilariasis in a cat. JAVMA 197:507–509.

Borgarelli M, Venco L, Piga PM, Bonino F, Ryan WG. 1997. Surgical removal of heartworms from the right atrium of a cat. JAVMA 211:68–69.

Cusick PK, Todd KS, Blake JA, Daly WR. 1976. *Dirofilaria immitis* in the brain and heart of a cat from Massachusetts. JAAHA 12:490–491.

Dillon AR, Brawner WR, Grieve RB, Buxton-Smith B, Schultz RD. 1987. The chronic effects of experimental *Dirofilaria immitis* infection in cats. Seminars Vet Med Surg (Small Anim) 2:72–77.

Donahoe JMR, Holzinger EA. 1974. *Dirofilaria immitis* in the brains of a dog and a cat. JAVMA 164:518–519.

Fei CY, Mo KM. 1997. Survey for endoparasitic zoonoses in stray dogs and cats in Taipei city. J Chin Soc Vet Sci 23:26–33.

Fukushima K, Hutsell D, Patton S, Patton CS. 1984. Aberrant dirofilariasis in a cat. JAVMA 184:199–201.

Kendall K, Collins GH, Pope SE. 1991. *Dirofilaria immitis* in cats from inner Sydney. Aust Vet J 68:356–357.

Labarthe N, Serrão ML, Melo YF, de Oliveira SJ, Lourenço-de-Oliveira R. 1998. Mosquito frequency and feeding habits in an enzootic canine dirofilariasis area in Niterói, state of Rio de Janeiro, Brazil. Mem Inst Oswald Cruz 93:145–154.

Lindquist WD, Winters KD. 1981. Cerebral feline dirofilariasis. Feline Pract 11:37–40.

Malik R, Church DB, Eade IG. 1998. Syncope in a cat. Aust Vet J 76:465–471.

Mansour AE, McCall JW, McTier TL, Supakorndej N, Ricketts R. 1995. Epidemiology of feline dirofilariasis. Infections induced by simulated natural exposure to *Aedes aegypti* experimentally infected with heartworms. Proc Heartworm Symp '95, Auburn, Alabama, pp 87–95.

Otto GF. 1974. Occurrence of the heartworm in unusual locations and in unusual hosts. Proc Heartworm Symp, pp 6–13.

Patnaik MM. 1989. On filarial nematodes in domestic animals in Orissa. Ind Vet J 66:573–574.

Railliet A, Henry A. 1911a. Sur une filaire péritonéale des porcins. Bull Soc Pathol Exot 4:386–389.

Railliet A, Henry A. 1911b. Remarques au sujet des deux notes de MM. Bauche et Bernard. Bull Soc Pathol Exot 4:485–488.

Roncalli RA, Yamane Y, Nagata T. 1998. Prevalence of *Dirofilaria immitis* in cats in Japan. Vet Parasitol 75:81–89.

Smith JW, Scott-Moncrieff C, Rivers BJ. 1998. Pneumothorax secondary to *Dirofilaria immitis* infection in two cats. JAVMA 213:91–93.

Stewart VA, Hepler DI, Grieve RB. 1992. Efficacy of milbemycin oxime in chemoprophylaxis of dirofilariasis in cats. Am J Vet Res 53:2274–2277.

Venco L, Calzolari D, Mazzocchi D, Morini S, Genchi C. 1998. The use of echocardiography as a diagnostic tool for the detection of feline heartworm (*Dirofilaria immitis*) infections. Feline Pract 26:6–9.

Venco L, Morini S, Pedemonte F, Sola LB. 1999. Cardio-pulmonary filariosis in the cat. Obiettivie Documenti Veterinari 20:39–46.

Zanotti S, Kaplan P. 1989. Feline dirofilariasis. Comp SA 11:1005–1018.

Dirofilaria repens Raillliet and Henry, 1911

Etymology

Diro = dread + *filaria* = thread along with *repens* = creeping.

Synonyms

Filaria acutiuscula Molin, 1858; *Dirofilaria conjunctivae* (Addario, 1885) Desportes, 1940.

History

The parasite first was described from the dog by Railliet and Henry (1911a, b). Desportes (1940) first recognized that the worm *Filaria conjunctivae* Addario, 1885, may have been the same species as that found in dogs. Skrjabin (1917) described a human case under the name of *Loa extraocularis,* and Skrjabin et al. (1930) attributed a second human case to *Dirofilaria repens.* In 1948, Skrjabin and Schikhobalova recognized *Loa extraocularis* as a synonym of *Dirofilaria repens.* Cancrini et al. (1990) felt that the laws of priority were such that the worm should be called *Dirofilaria conjunctivae* (Addario, 1885); but this designation has not been currently adopted.

Geographic Distribution

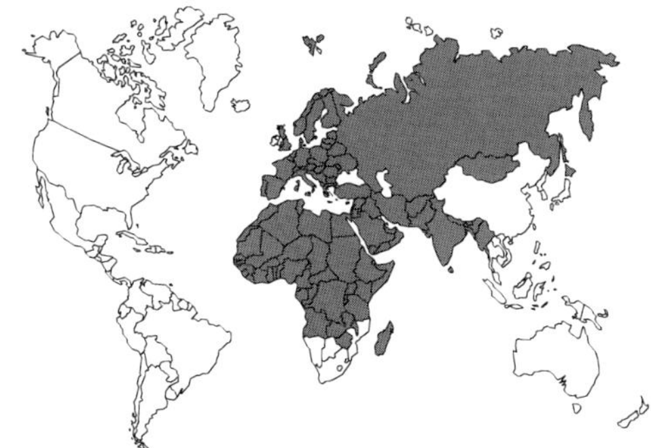

Fig. 4.86.

Chauve (1990) presented the distribution of *Dirofilaria repens* in dogs as including Nigeria and Uganda in Africa, along with Turkey, Italy, and France in Europe. Human cases have been reported from Italy, Greece, France, and other Mediterranean countries (Pampiglione et al., 1995; Pampiglione et al., 1996), as well as parts of Russia (Avdyukhina et al., 1997), Africa (O'Grady et al., 1962), Israel (Zweig et al., 1981), Sri Lanka (Dissanaike et al., 1982), and Okinawa (MacLean et al., 1979). Cats have been found to be infected in Malaysia (Chang et al., 1992; Mak et al., 1985; Rohde, 1962) and on the Pate Island off the coast of Kenya (Heisch et al., 1959). Cats and dogs have also been found infected in India (Patnaik, 1989) and Indonesia (Palmieri et al., 1985). Interestingly, the cats in the Mediterranean do not seem to support infections with this parasite in this locality, although Pampiglione et al. (1995) cited a personal reference from Dr. Genchi that a cat has been observed infected in Italy.

Location in Host

The adult worms are rather large (males are 5 to 7 cm long, and females are 10 to 17 cm long) and are found in the subcutaneous connective tissues of their hosts.

Parasite Identification

The females measure 13 to 17 cm, and the males measure 5 to 7 cm in length. The microfilariae are sheathless and are about 290 to 360 μm long by 6 to 8 μm wide.

Life Cycle

The adults live in the subcutaneous tissues. Microfilariae (about 300 μm long) are found in the blood and seem to be slightly periodic, being more common in the peripheral blood at night (Webber and Hawking, 1955). Mosquitoes of several different genera serve as the intermediate hosts (Bernard and Bauche, 1913; Fülleborn, 1908), and it takes about 9 to 21 days for the larvae to become infective, depending on the temperatures at which the mosquitoes are held. Gunewardene (1956) recovered infective larvae from mosquitoes (*Aedes albopictus*) by 12 days after infection. Mosquitoes incriminated as potential hosts (Manotovani and Restani, 1965) include *Aedes alpopictus, Aedes aegypti, Aedes albifasciatus, Psorophora cyanescens, Anopheles maculipennis, Anopheles petragnanii, Anopheles claviger, Anopheles atroparvus, Anopheles hyrcanus, Anopheles stephensi, Anopheles barbirostris, Mansonia uniformis, Mansonia annulifera, Mansonia titillans,* and *Armigeres obturbans.* Bain (1978) studied the development of the larvae in *Aedes detritus* and *Aedes caspius.* She described the morphology of the larval stages developing within these mosquitoes. Webber and Hawking (1955) inoculated dogs with infective larvae and found the prepatent period to be about 7 months, or 25 to 34 weeks. Microfilariae would circulate in the blood of infected dogs for 2 to 3 years.

Clinical Presentation and Pathogenesis

There are no reports regarding pathology or clinical presentation in cats infected with this parasite. Work has been presented for dogs.

Webber and Hawking (1955) stated, "No lesions caused by the worms could be detected in any of the dogs," referring to postmortem examination of 11 dogs that had been experimentally infected, of which 10 had been found to harbor adult worms. One of these dogs had as many as 137 adults. On rare occasions, dogs will present with a subcutaneous nodule (Huber, 1985). Pampiglione et al. (1995) stated that many cases in humans probably go unreported due to "the scant importance attached to the parasitic condition, for which we can vouch, at least as far as Italy is concerned."

Treatment

There have been no descriptions of treatment in the cat.

Epizootiology

The most intriguing aspect of the epizootiology of infections with this parasite is the fact that it seems much more common for cats to be infected in Southeast Asia than in southern Europe. This could be due to either different strains of the parasite or host being present in these two parts of the world, or it may be that the mosquitoes in Southeast Asian are more likely to feed on both dogs and cats and thus transmit the parasite between these two hosts.

Hazards to Other Animals

The cat really poses no threat to other animals. In Southeast Asia where cats have circulating microfilariae, it is possible that cats could serve as reservoirs for canine or human infections.

Hazards to Humans

There have been numerous infections with *Dirofilaria repens,* and Pampiglione et al. (1995) wrote an excellent review of human infections. There have been nearly 400 cases in people, with most cases, slightly less than half, occurring in Italy. Most of the cases have occurred as worms appearing in subcutaneous nodules on the head, thoracic wall, or upper limbs. Occasionally, worms may cause lesions in deeper tissues, and on rare occasions lesions in the lungs have been mistaken for malignancies. Of course, human infections are acquired by the bite of a mosquito in a fashion similar to that by which dogs and cats become infected.

Control/Prevention

Marconcini et al. (1993) showed that monthly ivermectin at the heartworm preventative dose of 6 μg/kg is capable of preventing dogs from becoming infected with *Dirofilaria repens.* Thus, it is to be expected that the use of monthly ivermectin in the cat would also prevent infection of with *Dirofilaria repens.*

REFERENCES

Anderson RC. 1952. Description and relationships of *Dirofilaria ursi* Yamaguti, 1941, and a review of the genus *Dirofilaria* Railliet and Henry, 1911. Trans Roy Can Inst Part II 29:35–65.

Avdyukhina TI, Supryaga VG, Postnnova VF, Kuimova RT, Micrnova NI, Muratov NE, Putintseva EV. 1997. Dirofilariasis in CIS countries. Analysis of cases from 1915–1996. Med Parazit Parazit Bol 1997(4):3–7.

Bain O. 1978. Dévelopment en Camargue de la filaire du chien, *Dirofilaria repens* Railliet et Henry, 1911, chex Aedes halophile. Bull Mus Nat Hist Nat 351:19–27.

Bernard PN, Bauche J. 1913. Conditions de propagation de la filariose sous-cutanée du chien, *Stegomyia fasciata* hôte intermédiaire de *Dirofilaria repens.* Bull Soc Pathol Exot 2:89–99.

Cancrini G, Mantovani A, Coluzzi M. 1979. Experimental infection of the cat with *Dirofilaria repens* of dog origin. Parassitologia 21:89–90.

Cancrini G, Mattiucci S, D'Amelio S, Coluzzi M. 1990. L'analisi elttroforetica di sistemi gene-enzima perr l'identificazione di forme larvali di Dirofilaria nell'uomo. Parassitologia 32(suppl 1):41.

Chang MS, Ho BC, Hardin S, Doraisingam P. 1992. Filariasis in Kota Saraarahan District Sarawak, East-Malaysia. Trop Biomed 9:39–46.

Chauve CM. 1990. *Dirofilaria repens* (Railliet and Henry, 1911), *Dipetalonema reconditum* (Grassi, 1890), *Dipetalonema dracunculoides* (Coabbold, 1870), and *Dipetalonema grassii* (Noé, 1907: Quatre filaires méconnues du chien. Prat Méd Chir Anim Comp Suppl 3:293–304.

Desportes C. 1940. *Filaria conjunctivae* Addario 1885, parasite accidentel de l'homme, est un *Dirofilaria.* Ann Parasitol Hum Comp 17:380–404, 515–532.

Dissanaike AS, Lykov VP, Sri Skanda R, Sivayoham I, Wijesekera SVI, Perera MCS. 1982. Four more cases of human infection with *Dirofilaria* (*Nochtiella*). Ceylon Med J 17:105–113.

Fülleborn F. 1908. Ueber Versuche an Hundefilarien un deren Uebertragung durch Müken. Arch Sch Trop Hyg Path Ther Exot Krakh 12:313–351.

Gunewardene K. 1956. Observations on the development of *Dirofilaria repens* in *Aedes* (*Stegomyia*) *albopictus* and other common mosquitoes in Ceylon. Ceylon J Med Sci 9:45–53.

Heisch RB, Nelson GS, Furlong M. 1959. Studies in filariasis in East Africa. 1. Filariasis on the Island of Pate, Kenya. Trans Roy Soc Trop Med Hyg 53:41–53.

Huber B. 1985. Cas cliniques: helminthoses canines à manifestations cutanées. Point Vét 17:43–48.

MacLean, JD, Beaver PC, Michalek H. 1979. Subcutaneous dirofilariasis in Okinawa, Japan. Am J Trop Med Hyg 28:45–48.

Mak JW, Lye MS, Sim BKL, Cheong WH, Lee CP. 1985. Studies on malaria and filariasis in Hilir Perak, Peninsular Malaysia. Trop Biomed 2:40–46.

Mantovani A, Restani R. 1965. Richerche sui possibili artropodi vettori di *Dirofilaria repens* in alcune provincie dell'Italia centrale. Parassitologia 7:109–116.

Marconcini A, Magi M, Hecht Contin B. 1993. The efficacy of ivermectin in the prophylaxis of *Dirofilaria repens* infection in dogs naturally exposed to infection. Parassitologia 35:67–71.

Nair CP, Roy R, Raghavan NGS. 1961. Susceptibility of *Aedes albopictus* to *Dirofilaria repens* infection in cats. Ind J Malariol 15:49–52.

Nelson GS. 1959. The identification of infective filaria larvae in mosquitoes: with a note on the species found in "wild" mosquitoes on the Kenya coast. J Helminthol 33:233–256.

O'Grady F, Fawcett AN, Buckley JJC. 1962. A case of human infection with *Dirofilaria* (*Nochtiella*) sp. Probably of African origin. J Helminthol 36:309–312.

Palmieri JR, Masbar S, Purnomo, Marwoto HA, Tirtokusumo S, Darwis F. 1985. The domestic cat as a host for brugian filariasis in South Kalimantan (Borneo), Indonesia. J Helminthol 59:277–281.

Pampiglione S, Canestri Trotti G, Rivasi F. 1995. Human dirofilariasis due to *Dirofilaria* (*Nochtiella*) *repens:* a review of world literature. Parassitologia 37:149–193.

Pampiglione S, Canestri Trotti G, Rivasi F, Vakalis N. 1996. Human dirofilariasis in Greece: a review of reported cases and a description of a new, subcutaneous case. Ann Trop Med Parasitol 90:319–328.

Patnaik MM. 1989. On filarial nematodes in domestic animals in Orissa. Ind Vet J 66:573–574.

Railliet A, Henry A. 1911a. Sur une filaire péritonéale des porcins. Bull Soc Pathol Exot 4:386–389.

Railliet A, Henry A. 1911b. Remarques au sujet des deux notes de MM. Bauche et Bernard. Bull Soc Pathol Exot 4:485–488.

Rohde K. 1962. Helminthen aus Katzen un Hunden in Malaya; Bemerkungen zu ihrer epideiologischen Bedeutung für den Menschen. Ztsch Parasitenk 22:237–244.

Scarzi M. 1995. Cutaneous dirofilariosis in dogs. Obiettivi e Documenti Veterinari. 16(6):11–15.

Skrjabin KI. 1917. *Loa extraocularis* n. sp. parasite nouveu de l'oeil de l'homme. CR Hebd Soc Biol Paris 80:759–762.

Skrjabin KI, Schikhobalova NP. 1948. Filariae of man and animals. 171–173 [in Russian].

Skrjabin KI, Althausen AJ, Schuilman ES. 1930. First case of *Dirofilaria repens* from man. Trop Med I Vet Moscow 8:9–11 [in Russian].

Webber WAF, Hawking F. 1955. Experimental maintenance of *Dirofilaria repens* and *D. immitis* in dogs. Exp Parasitol 4:143–164.

Yen PKF, Zaman V, Mak JW. 1982. Identification of some common infective filarid larvae in Malaysia. J Helminthol 56:69–80.

Zweig A, Karasik A, Hiss J. 1981. *Dirofilaria* in a cervical lymph node in Israel. Hum Pathol 12:939–940.

Dirofilaria striata (Molin, 1858) Railliet and Henry, 1911

Dirofilaria striata was first described from pumas in Brazil by Molin (1858) and redescribed by Anderson and Diaz-Ungria (1959) from ocelots and margay cats from Venezuela. These are very large worms that live in the subcutaneous tissue and fascia. The females may reach 28 to 36 cm in length, and the males are 8 to 10 cm long. *Dirofilaria striata* has also been found in Florida panthers (Forrester et al., 1985; Lamm et al., 1997). Orihel and Ash (1964) recovered this worm from bobcats in Louisiana and showed that larvae would develop to the infective stage in mosquitoes (*Anopheles quadrimaculatus*). When these mosquitoes were allowed to feed on kittens, examination of one kitten 90 days after infection revealed only nodules containing degenerating larvae at the sites of inoculation and deeper tissues of the trunk and legs. Two other kittens remained negative for microfilariae over the next 11 months after inoculation.

There have been several cases of human infection with *Dirofilaria striata* in the United States (Orihel and Eberhard, 1998; Orihel and Isbey, 1990). Typically, the worms have been recovered from subcutaneous nodules. Interestingly, microfilariae similar to that of *Dirofilaria striata* have been recovered from greyhounds in Florida (Courtney et al., 1985), although there has been no record of finding microfilariae in cats from that area.

Chitwood (1933) reported on the recovery of *Dirofilaria acutiuscula* from a Canadian lynx. The worms were originally reported from wild hogs in Brazil. Again, these forms have not been reported from domestic cats.

REFERENCES

Anderson RC, Diaz-Ungria C. 1959. Nematodes de Venezuela, VI. *Dirofilaria striata* (Molin, 1858) Railliet y Henry, 1911 en felinos suramericanos, con comentarios sobre las *Dirofilaria* en carnivoros. Bol Venez Lab Clin 4:3–15.

Chitwood BG. 1933. Note on a genus and species of nematode from *Lynx canadensis*. J Parasitol 20:63.

Courtney CH, Sundlof SF, Lane TJ. 1985. Impact of filariasis on the racing greyhound. JAAHA 21:421–425.

Forrester DJ, Conti JA, Belden RC. 1985. Parasites of the Florida panther (*Felis concolor coryi*). Proc Helm Soc Wash 52:95–97.

Lamm MG, Roelke ME, Greiner EC, Streible CK. 1997. Microfilariae in the free-ranging Florida panther (*Felis concolor coryi*). J Helm Soc Wash 64:137–141.

Molin R. 1858. Versuch eineu Mongographie der Filarien. Sitz Akad Wissensch Wien Math-naturw Cl 28:365–461.

Orihel TC, Ash LR. 1964. Occurrence of *Dirofilaria striata* in the bobcat (*Lynx rufus*) in Louisiana with observations on its larval development. J Parasitol 50:590–591.

Orihel TC, Eberhard ML. 1998. Zoonotic filariasis. Clin Microbiol Rev 11:366–381.

Orihel TC, Isbey EK. 1990. *Dirofilaria striata* infection in a North Carolina child. Am J Trop Med Hyg 42:124–126.

Redington BC, Jackson RF, Seymour WG, Otto GF. 1977. The various microfilariae found in dogs in the United States. Proc Heartworm Symp '77:14–21.

ADENOPHOREA

ENOPLIDA

The adenophorean nematodes of the cat are represented by the various members of the order Enoplida: capillarids, *Eucoleus, Aonchotheca,* and *Pearsonema* species; *Trichuris; Anatrichosoma;* and *Trichinella.* Other than some of the capillarids, most of these infections are rather rare in cats. The aphasmids differ from the Secernentea in that the stage typically infective to the final host is the first-stage larva.

Structurally, the aphasmids are also much different from the secernentean nematodes. The esophagus has a peculiar structure that appears as a chain of glandular cells with a small esophageal lumen. This type of esophagus is called a stichosome esophagus, with the individual cells being stichocytes. Another difference with the aphasmids is that the anal opening on both the male and female tends to be terminal. Thus, there is no tail that protrudes beyond the anal opening.

Eucoleus aerophilus (Creplin, 1839) Dujardin, 1845

Etymology

Eu = good + *coleus* = sheath and *aerophilus* for lung loving.

Synonyms

Capillaria aerophila (Creplin, 1839).

History

The worm was found in a fox and named *Trichosoma aerophilus* by Creplin in 1839. Dujardin changed the name to *Thominx aerophila* in 1845, and then in 1915, Travassos transferred the worm to the genus *Capillaria.* However, in recent years the work of Moravec (1982) has come to be accepted, and the worm has been assigned to the genus *Eucoleus.* This worm has been considered a major parasite of foxes, where it can cause severe pathology (Christenson, 1938).

Geographic Distribution

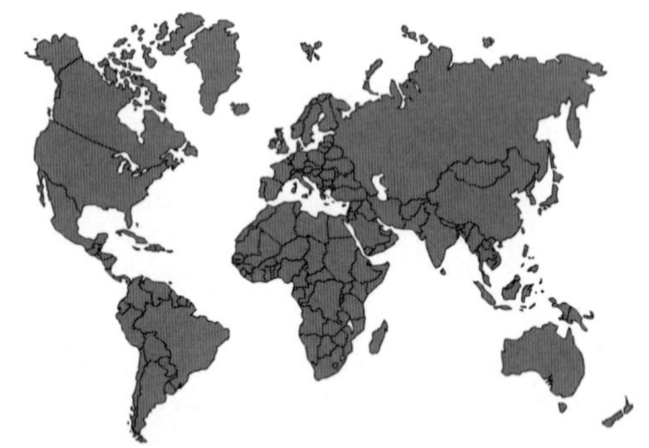

Fig. 4.87.

This worm has been described from around the world. There have been relatively recent reports from the United States (Corwin et al., 1984)), Belgium (Thienpoint et al., 1981), Germany (Schulz, 1981), Italy (Trotti et al., 1990), Argentina (Radman et al., 1986), Japan (Matoyoshi et al., 1996), and Tasmania (Milstein and Goldsmid, 1997).

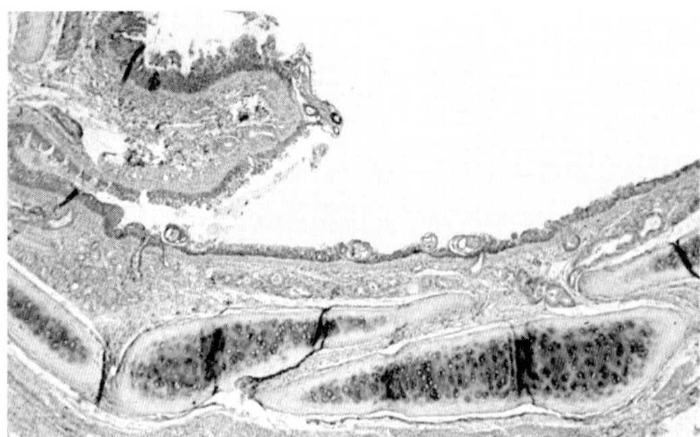

Fig. 4.88. *Eucoleus aerophilus.* Histological section through the bronchiolar mucosa showing sections of the worm embedded in the superficial epithelium.

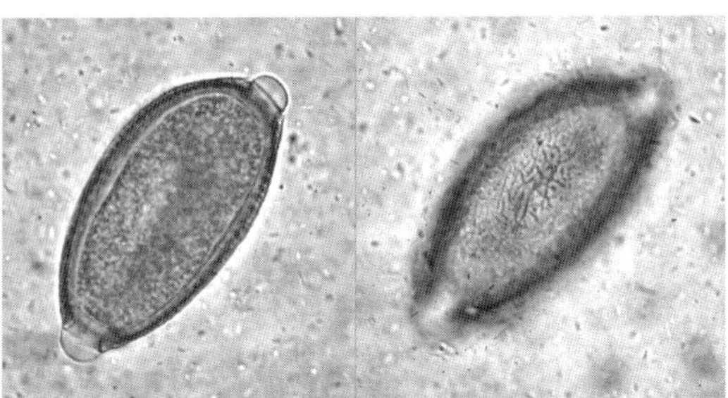

Fig. 4.89. *Eucoleus aerophilus.* Two views of the same egg of this worm. The left view shows the striations apparent in the eggshell when viewed at a focal plane near the center of the egg. The right view shows the surface of the eggshell with its fine lattice-work sculpturing. (Illustration courtesy of Dr. Barry Campbell)

Location in Host

These worms are found threaded through the mucosa of the trachea, bronchi, and bronchioles (Fig. 4.88).

Parasite Identification

The eggs are 59 to 83 μm long by 26 to 40 μm wide. The surface of the egg has a net-like ornamentation (Fig. 4.89). The adults are typically seen most commonly in histologic sections, but when whole worms are removed, the genus can be recognized by the long, spined spicular sheath of the male.

Life Cycle

The life cycle of *Eucoleus aerophilus* has not been well described, but it is believed that direct ingestion of the egg with an infective larva is the most common route of infection (Campbell and Little, 1991). The prepatent period is somewhere between 3 to 5 weeks. The eggs are deposited by the female within the tracts they have made in the mucosa, and the eggs slowly work their way to the surface. The eggs are then coughed up and swallowed to be passed in the feces. Once eggs are deposited on the soil, they take about 40 days to become infectious.

Clinical Presentation and Pathogenesis

The main clinical signs reported in the cat include coughing and wheezing due to bronchiole disease. A bronchial pattern may be present on chest radiographs.

Treatment

Levamisole has been successfully used to treat infected cats (Endres 1976; Norsworthy, 1975).

Epizootiology

Very little is known because of the poorly understood life cycle.

Hazards to Other Animals

The life cycle is believed to be direct, so cats could serve as sources of infection for other animals. This parasite can cause severe disease in foxes; thus, cats could serve as vectors of this agent under certain circumstances.

Hazards to Humans

Eucoleus has been reported as a human parasite in seven cases in Russia, one in Morocco, one in Iran, and one in the Ukraine (Beaver et al., 1984). In these cases the most common signs were acute bronchitis and bronchiolits, usually with asthma and a productive cough.

Control/Prevention

Because the life cycle is direct, good fecal control is essential to prevent the disease from becoming a serious problem. In catteries or shelters, the number of infected animals could reach very high levels; thus, it is imperative that under conditions of group housing that sanitation be well maintained, outdoors as well as indoors.

REFERENCES

Beaver PC, Jung RC, Cupp EW. 1984. Clinical Parasitology. 9th edition. Philadelphia, Pa: Lea and Febiger. 825 pp.

Campbell BG, Little MD. 1991. Identification of the eggs of a nematode (*Eucoleus boehmi*) from the nasal mucosa of North American dogs. JAVMA 198:1520–1523.
Christenson RO. 1938. Life history and epidemiological studies on the fox lungworm, *Capillaria aerophila* (Creplin, 1839). Livro Jub L Travassos, 119–136.
Corwin RM, Pratt SE, McCurdy HD. 1984. Anthelmintic effect of febantel/praziquantel paste in dogs and cats. Am J Vet Res 45:154–155.
Creplin FCH. 1839. Eingeweidewürmer, finnenwürmer, thierwürmer. Allg Encycl der Wissensch u Künste Ersch and Gruber, Lepzig 1st sect 32:277–302.
Dujardin F. 1845. Histoire naturelle des helminthes. Lib Encycl Roret, Paris. 655 pp.
Endres WA. 1976. Levamisole in treatment of *Capillaria aerophila* in a cat: a case report. Vet Med SA Comp 71:1553.
Matoyoshi M, Ameku Y, Keruma T, Kinjo E. 1996. Isolation of *Pasteurella dagmatis* from an Iriomote cat (*Felis iriomotensis*) with parasitic bronchopneumonia. J Jap Vet Med Assoc 49:879–883.
Milstein TC, Goldsmid JM. 1997. Parasites of feral cats from southern Tasmania and their potential significance. Aust Vet J 75:218–219.
Molin R. 1858. Versuch einer Monographic der Filarieu. Sitzungsb K Acad Wissensch Wien, Math-Naturw 28: 365–461.
Moravec F. 1982. Proposal of a new systematic arrangement of nematodes of the family Capillariidae. Folia Parasitol 29:119–132.
Norsworthy GD. 1975. Feline lungworm treatment case report. Feline Pract 5(3):14.
Radman N, Venturini L, Denegri G. 1986. Experimental confirmation of the presence in Argentina of *Capillaria aerophila* Creplin, 1839 (Nematoda, Capillaridae). Rev Iberica Parasitol 46:267–272.
Schulz HP. 1981. Three frequently seen nematode infections of cats: *Aelurostrongylus abstrusus, Capillaria aerophila, Ollulanus tricuspis.* Zeitschrift fur Versuchstierkunde 23:186.
Thienpoint D, Vanparijs O, Hermans L. 1981. Epidemiology of helminthiases of the cat in Belgium. The prevalence of *Ollulanus tricuspis.* Rec Med Vet l'Ecole d'Alfort 157:591–595.
Travassos LP. 1915. Contribuições para o conhecimento da fauna helmintolojica brasileira. V. Sohre as especies brasileiras do genero *Capillaria* Zeder, 1800. Mem Inst Oswaldo Cruz 7:146–172.
Trotti GC, Corradini L, Visconti S. 1990. Parasitological investigations in a cattery in Ferrara. Parassitologia 32:42–43.

Aonchotheca putorii (Rudolphi, 1819) López-Neyra, 1947

Etymology

a = un- + *oncho* = spined + *theca* = sheath (referring to the unspined sheath on the spicule of the male) and *putorii* for the original isolation from a ferret.

Synonyms

Trichosoma putorii Rudolphi, 1819; *Trichosoma erinacei* Rudolphi, 1819; *Trichosomum exigua* Dujardin, 1845; *Trichosomum entomelas* Dujardin, 1845; *Calodium alatum* Molin, 1858; *Capillaria erinacea* (Rudolphi, 1819) Travassos, 1915; *Capillaria mustelorum* Cameron and Parnell, 1933; *Capillaria putorii* (Rudolphi, 1819) Travassos, 1915.

History

Aonchotheca putorii was first described by Rudolphi in 1819 as *Trichosoma putorii* from the stomach of a ferret, *Mustela putorius.* Butterworth and Beverley-Burton (1980) felt that *Capillaria erinacei* of the European hedgehog and *Capillaria mustelorum* of the weasel in Scotland were synonymous with the species recovered from ferrets.

Geographic Distribution

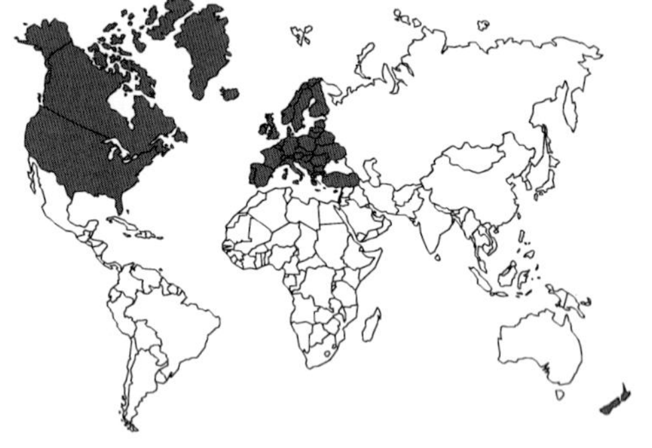

Fig. 4.90.

Aonchotheca putorii has been reported from domestic cats in Europe, North America, and New Zealand (Butterworth and Beverley-Burton, 1980). *Aonchotheca putorii* is a common parasite of the stomach and small intestine of such wild mammals as bobcats, raccoons, mink, and various other mustelids (Butterworth and Beverley-Burton, 1980; Campbell, 1991).

Location in Host

Aonchotheca putorii is usually observed in the gastric mucus, but some descriptions note its occurrence in the small intestine. In the Iowa report, the parasites were found in the gastric mucus, but only on occasions where there had been intestinal reflux (Greve and Kung, 1983).

Butterworth and Beverley-Burton (1980) found that the worms lived within the gastric mucosa and were easiest to identify in tissues when the mucosal surface was washed with 1 percent aqueous methylene blue, which gave the tissues a light blue appearance and made the unstained worms easier to visualize.

Parasite Identification

Particular morphologic details of adult *Aonchotheca putorii* are influenced by the definitive hosts that they parasitize. In the feline, the male stomach capillarids range in size from 2.52 to 5.29 mm (average 3.97 mm); the females range in size from 3.46 to 7.40 mm (average 5.04 mm). The gastric capillarids recovered from cats in New Zealand were approximately 8 mm in length (Collins and Charleston, 1972). The width at the posterior end of the stichosome of the male is from 24 to 38 µm (average 29), while that of the female is from 24 to 38 µm (average 33.4). The maximum width of the male ranges from 31 to 41 µm (average 33); that of the female is 34 to 51 µm (average 41.4). The distance from the vulva to the anterior end in the female is 2.01 to 3.18 µm (average 2.48). The vulvar flap of *Aonchotheca putorii* may or may not be covered by a cuticular flap; instead, the vulva is surrounded by varying amounts of corrugation. The males demonstrate a characteristic structure of the tip of the spicule and a distinct form of the lateral and caudal alae (Greve and Kung, 1983). The spicule length in the male is from 162 to 276 µm with an average length of 211 µm. The characteristic of this genus that allows easiest identification of these worms is the lack of spines on the cirrus, or spicular sheath, which surrounds the spicule.

The egg length of this capillarid is from 57 to 66 µm (average 61.3); the egg width is from 21 to 28 µm (average 23.3). The eggs are characterized by having a dark shell with thickened ridges on their surfaces (Fig. 4.91).

Life Cycle

It has been postulated that the New Zealand cats became infected by ingesting infective eggs of *Aonchotheca putorii* from soil contaminated with hedgehog feces. These capillarids reach maturity in the stomachs of cats and dogs as well as in hedgehogs (Collins, 1973).

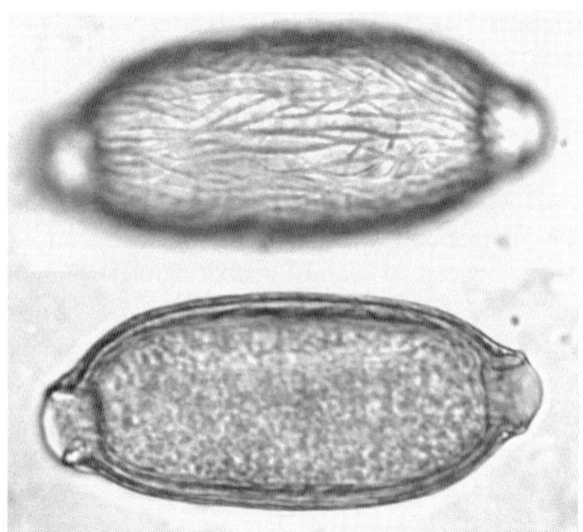

Fig. 4.91. *Aonchotheca purtorii.* Two views of the same egg of this worm. The top view shows the surface of the egg with its deep striations. The bottom view shows how the eggshell appears to have a rough surface at midsection. (Illustration courtesy of Dr. Barry Campbell)

Clinical Presentation and Pathogenesis

Until the reports by Curtsinger et al. (1993), the pathogenicity of *Aonchotheca putorii* in domestic cats was not known (Greve and Kung, 1983). It had not been associated with clinical illness in cats in the United States, but a European report documented it as a cause of feline gastritis (Wagner, 1936).

There are few reports on the clinical presentation of infection in cats with this parasite. One domestic cat presented with a 3-week history of partial anorexia and intermittent passage of bloody vomitus and tarry feces (Curtsinger et al., 1993). Physical examination revealed lethargy, dehydration, pale mucous membranes, and signs of pain when the cranial portion of the abdomen was palpated. A complete blood cell count revealed a normocytic, normochromic anemia. Serum biochemistry tests revealed hyperglycemia, hypocalcemia, and hypokalemia. Multiple fecal examinations were negative. Contrast radiography revealed delayed gastric emptying. Exploratory laparotomy revealed a 0.5 cm diameter perforation in the caudal aspect of the pylorus. There were adhesions between the pylorus and the surrounding structures. Histology of gastric tissue obtained by gastroduodenoscopy showed chronic, hyperplastic pyloric gastritis, dilation of numerous pyloric glands, regions of superficial mucosal fibrosis, and perforation of an ulcer in the caudal aspect of the pylorus. Adult nematodes, identified as *Aonchotheca putorii,* and their eggs were observed in the pyloric mucosa, near the perforation. The nematodes in tissue sections were between 26 and 40 mm in diameter. Some contained a linear arrangement of yellow-brown operculated eggs. The worms were surrounded by mucus that contained many red blood cells and a few neutrophils. Some parasites were observed in the lamina propria of the mucosae. Smaller worms ranging in size from 15 to 24 mm (hypothesized to be larvae) were noted in the deeper layers of the mucosa, within glandular lumens, and between the basement membrane and the epithelial cells of the glands. Regions of cellular necrosis and regeneration surrounded the worms. Eggs were noted in the pyloric mucus and in the lumens of the pyloric glands.

Treatment

When an infected cat was treated with levamisole (2 doses: 7.5 mg/kg at 2-week intervals, the first dose split 12 hours apart and the second dose given singly), eggs of *Aonchotheca putorii* disappeared from the feces (Greve and Kung, 1983).

Curtsinger et al. (1993) administered ivermectin (300 mg/kg body weight) *per os* 1 week following surgery and again 2 weeks later.

Epizootiology

Infected cats may serve as carriers. The exact role of wild animals in the epizootiology of gastric capillariasis has not been studied.

Hazards to Other Animals

Aonchotheca putorii has been recorded from the American black bear, European hedgehog, raccoon, swine, bobcat, and a variety of mustelids. Such a broad host range is typical for many capillarid species. Cross transmission is possible from host to host (Collins, 1973; Greve and Kung, 1983).

Hazards to Humans

There have been no reports of cross transmission of *Aonchotheca putorii* to humans.

Control/Prevention

Infection results from ingestion of soil contaminated by feces containing infective eggs. These feces could come from a variety of definitive hosts. Cats should not be allowed to roam freely.

REFERENCES

Butterworth EW, Beverley-Burton M. 1980. The taxonomy of *Capillaria* spp (Nematoda: Trichuridea) in carnivorous mammals from Ontario, Canada. Syst Parasitol 1:211–236.

Cameron TWM, Parnell IW. 1933. The internal parasites of land mammals in Scotland. R Phys Soc Edinb 22:133–154.

Campbell BG. 1991. *Trichuris* and other trichinelloid nematodes of dogs and cats in the United States. Comp Cont Educ Pract Vet 13:769–779, 801.

Collins GH. 1973. A limited survey of gastro-intestinal helminths of dogs and cats. NZ Vet J 21:175–176.

Collins GH, Charleston WAG. 1972. *Ollulanus tricuspis* and *Capillaria putorii* in New Zealand cats. NZ Vet J 20:82.

Curtsinger DK, Carpenter JL, Turner JL. 1993. Gastritis caused by *Aonchotheca putorii* in a domestic cat. J Am Vet Med Assoc 203:1153–1154.

Greve JH, Kung FY. 1983. *Capillaria putorii* in domestic cats in Iowa. J Am Vet Med Assoc 182:511–513.

López-Neyra CR. 1947. Los capillariinae. Memorias de la R. Academia de Ciencias exactas, físicas y naturales de Madrid 12:248 pp.

Rudolphi KA. 1819. Entozoorum synopsis cui accedunt mantissa duplex et indices locupletissimi. Berlin:813 pp.

Wagner O. 1936. Beitrage zu einer Revision der Nematoden-Gattungen *Capillaria, Hepaticola,* und *Eucoleus*. Senckenbergiana 18(5,6):245–269.

Pearsonema feliscati (Diesing, 1851) Freitas and Mendonça (1960)

Etymology

Pearsonema for Dr. Pearson and *feliscati* for the feline host.

Synonyms

Moravec (1982) accepted the species *Pearsonema feliscati* as being distinct from *Pearsonema plica.* After a long discussion of the history of the two species and their associated taxonomy, Butterworth and Beverley-Burton (1980) felt that the species in North American domestic cats should be considered as *Capillaria travassoi* (Freitas and

Lent, 1936; Ehrlich, 1947). Butterworth and Beverley-Burton described the only reliable means of distinguishing the two species as patterns on the surfaces of the respective eggshells, appearing as large depressions and ridges on *Pearsonema plica* and appearing striated on *Capillaria travassoi,* and by the terminal caudal alae of the males, triangular in *Pearsonema plica* and rounded in *Capillaria travassoi.* Thus, until such time as these worms are more carefully compared and the eggs in the urine of cats more carefully studied and illustrated, it will be difficult to determine whether or not these are indeed the same species or whether or not their geographical ranges overlap.

History

In 1819 Rudolphi was the first to report the presence of nematode worms in the urinary bladder and renal pelvis in dogs, cats, and foxes. He named the parasite *Capillaria plica.* In 1851, Diesing identified a species of *Capillaria* in the bladder of cats from Egypt and other locales and named it *Capillaria feliscati* (Wilson-Hanson and Prescott, 1982a). Lewis (1927) reported this capillarid from the urinary bladder of cats in Wales. Chen (1934) recorded it from cats in Canton, China. Enzie (1951) felt that *Pearsonema plica* was markedly different from the *Pearsonema feliscati* usually encountered in feline urine and questioned whether *Pearsonema plica* actually occurs in the cat. In 1953, Chitwood and Enzie published a report on *Pearsonema plica* in the urinary bladder of a cat, adding further credence to the fact that the two species are distinct.

Geographic Distribution

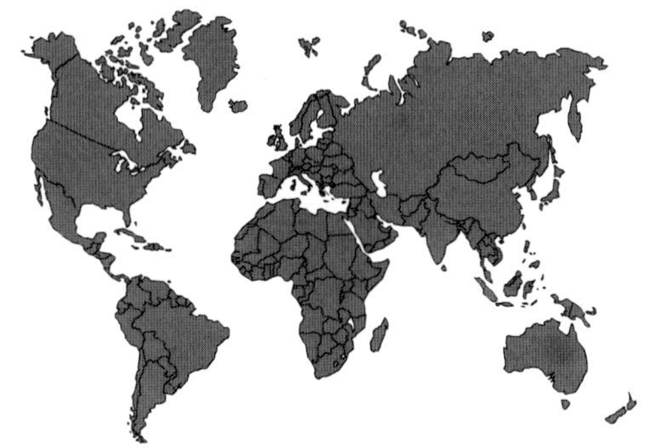

Fig. 4.92.

Pearsonema feliscati has been observed in cats from localities throughout the world. Subsequent to its original documentation in Egyptian cats by Diesing, Lewis (1927) reported this capillarid from the urinary bladder of cats in Wales, and Finnerup (1986) reported it in a cat from Denmark. Chen (1934) recorded it from cats in Canton, China. Waddell (1967, 1968a) reported infection rates in 34 percent and 31 percent of adult cats in Brisbane, Australia. A 12-month, Australian survey of 400 cats of varying ages revealed that 18.3 percent of cats aged 2 years and older were infected with *Pearsonema feliscati.* Younger cats demonstrated a lower infection rate. No cat under 2 years of age was infected (Wilson-Hanson and Prescott, 1982b). In North America, *Pearsonema feliscati* is either uncommon or overlooked (Lautenslager, 1976). Nevertheless, the occurrence of the feline bladder worm has been documented by veterinarians in the United States (Harris, 1981).

Location in Host

Adult *Pearsonema feliscati* are found within the urinary bladder of the cat. One source stated that these worms move freely within the urine in the bladder and tend not to attach to the bladder mucosa (Wilson-Hanson and Prescott, 1982a). Another source stated that the tiny adult worms are embedded in the bladder epithelium. In some cases, the worms have been found in the ureters and the renal pelvis (Campbell, 1991).

Parasite Identification

Male *Pearsonema feliscati* are 13 to 30 mm in length, while the females are from 28 to 32 mm in length. The spicule sheath of the male, like that of species of *Aonchotheca,* is not spined. The labia of the female's vulva are slightly protruding; they are located some distance from the termination of the esophagus. Both sexes possess a terminal anus that is surrounded by three slight lobes (Enzie, 1951).

The eggs of this parasite are passed in the urine. The eggs of *Pearsonema feliscati* have been illustrated by Enzie (1951), Waddell (1967), and Burgu and Doganay (1986). The eggs with bipolar plugs tend to have a pitted surface, but the surface does not appear to have pits as large as those illustrated for *Pearsonema plica* by Enzie (1951) and Butterworth and Beverley-Burton (1980). As

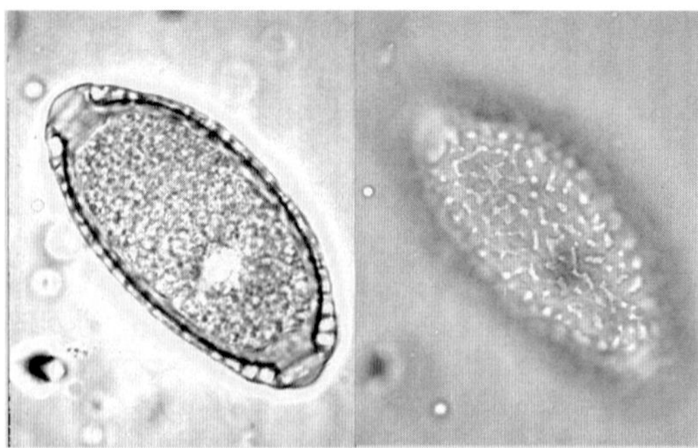

Fig. 4.93. *Pearsonema feliscati.* Two views of the egg of this worm that are found in the urine. The view on the left shows the large punctate pits that appear to be within the eggshell; the view on the right shows the bleb-like striations on the surface of the shell.

shown by Enzie (1951), the eggs of *Pearsonema feliscati* are markedly different than those of *Pearsonema plica.* When passed in the urine, the eggs of both species typically contain one or two cells, and they measure 51 to 65 by 24 to 32 μm (Enzie, 1951) (Fig. 4.93).

Life Cycle

The life cycle of *Pearsonema feliscati* is thought to be similar to that of *Pearsonema plica* as described by Enigk (1950). After passage in the urine, the eggs embryonate, and after ingestion by earthworms, the larvae develop to the infective stage within the coelomic cavity. In the case of *Pearsonema plica,* the earthworm is considered an obligate intermediate host. Following ingestion of infected earthworms by the final host, the larvae are found in the wall of the small intestine for the first 8 to 10 days after infection and then supposedly make their way via the circulatory system to the bladder. The prepatent period in experimentally infected foxes was 58 to 63 days.

Cats are not known to eat earthworms, and paratenic hosts (transport hosts, e.g., birds) have been suggested as the means by which cats become infected (Prescott, 1984). Some believe that the life cycle is direct, not involving an intermediate host.

Clinical Presentation and Pathogenesis

Pearsonema feliscati is generally regarded as producing little pathology (Waddell, 1967, 1968a). However, if the ureters become plugged with worms, cats may display the clinical signs of post–renal obstruction (Campbell, 1991). In many infected cats, the serosal surface of the bladder is discolored a brownish pink. This discoloration was observed in bladders containing four or more nematodes. The mucous membranes were not visibly inflamed; however, in histopathologic section, there were areas of dilated blood vessels, extravasated blood, and lifting transitional epithelium with some inflammatory cells. Within the incised bladders, all worms moved freely within the urine; none appeared to be attached to the bladder mucosa. The maximum number of adult worms recovered from a single urinary bladder was 25. Large numbers of eggs were found in all bladders containing 5 or more adults. Protein concentration of the urine increased as the adult population of *Pearsonema feliscati* increased. There was no relationship between the presence of adult capillarids in the bladder and cystitis (Wilson-Hanson and Prescott, 1982a).

Treatment

Urinary capillariasis has been treated with oral methyridine (200 mg/kg, once). Transitory side effects were noted. Appetite was normal within 12 hours following treatment (Waddell, 1968b; Georgi, 1975).

Harris (1981) noted the disappearance of *Pearsonema* eggs from the urine of a cat following treatment with levamisole (45 mg, subcutaneously, once a week for two injections). Ivermectin (0.2 mg/kg, subcutaneously) has been reported to be successful in treating urinary capillariasis in a dog (Kirkpatrick and Nelson, 1987).

Epizootiology

Older cats may serve as carriers. The exact role of wild animals in the epizootiology of urinary capillariasis is not known.

Hazards to Other Animals

As stated above, it is not clear whether this parasite has a direct life cycle or one utilizing an intermediate host. Thus, in a cattery situation it is difficult to determine the extent of environmental contamination with eggs shed in the urine.

Hazards to Humans

There have been no documented cases of the transmission of *Pearsonema feliscati* from cats to man.

Control/Prevention

Methods of control include keeping animals away from soil surfaces and discouraging contact with areas frequented by wild animals (Campbell, 1991).

REFERENCES

Burgu A, Doganay A. 1986. [Some difficulties in the identification of responsible species of urinary capillariose in cats.] [In Turkish]. A U Vet Fak Derg 33:38–51.

Butterworth EW, Beverley-Burton M. 1980. The taxonomy of *Capillaria* spp (Nematoda: Trichuridea) in carnivorous mammals from Ontario, Canada. Syst Parasitol 1:211–236.

Campbell BG. 1991. *Trichuris* and other trichinelloid nematodes of dogs and cats in the United States. Comp Cont Educ Pract Vet 13:769–779, 801.

Chen HT. 1934. Helminths of cats in Fukien and Kwangtung provinces with a list of those recorded from China. Lingnan Sci J 16:201–273.

Chitwood MB, Enzie FD. 1953. The domestic cat a new host for *Capillaria plica* in North America. Proc Helminthol Soc Wash 20:27–28.

Ehrlich I. 1947. [A revision of *Capillaria* species (Nematoda) from the urinary bladder of the domestic cat.] Glasnik Hrvatskoga prirodoslovnoga drustva. Zagreb 1:79–85.

Enigk K. 1950. Die Biologie von *Capillaria plica* (Trichuroidea. Nematodes). Z Tropenmed Parasitol 1:560–571.

Enzie FD. 1951. Do whipworms occur in domestic cats in North America? J Am Vet Med Assoc 119:210–213.

Finnerup E. 1986. *Capillaria feliscati*—urinblëreorm hos kat. Dansk Vett Tidsskr 69:60–61.

Freitas JFT, Lent H. 1936. Estudo sobre os Capillariinae parasitos de mammiferos. Memórias do Instituto Oswaldo Cruz 31:85–160.

Georgi JR. 1975. Feline lungworm treatment. Feline Pract 5:16, 20.

Harris LT. 1981. Feline bladderworm. VM/SAC 76:844.

Kirkpatrick CE, Nelson GR. 1987. Ivermectin treatment of urinary capillariasis in a dog. J Am Vet Med Assoc 191:701–702.

Lautenslager JP. 1976. Internal helminths of cats. Vet Clin North Am 6:353–365.

Lewis EA. 1927. A study of the helminths of dogs and cats of Aberyswyth, Wales. J Helminthol 5:171–182.

Moravec F. 1982. Proposal of a new systematic arrangement of nematodes of the family Capillariidae. Folia Parasitol 29(2):119–131.

Prescott CW. 1984. Parasitic Diseases of the Cat in Australia. Sydney, Australia: Postgraduate Foundation in Veterinary Science. 112 pp.

Rudolphi KA. 1819. Entozoorum synopsis cui accedunt mantissa duplex et indices locupletissimi. Berlin. 813 pp.

Waddell AH. 1967. *Capillaria feliscati* in the bladder of cats in Australia. Aust Vet J 43:297.

Waddell AH. 1968a. Further observations on *Capillaria feliscati* in the cat. Aust Vet J 44:33–34.

Waddell AH. 1968b. Anthelmintic treatment for *Capillaria feliscati* in the cat. Vet Rec 82:598.

Wilson-Hanson S, Prescott CW. 1982a. *Capillaria* in the bladder of the domestic cat. Austral Vet J 59:190–191.

Wilson-Hanson S, Prescott CW. 1982b. A survey for parasites in cats. Aust Vet J 59:192.

Calodium hepaticum (Bancroft, 1893) Moravec, 1982

Calodium hepaticum is better known by its synonym *Capillaria hepatica.* This parasite lives within the parenchyma of the liver of rodents. The female worm deposits eggs in the liver where they remain until the host dies or is eaten. The eggs are not infective for another host, however, until they have spent more than a month undergoing embryonation in the soil. Rats become infected when they ingest embryonated eggs. Three weeks after infection, the females begin to lay eggs in the liver of the rat (Campbell, 1991).

The predatory nature of the cat is such that the eggs of *Calodium hepaticum* are not uncommonly found in cat feces (Fig. 4.94). The eggs can be recognized by their porous surface (giving them a striated appearance in sections) and by their size 51 to 68 μm by 30 to 35 μm (Campbell, 1991) (Fig. 4.95). Thus, these eggs can be readily distinguished from the eggs of *Eucoleus aerophilus* and *Aonchotheca putorii,* which will also appear in feline feces.

Calodium hepaticum occurs on rare occasions in the livers of other hosts. It has been reported from dogs, horses, humans, and other primates. Reports on infection in the liver of cats are rare. There is one report from Slovakia (Mituch, 1968) and one from Brazil (Santos and Barros, 1973).

REFERENCES

Campbell BG. 1991. *Trichuris* and other trichinelloid nematodes of dogs and cats in the United States. Comp Cont Educ Pract Vet 13:769–799, 801.

Mituch J. 1968. Die Helminthenfauna der Hauskatze (Felis domestica L.) in der Slowakei (USSR). Folia Vet 12:165.

Moravec F. 1982. Proposal of a new systematic arrangement of nematodes of the family Capillariidae. Folia Parasitol 29 (2):119–131.

Santos MN, Barros CSL. 1973. *Capillaria hepatica:* parasite of dog and cat in Rio Grande do Sol State. Rev Med Vet Sao Paulo 9:133–140.

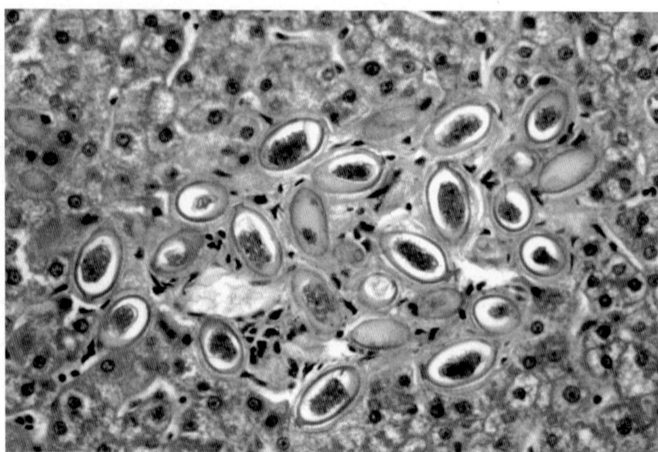

Fig. 4.94. *Calodium hepaticum.* The highly striated appearing eggs of this worm as they would appear in the feces of a cat that had eaten an infected rodent.

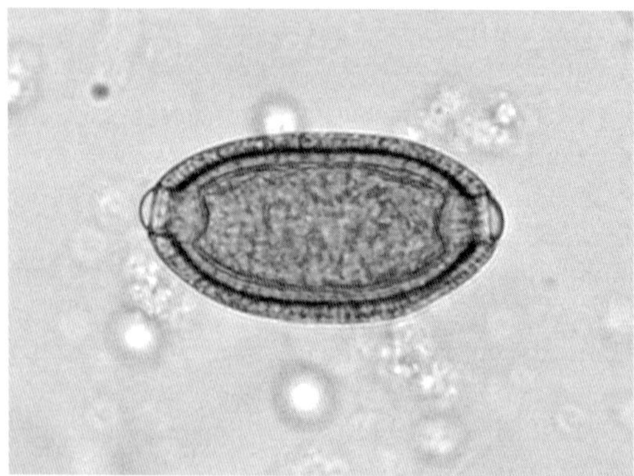

Fig. 4.95. *Calodium hepaticum.* The typical egg of this capillarid, with its highly striated shell.

Anatrichosoma Species

This genus of rarely encountered, capillarid-like worms was first discovered in the skin and nasal mucosa of monkeys in Asia and Africa and was named *Trichosoma cutaneum* by Swift, Boots, and Miller (1922). The genus *Anatrichosoma* was created in 1954 for a second species, *Anatrichosoma cynomolgi,* also from monkeys (Smith and Chitwood, 1954; Chitwood and Smith, 1958). In the genus *Anatrichosoma,* there are now eight recognized species that have been reported from a wide variety of tissue sites in primates, rodents, shrews, and marsupials. *Anatrichosoma cutaneum* and *Anatrichosoma cynomolgi* have been detected in the skin and nasal mucosa of Asian monkeys (Allen, 1960; Orihel, 1970) (Fig. 4.96). *Anatrichosoma rhina* and *Anatrichosoma nacepobi* have been reported from the nasal mucosa of Indian monkeys (Conrad and Wong, 1973). *Anatrichosoma gerbilis* was described from specimens collected from the stomach mucosa of a north African gerbil (Bernard, 1964). *Anatrichosoma ocularis* was described from the eye of the common Thai tree shrew (File, 1974). *Anatrichosoma haycocki* has been described from the dasyurid marsupials, *Antechinus swainsonii* and *Antechinus stuartii,* where it lives in the paracloacal glands (Spratt, 1982). *Anatrichosoma buccalis* was described from the buccal mucosa of common opossums, *Didelphis marsupialis,* that were collected in Louisiana, Costa Rica, and Colombia (Pence and Little, 1972).

The only report of anatrichosomiasis from the cat occurred in South Africa (Lange et al., 1980). The affected cat appeared listless and depressed at the time of clinical presentation. The cat was disinclined to move due to complete or partial sloughing of the epidermis of the footpads of all four feet. The lesions resembled burn wounds, with necrosis of the epidermis and exudation that caused caking of the hair on the feet and between the toes. With sloughing of the epidermis of a particular footpad, the underlying tissue appeared soft and red. The dorsal surface of both carpal

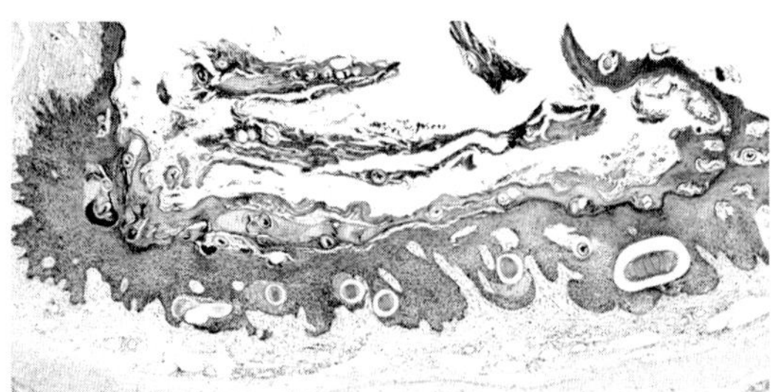

Fig. 4.96. *Anatrichosoma cynomolgi.* This is a section through the skin of a monkey showing various sections through the worm that is embedded in the epithelium.

joints had pressure sores characterized by alopecia, scab formation, and thickened skin. The cat was euthanatized due to a diagnosis of chronic interstitial nephritis. On postmortem examination, all five pads of the left front paw had no epidermis. The center pad of the right front paw demonstrated almost complete detachment of the epithelium. The detached part was dry, discolored, and hard. Both hind feet showed similar lesions of the center pads and the lateral toe pads. A single intact female worm and fragments of three others were recovered from the cat's footpads. The total length of the female worm was slightly over 4 cm. The stichosome esophagus made up about 10 percent of the total body length, and the vulva was just behind the termination of the esophagus. The uterus was filled with bioperculate brown eggs, each of which was larvated. The eggs were 63–72 μm by 35–44 μm.

There have been no successful experimental infections of any host with any species of *Anatrichosoma.* In the case of *Anatrichosoma buccalis* of the common opossum of North and South America, the adult female nematodes make extensive tunnels through the superficial layers of the hard palate, gum, and tongue (Pence and Little, 1972; Little and Orihel, 1972). Male nematodes are usually found in the deeper layers of the dermis and, more rarely, in the outer epidermal layers associated with the females. Males reside in tunnels that are not so well defined. The males are about the same length as the females but are much thinner, and during copulation, the posterior end of the male worm is inserted into the uterus of the female. When they are not copulating, the males leave the females and migrate from the mucosal epithelium to the deeper tissues. The females make extensive tunnels through the superficial layers of the stratified squamous epithelium and leave a trail of embryonated eggs as they wander through the tissue.

Other than the cat, species besides primates, marsupials, and shrews that have been host to rare infections include dogs in Alabama and Arizona and human beings in Japan, Vietnam, and Malaysia. In the first report of *Anatrichosoma* infection in a dog, the initial diagnosis was made by observing typical eggs on fecal flotation (Hendrix et al., 1987); the dog had presumably licked the skin lesion, and the eggs were swallowed and passed out in the feces. In the second canine infection, the diagnosis of infection in the dog in Arizona was made when the eggs were recognized to be present in the hundreds in the washed detritus from both ears (Hendrix et al., 1990). In the case in the human being infected in Japan, single lesions, red zigzag tracks, appeared on the left middle finger and on the right ankle of a businessman (Morishita and Tani, 1960). The tracks grew about 5 to 10 mm each day. A single female worm was removed from the end of each tract, and the worms were about 25 mm long. In the Vietnamese case (Lê-van-hoa et al., 1963) lesions containing worms or eggs were observed between fingers of the hands, on the left foot, and on the scrotum. In the Malaysian case, the discovery of *Anatrichosoma* eggs was an incidental finding in an asymptomatic person whose face was scraped as part of a survey on the prevalence of *Demodex* within the aboriginal Malaysian population (Marwi et al., 1990).

REFERENCES

Allen AM. 1960. Occurrence of the nematode, *Anatrichosoma cutaneum,* in the nasal mucosae of *Macaca mulatto* monkeys. AJVR 21:389–392.

Bernard J. 1964. *Trichosomoides gerbilis* n. sp. parasite stomacal d'un gerbille d'Afrique du Nord. Arch Inst Past Tunis 41:33–38.

Chitwood MB, Smith WN. 1958. A redescription of *Anatrichosoma cynomolgi* Smith and Chitwood, 1954. Proc Helm Soc Wash 25:112–117.

Conrad HD, Wong MM. 1973. Studies on *Anatrichosoma* (Nematoda: Trichinellida) with descriptions of *Anatrichosoma rhina* sp. n. and *Anatrichosoma nacepobi* sp. n. from the nasal mucosa of *Macaca mulatta.* J Helminthol 47:289–302.

File SK. 1974. *Anatrichosoma ocularis* sp. n. (Nematoda: Trichosomoididae from the eye of the common tree shrew, *Tupaia glis.* J Parasitol 60:985–988.

Hendrix CM, Blagburn BL, Boosinger TR, Logan RT, and Lindsay DJ. 1987. *Anatrichosoma* sp infection in a dog. J Am Vet Med Assoc 191:984–985.
Hendrix CM, Greve JH, Jeffers MD, Glock RD. 1990. Observation of *Anatrichosoma*-like eggs from otic irrigations of a dog. Canine Pract 15:34–36.
Lange AL, Verster A, Van Anstel SR, De La Rey R. 1980. *Anatrichosoma* sp. infestation in the footpads of a cat. J S Afr Vet Assoc 51:227–229.
Lê-van-hoa, Duong-hong-mo, and Nguyên-luu-viên. 1963. Premier cas de Capillariose cutanêe humaine. Bull Soc Pathol Exot 56:121–126.
Little MD, Orihel TC. 1972. The mating behavior of *Anatrichosoma* (Nematoda: Trichuroidea). J Parasitol 58:1019–1020.
Marwi MA, Omar B, Mahammod CG, Jeffery J. 1990. *Anatrichosoma* sp. egg and *Demodex folliculorum* in facial skin scrapings of Orang Aslis. Trop Biomed 7:193–194.
Morishita K, Tani T. 1960. A case of *Capillaria* infection causing creeping eruption in man. J Parasitol 46:79–83.
Orihel TC. 1970. Anatrichosomiasis in African monkeys. J Parasitol 56:982–985.
Pence DB, Little MD. 1972. *Anatrichosoma buccalis* sp. n. (Nematoda: Trichosomoididae) from the buccal mucosa of the common opossum, *Didelphis marsupialis* L. J Parasitol 58:767–773.
Smith WN, Chitwood MB. 1954. *Anatrichosoma cynomolgi,* a new trichurid nematode from monkeys. J Parasitol 40(suppl):12.
Spratt DM. 1982. *Anatrichosoma haycocki* sp. n. (Nematoda: Trichuridae) from the paracloacal glands of *Antechinus* spp., with notes on *Skrjabinocapillaria skaarbilovitsch.* Ann Parasitol Hum Comp 57:63–71.
Swift HF, Boots RH, Miller CP. 1922. A cutaneous nematode infection in monkeys. J Exp Med 35:599–620.

Trichuris felis (Diesing, 1851) Diaz-Ungria, 1963

Etymology

The genus name *Trichuris,* which may be translated as "hair tail," is actually a misnomer. A more appropriate name is *Trichocephalus* or *Trichocephalos* ("hair head"), nomenclature that has been employed in Russia and in certain countries of eastern Europe.

History

In 1851, Diesing described a species of *Trichocephalus* (*Trichuris*) from a tiger-cat in Brazil. He named the parasite *Trichocephalus felis;* however, the only description that he gave was that it was about 2 cm in length. Almost all other authors either ignore this species or regard it as differing from the trichurid of the domestic cat. Two species of *Trichuris, Trichuris campanula* and *Trichuris serrata,* were described from the domestic cat in Brazil by von Linstow in 1879 and 1889, respectively. In the case of *Trichuris campanula,* no complete male worm was recovered. In 1923 Urioste, a Brazilian, concluded that *Trichuris serrata* was the only valid species; however, Baylis (1931) pointed out that there were considerable discrepancies between von Linstow's measurements of *Trichuris serrata* and those of Urioste. Urioste's measurements agreed very closely with the original description of *Trichuris campanula.* Urioste included a complete description of the male worm (Clarkson and Owen, 1960). Diaz-Ungria (1963), after finding worms in a *Felis tigrina* in Venezuela, compared what had been described up to this point in time. Until the worms are better described, there seems to be no reason not to give the name *Trichuris felis* priority. Arenas et al. collected *Trichuris serrata* from Cuba in 1934, and Vogelsang reported the infrequent finding of *Trichuris campanula* in Venezuela (Enzie, 1951).

More recently, reports of adult feline whipworms have been made in Australia (Holmes and Kelly, 1972; Kelly, 1973; Ng and Kelly, 1975a). Whenever others have reported finding eggs of *Trichuris* in the feces of cats in various localities throughout the world, it is highly probable that these reports were due to mistaken identification of capillarid eggs (Enzie, 1951).

Geographic Distribution

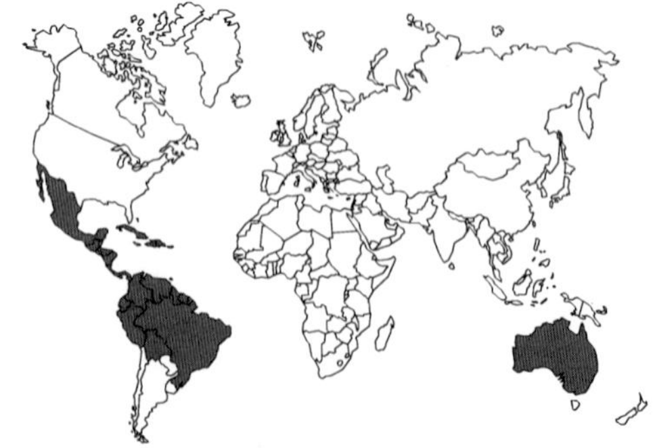

Fig. 4.97.

The feline whipworm is an extremely rare parasite, demonstrating a diverse geographic range. Sporadic reports of feline trichuriasis have been made from across the United States (Lillis, 1967; Burrows, 1968; Hass, 1973). Adult feline whipworms have been recovered from Madison, Wisconsin (Hass 1976), Miami, Florida (Hass, 1978; Hass and Meisels, 1978), the Bahama Islands (Clarkson and Owen, 1959), Cuba, and Venezuela in the Americas; from Switzerland and Poland (the former East Prussia) in Europe (Enzie, 1951); and from Australia (Holmes and Kelly, 1972; Kelly, 1973; Ng and Kelly, 1975a).

Location in Host

Members of the genus parasitize the cecum and colon.

Parasite Identification

The whipworm is composed of a thin, filamentous anterior end (the "lash" of the whip) and a thick posterior end (the whip's handle). Adult feline whipworms possess this unique whip shape (Hendrix et al., 1987). *Trichuris campanula* has been reported to be 20.5 to 38 mm long, while *Trichuris serrata* has been reported to be 38 to 49.5 mm long (Hass and Meisels, 1978; Ng and Kelly, 1975a). However, for the present, it is best to just consider that these worms are probably less than 5 cm in length.

The egg of the feline whipworm may be described as being "trichinelloid" (Campbell, 1991) or "trichuroid," possessing a thick, yellow-brown, symmetrical shell with polar plugs at both ends and is unembryonated (not larvated) when laid (Hendrix et al., 1987). The eggs of *Trichuris campanula* described by Hass and Meisels (1978) averaged 63 to 85 μm by 34 to 39 μm; while those of *Trichuris serrata* described by Ng and Kelly (1975a) averaged 54 by 40 μm.

It is important to remember that *Trichuris felis* eggs may be easily confused with those of *Eucoleus aerophilus, Aonchotheca putorii,* and *Pearsonema feliscati.* It is also easy to confuse the eggs of the feline trichurids with the eggs of members of the genus *Anatrichosoma.* The eggs of *Trichuris* and the capillarids are unembryonated, while those of *Anatrichosoma* contain larvae.

Life Cycle

Nematodes of the genus *Trichuris* are parasites of the large intestinal mucosal epithelium. In this site, the adult worms live, feed, and move slowly. Adult female whipworms are oviparous, producing typical double-operculated eggs that pass to the external environment each day in the host's feces. In spite of adverse environmental conditions, whipworm eggs are markedly resistant to the elements and may remain viable in the soil for months or even years under optimal conditions. While in the external environment, the egg develops to the stage that contains the infective larva.

The eggs of *Trichuris campanula* embryonate within a 3-week period (Hass and Meisels, 1978). Using eggs from a case in Miami, Florida, Hass and Meisels experimentally infected four cats, and three eventually shed eggs in their feces, with prepatent periods of 62, 76, and 91 days. We know almost nothing about how or where these worms develop within the intestine of the cat, although based on work with the mouse and canine forms, it is assumed that development all takes place within the intestinal mucosa.

Clinical Presentation and Pathogenesis

There have been numerous reports of whipworm infections in cats; however, these reports were primarily the results of fecal flotation procedures. There have been no descriptions of clinical signs or pathology associated with feline trichuriasis. Prescott (1984) stated that the pathogenesis of *Trichuris* species in the cat is unknown since heavy infections have not been recorded. Actual recovery of feline whipworms from cats at necropsy is rare; the maximum number of worms recovered from any one cat is reported as six (Ng and Kelly, 1975a).

Diagnosis

The egg of the feline whipworm possesses a thick, yellow-brown, symmetrical shell with polar plugs at both ends and is unembryonated (not larvated) when laid. The eggs of *Trichuris campanula* average 63 to 85 μm by 34 to 39 μm; those of *Trichuris serrata* average 54 by 40 μm (Hass and Meisels, 1978; Ng and Kelly, 1975a).

Treatment

Prescott (1984) recommended the use of fenbendazole (50 mg/kg once a day for 3 consecutive days) to treat whipworms in the cat. This dosage was extrapolated from the dosage for the dog.

Epizootiology

Infected domestic cats may serve as carriers. The exact role of wild Felidae (Cameron, 1937; Prescott, 1984) in the epizootiology of feline trichuriasis has not been determined.

Hazards to Other Animals

Although whipworms parasitize the lower bowel of a variety of both domestic and wild animals, these helminths are extremely host specific. There have been reports of the presence of the feline trichurids in larger members of the Felidae family (Cameron, 1937; Prescott, 1984).

Hazards to Humans

Human infections with feline trichurids have not been recorded in the literature (Ng and Kelly, 1975b). Although canine trichurids have been associated with human infections worldwide, the rarity of infection and low parasite numbers in cats make the role of the cat of little importance in this zoonosis (Prescott, 1984).

Control/Prevention

Effective control of feline whipworms involves proper diagnoses, therapy, and sanitation of the cattery. To prevent reinfection, one must remove feces daily from the litter box. Overcrowding of cats should be avoided in the cattery. Confining many animals to a small area increases environmental contamination and encourages transmission.

REFERENCES

Arenas R, Kouri P, and Basnuevo JG. 1934. Sobre parasitismo en los animales domesticos. Bol Mens Coll Vet NAC Habana 3:764–768.

Baylis HA. 1931. On the structure and the relationships of the nematode *Capillaria* (Hepaticola) *hepatica* Bancroft. Parasitology 23:533–543.

Burrows RB. 1968. Internal parasites of dogs and cats from central New Jersey. Bull NJ Acad Sci 13:3–8.

Cameron TWM. 1937. Studies on the endoparasitic fauna of Trinidad mammals V. Further parasites from the ocelot. Can J Res 15:24–27.

Campbell BG. 1991. *Trichuris* and other trichinelloid nematodes of dogs and cats in the United States. Comp Cont Educ Pract Vet 13:769–779, 801.

Clarkson MJ, Owen LN. 1959. The parasites of domestic animals in the Bahama Islands. Ann Trop Med Parasitol 53:341–346.

Clarkson MJ, Owen LN. 1960. The species of *Trichuris* in the domestic cat. J Helminthol 34:319–322.

Diaz-Ungria C. 1963. Nématodes parasites, nouveaux ou intéressants, du Vénézuéla. Ann Parasitol 38:893–913.

Diesing KM. 1851. Systema Helminthum. Vols 1 and 2. Vindobonae. 679 and 588 pp.

Enzie FD. 1951. Do whipworms occur in domestic cats in North America? J Am Vet Med Assoc 119:210–213.

Hass DK. 1973. Do whipworms occur in cats? Feline Pract 3(4):36–37.

Hass DK. 1976. Whipworm reports requested (letter). Feline Pract 6(1):5.

Hass DK. 1978. Feline whipworms do exist. Feline Pract 8(2):31–32.

Hass DK, Meisels LS. 1978. *Trichuris campanula* infection in a domestic cat from Miami, Florida. Am J Vet Res 39:1553–1555.

Hendrix CM, Blagburn BL, Lindsay DS. 1987. Whipworms and intestinal threadworms. Vet Clin North Am 17:1355–1375.

Holmes PR, Kelly JD. 1972. Occurrence of the genus *Trichuris* in the domestic cat. Aust Vet J 48:535.

Kelly JD. 1973. Occurrence of *Trichuris serrata* von Linstow, 1879 (Nematoda: Trichuridae) in the domestic cat (*Felis catus*) in Australia. J Parasitol 59:1145–1156.

Lillis WG. 1967. Helminth survey of dogs and cats in New Jersey. J Parasitol 53:1082–1084.

Linstow OFB. 1879. Helminthologischen Studien. Arch Naturg, Berlin 45:165–188.

Linstow OFB.1989. Helminthologisches. Arch Naturg, Berlin 54:235–246.

Ng BKY, Kelly JD. 1975a. Isolation of *Trichuris campanula* von Linstow, 1889 from Australian cats. Aust Vet J 51:450–451.

Ng BKY, Kelly JD. 1975b. Anthropozoonotic helminthiases in Australasia: Part 3—Studies on the prevalence and public health implications of helminth parasites of dogs and cats in urban environments. Int J Zoo 2:76–91.

Prescott CW. 1984. Parasitic Diseases of the Cat in Australia. Sydney, Australia: Postgraduate Foundation in Veterinary Science. 112 pp.

Urioste O. 1923. Contribucão aoestudo do *Trichuris*. These (Rio de Janeiro). 57 pp.

Trichinella spiralis (Owen, 1835) Railliet, 1896

Etymology

Trichinella = hair-like and *spiralis* for the spiral nature of the larval stage.

Synonyms

Trichina spiralis Owen, 1835.

History

The worm was first recovered at necropsy from the tissues of an Italian male patient in England.

In 1851, Herbst found larvae in the muscles of a cat. In 1860, Leuckart showed that when larvae were fed to cats, they developed to adults within the intestinal mucosa.

Geographic Distribution

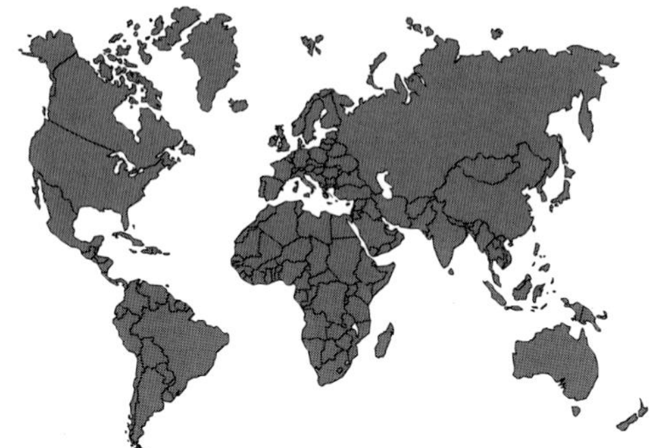

Fig. 4.98.

There are currently five recognized species of *Trichinella* (Pozio et al., 1992). *Trichinella spiralis* is considered the domesticated species that is found throughout the world in pigs and associated wildlife. *Trichinella britovi* Pozio, La Rosa, Murrell, and Lichtenfels, 1992, is found in the Palearctic where it infects various mammalian hosts. *Trichinella nativa* Britov and Boev, 1972, is found in the Holarctic where it infects sylvatic mammals. *Trichinella pseudospiralis* Garkavi, 1972, is found throughout the world and uses both avian and mammalian hosts; this species differs from the others in that the larvae do not develop surrounding nurse cells within muscle tissue. The fifth species, *Trichinella nelsoni* Britov and Boev, 1972, is restricted to equatorial Africa. All these species are capable of infecting cats, and wild cats can probably fall prey to any of these species when they capture and eat infected animals. Due to the fact that *Trichinella pseudospiralis* will infect either avian or mammalian hosts, it would seem that cats are liable to rather commonly become infected with this species when it is present in their environment.

Holzworth and Georgi (1974) gave an excellent and complete summary of the reported cases of trichinosis in cats. More recently, infections have been reported from Chile (Bonilla Zepeda, 1980; Alcaino et al., 1981), Egypt (Morsy et al., 1981), Finland (Hirvela Koski et al., 1985), Italy (Pozio et al., 1987), and China (He et al., 1995; Liu et al., 1997; Zhu et al., 1998).

Location in Host

The larval stages are within muscle fibers where they tend to form cyst-like stages called nurse cells. The adults occur within the small intestine of the host.

Parasite Identification

When they have finished development to the infective stage, the larvae in muscles are about 0.8 mm to 1 mm in length. The adults that are present in the intestine have lengths of 1.2 and 2.2 mm, respectively, for the males and females. All stages of these worms, like those of *Trichuris,* the capillarids, and *Anatrichosoma,* have a stichosome esophagus that is composed of a linear arrangement of cells with large nuclei. The male of *Trichinella* species does not have a spicule, and the tail terminates with two lateral lobes that give it a characteristic appearance. The mature patent female of *Trichinella* can be recognized by the prelarvae that she contains. Each prelarva is about 100 μm long.

Life Cycle

The life cycle is basically the same for all species of *Trichinella.* The host becomes infected when it eats meat containing infective muscle-stage larvae. The larvae are digested out of the muscle, and development takes place within the mucosa of the small intestine (Fig. 4.99). The larvae rapidly undergo four molts to form adults, which are present a little over 1 day after infection. The adults then mate, and beginning about 6 days after the infected meat was ingested, the females begin to deposit small larvae into the mucosa (Figs. 4.100 and 4.101). The females can produce

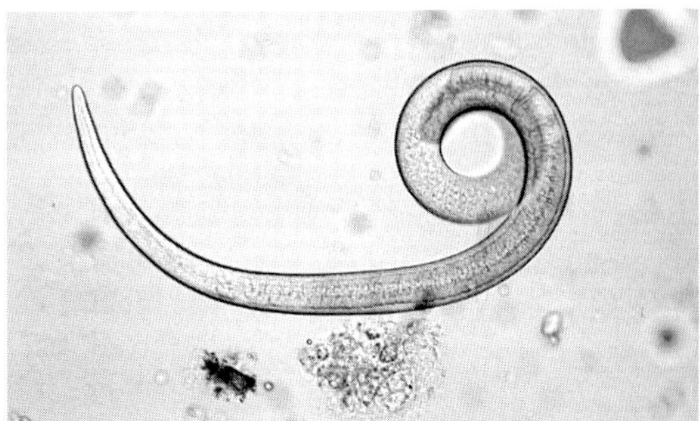

Fig. 4.99. *Trichinella spiralis.* Free infective first-stage larva experimentally digested out of rat muscle by the use of artificial digestion fluid. (Infected muscle supplied by Dr. Judith Appleton)

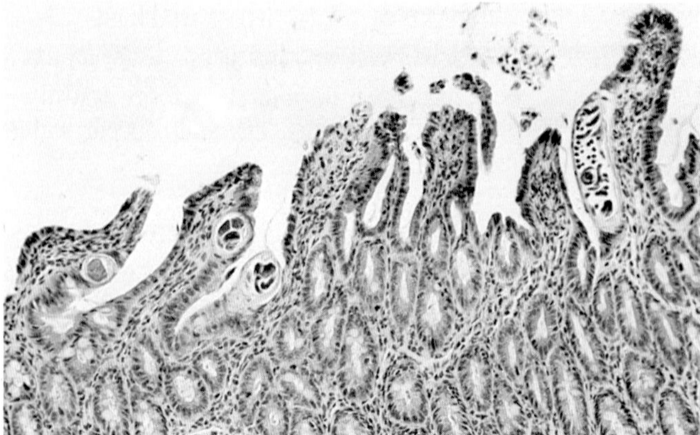

Fig. 4.100. *Trichinella spiralis.* Histological section with adult worms in the intestinal mucosa of an experimentally infected rat 7 days after infection. Note the section through a female filled with prelarvae. (Tissue supplied by Dr. Judith Appleton)

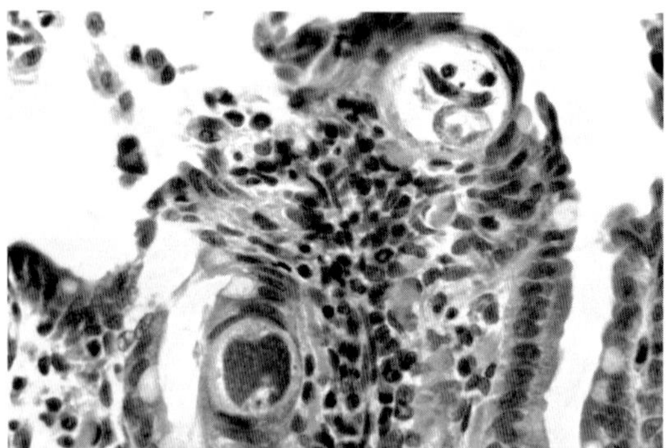

Fig. 4.101. *Trichinella spiralis.* Histological section through the intestinal mucosa of an experimentally infected rat showing two transverse sections through an adult female. (Tissue supplied by Dr. Judith Appleton)

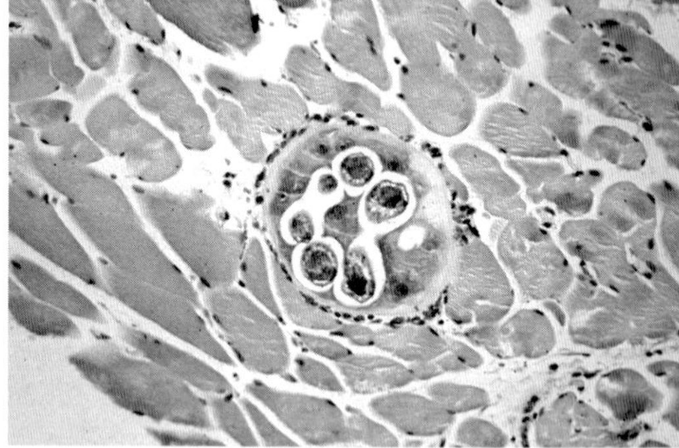

Fig. 4.102. *Trichinella spiralis.* Histological section of a muscle biopsy from an experimentally infected cat.

larvae for anywhere from 4 to 16 weeks. Larvae enter the bloodstream and make their way to the muscles, and here, the larvae penetrate individual striated muscle fibers. In all cases but *Trichinella pseudospiralis,* the larvae become encapsulated in the muscle cell in a structure called a nurse cell (Figs. 4.102 and 4.103). Typically, the larvae have completed their development before the completion of nurse cell formation, which can take place anywhere from 16 to 60 days after initiation of infection depending on the species involved. Larvae within the tissues can remain viable for years, although calcification often begins after 6 to 9 months of infection. Cats serve as rather good

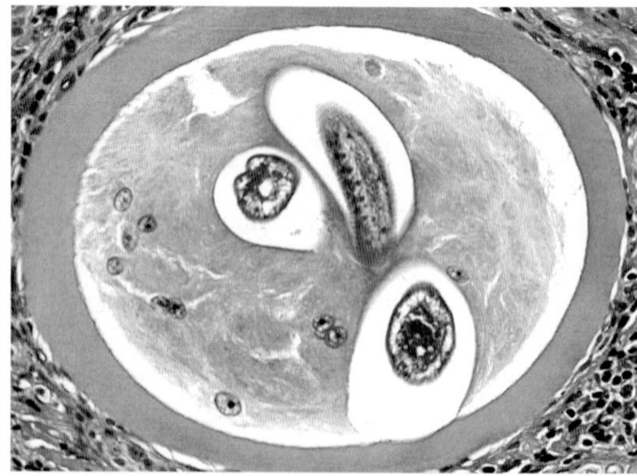

Fig. 4.103. *Trichinella spiralis.* Histological section of a muscle biopsy from an experimentally infected cat. Note the thick nature of the enclosing capsule.

hosts for *Trichinella spiralis* and can support relatively large numbers of muscle larvae per gram of muscle (Holzworth and Georgi, 1974).

Clinical Presentation and Pathogenesis

After experimental infections, cats show signs referable to muscle damage including lethargy, weakness, weight loss, and hypersalivation. Other signs may include diarrhea that may or may not include bloody feces. In other cases, cats have shown very little in the way of signs of infection, even though they have ultimately supported rather high loads of muscle larvae (about 300 larvae per gram of muscle). Akhmurtova (1987) experimentally infected cats with *Trichinella spiralis, Tichinella nativa,* and *Trichinella nelsoni* and found that *Trichinella nativa* caused the most serious inflammation of the muscle tissue and that *Trichinella nelsoni* was the least pathogenic for cats.

Experimentally infected cats with *Trichinella spiralis* do not develop significantly increased numbers of circulating eosinophils as have been reported in human cases (Fourestié et al., 1988). However, in a naturally infected cat, the highest eosinophil count reported during a 5-month period the cat was studied was 22 percent of the total white cell count (Holzworth and Georgi, 1974).

In the one naturally acquired infection in a cat that was carefully followed (Holzworth and Georgi, 1974), the initial presentation was puddles of fresh, gelatinous, bloody feces in the litter box. The bloody feces were produced for about 6 days and were found to contain large numbers of adult *Trichinella.* In this case, although a larva was recovered from the blood of the cat, there were no signs of myocardial involvement as observed by electrocardiac examination 2 weeks after the appearance of the first bloody stool. The cat developed a moderate eosinophilia. About 3 weeks after the initial bloody stool, the cat did appear to undergo an episode of disorientation based on unusual behavior, but the relationship of this sign to the underlying trichinosis can only be conjectured.

Treatment

Cats treated with albendazole (50 mg/kg twice daily for 7 days) had reduced numbers of larvae in their muscles about 1 week after the administration of the last treatment. However, the number of larvae in the muscles was reduced to zero in only one of four treated cats, and this number was based only on a single small biopsy specimen from each animal.

Epizootiology

There is a great deal to be learned about the epizootiology of trichinosis in cats, especially in light of the fact that several species are involved. There have been no serious surveys performed among urban or suburban cats in most developed nations in recent years, and there has been little done to identify the serological status of cats around the world.

Hazards to Other Animals

Cats probably pose no serious threat to other animals due to their probably seldom being eaten.

Hazards to Humans

Cats pose no threat to humans.

Control/Prevention

Cats can be prevented from becoming infected only by keeping them from eating captured prey. In a case from the Altai region of Siberia, a man became ill after having eaten raw badger meat. The family cat that had been fed on leftovers and offal also became infected (Krainyaya et al., 1979).

REFERENCES

Akhmurtova, TL. 1987. Infective process in domestic cats infected with different species of *Trichinella.* Izvest Akad Nauk Kazak SSR, Biol 2:41-45 [Russian].

Alcaino HA, Gorman TR, Santibanez M, Vilches G. 1981. Trichinellosis en gatos y perros del area metropolitana de Chile. Rev Iberica Parasitol 41:461–462.

Bonilla Zepeda C. 1980. Estudio de la fauna helmintologica del gato en la ciudad de Valdivia, Chile. Arch Med Vet 12:277.

Bowman DD, Darrigrand RA, Frongillo MK, Barr SC, Flanders JA, Carbone LG. 1993. Treatment of experimentally induced trichinosis in dogs and cats. AJVR 54:1303–1305.

Fourestié V, Bougnoux ME, Ancelle T, Liance M, Roudot-Thoraval F, Naga H, Pairon-Pennachioni M, Rauss A, Lejonc JL. 1988. Randomized trial of albendazole versus tiabendazole plus flubendazole during an outbreak of human trichinellosis. Parasitol Res 75:36–41.

He ZP, Chen PH, Xie Y, Lu SQ, Wang FY. 1995. Study on the genomic DNA of 7 isolates of *Trichinella spiralis* in China. Acta Parastiol Med Ent Sinica 2:218–222 [Chinese].

Herbst G. 1851. Beobactungen über *Trichina spiralis* in Betreff der Uebertragung der Eigenweidewürmer. Nachrichten Georg-Augusts Unir Konig Gesselsch Wissensch Göttingen 260–264.

Hirvela Koski V, Aho M, Asplund K, Hatakka M, Hirn J. 1985. *Trichinella spiralis* in wild animals, cats, mice, rats and farmed fur animals in Finland. Nord Vet 37:234–247.

Holzworth J, Georgi JR. 1974. Trichinosis in a cat. JAVMA 165:186–191.

Krainyaya VS, Gorbunov NS, Ivanov AS. 1979. A case of group human infection with a natural strain of *Trichinella* in the Altai. Med Parazit Parazit Bol 48:87–88 [Russian].

Leuckart R. 1860. Der Geschlechstreife Zustand der *Trichina spiralis.* Eine vorlaufige Mittheilung. Zeitsch rationeile Med 8:259–262, 334–335.

Liu MY, Song MX, Yang RF, Chen PH, An CL, Liu ZS, Guo ZB, Hou SL, Lu YX, Zhu XP. 1997. Identification of some Chinese isolates of Trichinella spiralis by RAPD. Chin J Vet Sci Technol 27:18–20 [Chinese].

Morsy TA, Sadek MSM, Abdel Hamid MY. 1981. Intestinal parasites of stray cats in Cairo, Egypt. J Egypt Soc Parasitol 11:331–345.

Pozio E, Rossi P, Amati M. 1987. Epidemiologie de la trichinellose en Italie: correlation entre le cycle sauvage et l'homme. Ann Parasitol Hum Comp 62:456–461.

Pozio E, LA Rosa G, Murrell KD, Lichtenfels JR. 1992. Taxonomic revision of the genus *Trichinella.* J Parasitol 78:654–659.

Zhu XP, Liu MY, Wang FY, Zhou L, Song MX. 1998. Identification of three isolates of *Trichinella* in China on the basis of restriction fragment length polymorphisms (RFLP) analysis. Acta Parasitol Med Ent Sinica 5:101–105 [Chinese].

5 THE ARTHROPODS

The arthropods (meaning: jointed feet) form a large group of organisms that includes the horseshoe crabs, crustacea, millipedes, centipedes, arachnids (spiders, scorpions, ticks, and mites), and insects (flies and lice). This is a huge group of organisms, but fortunately, only a few are important as pathogens of cats and other animals. In this chapter, we will discuss some of the arachnids (ticks and mites) and some of the insects (lice, fleas, and flies) that cause or transmit diseases of cats. Another small group of the arthropods that is given a cursory coverage is the pentastomids.

ARACHNIDS

The ticks and mites compose a group of organisms that is part of a larger group of arthropods known as the Arachnida. Included in this group are the scorpions (Scorpiones) and the spiders (Araneae). The ticks and mites are actually composed of four groups of organisms, most of which are free-living. The Metastigmata is the group representing the ticks (composed of the "hard ticks" of the Ixodidae and the "soft ticks" of the Argasidae), and all the representatives in this group are parasitic in some part of the life cycle. The Mesostigmata contains the chigger mites (trombiculids) and the two fowl mites (*Dermanyssus* and *Ornithonyssus*); this group also contains many free-living species. The Prostigmata contains the follicular mites (*Demodex*) and several hair-clasping mites (*Cheyletiella*). The Astigmata contains many parasitic forms, including the burrowing mites (*Notoedres* and *Sarcoptes*), the ear mite (*Otodectes*), and another hair-clasping mite (*Lynxacarus radovskyi*).

Ticks and mites are characterized as adults by having four pairs of legs and a fused anterior and posterior body (unlike spiders and scorpions) that appears to lack segmentation. The mouthparts are found on an anteriorly projected structure called the gnathosoma. The ticks and mites breathe either through tracheae or directly through the cuticle. The position of the opening of the major lateral trunks of the tracheal system is used to distinguish the different groups. In the Metastigmata (ticks) the lateral openings of the tracheal system are through stigmata that are found behind the fourth pair of legs. In the case of the Mesostigmata, the lateral stigmatal openings are between the third and fourth pair of legs. In the Prostigmata, the stigmatal openings (although difficult to visualize or absent) are located at the base of the mouthparts. The Astigmata has no trachea and, hence, no stigmatal opening. Krantz (1978) presented a classification of ticks and mites that differs from that used here, which is based on that of Baker and Wharton (1952) and Nutting (1984). In the classification of Krantz, the Metastigmata is equivalent to the suborder Ixodida, the Mesostigmata are placed in the suborder Gamasida, the Prostigmata are placed in the suborder Actinedida, and the Astigmata are placed in the suborder Acaridida.

The basic life cycle of a tick or mite includes an egg, a larval stage (with three pairs of legs), a nymphal stage, and the adult. In some cases, there may be more than one nymphal stage, and often these have discrete names. For example, in the case of *Otodectes cynotis,* the stage that comes out of the egg is called a larva, the first nymphal stage is called a protonymph, the second nymphal stage is called a deutonymph, and this is followed by the adult stage. Some mites have a third nymphal stage that is called a tritonymph. Some of the soft ticks will go through as many as five nymphal stages. The hard ticks tend to have the fewest stages: a larva, a nymph, and the adult.

REFERENCES
Baker EW, Wharton GW. 1952. An Introduction to Acarology. New York, NY: Macmillan Co.
Krantz GW. 1978. A Manual of Acarology. 2d edition. Corvallis, Ore: Oregon State University Book Stores. 509 pp.
Nutting WB. 1984. Mammalian Diseases and Arachnids. Vols I and II. Boca Raton, Fla: CRC Press.

METASTIGMATA

The Metastigmata represents the ticks. Members of the Metastigmata tend to be over 2 mm in length as adults. The respiratory openings, stigmata, are without peritremes and near the base of the fourth pair of legs. This group is divided into three smaller groups, the soft ticks, which compose the Argasidae; the hard ticks, which compose the Ixodidae; and a poorly known intermediate group, the Nutallidae. Cats are known to be parasitized by both the Argasidae and the Ixodidae. All ticks feed by sucking blood and tissue fluids from a vertebrate host. Members of the Ixodidae are called hard ticks because they bear a cuticularized protective dorsal scutum or shield. This shield is lacking in the Argasidae, and therefore, members tend to be called soft ticks. The soft ticks tend to live in nesting areas, and when the host is in or on the nest, the soft ticks crawl onto the host and feed rapidly. The hard ticks, on the other hand, tend to await hosts more in the open and to feed more slowly, which causes them to be attached to the host for longer periods.

Argasidae

Members of the Argasidae, or soft ticks, are obligate ectoparasites of a wide variety of flying and land vertebrates. Most soft ticks reside in the dens, burrows, caves, and nests of their hosts and require multiple hosts to complete the prolonged, physiologically slow life cycle. Argasid ticks have existed since the late Paleozoic to early Mesozoic eras. The genera *Ornithodoros* and *Argas* were original genera and existed partially as we know them today. Other genera and species of soft ticks have become extinct. Prehistoric reptiles were probably the first natural host of the early soft ticks. In the early Tertiary period, primitive bird and mammal lines expanded into many specialized orders that replaced reptiles as the dominant terrestrial hosts. The argasid ticks became adapted to microhabitats associated with the nests, roosts, dens, caves, and lairs inhabited by birds or mammals. The large argasid ticks survived in association with porcupines, warthogs, wild pigs, and hyenas. The smaller argasid ticks evolved along with birds, rodents, bats and insectivores (Hoskins and Cupp, 1988).

In general, the argasids are likely to have several nymphal stages as part of their life cycle and may have as many as five to eight nymphal instars before they mature into adults. If the adult ticks are blood feeders, it is possible that they will take several blood meals after they reach sexual maturity. Two genera have been found to bother cats. Species of *Ornithodoros* have been observed to attack cats; this tick is parasitic in all life stages. Although some 100 species of *Ornithodoros* have been described, only two are known to attack cats. Only two species of *Otobius* have been described, but both have been recovered from cats. Adults of *Otobius* are not parasitic.

REFERENCES
Hoskins JD, Cupp EW. 1988. Ticks of veterinary importance. Part II. The Argasidae family: Identification, behavior, and associated diseases. Comp Cont Educ Pract Vet 10:699–709.

Ornithodoros talaje (Guèrin-Méneville, 1849) Neumann, 1911

Etymology

Ornitho = bird and *doros* = leather bag.

Synonyms

Argas talaje Guèrin-Méneville, 1849; *Alectorobius talaje* (Guèrin-Méneville, 1849) Pocock, 1907.

History

Ornithodoros talaje was originally described by Guèrin-Méneville in 1849 for ticks collected from Guatemala.

Geographic Distribution

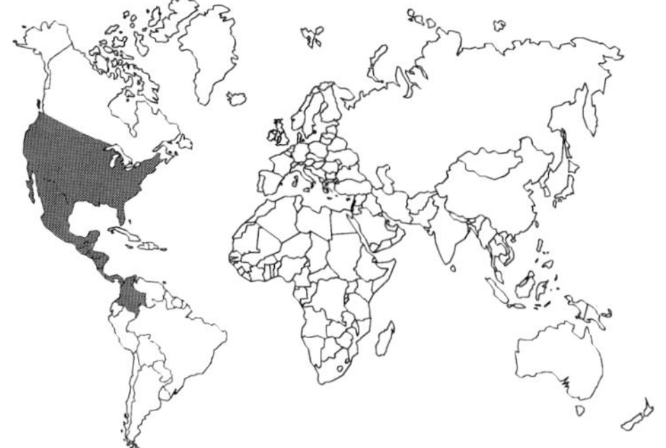

Fig. 5.1.

The range of *Ornithodoros talaje* extends from California and Kansas to Argentina. In the United States, it is known to be from California, Arizona, Nevada, Kansas, Texas, and Florida. This tick has been reported from the "hot country" of Mexico and has been found on the peninsula of Yucatán, Campeche, Tabasco, Chiapas, and the isthmus and state of Veracruz and extending along the Gulf Coast toward Texas; on the Pacific Coast the species has not been found except to the north in the region of the isthmus (Cooley and Kohls, 1944). *Ornithodoros talaje* is also widely distributed in Panama (Dunn, 1933).

Location in Host

Of 100 Panamanian cats, 26 were infested with *Ornithodoros talaje.* The specific collection site in the feline haircoat was not noted (Dunn, 1933). Tiny argasid larvae may localize on the cat's body, head, and neck. Nymphs and adults are often found in the host's environment (Hoskins and Cupp, 1988).

Parasite Identification

In members of the genus *Ornithodoros,* the capitulum is either subterminal or distant from the anterior margin; the hypostome is well developed, essentially similar in adults of both male and female soft ticks (Fig. 5.2) and in the nymphal stages. The integument has discs and mamillae that blend in a wide variety of patterns. This integumental pattern is continuous over the sides from dorsal to ventral surfaces. Dorsal humps and subapical dorsal protuberances on the legs are progressively more prominent in successive nymphal stages. The body is more or less flattened but strongly convex dorsally when distended. In *Ornithodoros talaje,* cheeks (the paired flaps at the sides of the camerostome) are present (Hoskins and Cupp, 1988). The hood (the anterior projection of the integument) is present but small. The camerostome (the cavity in which the capitulum is located) is indefinite and obscured by the large cheeks (Cooley and Kohls, 1944). The genus *Ornithodoros* includes 100 species in eight subgenera (Hoogstraal, 1985). Cooley and Kohls (1944) provided detailed descriptions of the adult and larval stages of *Ornithodoros talaje.*

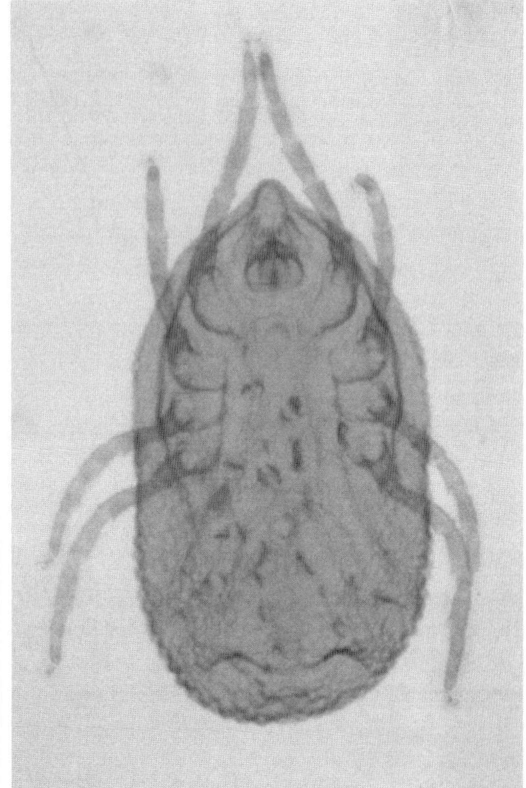

Fig. 5.2. *Ornithodorus* species. Ventral view of female tick.

Life Cycle

There are four developmental stages in the life cycle of *Ornithodoros talaje:* egg, larva, nymph, and adult male and female. This tick has been collected from a wide variety of hosts. In the United States, it has been found only on wild rodents or in association with them. In Mexico, natural hosts are small, wild rodents and other mammals that inhabit underground nests (Cooley and Kohls, 1944). Mating occurs off the host and is facilitated by pheromones. Reception of the pheromone is handled by sensillae on palps located lateral to the mouthparts. These pheromones act to assemble members of the population. All stages respond; however, males respond to females more vigorously than females respond to males. Adults feed and mate several times. Females oviposit several times (Hoskins and Cupp, 1988).

Clinical Presentation and Pathogenesis

Of 100 cats examined by Dunn (1933) in Panama, 26 were infested with primarily the larval stage of *Ornithodoros talaje*. A second-stage nymph was found on one cat. This author attributed no clinical signs in the infested cats, although the bite of *Ornithodoros talaje* has been reported to be painful (Harwood and James, 1979).

Diagnosis

This tick is best diagnosed by identification of its unique morphologic characteristics. Credible criteria for identifying *Ornithodoros talaje* are now determined by trained entomologists. Blood tubes or screw-cap vials containing 70 percent isopropyl alcohol are used for preserving collected stages. A definitive diagnosis is usually performed by an area, state, or federal veterinarian; local cooperative extension service; or university with a school of veterinary medicine or a department of entomology (Hoskins and Cupp, 1988).

Treatment

Any of the popular acaricides used for treating infestation of hard ticks on cats should prove effective in treating *Ornithodoros talaje*.

Epizootiology

This tick is usually diagnosed in cats who are allowed to roam freely. The tick is seldom observed in dwellings, so it is rarely found in house cats (Cooley and Kohls, 1944).

Hazards to Other Animals

This species has been collected from a wide variety of hosts throughout the Americas. In the United States, it has been found only on wild rodents or in association with them. In Mexico, the natural hosts are small, wild rodents and probably other mammals that inhabit subterranean nests (Cooley and Kohls, 1944). Among the hosts in Panama listed by Dunn (1933) were man; several species of mice; several species of monkeys, dogs, chickens, and opossums; and a snake.

Hazards to Humans

This tick is a vector of Mexican-American relapsing fever of humans (Hoskins and Cupp, 1988).

Control/Prevention

Accurate identification of soft ticks from the parasitized host or from the environment is a prerequisite to their control (Hoskins and Cupp, 1988). The cat's ability to roam freely to areas frequented by rats and mice (alleys, deserted lots, etc.) should be restricted. Rodent control should also prove effective (Harwood and James, 1979).

REFERENCES

Cooley RA, Kohls GM. 1944. The Argasidae of North America, Central America and Cuba, Monograph 1. Am Midl Nat 37–117, 142.

Dunn LH. 1933. Observations on the host selection of *Ornithodoros talaje* Guèrin, in Panama. Am J Trop Med 13:475–483.

Harwood RF, James MT, Jr. 1979. Entomology in Human and Animal Health. 7th ed. New York, NY: Macmillan, pp 389–391, 400.

Hoogstraal H. 1985. Argasid and Nuttalliellid ticks as parasites and vectors. Adv Parasitol 24:135–238.

Hoskins JD, Cupp EW. 1988. Ticks of veterinary importance. Part II. The Argasidae family. Identification, behavior, and associated diseases. Comp Cont Educ Pract Vet 10:699–709.

Ornithodoros puertoriciensis Fox, 1947

Ornithodoros puertoriciensis was originally described from the nests of rats in Puerto Rico. Dr. Fox (1977) found two engorged larvae on a kitten from the Santurce section of San Juan, Puerto Rico. The next day, three more larvae were collected. From the larvae, adults were reared for identification. This tick is mainly a parasite of wild rats and mice, but the larvae will bite other hosts including skunks, opossums, lizards, and even humans. This tick was redescribed in 1989 by Endris et al. using specimens that were collected from rodent burrows by a vacuum sampling technique and showed that the range of this tick extended through Jamaica, Haiti, the Dominican Republic, Puerto Rico, St. Croix, the U.S. Virgin Islands, Guadeloupe, and Trinidad and into Mexico, Nicaragua, Panama, Colombia, Venezuela, and Surinam.

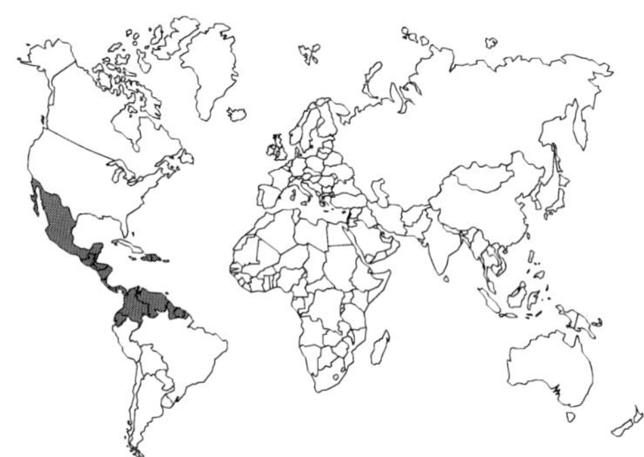

Fig. 5.3.

REFERENCES

Endris RG, Keirans JE, Robbins RG, Hess WR. 1989. *Ornithodoros (Alectorobius) puertoriciensis* (Acari: Argasidae): Redescription by scanning electron microscopy. J Med Entomol 26:146–154.

Fox I. 1947. *Ornithodoros puertoriciensis,* a new tick from rats in Puerto Rico. J Parasitol 33:253–259.

Fox I. 1977. The domestic cat, *Felis catus* L., a new host recorded for the tick *Ornithodoros puertoriciensis* Fox. J Agric Univ Puerto Rico 61:509.

Otobius megnini (Dugès, 1844) Banks, 1912

Etymology

Oto = ear and *bius* = way of life, along with *megnini* for Dr. Megnin.

Synonyms

Argas megnini Dugès, 1884; *Rhyncoprium spinosum* Marx; *Ornithodoros megnini* (Dugès, 1844) Neumann, 1911.

History

Otobius megnini was originally described by Dugès in 1884 in Guanajuato, Mexico. This tick is an American species which has spread to such far-reaching areas as India and South Africa (Munaó Diniz et al., 1987).

Geographic Distribution

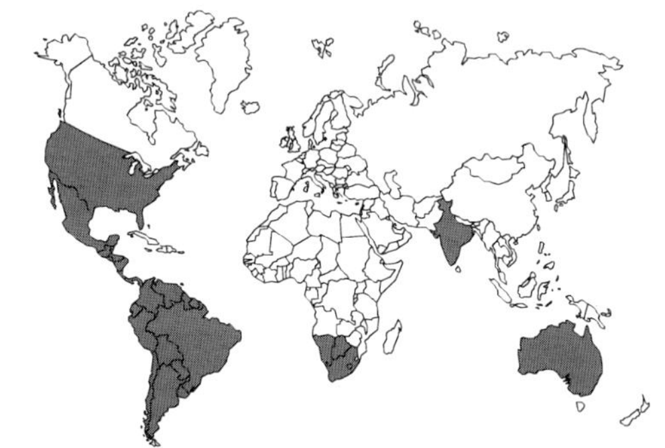

Fig. 5.4.

Otobius megnini is distributed throughout much of the western United States and is especially prevalent in the arid regions of the southwestern United States. Many of the reports of this parasite in northern, central, and eastern states are probably the result of infested livestock shipments (Cooley and Kohls, 1944). In the United States, the eastern boundary for the natural occurrence of *Otobius megnini* is approximately the 97th meridian (Bishopp and Trembley, 1945). This soft tick has been reported in Central and South America (Argentina, Brazil, and Chile), Australia, South Africa, and India (Cooley and Kohls, 1944). There have been only two reports of this soft tick in domestic cats (Brumpt, 1936; Cooley and Kohls, 1944).

Location in Host

The larval and nymphal stages of members of the genus *Otobius* most often parasitize the ears of their hosts.

Parasite Identification

The unfed larva is 0.66 mm from the tip of the hypostome to the posterior extremity. Its body is oval. There are two pairs of hemispherical, ocellus-like eyes. The integument is thin and striated

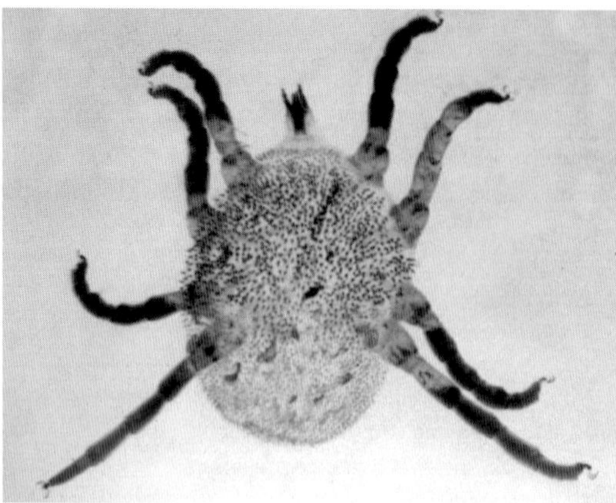

Fig. 5.5. *Otobius megnini.* First nymphal stage, preserved and cleared specimen.

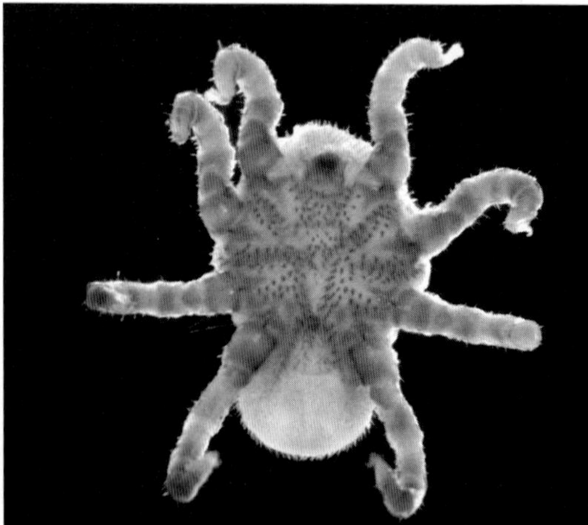

Fig. 5.6. *Otobius megnini.* First nymphal stage, alcohol-preserved specimen.

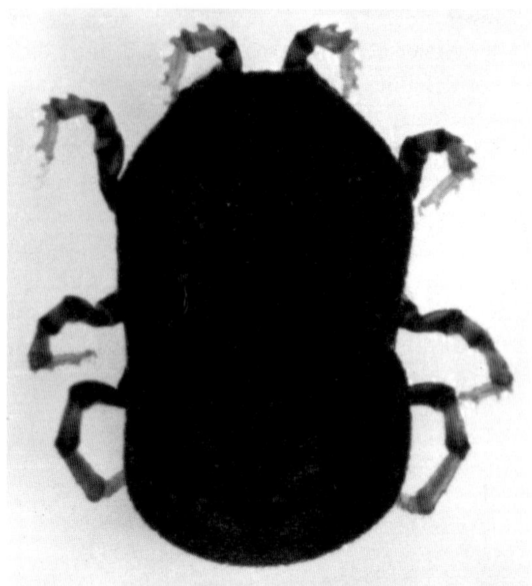

Fig. 5.7. *Otobius megnini.* Second nymphal stage.

with a few bristle-like hairs arranged symmetrically. The capitulum is visible in both dorsal and ventral views. The hypostome and palps are very long. The six legs are long. The engorged larva is much distended, broader in front. The capitulum is also distended as a conical anterior projection. The engorged larva is 4 by 2.5 mm (Cooley and Kohls, 1944).

The first nymphal stage is very much like the newly emerged second stage. However, it is smaller, and has more slender legs (Figs. 5.5 and 5.6). Its hypostome measures only 0.195 mm (Brumpt, 1936; Cooley and Kohls, 1944).

The second nymphal stage is the stage that is commonly found in the ears of the infested host (Cooley and Kohls, 1944) (Fig 5.7). The nymphs are widest at the middle. Their skin is mamillated and has numerous spine-like processes. The body is bluish gray, while the legs, mouthparts, and spines are pale yellow. There are four pairs of legs.

Adults, which are nonparasitic, have a constriction at the middle, giving the body a violin shape. The adults have a skin that is not spiny. This stage can be recovered from the environment of the host and is not collected from the host.

Life Cycle

Eggs of *Otobius megnini* are laid on or near the ground. They hatch in 18 days or more. The larvae then crawl up vegetation, fence posts, and feed bunks to await hosts. Unfed larvae may live off the host for more than 2 months. If they find a host, they locate in the ears where they engorge for 5 to 10 days. The larvae molt to the nymphal stage in the ears. Here they engorge for about a month. However, the nymphs may remain in the ear for as long as 7 months. When ready to molt, they crawl out of the ears to the ground where they molt to adults. The females may lay eggs for as long as 6 months. While ixodid (hard) ticks are often referred to as one-, two-, or three-host ticks, argasids are often referred to as many-host or multihost ticks. *Otobius megnini* is the exception to this rule. It is a single-host tick (Hoskins and Cupp, 1988).

Clinical Presentation and Pathogenesis

Although clinical signs have not been reported in domestic cats, lions have been reported to develop pruritis (manifested by shaking of the head, ear scratching, and holding the head to one side) as a result of the larvae and nymphs moving and feeding within the external ear canal. The condition may advance such that the inflammatory response and secondary infection may penetrate the tympanic membrane, causing otitis media and interna, and ultimately encephalitis. Usually infestation in lions is asymptomatic.

Diagnosis

The otoscope may be used to visualize the ticks within the external ear canal. A cotton swab or blunt forceps may be used to remove the waxy exudate. This exudate must be examined for the presence of larvae and nymphs. *Otobius* can be distinguished from *Ornithodoros* by the fact that the nymphal stage is beset with spines. The nymphs of *Ornithodoros* may be mamillated or tuberculated, but they lack spines as are present in *Otobius*. *Otobius megnini* nymphs may be distinguished from the nymphs of *Otobius lagophilus* by the fact that in *Otobius megnini* the integument has numerous heavy spines anteriorly and thinner spines posteriorly while the spines on *Otobius lagophilus* are all of one size. Also, if the ventral surface of the hypostome of *Otobius megnini* is examined, it will be found that there are four teeth (denticles) on each side of the midline while there are only three on each side of the midline in *Otobius lagophilus*. The adults differ in that the pits on the dorsal surface of *Otobius megnini* are separated by a distance that is twice or more the diameter of one pit while the pits on the dorsal surface of *Otobius lagophilus* are closer together than the diameter of a single pit.

Treatment

Any of the popular acaricides used for treating infestation of hard ticks on cats should prove effective in treating *Otobius megnini*. When applying any medication to the ear, great care should be taken to avoid damaging the external ear canal.

Epizootiology

This tick is usually diagnosed in cats who are allowed to roam freely and is seldom found in house cats. This tick is usually acquired from a pen, corral, or limited range area where larvae migrate onto the host animal. This tick may be found on hosts throughout the year, but its destructive effects are particularly recognizable during winter and spring, especially following long periods of drought when both range and livestock are poor (Bishopp and Trembley, 1945).

Hazards to Other Animals

The larvae and nymphs of *Otobius megnini* may occur on domestic animals such as cattle, sheep, horses, and dogs and on a wide range of wild animals (Eads and Campos, 1984). These animals include mules, asses, goats, hogs, coyotes, deer, mountain sheep, cottontail rabbits, jackrabbits, ostriches (Cooley and Kohls, 1944), collared peccaries, and pronghorns (Eads and Campos, 1984). This tick is a suspected vector of *Coxiella burnetii,* the etiologic agent of Q fever (Munaó Diniz et al., 1987; Hoskins and Cupp, 1988).

Hazards to Humans

Human parasitism by *Otobius megnini* is a potential health problem in the southwestern United States, especially in rural areas where people live in close contact with domesticated animals (Eads and Campos, 1984). As with domesticated and wild hosts, the ticks infesting the human cases had a predilection for the ear canal (Bishopp and Trembley, 1945; Eads and Campos, 1984).

Control/Prevention

Accurate identification of soft ticks from the parasitized host or from the environment is a prerequisite to their control (Hoskins and Cupp, 1988). The cat's ability to roam freely to areas frequented by livestock (sheds, yards, or kraals) should be restricted.

REFERENCES

Bishopp FC, Trembley HL. 1945. Distribution and hosts of certain North American ticks. J Parasitol 31:1–53.

Brumpt E. 1936. Contribution a l'étude de l'évolution des Ornithodores. Biologie et longévité de l'*Ornithodoros megnini*. Ann Parasitol 14:647–651.

Cooley RA, Kohls GM. 1944. The Argasidae of North America, Central America and Cuba, Monograph 1. Am Midl Nat. Notre Dame, Ind, University of Notre Dame, 21–36.

Eads RB, Campos EG. 1984. Human parasitism by *Otobius megnini* (Acari: Argasidae) in New Mexico, US. J Med Entomol 21:244.

Hoskins JD, Cupp EW. 1988. Ticks of veterinary importance. Part II. The Argasidae family: Identification, behavior, and associated diseases. Comp Cont Educ Pract Vet 10:699–709.

Munaó Diniz LS, Belluomini HE, Travassos Filho LP, da Rocha MB. 1987. Presence of the ear mite *Otobius megnini* in the external ear canal of lions (*Panthera leo*). J Zoo Anim Med 18:154–155.

Otobius lagophilus Cooley and Kohls, 1940

Etymology

Oto = ear and *bius* = way of life, along with *lago* = hare and *philus* = loving.

Synonyms

None.

History

Otobius lagophilus was first described by Cooley and Kohls in 1940. It is another soft tick that may parasitize cats (Cooley and Kohls, 1944).

Geographic Distribution.

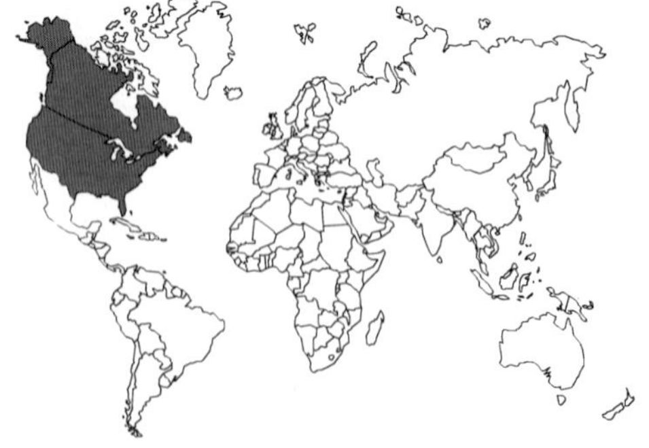

Fig. 5.8.

Otobius lagophilus is known from Alberta, Canada, and from the following states: California, Colorado, Idaho, Montana, Nevada, Oregon, and Wyoming. There has been a single, isolated case report of this tick from a cat in Alberta, Canada (Cooley and Kohls, 1944).

Location in Host

Cooley and Kohls (1944) found that the nymphs were attached in the fur on the face of rabbits near the vibrissae.

Parasite Identification

Cooley and Kohls (1944) stated that "This species resembles the well-known spinose ear tick, *Otobius megnini,* but it is readily separated by the following characters: its smaller size; the heavy V-shaped spines found on the anterior surfaces in *megnini* are replaced in *lagophilus* by slender spines which are the same as those on the posterior parts; denticles on the hypostome in a 3/3 pattern instead of 4/4; legs more slender; spiracles of the nymph mildly convex instead of conically protuberant."

Life Cycle

As with *Otobius megnini* the adults of *Otobius lagophilus* are not parasitic. The nymphs are found on the fur of the face of rabbits. Adults have been found at the entrance of rabbit burrows or well down in burrows.

Clinical Presentation and Pathogenesis

Except for a single collection from a cat in Lethbridge, Alberta, Canada, in 1941, the only known hosts for *Otobius lagophilus* are cottontail rabbits and jackrabbits. No clinical signs have been attributed to infestation of cats with this tick.

Diagnosis

Finding the spinose nymphal stage on the cat.

Treatment

Any of the popular acaricides used for treating infestation of hard ticks on cats should prove effective in treating *Otobius lagophilus.*

Epizootiology

Little is known about the epizootiology of this parasite relative to its association with the cat. Cats probably come into contact with the nymphs at either the burrows used by rabbits or by direct contact with infested rabbits.

Hazards to Other Animals

Other than the single report from the cat, the only known hosts for *Otobius lagophilus* are cottontail rabbits and jackrabbits (Cooley and Kohls, 1944).

Hazards to Humans

This tick is not known to attack humans.

Control/Prevention

Accurate identification of soft ticks from the parasitized host or from the environment is a prerequisite to their control (Hoskins and Cupp, 1988). The cat's ability to roam freely to areas frequented by rabbits should be restricted if infestations with this parasite are observed to be a problem.

REFERENCES

Cooley RA, Kohls GM. 1940. Two new species of Argasidae (Acarina: Ixodoidea). Publ Health Rep 55:925–933.

Cooley RA, Kohls GM. 1944. The Argasidae of North America, Central America and Cuba, Monograph 1. Am Midl Nat. Notre Dame, Ind, University of Notre Dame, 21–36.

Hoskins JD, Cupp EW. 1988. Ticks of veterinary importance. Part II. The Argasidae family: Identification, behavior, and associated diseases. Comp Cont Educ Pract Vet 10:699–709.

Ixodidae

The hard ticks represent some 13 genera and about 650 species. Most of the hard ticks are tropical; thus, infestations with these parasites more commonly occur in warmer climates. The different stages of hard ticks are often less fastidious in their choice of hosts than are the soft ticks, and often cats can become infested with larvae, nymphs, or adults of species of these parasites that are more commonly found on other domestic animals or wildlife. Due to the large number of species involved, the ticks will often not be identified beyond being recognized as a hard tick or as being one of the more common genera.

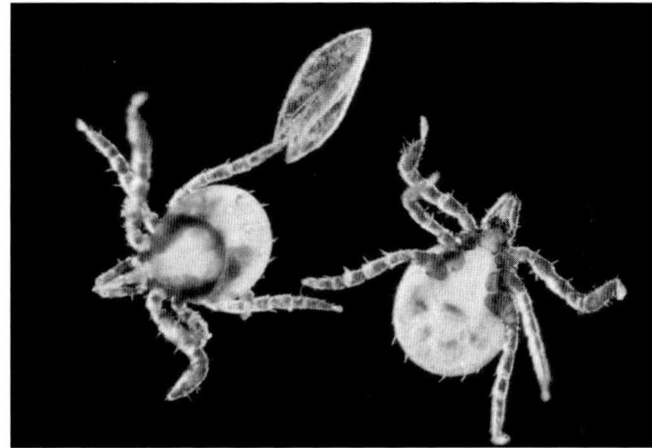

Fig. 5.9. *Ixodes dammini.* Two larvae that have just hatched from eggs.

The fact that ticks feed on the tissue fluids of their hosts allows them to serve as vectors of disease. Cats are sometimes infected with other pathogens by the bite of a tick, for example, *Cytauxzoon,* which the tick obtains while feeding as a larva or nymph.

The common ticks parasitic on dogs and humans often are also found on cats. Those genera that are most often observed are *Ixodes, Dermacentor,* and *Rhipicephalus.* Other genera that sometimes occur on cats are *Haemaphysalis* and *Amblyomma.* Some of these are one-host ticks, some are two-host ticks, and some are three-host ticks. This terminology deals with hosts relative to the occurrence of molting. In the case of hard ticks, there are three distinct stages: the larva that hatches from the egg (Fig. 5.9) (it feeds one time), the nymph that develops from the larva (it feeds one time), and the adult that develops from the nymph (the adult female feeds only one time; the adult male feeds little if any usually). Thus, in the case of one-host ticks, all stages feed on the same host without falling off to molt. In the case of two-host ticks, the larva and nymph feed on one host, and the adult on a second host. Finally, in the case of three-host ticks, the larva feeds on one host and falls off, the nymph feeds on a second host and falls off, and the adult feeds on a third host. For cats, almost all the species of importance are three-host ticks. *Rhipicephalus sanguineus,* the brown dog tick, which will feed

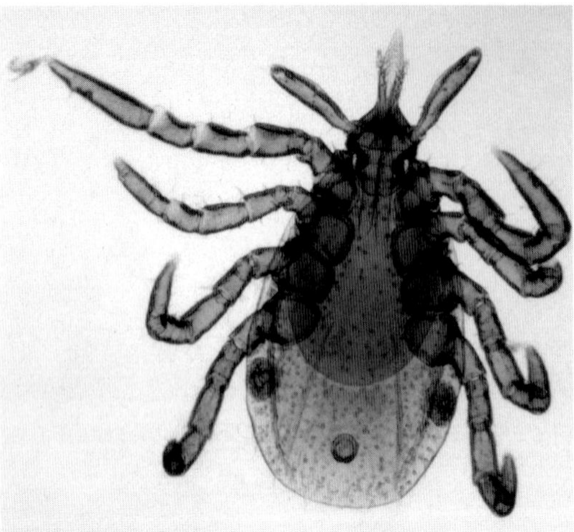

Fig. 5.10. *Ixodes dammini.* Nymph.

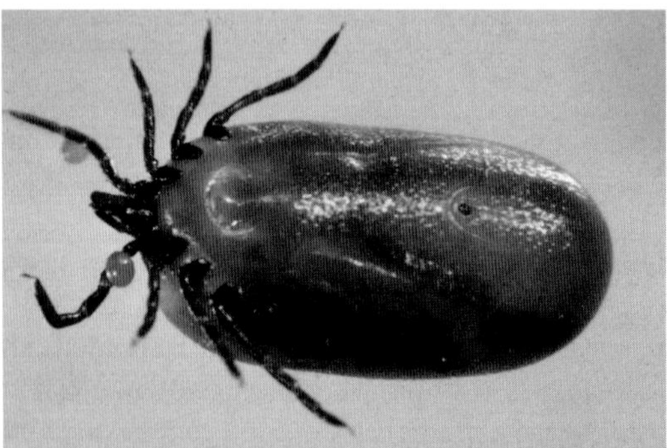

Fig. 5.11. *Ixodes dammini.* Engorged female. There are eggs sticking to each of the two most anterior legs.

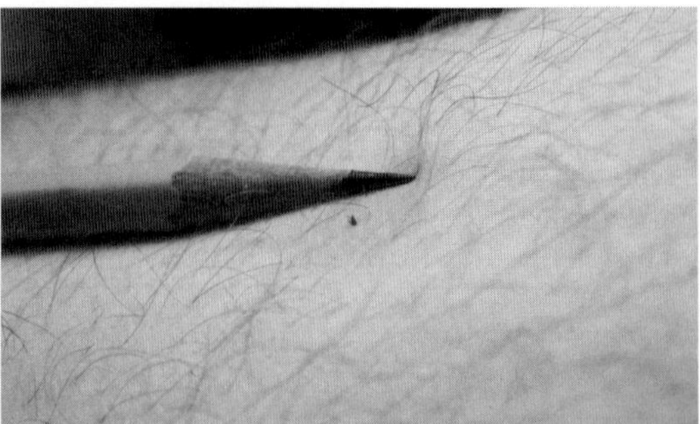

Fig. 5.12. *Ixodes dammini.* Nymph feeding in a persons arm.

on cats, is a three-host tick, but all stages in the life cycle prefer to get back on a dog to feed after they have molted.

Ixodes Species

There are some 250 species of ticks in this genus. Ticks of the genus *Ixodes* have a preanal groove or arch, the scutum is not ornamented, and they have neither eyes nor festoons. Examples include *Ixodes dammini,* with larvae (Fig. 5.9) and nymphs (Fig. 5.10) that feed on rodents and adults that feed on deer (Fig. 5.11). *Ixodes dammini* is found in the northeastern United States (many consider this species a synonym of *Ixodes scapularis*). It is often the nymph of this species that bites people to transmit Lyme disease (Fig. 5.12). The European counterpart is *Ixodes ricinus.* This tick transmits various *Babesia* and *Borrelia* species. *Ixodes scapularis* has larvae that feed on lizards, nymphs that feed on lizards and rodents, and adults that feed on deer. This tick is found in the southeastern United States. In the western United States the counterpart tick is *Ixodes pacificus,* which feeds on rodents as larvae and nymphs and mule deer as adults.

Dermacentor Species

There are only about 30 species of tick in this genus. The scutum of a typical *Dermacentor* is ornamented. (One species, *Dermacentor nitens,* the tropical horse tick of the southeastern United States, has a scutum that is not ornamented.) Ticks that are members of the genus *Dermacentor* have eyes and festoons along with a rectangular basis capituli (Figs. 5.13 to 5.16). *Dermacentor variabilis,* the American dog tick, has larvae and nymphs (Fig. 5.17) that feed on rodents and adults that prefer dogs but will attack cats or people. This tick is mainly found in the eastern United States and serves as the vector of Rocky Mountain spotted fever. In the Rocky Mountains, this tick is replaced with *Dermacentor andersoni,* which transmits the rickettsia in that area.

Amblyomma Species

This genus of 100 or so species of ticks is mainly found in the tropics. These ticks have an orna-

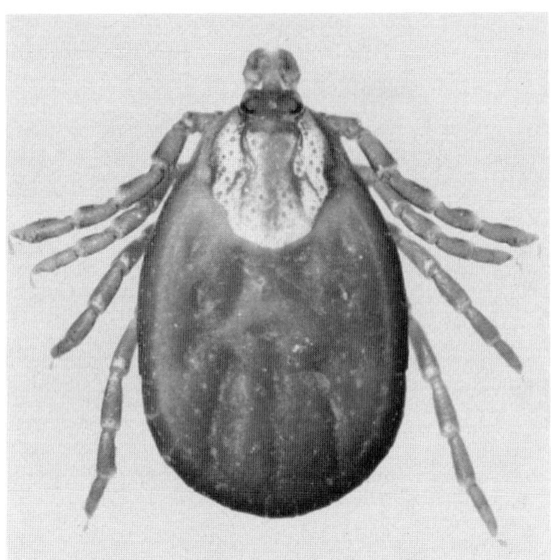

Fig. 5.13. *Dermacentor variabilis.* Dorsal view of adult female.

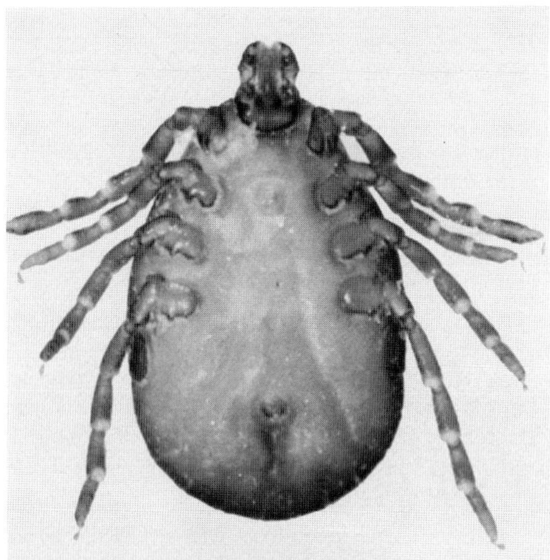

Fig. 5.14. *Dermacentor variabilis.* Ventral view of adult female.

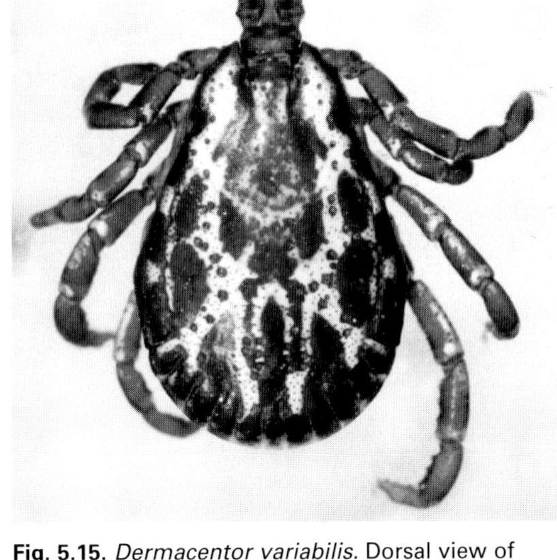

Fig. 5.15. *Dermacentor variabilis.* Dorsal view of adult male.

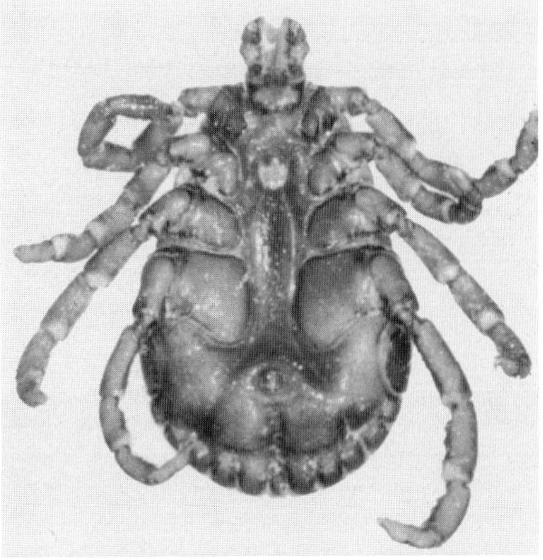

Fig. 5.16. *Dermacentor variabilis.* Ventral view of adult male. Note that the first coxa, segment of the leg that attaches to the body, gets larger with each leg from the anterior to the posterior of the body.

mented scutum, eyes, and festoons and relatively long mouthparts. *Amblyomma americana,* the lone star tick, is found in the southern United States and is a three-host tick that shows very little host preference in any stage. The common name, the lone star tick, is derived from the single white spot that appears on the back of the female (Fig. 5.18). These ticks are sometimes found quite far north and have been recovered from dogs in New York and New Jersey. Some of the tropical species such as *Amblyomma variegatum,* which is found in Africa and the Caribbean islands, have a very ornate and colorful scutum (Fig. 5.19).

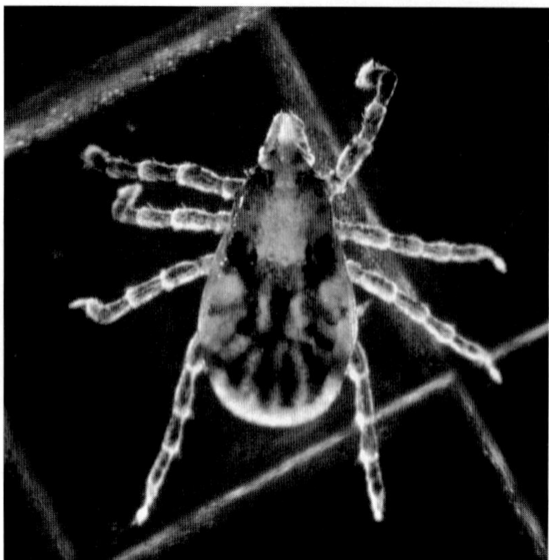

Fig. 5.17. *Dermacentor variabilis.* Nymph.

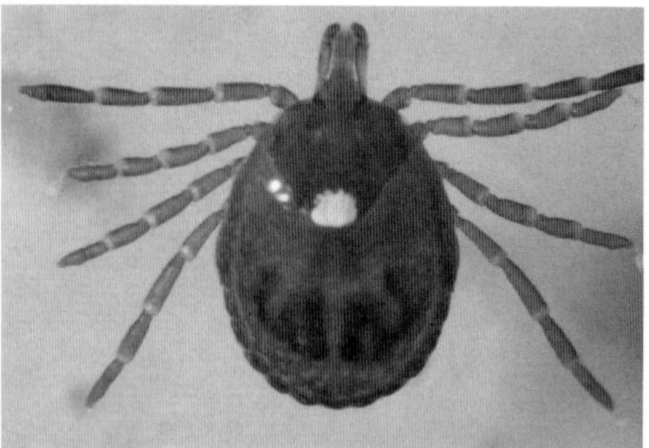

Fig. 5.18. *Amblyomma americana.* Adult female showing the scutum with a single white mark.

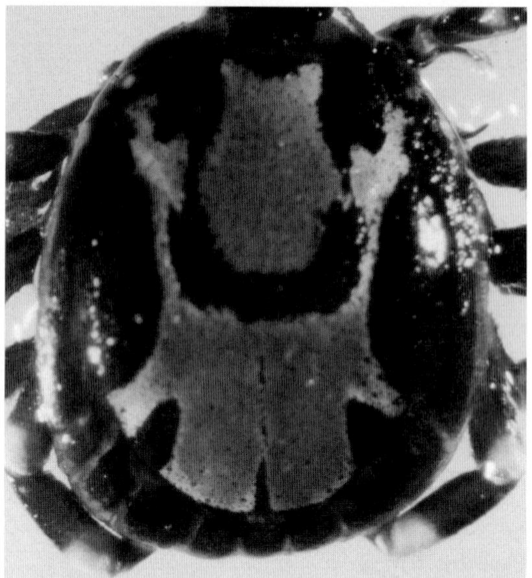

Fig. 5.19. *Amblyomma variegatum.* Scutum of adult male showing the highly ornate scutum. The black and white image does not do justice to the beautiful colors present on this tick.

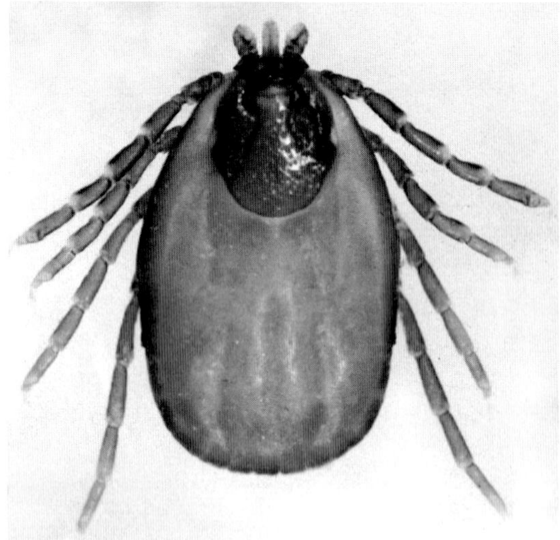

Fig. 5.20. *Rhipicephalus sanguineus.* Adult female.

Rhipicephalus Species

This group of around 60 species is mainly found in Africa. However, the brown dog tick, *Rhipicephalus sanguineus,* has traveled from East Africa to almost everywhere dogs have. This has been accomplished by the ability and desire of the larvae and nymphs to feed on dogs. Thus, this three-host tick has all hosts represented by the same species. This tick will, however, also feed on cats if they are within the same household. Species of *Rhipicephalus* have no ornamentation, have eyes and festoons, and have a basis capituli that is hexagonal (giving the tick its name "fan head") (Figs. 5.20 and 5.21). The males of this genus also have an adanal shield that is quite obvious on living, uncleared specimens (Fig. 5.22). This tick does not do well in cold weather but has been

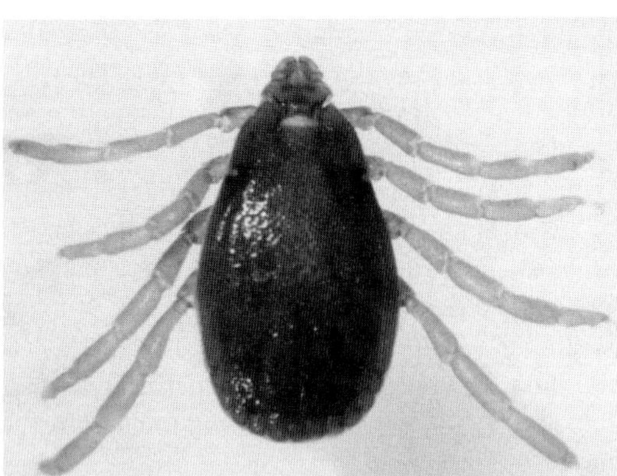

Fig. 5.21. *Rhipicephalus sanguineus.* Dorsal view of adult male.

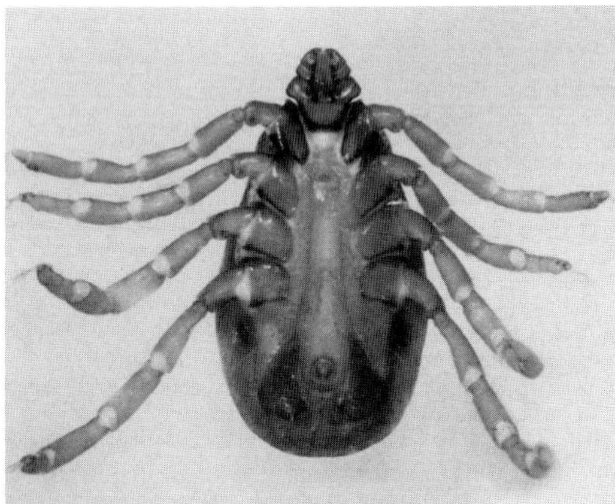

Fig. 5.22. *Rhipicephalus sanguineus.* Ventral view of adult male. Note the two dark adanal plates on each side of the anus at the posterior of the body. The first coxa of each leg is about the same apparent size (compare with Fig. 5.16).

domesticated to the point where it can happily undergo its entire life cycle within a house as long as there is a dog present to supply meals.

Haemaphysalis Species

This is a rather large group of 150 or so species. Only two of these species are found in the United States. Both these species are characterized by having no ornamentation of the scutum, having festoons but no eyes, and a characteristic flaring of the second palpal segment that gives the head a rather triangular appearance. *Haemaphysalis leporipalustris* is typically found on rabbits, but occasionally it gets on cats. Similarly, *Haemaphysalis chordeilis* usually infests birds, but it will also occasionally get onto cats.

Tick Paralysis

History

Tick paralysis is a well-known paralytic syndrome that occurs in many vertebrate hosts throughout the world and may be induced by at least 46 species of ticks (Stone, 1988). In North America, cats appear to be resistant to tick paralysis and show no clinical signs other than prolonged attachment of numerous ticks (Malik and Farrow, 1991). According to the Veterinary Medical Data Base, West Lafayette, Indiana, no cases of tick paralysis in the feline have been documented from the reporting member institutions (colleges/schools of veterinary medicine) across North America; however, a single case of tick paralysis due to an engorged female tick of the genus *Dermacentor* has been reported from a cat in Georgia (Anderson, 1985).

However, tick paralysis due to an Australian tick, *Ixodes holocyclus,* presents as a far more harmful syndrome than that produced by its North American counterpart (Malik and Farrow, 1991). *Ixodes holocyclus,* which is indigenous to Australia, was first described by Captain W. H. Howell in a diary reporting his expedition from Lake George to Port Phillip in 1824–1825. This tick is the most common cause of tick paralysis in eastern Australia (Prescott, 1984). A case of tick paralysis due to *Ixodes cornuatus* in a cat from Tasmania was reported in 1974 (Mason et al., 1974). Mason et al. (1974) also noted an additional case of paresis in a cat from northern Tasmania; other cases of feline tick paralysis had been previously reported by Roberts (1970). Early experimental studies of tick paralysis in the canine were performed by Ross (1927). Later, Ilkiw et al. (1987, 1988) and Ilkiw and Turner (1987a, b, 1988) provided an extensive treatise on the clinical, histologic, blood-gas, hematologic, biochemical findings and cardiovascular and respiratory effects and treatment of *Ixodes holocyclus* infestations in dogs. However, similar controlled studies have not been performed in cats.

Geographic Distribution

Although several species of ticks in North America are able to produce tick paralysis, *Dermacentor andersoni* (the Rocky Mountain wood tick) and *Dermacentor variabilis* (the American dog tick) are most often identified as causative agents of tick paralysis in cattle, sheep, and humans (Malik and Farrow, 1991). The tick that produced the isolated case of feline tick paralysis in North America was a *Dermacentor* species (Anderson, 1985).

Three different species of ticks comprise the *Ixodes holocyclus* group. These are *Ixodes myrmecobii* in Western Australia; *Ixodes cornuatus* in Tasmania, Victoria, and the southern coastal areas of New South Wales bordering Victoria and overlapping with this distribution; and *Ixodes holocyclus* in the coastal area of Victoria to the Tambo River and the coastal areas of New South Wales and Queensland (Kemp, 1979). The distribution of *Ixodes holocyclus* is largely determined by that of its principal hosts, the short-nosed bandicoot, *Isoodon macrourus,* and the long-nosed bandicoot, *Perameles nasuta.* This tick commonly occurs in moist environments, in areas of dense undergrowth with abundant leaf litter (Stone and Wright, 1979). Beveridge (1991) noted the occurrence of *Ixodes holocyclus* in the western suburbs of Melbourne, a report that extended the known geographic range of this tick 250 km to the west. *Ixodes hirsti* has also been associated with tick paralysis (Malik and Farrow, 1991) and is restricted to South Australia, Western Australia, southern New South Wales, Victoria, and Tasmania. *Ixodes cornuatus* is restricted to southern New South Wales, Victoria, and Tasmania (Stone, 1988). In Tasmania, *Ixodes cornuatus* has been associated with tick paralysis in cats (Mason et al., 1974).

Location in Host

Paralysis results from the engorgement of members of the genus *Ixodes,* most commonly *Ixodes holocyclus,* although *Ixodes cornuatus, Ixodes myrmecobii,* and *Ixodes hirsti* have been implicated in some cases of paralysis (Kemp, 1979). The syndrome will not develop until the ticks have been attached for at least 4 days. Attachment to the skin of the definitive host is most common in the spring and summer. Most cases of tick paralysis are seen during this period. The syndrome usually occurs after infestation with adult female ticks; however, heavy infestations with nymphs or larvae may produce paralysis (Malik and Farrow, 1991). Male ticks usually do not become attached to the host but may be found free in the coat (Prescott, 1984). The tick from the North American case was attached over the cranial thoracic vertebrae (Anderson, 1985), an area that is difficult to impossible for a cat to reach during the grooming process.

Parasite Identification

Ross provided extensive gross descriptions of the larval, nymphal, and adult male and female stages of *Ixodes holocyclus* (Ross, 1924). *Ixodes holocyclus, Ixodes cornuatus,* and *Ixodes hirsti* are members of the subgenus *Sternalixodes.* Homscher et al. (1988) utilized scanning electron microscopy to study the structure of Haller's organ in eight of the nine members of the subgenus *Sternalixodes.* Among the ticks examined, these researchers found the morphology of Haller's organ to be remarkably uniform. The general shape of the organ; shape and depth of the anterior trough; type, number, and arrangement of the anterior trough setae and tarsal hump setae; and location, size, and shape of the capsular aperture are virtually identical in the eight species examined. Some differences are evident, especially in the prominence of the tarsal hump and the steepness of the tarsal hump walls. *Ixodes holocyclus* was the most variable species in this study. The differences between male and female specimens of this species are as great as those observed when separate sexes are compared. It was concluded that more specimens of *Ixodes holocyclus* should be examined to discern if these differences are consistent.

Members of the adult *Ixodes holocyclus* group demonstrate small and not always constant structural differences. These differences lie in the shape of the cornuae, palpal article I, and the spur on coxa I. *Ixodes holocyclus* is identified by the characteristic circle around its anus. Larvae of *Ixodes holocyclus* and *Ixodes cornuatus* are more easily identified than their adult counterparts. Some of the structures, particularly the pattern of hairs, are distinctly different (Kemp, 1979).

Life Cycle

The adult *Ixodes holocyclus* is a flat, oval tick with prominent mouthparts and brown legs. There are four developmental stages in its life cycle: egg, larva, nymph, and adult. The female is a productive egg layer, laying 2,000 to 3,000 eggs, which hatch in 49 to 61 days. The larvae (or seed ticks) become active in about 1 week and attach themselves to a host where they feed for 4 to 6 days. Suitable hosts may be the bandicoot, the echidna, the opossum, all domesticated animals, and even man. Following engorgement, the larva drops off and, during a period of 19 to 41 days, molts and develops to the nymphal stage. The engorged nymph develops to the adult stage in 3 to 10 weeks and, after molting to the adult stage, attaches itself to the third host where it engorges for 6 to 21 days (Prescott, 1984). Large numbers of larvae, nymphs, and adults may be found on the same animal (Ross, 1924). Although all feeding stages of the tick can cause paralysis, adult females are responsible for most of the cases.

Clinical Presentation and Pathogenesis

Most information concerning tick paralysis in small animals has been gathered from observations of dogs. Clinical signs are usually observed 5 to 7 days following attachment of the tick. The rate of engorgement of the parasites will determine the length of time prior to the onset of symptoms. This period may be prolonged up to 2 weeks in colder weather. In massive infestations, clinical signs may appear until as early as the fourth day (Malik and Farrow, 1991). Tick paralysis presents initially with loss of appetite and voice, incoordination, following by ascending flaccid paralysis, ocular irritation, excessive salivation, and asymmetric pupillary dilatation. Tetraplegia and respiratory distress occur later and are almost inevitably followed by death if treatment is not instituted (Stone, 1988).

Affected cats typically are distressed and agitated. Initially there is a change in voice that is especially noticeable in Siamese and Burmese cats. Retching or coughing may accompany this sign. Pupillary dilatation is common; however, vomiting is rare in comparison with that observed in the dog (Malik and Farrow, 1991). Roberts noted two cases of tick paralysis in cats. Both cats were exhibiting signs of tick paralysis, one cat "crawling with its front legs and dragging its hind legs on the ground" and the other "walking as though it was properly drunk." The cats died 7 and 10 days respectively after the signs were observed. The causative agent was *Ixodes hirsti* (Roberts, 1961). A cat from Tasmania presented with a flaccid paralysis and dilated pupils. On the second day of illness, it exhibited obvious signs of respiratory distress. On the third day, the cat died and was submitted for postmortem examination. At necropsy, the cat exhibited a cyanosed tongue and nose. Behind the ear was an engorged female *Ixodes cornuatus*. At the attachment site, the subcutaneous tissues were locally edematous and stained by blood pigments. Other gross lesions were endocardial and epicardial hemorrhages. The endocardial hemorrhage was especially severe on the papillary muscles of the left ventricle. Histologically, the subcutaneous tissue was characterized by hemorrhage and edema with extensive local infiltration by polymorphonuclear leukocytes, lymphocytes, and plasma cells (Mason et al., 1974).

In the case of tick paralysis in the North American cat, the cat presented with a history of acute listlessness and paresis, anorexia, but no vomition or diarrhea. On physical examination, the cat was markedly depressed and nonresponsive. Both hindlimbs demonstrated flaccid paralysis. Respiratory distress was not evident. The cat was 7 to 8 percent dehydrated. Within 8 hours of tick removal, improvement was noted. The cat became more alert and responsive and made attempts to move about. Within 24 hour, all evidence of flaccid paralysis had subsided.

Diagnosis

Identification of larval, nymphal, and adult male and female ticks of the genus *Ixodes* infesting the skin and haircoat of affected cats is the best method of definitive diagnosis of tick paralysis. Diagnosis is confirmed following rapid improvement of the affected cat following removal of the ticks. The diagnosis is certain in classical cases of rapidly ascending flaccid motor paralysis associated with identification of engorged female ticks of the genus *Ixodes*. The change in voice, referable to laryngeal paresis is suggestive of tick paralysis. Detailed neurologic testing reveals reduced muscle tone and diminished to absent myotactic reflexes early in the course of the disease. Although withdrawal reflexes are initially normal, they become progressively slower and weaker as the syndrome advances. Although proprioception and cutaneous sensation are thought to be preserved, diminished perception of noxious tactile stimuli occasionally has been noted. The gag reflex is constantly depressed, and the inability to swallow results in drooling of saliva. Rapid commencement of clinical signs is associated with more severe disease and an increased likelihood of death (Malik and Farrow, 1991).

Treatment

There are three stages in the treatment regimen for tick paralysis caused by *Ixodes holocyclus:* removal of offending tick(s), counteraction of circulating toxin, and commencement of symptomatic and supportive therapy.

After a diagnosis of tick paralysis is made, a thorough search of the cat's haircoat is indicated. Ticks can be found on almost any part of the body. In cats, they are usually found in areas that are inaccessible to grooming (e.g., under the chin, on the neck, or between the shoulder blades). If only one tick is found, the search should be continued and be as thorough as possible. If all ticks are not removed, recovery may not occur. In longhaired cats, clipping the haircoat often expedites the detection of additional ticks.

Ticks are best removed by sliding the blades of a partially opened pair of scissors between the tick and the cat's skin. Using a levering action, the tick can be maneuvered from the attachment site with its mouthparts intact. This strategy prevents additional release of toxin into the cat. Efforts should be made to determine if the tick is one of the species that produces tick paralysis. Removal of the offending tick may prevent the development of tick paralysis, if the cat has not yet begun to demonstrate clinical signs. Nevertheless, if the cat is exhibiting signs, removal of the tick is not adequate. The syndrome is likely to advance for up to 48 hours without proper therapy.

Hence, hyperimmune serum should be administered intravenously in cats to neutralize the effects of the circulating tick toxins. Since hyperimmune serum is derived from canine sources, risk is associated with its administration to other species (anaphylaxis is rare in cats initially receiving antitick serum). Intravenous hydrocortisone (30 mg/kg) can be routinely administered just prior to the slow intravenous injection of antitick serum (5–10 ml) to seriously affected cats. Epinephrine (1 ml of a 1:10,000 solution) should be accessible in the event of anaphylaxis. An alternate regimen is to administer hyperimmune sera to cats either intraperitoneally or intravenously following premedication with acepromazine or an antihistamine. Canine hyperimmune serum should initially be withheld from mildly affected cats, pending their response to tick extraction.

In mildly affected cats with a definitive ascending paralysis, removal of ticks and administration of hyperimmune serum usually result in obvious clinical improvement within 24 to 48 hours; however, there is little clinical change during the first 12 hours. If the cat fails to respond to hyperimmune serum after a suitable time, the cat should be reexamined for undetected ticks.

Cats with more-advanced tick paralysis gain from administration of drugs that decrease peripheral vascular resistance, thereby easing respiratory distress associated with pulmonary congestion and edema. The alpha-adrenoreceptor antagonist phenoxybenzamine (1 mg/kg diluted into at least 20 ml of 0.9 percent sodium chloride and repeated every 12–24 hours if necessary) and the phenothiazine tranquilizer acepromazine (0.05–0.10 mg/kg every 6–12 hours) given slowly intravenously have been used most often in this situation. A vasodilator should be administered to cats with clinical signs related to pulmonary congestion and edema. Both phenoxybenzamine and phenothiazine produce effective sedation as well as alleviating the respiratory distress. Afterload reducers, such as hydralazine and sodium nitroprusside, have not been tested clinically or experimentally in cats with tick paralysis. Furosemide may be used as an aid to remove fluid from the lungs. Cats with pulmonary edema may benefit from supplementary oxygen. This is easily provided by piping 100 percent oxygen into a cat induction chamber through a disposable plastic nebulizer. It is imperative to avoid hypothermia in affected animals.

Persistent nursing care is essential in animals with tick paralysis. Since any stress adversely affects the course of the disease, cats should be attended with minimal interference in the quietest part of the hospital. They should be maintained in a cool, air-conditioned environment since neuromuscular blockade is aggravated by any increased temperatures. To minimize ventilation/perfusion mismatch, animals should be placed in sternal recumbency on a well-padded surface using towels and sandbags. Following episodes of vomiting or regurgitation, the pharynx should be swabbed clean to reduce the risk of aspiration.

Submaintenance fluid requirements should be provided after the first day (0.45 percent sodium chloride containing 16 mmol potassium chloride/L; 20–40 ml/kg/day), especially in animals in which recovery is prolonged. Fluids must be given slowly because of the predisposition of affected animals to develop pulmonary congestion and edema.

Prophylactic antibiotics are inappropriate in tick paralysis, and atropine is contraindicated. Cardiac arrhythmias directly or indirectly result from sympathetic overactivity and tend to resolve following the administration of phenoxybenzamine and acepromazine and require no specific treatment. Although high doses of glucocorticosteroids (0.5 mg/kg dexamethasone every 12 hours) have been shown to be advantageous in advanced cases of tick paralysis, their conventional use is unwarranted due to the threat of aspiration pneumonia. The role and efficacy of antiemetics have not been adequately described.

Food and water should be withheld from paralyzed animals because pharyngeal dysfunction, megaesophagus, laryngeal paresis, and a weak cough create a tendency for aspiration pneumonia. They should be withheld until the patient is mobile and has not vomited for 24 hours. Small volumes of water can then be given; food can be offered subsequently if there is no vomiting. Following recovery, a convalescence phase should be imposed with restriction of exercise and avoidance of high temperatures. Strenuous exercise within a day of complete recovery from tick paralysis has resulted in collapse and sudden death. Extreme temperature may cause recovered animals to relapse into paralysis (Malik and Farrow, 1991).

Epizootiology

Tick paralysis is seen in man and domesticated animals who either reside in or have had a history of visiting the bush and scrub country along the coastal fringe of eastern Australia. Long-haired cats are at a definite disadvantage with regard to the owner's ability to detect ticks within the haircoat. Facts on the seasonal incidence of *Ixodes holocyclus* are patchy, but there are indications that female ticks are most common in spring and early summer, larval ticks in summer and autumn, and nymphs in autumn and winter. Regardless, adults occur in low numbers at all times during the year. The host-seeking behavior of females is said to be more aggressive during warm, moist weather that follows spring storms. Adult male and female ticks are abundant in areas of overgrowth or regrowth, especially around the base of small trees or shrubs surrounded by low vegetation (e.g., wild raspberry, crofton weed, and lantana). Ticks occur on the mat of vegetation and in the lower foliage and leaf litter. These are areas frequented by bandicoots, which are of most importance in the ecology of the paralysis tick (Doube, 1975).

Hazards to Other Animals

The normal hosts of Australian tick paralysis ticks include bandicoots, brush-tailed opossums, macropods, and koalas. These native mammals are relatively resistant to the toxins produced by the ticks, often carrying heavy burdens of ticks without showing evidence of harm (Stone and Wright, 1979; Stone, 1988).

Ixodes holocyclus has been reported to be the most consistently toxic paralyzing tick in the world. Not only does it cause serious economic loss to the Australian livestock industry, it is also of significant importance to pet owners. It has been reported that there may be at least 20,000 domestic animals in Australia affected by tick paralysis each year. Of these, at least 10,000 may have been companion animals referred to veterinarians for treatment. Livestock are also vulnerable to tick paralysis toxin: as many as 10,000 calves have died in New South Wales alone. Adult cattle, horses, sheep, goats, and deer are affected by heavier infestations. However, juvenile piglets, foals, kids, lambs, and fawns in deer-farming programs are at greatest risk. It has been estimated that tick paralysis affects as many as 100,000 animals or more each year. *Ixodes cornuatus* and *Ixodes hirsti* can produce a similar paralysis. *Ixodes cornuatus* has been incriminated in paralysis of dogs in Victoria and Tasmania and of sheep and calves in Victoria (Stone, 1988).

In North America, dogs, sheep, and cattle have fallen victim to the paralytic effects of *Dermacentor andersoni* (the Rocky Mountain wood tick), *Dermacentor variabilis* (the American dog tick), and several other species of ticks in North America (Malik and Farrow, 1991).

Hazards to Humans

Ixodes holocyclus has been reported to produce paralysis in humans, notably infants. Human infestations with this tick are occurring with increasing frequency, even in areas once not considered to be in its geographic distribution (Beveridge, 1991). The symptoms of tick paralysis in human beings are similar to those observed in animals. They include ascending paralysis characterized by unsteadiness in walking and/or lethargy, weakness in upper limbs, difficulty in swallowing, respiratory distress, and even death in the absence of treatment. Other effects may be photophobia, double vision, pupillary dilatation and occasionally myocarditis. Localized paralysis, particularly of the face, occasionally occurs.

Ixodes cornuatus infestations of humans have caused abdominal pain, vomiting, and headache as well as severe pain at the bite site. A single case of tick paralysis in a human that was attributable to *Ixodes cornuatus* has been reported (Stone, 1988).

Control/Prevention

Daily examination is the least expensive and most effective form of prevention. The syndrome will not develop until the ticks have been attached for at least 4 days. In the future, it may be possible to vaccinate cats using toxoids derived from the different toxins of *Ixodes holocyclus* (Malik and Farrow, 1991). Cats should be restricted from roaming in heavily wooded areas and areas with thick underbrush. This control technique is difficult to accomplish with outdoor cats. In areas of heavy tick numbers, cats should be placed on a monthly treatment regimen of fipronil.

REFERENCES

Anderson WI. 1985. Tick paralysis in a cat. Mod Vet Pract 66:1006.

Beveridge I. 1991. *Ixodes holocyclus* in the Melbourne metropolitan area. Aust Vet J 68:214.

Doube BM. 1975. Cattle and the paralysis tick *Ixodes holocyclus*. Aust Vet J 51:511–515.

Homscher PJ, Keirans JE, Robbins RG, Irwin-Pinkley L, Sonenshine DE. 1988. Scanning electron microscopy of ticks for systematic studies: Structure of Haller's organ in eight species of the subgenus *Sternalixodes* of the genus *Ixodes* (Acari: Ixodidae). J Med Entomol 25:348–353.

Ilkiw JE, Turner DM. 1987a. Infestation in the dog by the paralysis tick, *Ixodes holocyclus* 2. Blood gas and pH, haematological and biochemical findings. Aust Vet J 64:139–142.

Ilkiw JE, Turner DM. 1987b. Infestation in the dog by the paralysis tick, *Ixodes holocyclus* 3. Respiratory effects. Aust Vet J 64:142–144.

Ilkiw JE, Turner DM. 1988. Infestation in the dog by the paralysis tick, *Ixodes holocyclus* 5. Treatment. Aust Vet J 65:236–238.

Ilkiw JE, Turner DM, Howlett CR. 1987. Infestation in the dog by the paralysis tick *Ixodes holocyclus* 1. Clinical and histological findings. Aust Vet J 64:137–139.

Ilkiw JE, Turner DM, Goodman AH. 1988. Infestation in the dog by the paralysis tick, *Ixodes holocyclus* 4. Cardiovascular effects. Aust Vet J 65: 232–235.

Kemp DH. 1979. Identity of Australian paralysis ticks. Proc 56th Annu Conf Aust Vet Assoc 1979. Pp 73–74.

Malik R, Farrow BRH. 1991. Tick paralysis in North America and Australia. Vet Clin N Am 21:157–171.

Mason RW, Kemp DH, King SJ. 1974. *Ixodes cornuatus* and tick paralysis. Aust Vet J 50:580.

Prescott CW. 1984. Ticks, spiders, insects, cane toads, platypus venom intoxications—II. Aust Vet Pract 14:111–116.

Roberts FHS. 1961. Tick paralysis in South Australia. Aust Vet J 37:440.

Roberts FHS. 1970. Australian Ticks. Melbourne, Australia: CSIRO, p. 59.

Ross IC. 1924. The bionomics of *Ixodes holocyclus* Neumann, with a redescription of the adult and nymphal stages and a description of the larvae. Parasitol 16:365–381.

Ross IC. 1927. An experimental study of tick paralysis in Australia. Aust Vet J 3:71–74.

Stone BF. 1988. Tick paralysis, particularly involving *Ixodes holocyclus* and other *Ixodes* species. In Advances in Disease Vector Research, vol 5, ed KF Harris, pp 61–85. New York, NY: Springer-Verlag.

Stone BF, Wright IG. 1979. Toxins of *Ixodes holocyclus* and immunity to paralysis. Proc 56th Annu Conf Aust Vet Assoc 1979. Pp 75–78.

MESOSTIGMATA

Mesostigmatid mites are characterized by appearing as small tick-like arachnids. They differ from ticks in that the stigmata are located between the third and fourth pairs of legs, and each stigma is associated with an anteriorly directed peritreme. Mesostigmatid mites tend to have long legs and bodies that are covered with small hairs. There are some 19 superfamilies of mesostigmatid mites (Desch, 1984; Baker et al., 1956). Most of the mites in this group are actually free-living predators associated with soils and vegetation. Most adult mesostigmatid mites are 0.5 to 0.7 mm long with an oval to oval-oblong body shape. Families of general medical importance include the Macronyssidae, which is found mainly on bats, the Dermanyssidae, which parasitizes birds and mammals, the Laelapidae, which includes free-living forms and species parasitic on rodents, and the Halarachnidae, which includes the parasitic respiratory mites *Pneumonyssus simicola* of primates and *Pneumonyssoides caninum* of dogs.

There is only a single mesostigmatid mite, *Dermanyssus gallinae,* that is of importance in feline medicine. Many of the parasitic mesostigmatid mites tend to be nest-dwelling species, and there are numerous species that are found in rodent nests, such as *Ornithonyssus bacoti* (the tropical rat mite) and *Laelaps nutalli* (the domestic rat mite), that one would expect to occasionally be found on cats. However, as of this time the authors are not aware of these mites being reported as causing lesions on feline hosts.

REFERENCES

Baker EW, Evans TM, Gould DJ, Hull WB, Keegan HL. 1956. A Manual of Parasitic Mites of Medical or Economic Importance. New York, NY: National Pest Control Association.

Desch CE. 1984. Biology of biting mites (Mesostigmata). In Mammalian Diseases and Arachnids, vol I, ed WB Nutting, pp 83–109. Boca Raton, Fla: CRC Press.

Dermanyssus gallinae (DeGeer, 1778)

Etymology

Derma = skin and *nyssus* = to prick, along with *gallinae* for the chicken host.

History

Dermanyssus gallinae, which primarily affects avians, was first described by DeGeer in 1778. This mite infests cats only occasionally (Grant, 1985).

Geographic Distribution

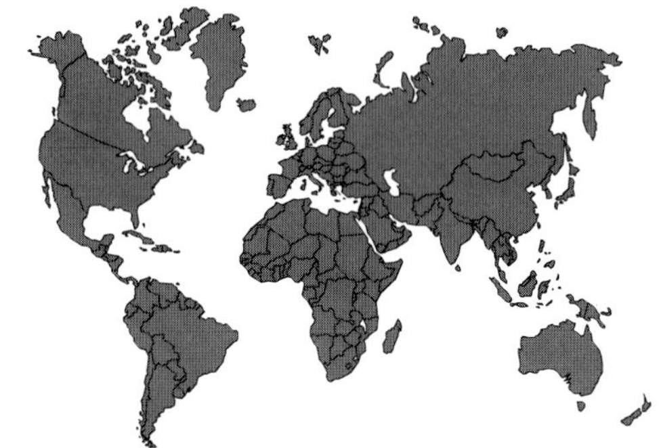

Fig. 5.23.

The mite is worldwide in its distribution, attacking the fowl, the pigeon, the canary, and other cage birds (Harwood and James, 1979).

Location in Host

Dermanyssus gallinae is a nonburrowing, bloodsucking mite that usually infests birds or their domiciles (Regan et al., 1987). This mite on rare occasions is found within the haircoat of cats (Grant, 1985). A case of this mite infesting the cat in the United States revealed lesions consisting of erosions, crusts, and excoriations on the head (Muller et al., 1983). Grant (1989) reports lesions on the dorsum and the extremities of the cat.

Parasite Identification

Dermanyssus gallinae is often referred to as the red mite of poultry, but it is only red if it has recently fed on its host's blood. In the unfed state, this mite is white, gray, or black. The fully engorged adult female is about 1 mm long or longer (Fig. 5.24). All other developmental stages are smaller. This mite possesses a very prominent dorsal shield. The shield does not quite extend to the posterior end of the body, and its posterior end is truncated. The hairs on the dorsal shield are smaller than those on the carapace that surrounds the shield. On the posterior ventral surface of the mite is a prominent anal plate; the anus is located

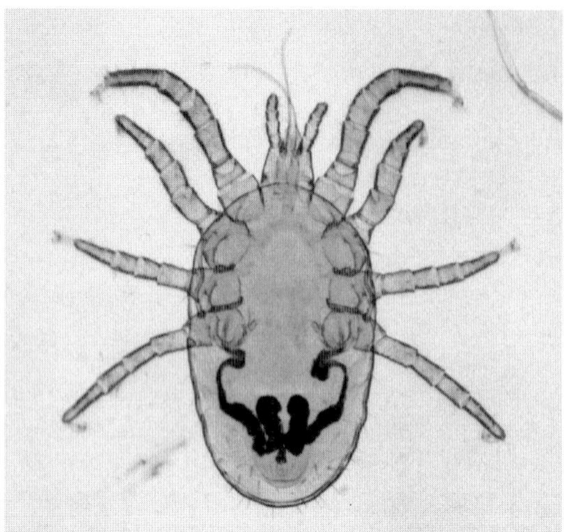

Fig. 5.24. *Dermanyssus gallinae.* Adult mite. Notice the long, narrow, chelicerae.

on the posterior aspect of this plate. This mite possesses long, whip-like chelicerae. Many of these key morphologic features can only be visualized after the mites have been cleared in lactophenol and examined under a compound microscope.

Life Cycle

The majority of this mite's life cycle takes place in the domicile of the avian definitive host. Following a blood meal, eggs are laid in the nests of birds or in the cracks and crevices in the walls of poultry houses. Up to seven eggs are laid at a time. At outdoor summer temperatures, the eggs hatch in 2 to 3 days, releasing the six-legged larvae, which do not feed. The larvae molt to the eight-legged protonymph stage, which will feed on the host's blood. After another 1 to 2 days, they develop into deutonymphs. These feed on blood and, after another 1 to 2 days, molt to adults. Under optimum conditions, the entire life cycle can be completed in 7 days to 5 months (Grant, 1989). Under experimental conditions, the adult mites have been able to live for 34 weeks without a blood meal.

Clinical Presentation and Pathogenesis

Mites often infest wild birds nesting in the eaves of homes. These mites may enter open windows and infest the people or their pets living there. Most cases associated with pets are found in cats or dogs that have access to or live in recently converted poultry houses. Clinical signs include erythema and papulocrustous eruptions that are intensely pruritic. These lesions are often distributed over the back and extremities (Muller et al., 1983).

Diagnosis

Infestations with *Dermanyssus gallinae* are often diagnosed by a history of contact with poultry houses or by close examination of environmental conditions (e.g., eaves, air conditioners, open windows, etc.) associated with a building that birds use for nesting (Muller et al., 1983; Regan et al., 1987). The mites are visible to the naked eye, particularly if they have fed recently on blood, and as a result, they are red in color. Diagnosis is by finding the mites on skin scraping (Muller et al., 1983). When suspected mites are removed from an infested host, cleared in lactophenol, and examined under a compound microscope, they will demonstrate the key morphologic features necessary for identification: size, number of legs, the very prominent dorsal shield with its truncated posterior end, and the ventral anal plate with the anus located on the posterior aspect.

Treatment

Dermanyssus gallinae is susceptible to most insecticidal preparations; almost any bath, dip, or spray will eliminate the mites (Muller et al., 1983).

Epizootiology

Most cases of *Dermanyssus gallinae* in the cat occur when there is an association of cats with poultry houses. The possibility of spread from pigeons or pigeon nests around houses also exists (Muller et al., 1983).

Hazards to Other Animals

Ramsay and Mason (1975) reported a case in a dog that was so infested that the numbers of mites crawling through the haircoat resembled the dandruff produced in infestations with *Cheyletiella* species.

Hazards to Humans

When pigeons nest near human dwellings, these mites may attack humans. *Dermanyssus gallinae* is only one of six mites that may produce fowl mite dermatitis in humans. In the absence of an avian host, this mite will attack humans, producing a pruritic, macular, papular, vesicular, or urticarial rash. It may also serve as a potential vector for the viruses of eastern and western equine encephalomyelitis and Saint Louis encephalitis (Regan et al., 1987). Laboratory and epidemiologic studies suggest that these mites play no important role in the maintenance of these pathogens. Field isolation probably means that the mite has recently fed on viremic birds (Harwood and James, 1979).

Control/Prevention

Treatment of the infested premises that serve as the source of infestation should be accomplished to prevent reinfestation (Muller et al., 1983).

REFERENCES

Grant DI. 1985. Notes on parasitic skin disease in the dog and cat. Br Vet J 141:447–462.

Grant DI. 1989. Parasitic diseases in cats. J Sm Anim Pract 30:250–254.

Harwood RF, James MT. 1979. Helminths, Arthropods, and Protozoa of Domesticated Animals. 7th ed. New York, NY: Macmillan. P 347.

Muller GH, Kirk, RW, Scott, DW. 1983. Small Animal Dermatology. 3rd ed. Philadelphia, Pa: WB Saunders. P 317.

Ramsay GW, Mason PC. 1975. Chicken mite (*D. gallinae*) infesting a dog. N Zealand Vet J 62:701.

Regan AM, Metersky ML, Craven DE. 1987. Nosocomial dermatitis and pruritus caused by pigeon mite infestation. Arch Intern Med 147:2185–2187.

PROSTIGMATA

There are over 10,000 described species of prostigmatid mites, but very few are actually known to cause disease. These mites are divided into 120 families, but only members of 16 of these families are reported as having caused disease in mammals (Nutting, 1984). The most widely known species in this group are the spider mites that attack houseplants and the red (or velvet) mites that are micropredators in gardens. The cat can serve as a host for three markedly different prostigmatid genera. The genus *Cheyletiella* contains mites whose labial structures are highly adapted for hair clasping, and these mites glue their eggs to the hairs of their feline host. The genus *Demodex* is represented by a group of mites with elongated bodies that have adapted to living within hair follicles. The trombiculid mites or chiggers are mites that are free-living predators as adults but the larval stage requires a meal from a vertebrate host.

REFERENCES

Nutting WB. 1984. Bioecology of prostigmatic mites (Prostigmata). In Mammalian Diseases and Arachnids, vol I, ed WB Nutting, pp 143–166 Boca Raton, Fla: CRC Press.

Cheyletiella blakei Smiley, 1970

Etymology

Cheyle = lips and *tiella* = a diminutive meaning that this is smaller than *tia* or *tea,* along with *blakei* for Dr. D.F. Blake, Department of Biology, Walla Walla College, Washington.

Synonyms

None.

History

In 1878, Mégnin was the first to describe adult *Cheyletiella* mites, and he theorized that these mite preyed on other mites (Merchant, 1990); hence, he gave them *Cheyletus parasitivorax* as their scientific name (Bronswijk and Kreek, 1976). It has been demonstrated, however, that members of this genus are true "mange" mites and not predatory on other mites (Merchant, 1990). The mite genus *Cheyletiella* was erected by Canestrini in 1885 to contain the genus described by Mégnin in 1878 as *Cheyletus parasitivorax.* In the beginning, there were some inconsistencies in the spelling of the generic name: *Cheletiella, Cheiletiella,* and *Cheyletiella* (Bronswijk and Kreek, 1976). Eggs of *Cheyletiella* species were not described until 1917. They were "fixed to a hair . . . elongated, resembling the eggs of a louse in general appearance, but minute, and with a very delicate cuticle" (Hirst,

1917). Reed (1961) reported "nit-like objects" on the hair that could be interpreted as being either mites or eggs (Ewing et al., 1967). Hirst (1917) was the first to report that *Cheyletiella* occurred on cats. This was followed by several other reports (Smiley, 1970) that recognized *Cheyletiella,* as *Cheyletiella parasitivorax,* occurring on cats. Ewing et al. (1967) noted that the sensory organ on the leg of the mite from cats differed morphologically from that present on the mite from dogs, and Smiley (1970) described *Cheyletiella blakei* from cats as a new species (using as types specimens recovered from a cat in Ithaca, New York). Human involvement with this mite was first reported by Lomholt in 1918.

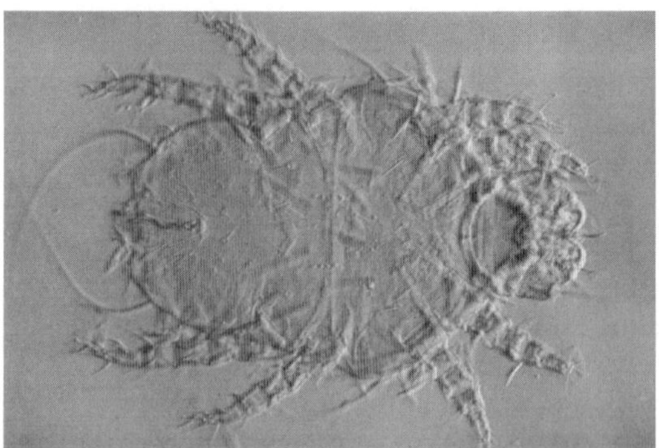

Fig. 5.26. *Cheyletiella* species. Note the large palpal claws.

Geographic Distribution

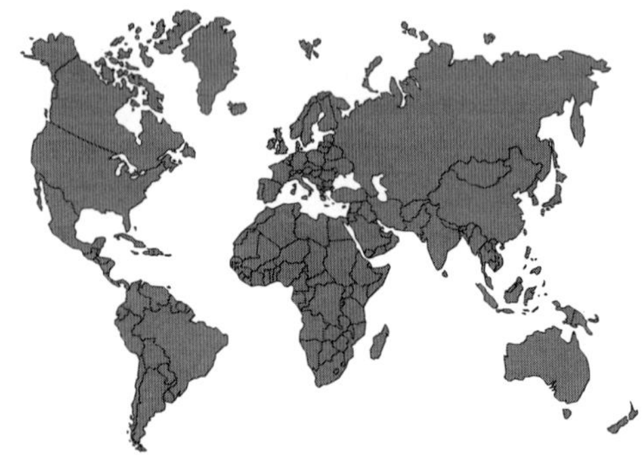

Fig. 5.25.

Bronswijk and Kreek (1976) provided a synopsis of the worldwide distribution of cheyletiellosis in the rabbit, dog, and cat. Reports of feline infestation have originated from every continent. Recent reports of feline infestation have come from the United States (Keh et al., 1987), Italy (Faravelli and Genchi, 1984; Faravelli and Traldi, 1985; Dal Tio et al., 1990), Turkey (Dinçer and Karaer, 1985), and Yugoslavia (Wikerhauser and Pinter, 1987).

Location in Host

Mites of the genus *Cheyletiella* are surface dwelling (nonburrowing), feeding on the keratin layer of the skin and in the haircoat of the definitive host. These mites thrive on keratin debris and tissue fluids. Cats typically exhibit scaling on the head, neck, and dorsum, lesions easily confused with those of flea-allergy dermatitis and miliary dermatitis (Smith, 1988). Kwochka (1987) reported that these mites have also been observed to crawl in and out of the nostrils of cats.

Parasite Identification

Cheyletiellosis has been referred to as "walking dandruff" because the mites often resemble large, mobile flakes of dandruff. Cheyletiellid mites are unique among mites that parasitize domestic cats, possessing distinct key morphologic features. These are large (500 by 265 μm [Foley, 1991]) mites, visible to the naked eye. Utilizing the compound microscope, one can discern their most characteristic key morphologic feature: their enormous hook-like accessory mouthparts (palpi) (Fig. 5.26). These palpi assist the mite in attaching to the host as it feeds on tissue fluids (Schmeitzel, 1988). Kwochka (1987) reported that these mites also feed on skin surface debris. Members of the genus are also known for their characteristic body shape, a shape that has been reported as being like that of a "shield" (Kwochka, 1987) or that of a "bell pepper" or a "western horse's saddle" when viewed from above.

Three species of *Cheyletiella* have been suspected of infesting cats: *Cheyletiella blakei* (most commonly), *Cheyletiella yasguri* (common on dogs), and *Cheyletiella parasitivorax* (common on rabbits) (Grant, 1989). One of the characteristic features used to differentiate the various species in the genus *Cheyletiella* is the shape of the sense organ on the first pair of legs. This organ is reported to be conical in *Cheyletiella blakei,* heart shaped in *Cheyletiella yasguri,* and globose in *Cheyletiella parasitivorax.* Species identification, however, is often difficult due to the individual variation in the shape of this organ and to distortion during fixation and mounting for light microscopy (Schmeitzel, 1988). The male organ of sperm transfer, the aedeagus or penis, extends from between the third and fourth pair of legs to the posterior of the body of the male mite and is a straight structure. The aedeagus of *Cheyletiella parasitivorax* is highly curved and resembles the blade of a scythe. Scanning electron microscopy can be of considerable help in the identification of species (Marchiondo and Foxx, 1978).

The eggs of *Cheyletiella* are often the means by which a diagnosis of cheyletiellosis is made, eggs being attached to the hair shaft at the pole (Grant, 1989). Eggs are 235 to 245 μm long by 115 to 135 μm wide (smaller than louse nits) and supported by cocoon-like structures bound to the hair shaft by strands of fibers (Ewing et al., 1967). Two or three eggs may be bound together on one hair shaft (Grant, 1989).

Life Cycle

The life cycle is spent entirely on the cat. These are nonburrowing mites, feeding on the keratin layer of the epidermis. There are five developmental stages in the life cycle of this surface-dwelling mite: egg, larva, nymph I, nymph II, and adult (Kwochka, 1987). The adult mite attaches eggs to hair (Foley, 1991). The larvae that emerge from the eggs have three pairs of legs, while each subsequent nymphal stage and the adult stages possess four pairs. Should the motile stages of this mite leave the definitive host, they usually die within 48 hours; however, female mites have been known to survive for as long as 10 days off the host under refrigerated conditions (Schmeitzel, 1988). The prepatent period for *Cheyletiella* species has been reported to range from 21 (Kwochka, 1987; Scheidt, 1987) to 35 days (Scott and Horn, 1987; Schmeitzel, 1988; Paradis et al., 1990; Foley, 1991).

The mites are very mobile and, as a result, are very contagious by direct contact. "Walking dandruff" can spread easily through a cattery (Foley, 1991). Mites of *Cheyletiella* species have been found on fleas, flies, and lice; Kwochka (1987) and Scott and Horn (1987) hypothesized that these larger ectoparasites may play a significant role in the animal-to-animal spread of cheyletiellosis.

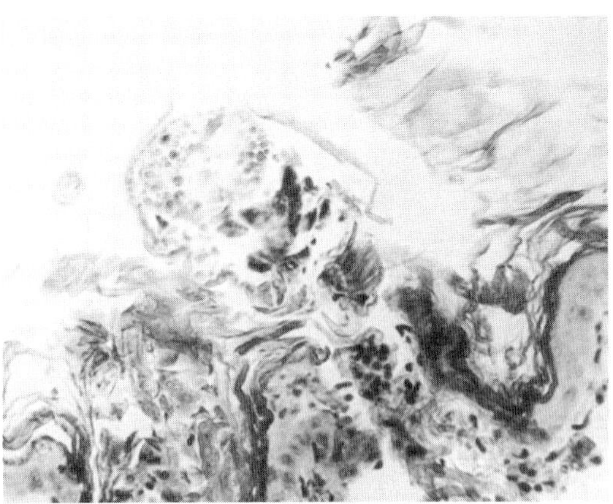

Fig. 5.27. *Cheyletiella* species. Histological section through a *Cheyletiella blakei* feeding on cat skin; the large palpal claw is evident in the section.

Clinical Presentation and Pathogenesis

The mites feed relatively superficially on the skin of their feline host (Fig. 5.27). The most characteristic clinical sign of an infestation with *Cheyletiella* species is the moving white flakes along the dorsal midline and head of the cat (Foley, 1991). Cheyletiellosis in cats has been described as a more localized dorsal crusting along the back with minimal or no pruritus. Cats will occasionally exhibit a diffuse miliary dermatitis that is characterized by reddish yellow crusted lesions. Scaling may be present (Kwochka, 1987).

Cats are often asymptomatic carriers. This feature may be due to the meticulous grooming habits of the feline that may reduce the level of infestation (Schmeitzel, 1988; Paradis et al., 1990). Frequently the first sign of cheyletiellosis is the development on the owner of an erythematous, papular, pruritic dermatitis. The lesions typically affect areas of close contact with the cat, particularly on the arms or trunk (Grant, 1989). Infested cats may manifest variable degrees of dermatitis or be asymptomatic carriers.

Diagnosis

Magnifying loupes and selective removal of questionable flakes or hairs is perhaps the quickest method of diagnosing cheyletiellosis (Foley, 1991). Multiple, repeated skin scrapings may be required as the mites are especially difficult to demonstrate (Scheidt, 1987; Paradis et al. 1990).

The "flea comb and potassium hydroxide (KOH) technique" has proven to be a reliable diagnostic technique. In this procedure, a flea comb is used to collect epidermal debris from a 10 cm by 10 cm area over the lumbosacral area. Material is placed in a 15 ml centrifuge tube with 1 ml of 10 percent KOH and heated in a water bath until hair and remains are dissolved (approximately 30 minutes). Saturated sugar solution is added to form a meniscus, a coverslip is applied, and the tube centrifuged at 1,500 rotations per minute for 10 minutes. The coverslip is then removed, placed on a glass slide, and examined microscopically under low power for eggs and the varied developmental stages of *Cheyletiella* species (Paradis et al., 1990).

Combing dandruff-like debris onto black paper often facilitates visualization of these highly mobile mites. Using clear cellophane tape to entrap mites collected from the haircoat often simplifies localization and viewing under the compound microscope (Merchant, 1990). Epidermal debris may be collected using a small vacuum cleaner and the debris subjected to examination (Schmeitzel, 1988).

Some fastidious cats may demonstrate mites and/or eggs on fecal flotation (Scheidt, 1987; Foley, 1991). Eggs observed in fecal flotation are large (230 by 100 μm) and embryonated. They are three to four times as large as hookworm eggs. The egg is characteristic in that high-powered microscopical examination of the pole of the egg in which the anterior of the mite is developing will reveal two small arrowheads or harpoons protruding from the surface of the eggshell.

Skin biopsy reveals a perivascular dermatitis that is spongiotic and hyperplastic. The perivascular dermal infiltrate contains neutrophils, mononuclear cells, and a few too many neutrophils. Sections of mites may be observed (Schmeitzel, 1988).

Treatment

Cheyletiella species are very sensitive to most insecticides. In warmer ecosystems where conventional, year-round flea control is practiced on animals, *Cheyletiella* infestations have been inadvertently eradicated. However, since these mites can live in the environment for up to 10 days, complete eradication in enzootic areas may be difficult, demanding the services of a professional exterminator (Scheidt, 1987).

Antiseborrheic shampoos are helpful in removing heavy scales and crusts prior to using an acaricide on the cat (Kwochka, 1987). Cheyletiellosis is usually treated by applications of topical acaricides in dip, powder, or shampoo forms. Treatment must be repeated four to eight times at weekly intervals (Paradis et al., 1990). Pyrethrins, carbaryl, rotenone powder, and lime sulfur dip are safe for use on cats (Foley, 1991). Due to the high degree of contagiousness with cheyletiellid mites, all of the animals in the household or cattery must be treated (Schmeitzel, 1988). The environment must be cleaned and treated with a residual acaricide to prevent reinfestation by any mites that might survive off the host. The services of a professional exterminator may be indicated (Scheidt, 1987).

Ivermectin has demonstrated good efficacy against *Cheyletiella* species in clinical trials at a dosage of 300 μg/kg body weight once by subcutaneous injection. This dosage should be repeated in 5 weeks (Paradis et al., 1990). The owner must be made aware of the fact that ivermectin is not currently licensed for use in cats and a release agreement or owner's consent form should be signed prior to its administration (Jackson, 1977). The product should not be given to kittens (O'Dair and Shaw, 1991). Ivermectin may be especially effective in controlling infestations of *Cheyletiella* species in households with many cats, when used by owners who are physically disabled, or when conventional therapies fail (Paradis et al., 1990).

Selamectin and fipronil both may be highly efficacious in treating infestations with this mite.

Epizootiology

Sporadic outbreaks of cheyletiellosis are common. Severe infestations can occur in litters, catteries, breeding farms, or pet shops (Merchant, 1990). Cheyletiellosis demonstrates no perceptible age, breed, or sex predilection (Scott and Horn, 1987). It has been suggested that the incidence and severity of clinical signs in the feline are greater in long-haired cats (Scheidt, 1987). In a survey of feline skin disorders seen in a university practice, Scott and Paradis (1990) noted that Himalayan cats accounted for 50 percent of the cases of cheyletiellosis. These mites are transmitted by both direct and indirect contact. It has been hypothesized that fleas, flies, and lice may play a transport role in the spread of *Cheyletiella* species from animal to animal (Scott and Horn, 1987). Fomites (e.g., grooming tools) have also been implicated in this transmission (Kwochka, 1987). With regard to age incidence, puppies and kittens appear to be most susceptible (Foley, 1991).

Hazards to Other Animals

This mite is extremely contagious and can affect rabbits, dogs, and humans (Grant, 1989); however, it is highly likely that the species on the cat prefers a feline host even though these mites are not host specific (Prescott, 1984; Foley, 1991).

Hazards to Humans

As mentioned previously, human infestation with *Cheyletiella* species was first reported in 1918 (Lomholt, 1918). Humans, especially cattery personnel, are highly susceptible to infestation by *Cheyletiella* species (Foley, 1991).

Human involvement has been reported to occur in 20 to 80 percent of the cases in cats and dogs. Human cheyletiellosis lesions may begin as single or grouped erythematous macules. These rapidly evolve into papules. The lesions frequently become vesicular or pustular and in time develop a central necrotic area. Pruritus is intense. Parts of the body that may be affected include the arms, legs, and torso. The face is rarely affected. Other lesions may include bullae, urticaria, erythema multiforme, and generalized pruritus without dermatitis (Scott and Horn, 1987). Skin scrapings from humans with *Cheyletiella* species are rarely positive. Diagnosis is often based on demonstration of mites or eggs, clinical history, clinical signs, and response to elimination of the mites. *Cheyletiella blakei* cannot complete its life cycle on humans. The induced dermatitis spontaneously regresses within 3 weeks following elimination of the mites (Scott and Horn, 1987).

Control/Prevention

Since the mites are easily destroyed by most common insecticides, the owner often "cures" the pet when he or she treats it with flea control products. All in-contact animals must be treated (Kwochka, 1987).

Because the female mite can survive up to 10 days off of the host (Schmeitzel, 1988), the premises must be thoroughly cleaned and sprayed with a residual insecticide (acaricide) such as microencapsulated pyrethrins and microencapsulated chlorpyrifos. A professional exterminator should be consulted to ensure complete application. Foggers may be used to ensure that the furniture where cats may jump and sleep is properly treated (Kwochka, 1987).

REFERENCES

Bronswijk JEMH, Kreek EJ. 1976. *Cheyletiella* (Acari: Cheyletiellidae) of dog, cat and domesticated rabbit, a review. J Med Entomol 13:315–327.

Dal Tio R, Taraglio S, Tomidei M, Vercelli A. 1990. Dermatite da *Cheyletiella*. Descrizione di otto casi e revisione della letteratura. G Ital Dermatol Venerol 125:19–24.

Dinçer S, Karaer Z. 1985. The first report on *Cheyletiella blakei* Smiley, 1970 (Acari: Cheyletiellidae) on a cat in Turkey. A U Vet Fac Derg 32: 250–257.

Ewing SA, Mosier JE, Foxx TS. 1967. Occurrence of *Cheyletiella* spp. on dogs with skin lesions. J Am Vet Med Assoc 151:64–67.

Faravelli G, Genchi C. 1984. Dermatitis, due to *Cheyletiella parasitivorax* Megnin, 1878 (Acarina, Cheyletidae) in man contracted from cat. G Malat Infet Parassit 36:831–833.

Faravelli G, Traldi G. 1985. La cheyletiellosi del gatto. Bollettina AIVPA 24:225–228.

Foley RH. 1991. Parasitic mites of dogs and cats. Comp Cont Educ Pract Vet 13:783–801.

Grant DI. 1989. Parasitic diseases in cats. J Sm Anim Pract 30:250–254.

Hirst S. 1917. On the occurrence of a pseudoparasitic mite (*Cheyletiella parasitivorax,* Mégnin) on the domestic cat. Ann Nat Hist Ser 8 20:132–133.

Jackson RF. 1977. The activity of levamisole against the various stages of *Dirofilaria immitis* in the dog. Proc Heartworm Symp, '77, pp 111–116.

Keh B, Lane RS, Shachter SP. 1987. *Cheyletiella blakei,* an ectoparasite of cats, as cause of cryptic arthropod infestations affecting humans. West J Med 146:192–194.

Kwochka KW. 1987. Mites and related disease. Vet Clin N Am 17:1263–1284.

Lomholt S. 1918. To tilfaelde af dyrefnat hos memmesket (*Cheiletiella parasitivorax*). Hospitaltidende 61:1098–1099.

Marchiondo AA, Foxx TS. 1978. Scanning electron microscopy of the solenidion on genu I of *Cheyletiella yasguri* and *C. parasitivorax.* J Parasitol 64:925–927.

Mégnin JP. 1878. Mémorie sur les cheylétides parasites. J Anat Physiol, Paris 14:416–441.

Merchant SR. 1990. Zoonotic diseases with cutaneous manifestations—Part I. Comp Cont Educ Pract Vet 12:371–378.
O'Dair HA, Shaw SE. 1991. Mite treatment of cats. Vet Rec 129:272.
Paradis M, Scott D, Villeneuve A. 1990. Efficacy of ivermectin against *Cheyletiella blakei* infestation in cats. J Am Anim Hosp Assoc 26:125–128.
Prescott CW. 1984. Parasitic Diseases of the Cat in Australia. Sydney, Australia: Post-graduate Foundation in Veterinary Science. Pp 69–71.
Reed CM. 1961. *Cheyletiella parasitivorax* [sic] infestation of pups. J Am Vet Med Assoc 138:306–307.
Scheidt VJ. 1987. Common feline ectoparasites part 2: *Notoedres cati, Demodex cati, Cheyletiella* spp. and *Otodectes cynotis*. Feline Pract 17(3):13–23.
Schmeitzel LP. 1988. Cheyletiellosis and scabies. Vet Clin N Am 18:1069–1076.
Scott DW, Horn RT, Jr. 1987. Zoonotic dermatoses of dogs and cats. Vet Clin N Am 17:117–144.
Scott DW, Paradis M. 1990. A survey of canine and feline skin disorders seen in a university practice: Small Animal Clinic, University of Montréal, Saint-Hyacinthe, Québec (1987–1988). Can Vet J 31:830–835.
Smiley RL. 1970. A review of the family Cheyletiellidae Acarina. Ann Entomol Soc Am 63:1056–1078.
Smith EK. 1988. How to detect common skin mites through skin scrapings. Vet Med 83:165–170.
Wikerhauser T, Pinter L. 1987. Parasitic mite *Cheyletiella blakei* in a cat. First case report in Yugoslavia. Vet Arhiv 57:63–70.

Demodex cati Hirst, 1919

Etymology

Demos = tallow and *dex* = woodworm, along with *cati* for the feline host.

Synonyms

Demodex folliculorum var. *cati* Megnin, 1877.

History

In 1859, Leydig stated that the cat was host to a species of *Demodex*. In 1877, Megnin described the species in the cat as *Demodex folliculorum* var. *cati* and gave the description: "This is a diminutive of the caninus variety having exactly its features with all dimensions reduced by one fourth." Hirst (1919) elevated the mite to specific status and presented a brief description of the species. In 1979, Desch and Nutting redescribed *Demodex cati* Hirst, 1919, and provided illustrations of all life cycle stages.

Geographic Distribution

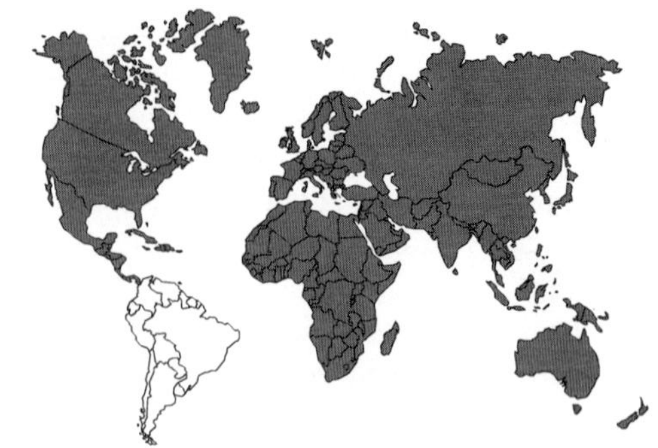

Fig. 5.28.

Cases of feline demodicosis due to *Demodex cati* have been described from North America, Europe, Australia, New Caledonia, Africa, and India (Beugnet and Chardonnet, 1993; Chesney, 1989; Yathiraj et al., 1994). Foley (1995) described feline demodicosis as "the least commonly diagnosed disease associated with mites in cats."

Location in Host

The mites live within the hair follicles of the cat (Fig. 5.29). The hair follicles that are most often infested include those of the eyelids, face, chin, or neck.

Parasite Identification

The mites are cigar shaped with very short legs (Desch and Nutting, 1979) (Fig. 5.30). The adult mites and nymphs possess eight very short legs, while the larval stage and protonymph possess six legs. The adult male mite is 182 μm long and 20 μm wide. The adult female is 220 μm long and about 30 μm wide. The eggs are 70.5 μm long and about 21 μm wide. In both the male and female, the opisthosoma makes up two-thirds of the total body length—the body is composed of the opisthoma (tail), the podosoma (body with legs), and the gnathosoma (anterior end with jaws). The other species of *Demodex* that occurs in the cat has a much shorter opisthosoma relative to the total body length.

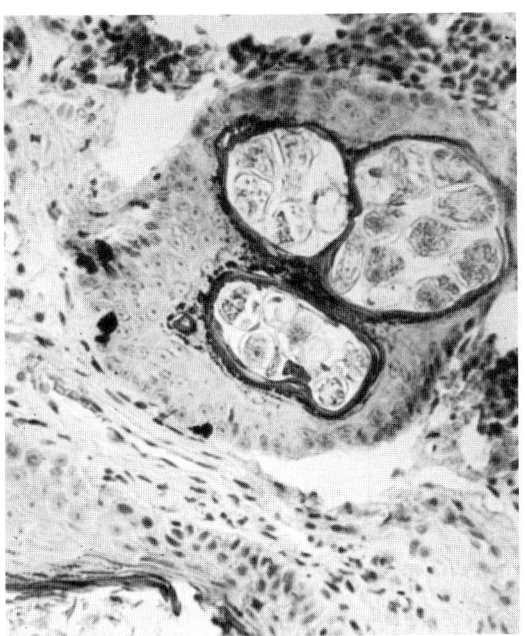

Fig. 5.29. *Demodex cati.* Section through a hair follicle containing numerous sections through mites.

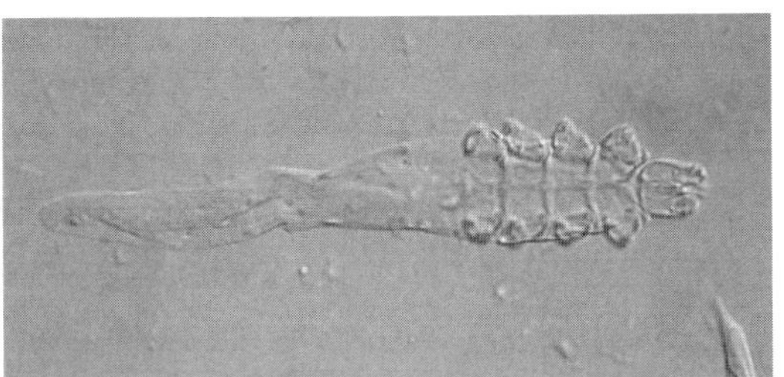

Fig. 5.30. *Demodex* species. Note the elongate body and very short legs.

Life Cycle

Although all life-cycle stages were described by Desch and Nutting (1979), there has been no specific work on the life cycle of *Demodex cati.* It is assumed that it is similar to that of *Demodex brevis* of humans. Basically, eggs are laid within the epidermal cavity, and the eggs hatch to produce a six-legged larval stage. The larva then develops to a six-legged protonymph, and finally to an eight-legged nymph. The adults also have eight legs, and it appears that the female is diploid and the male is haploid.

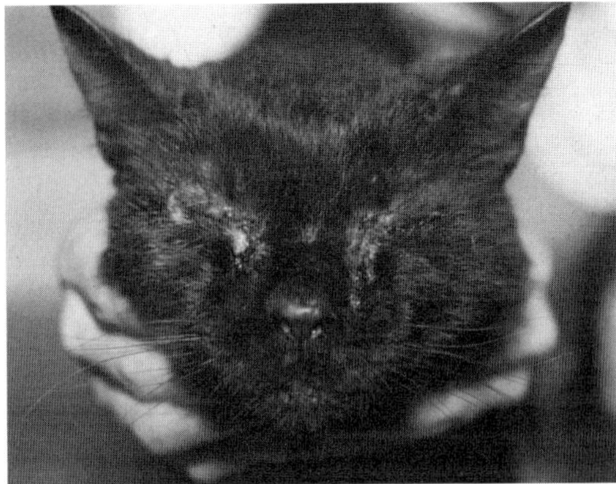

Fig. 5.31. Feline demodicosis. (Image provided by Dr. Robert Foley)

Clinical Presentation and Pathogenesis

Two forms of feline demodicosis, localized and generalized, are recognized (Foley, 1995). The localized form typically is associated with lesions that appear as acne or as erythematous patches of alopecia on the eyelids, face, chin, or neck (Fig. 5.31). The generalized form of the disease is considered by Foley (1995) to be represented by cats that have more than five lesion sites or more than one affected body region. Chesney (1989) reviewed 35 published cases of demodicosis in cats. Cases were reported in cats between 1 to 18 years of age, and there was no apparent predisposition for the disease to develop in young animals. There seemed to be no correlation with breed or sex, although it is possible that demodicosis may be slightly more common in Siamese and Burmese cats. Unlike dogs, in cats pyoderma is rare in generalized demodicosis.

It is believed that generalized demodicosis is more apt to appear in cats with underlying immunologic disorders or as sequelae to other infections (Chalmers et al., 1989). Systemic illnesses associated with generalized demodicosis include diabetes mellitus, Cushing's disease, feline leukemia virus infection, systemic lupus erythematosus, feline immunodeficiency virus infection, and toxoplasmosis (Guaguère, 1993).

Treatment

Treatment of feline demodicosis is usually successful (Foley, 1991). Treatments include 2.5 percent lime-sulfur dips, carbaryl shampoos, and malathion dips. Half-strength amitraz dips (0.0125 percent) have been found effective against feline demodicosis (Cowan and Campbell, 1988). Foley (1995) found that localized infestation with *Demodex cati* responds well to parenteral ivermectin (300 µg ivermectin/kg body weight) and 2.5 percent lime-sulfur immersion in the same protocol. In addition, he has treated with topical follicular flushing with 5 percent benzoyl peroxide gel, which he believes hastens resolution of the infestation. Foley (1995) believes generalized *Demodex cati* infestations have a more guarded prognosis if the cat is immunocompromised or has underlying severe disease. Therapy for the generalized form includes parenteral ivermectin again at 300 µg ivermectin per kilogram body weight. It has also been shown that extralabel amitraz immersion can be used in cats at half-strength (0.0125 percent) at weekly intervals to minimize the toxic side effects of sedation, salivation, hyperglycemia, and insulin resistance. The side effects of amitraz preclude its use in diabetic cats or in cats owned by diabetic clients without appropriate gloves and barriers being used during dipping (Foley, 1995). In one case of generalized demodicosis, ivermectin seemed to reduce mite numbers, but fresh lesions continued to appear in spite of ivermectin treatment (Yathiraj et al., 1994). In this case, treatment with 0.0125 percent amitraz baths (three treatments, at weekly intervals) caused the lesions to regress and the resolution of lesions by 50 days after the beginning of weekly amitraz therapy.

Epizootiology

Very little is known about the epizootiology of feline demodicosis. It is suspected that the mite is highly host specific and that most cats obtain their infections while nursing as kittens. However, none of these questions have been carefully analyzed experimentally.

Hazards to Other Animals

The mite is believed to be highly host specific and to be restricted to the domestic cat. Demodicosis in snow leopards, *Panthera uncia,* has recently been described as a new species, *Demodex uncii,* which is said to closely resemble *Demodex cati* (Desch, 1993).

Hazards to Humans

It is not believed that *Demodex cati* is transmissible to humans.

Control/Prevention

It is believed that many cats are infested with these mites at birth and that transmission between cats is unlikely.

REFERENCES

Beugnet F, Chardonnet L. 1993. Otite demodecique chex un chat. Rev d'Elev Med Vet Nouvelle Caledonie. 17:5–7.

Chalmers S, Schick RO, Jeffers J. 1989. Demodicosis in two cats seropositive for feline immunodeficiency virus. JAVMA 194:256–257.

Chesney CJ. 1989. Demodicosis in the cat. J Sm Anim Pract 30:689–695.

Cowan LA, Campbell K. 1988. Generalized demodicosis in a cat responsive to amitraz. JAVMA 192: 1442–1444.

Desch CE. 1993. A new species of hair follicle mite (Acari: Demodecidae) from the snow leopard, *Pathera uncia* (Schreber, 1775) (Felidae). Int J Acarol 19:63–67.

Desch C, Nutting WB. 1979. *Demodex cati* Hirst 1919: a redescription. Cornell Vet 69:280–285.

Foley RH. 1991. Parasite mites of dogs and cats. Comp Cont Educ Pract Vet 13:783–800.

Foley RH. 1995. Feline demodicosis. Comp Cont Educ Pract Vet 17:481–487.

Guaguère E. 1993. Démodécie féline: étude réetrospective de 9 cas. Prot Med Chir Anim Comp 28: 31–36.

Hirst S. 1919. Studies on Acari. I. The genus *Demodex,* Owen. Br Mus (Nat Hist). 53 pp.

Leydig F. 1859. Ueber Haarsakmilben und Krätzmilben. Arch Natur Berlin 1:338–354.

Megnin P. 1877. Memoire sur le *Demodex folliculorum* Owen. J Anat Physil 13:97–122.

Yathiraj S, Thimmappa Rai M, Madhava Rao P. 1994. Treatment of generalised demodicosis in a cat—a case report. Ind Vet J 71:393–395.

Demodex gatoi Desch and Stewart, 1999

A cat in Louisiana, was recently found to harbor a new species of *Demodex* that was different from *Demodex cati* and that is different from the species that has not yet been described (see the next section). The cat from which these mites were recovered was infested with both *Demodex cati* and the new species, *Demodex gatoi*. The cat was believed to be suffering from some form of immunodeficiency, and it had alopecia and scaly, crusty dermatitis of the face, neck, and ears. *Demodex gatoi*, like the unnamed species reported from the cat, lives on the epidermal surface rather than in hair follicles.

REFERENCES

Desch CE, Stewart TB. 1999. *Demodex gatoi:* new species of hair follicle mite (Acari: Demodecidae) from the domestic cat (Carnivora: Felidae). J Med Entomol 36:167–170.

Demodex Species

Etymology

Demos = tallow and *dex* = woodworm; this mite has not been assigned a specific name.

Synonyms

This mite has been recognized as separate from *Demodex cati*, but no specific name has been given.

History

Conroy et al. (1982) sent specimens of a *Demodex* recovered from a cat to Drs. Nutting and Desch for identification. They were informed that the specimens appeared distinct from *Demodex cati* and were similar in appearance to *Demodex criceti*, which resides in the stratum corneum of the hamster. Chesney (1989) in his review of feline demodicosis summarized seven reports of feline infestations with this mite. Chesney also felt that the reports by Gabbert and Feldman (1976) and White and Ihrke (1983) probably dealt with this unnamed species based on the photographs of the mite that accompanied these case presentations. Chesney went on to discuss the report of Keep (1981) and stated that these mites were also likely to be the unnamed species based on the description of the mites provided by Keep. Since the review of Chesney, additional cases of demodicosis due to this unnamed species have been reported: three cases by Guaguère (1993) and three cases by Morris (1996).

Geographic Distribution

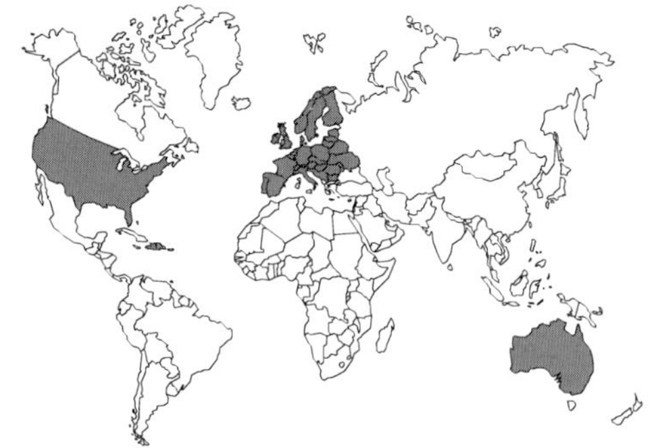

Fig. 5.32.

This unnamed species of mite has been reported from the United States (eight cases), from Europe (five cases), and from Australia (one case). Chesney (1989) reported that the unnamed species occurred in the United States in a domestic longhaired cat (Trimmier, 1966), a Siamese cat (Gabbert and Feldman, 1976), a Siamese cat (Conroy et al., 1982), a domestic shorthaired cat (Muller, 1983), a domestic shorthaired cat (McDougal and Novak, 1986), and two domestic shorthaired cats (Medleau et al., 1988). Morris (1996) described infection in three Siamese cats in the United States. Chesney (1989) described two cases from Europe: one from France in a domestic shorthaired cat (Carlotti et al., 1986) and one from England in a domestic longhaired cat (Chesney, 1988). Guaguère (1993) described three additional cases in domestic shorthaired cats in France. One Australian case is that of Wilkinson (1983) in a domestic shorthaired cat. Thus, of the 14 cases described, 5 have been described in Siamese cats, and all cases in Siamese cats have occurred in North America.

Location in Host

The unnamed *Demodex* that occurs in cats is found in the stratum corneum rather than in hair follicles. Two other species of *Demodex* that have been described from this location in their host include *Demodex criceti* of the hamster (Nutting and Rauch, 1958) and a species of *Demodex* that parasitizes *Onychomys leucogaster*, the grasshopper mouse (Nutting et al., 1973).

Parasite Identification

Chesney (1988) described two forms of the parasite. The longer form measured about 143 to 148 μm in total length (gnathosoma, 17 to 19 μm; podosoma, 56 to 58 μm; and opisthosoma, 66 to 73 μm) with a maximum width of 37 to 41 μm. The shorter form was about 110 μm long and 28 μm wide (gnathosoma, 16.5 μm; podosoma, 47 μm; opisthosoma, 47 μm). Foley (1995) gave measurements of 80 to 90 μm by 30 to 35 μm. In the unnamed *Demodex* of the cat, the opisthosoma makes up around 40 percent of the total body length, and in some of the illustrations it appears that significantly less than 40 percent of the total body length is made up of the opisthosoma. In *Demodex cati,* the opisthosoma makes up about two-thirds of the total body length. There is no anus on any of the life cycle stages in the genus *Demodex.*

Life Cycle

Based on the location of the mite in the stratum corneum and the morphological resemblance to *Demodex criceti,* it has been suggested that the biology is similar to that described for *Demodex criceti.* Studies with *Demodex criceti* have indicated that this mite is transferred from mother to young during suckling. Very little else is known concerning this mite, and the different life-cycle stages have not been described in detail. It is assumed that the life cycle is similar to that described for *Demodex brevis.* Thus, a six-legged larva hatches from the egg, develops to a six-legged protonymph, matures to a nymph, and then matures to an adult male or female (Nutting, 1983). Work with *Demodex caprae* of the goat has revealed that only males will develop from fertilized females and that the males are haploid and the females diploid. It is believed that this form of development may be considered advantageous to transfer because a single female, fertilized or not, could ultimately establish a complete colony of mites on a new host. The span of time per stage or for the entire life cycle varies for any given species of *Demodex* (Nutting, 1983). *Demodex auratus* of the golden hamster, *Mesocricetus auratus,* can build up large numbers of all life stages in 35 days; *Demodex folliculorum* has been estimated to complete its cycle in 14.5 days; and *Demodex caprae* has been estimated to undergo a complete cycle in several to 15 weeks (Nutting, 1983). Morris (1996) suggested that a cat that began to cohabitate with two infested cats contracted its infestation from these already infested cats.

Clinical Presentation and Pathogenesis

In the 14 cases of demodicosis due to the unnamed species of *Demodex,* Chesney (1989) considered 10 of the cases to represent generalized demodicosis. The 3 cases described by Guaguère (1993) were all of the localized type, while in the 3 cases described by Morris (1996), numerous mites were obtained from superficial skin scrapings of multiple sites on all animals. This mite typically induces pruritis, excessive grooming, alopecia, scaling, hyperpigmentation, erythema, and excoriation associated with self-abuse with signs suggestive of flea allergy dermatitis, atopy, immune-mediated or eosinophilic skin disease, food allergy, contact dermatitis, notoedric mange, or diabetic neurodermatitis (Foley, 1995).

Many of the cases of infestation with the unnamed species of *Demodex* have been diagnosed after treatment with corticosteroids for the initial presentation of skin lesions, for example, Chesney (1988), Conroy et al. (1982), Medleau et al. (1988), Morris (1996), and Wilkinson (1983). Morris (1996) felt that exogenous corticosteroid therapy as an immunosuppressive factor must remain speculative. Signs in one of his three cases appeared prior to the corticosteroid injections, and the signs resolved after lime-sulfur treatment. Two other cases were shown to actually have developed in cats that had an underlying food allergy. Human cases of demodicosis have developed following the long-term administration of corticosteroid therapy (Hakugawa, 1978; Sato et al., 1965), and rosacea-like demodicosis has been reported in HIV-positive children (Barrio et al., 1996). It is assumed that the mites are already present in these cases and that the immunotherapy causes the mites to increase in numbers.

Treatment

Foley (1995) recommended that cats infested with the unnamed species of feline *Demodex* be treated with parenteral ivermectin (300 μg ivermectin per kilogram bodyweight) along with 2.5 percent lime-sulfur immersion. He believes the mite is vulnerable to treatment with the lime-sulfur regimen alone in many cases because of this mite's localization in the stratum corneum. Foley stated that the prognosis for cats infested with this mite is good.

Epizootiology

Very little is known about the epizootiology of these mites. The report by Morris (1996) would suggest that infestations can be transferred between cats, but this has not been demonstrated in other situations.

Hazards to Other Animals

It is believed that this mite is specific for the feline host.

Hazards to Humans

It is believed that this mite does not infest humans.

Control/Prevention

Control is by the isolation and treatment of infested cats. It is expected that cats are infested while nursing although there is no direct evidence that this occurs.

REFERENCES

Barrio J, Lecona M, Hernanz JM, Sanchez M, Gurbindo MD, Lazaro P, Barrio JL. 1996. Rosacea-like demodicosis in an HIV-positive child. Dermatology (Switzerland) 192:143–145.

Carlotti D, Lemaire C, Lavayssiere J, Magnool JP. 1986. Le demodecie feline. A propos de trouis cas. Prat Med Chir Anim Comp 21:203–208.

Chesney CJ. 1988. An unusual species of *Demodex* mite in a cat Vet Rec 123:671–673.

Chesney CJ. 1989. Demodicosis in the cat. J Sm Anim Pract 30:689–695.

Conroy JD, Healey MC, Bane AG. 1982. New *Demodex* sp. infesting a cat: a case report. J Am Anim Hosp Assoc 18:405–407.

Foley RH. 1995. Feline demodicosis. Comp Cont Educ Pract Vet 17:481–487.

Gabbert N, Feldman BF. 1976. Feline demodex. Feline Pract 6:32–33.

Guaguère E. 1993. Démodécie féline: étude réetrospective de 9 cas. Prot Med Chir Anim Comp 28:31–36.

Hakugawa S. 1978. *Demodex folliculorum* infection on the face—abnormal parasitis of *Demodex folliculorum* observable with persons using topical steroid preparation habitually on the face. W Jap Dermatol 40:275.

Keep JM. 1981. Feline Dermatoses. Sydney, Australia: University of Sydney Post-Graduate Federation in Veterinary Science.

McDougal WJ, Novak CP. 1986. Feline demodicosis caused by an unnamed *Demodex* mite. Comp Cont Educ Pract Vet 8:820–822.

Medleau L, Brown CA, Brown SA, Jones CS. 1988. Demodicosis in cats. J Am Anim Hosp Assoc 24:85–91.

Morris DO. 1996. Contagious demodicosis in three cats residing in a common household. J Am Anim Hosp Assoc 32:350–352.

Muller GH. 1983. Feline demodicosis. In Current Veterinary Therapy, vol VIII, p 487. Philadelphia, Pa: WB Saunders.

Nutting WB. 1983. Biology and pathology of hair follicle mites (Demodicidae). In Cutaneous Infestations of Man and Animal, ed LC Parsih, WB Nutting, RM Schwartsman, pp 181–199. New York, NY: Praeger.

Nutting WB, Rauch H. 1958. *Demodex criceti* n. species (Acarina: Demodicidae) with notes on its biology. J Parasitol 44:328–333.

Nutting WB, Satterfield LC, Cosgrove GE. 1973. *Demodex* sp. infesting tongue, esophagus, and oral cavity of *Onychomys leucogaster,* the grasshopper mouse. J Parasitol 59:893–896.

Sato Y, Higuchi H, Saito U. 1965. Demodectic eczematoid eruption on the face of a boy receiving a long-term corticosteroid treatment. Jap J Dermatol 75:331.

Trimmier WR. 1966. Demodicosis in a cat. Southwest Vet 20:57–58.

White SD, Ihrke PJ. 1983. Feline Medicine. Ed. PW Pratt, p 541. Santa Barbara, Calif: American Veterinary Publications.

Wilkinson GT. 1983. Demodicosis in a cat due to a new mite species. Feline Pract 13:32–35.

Trombiculid Mites: Chiggers

Synonyms

Chiggers, red bugs, harvest mites, itch mites, scrub mites, bichos colorados, bêtes rouges, rouget, herbstmilben, akamushi, tsutsugamushi, kedani, (Wharton and Fuller, 1952), heel-bugs, black soil itch mites, lepte automnale, aoutat, scrub itch mites, and duck-shooters itch mites (Prescott, 1984).

History

Trombiculid mites (chiggers) are pestiferous mites that attack man, his domestic animals, and wild animals. Knowledge of chiggers probably extends back to prehistoric times. Reference to chiggers in the Western Hemisphere does not occur prior to 1733; however, there are references to this mite as early as the sixth century in China. In 1758, Linnaeus described a single species of chigger *Acarus batatas* (*Trombicula batatas*). Most of the information concerning chiggers and the problems they cause in man was garnered during and following World War II. Wharton and Fuller (1952) noted the cat has served as host to eight species of chiggers: *Trombicula* (*Eutrombicula*) *alfreddugesi*, *Trombicula* (*Leptotrombidium*) *akamushi*, *Trombicula* (*Leptotrombidium*) *legacy*, *Trombicula* (*Neotrombicula*) *autumnalis*, *Trombicula* (*Neotrombicula*) *shannoni*, *Euschöngastia westraliense*, *Acomatacarus* (*Acomatacarus*) *adelaideae*, and *Acomatacarus* (*Acomatacarus*) *australiensis*. *Walchia americana* has also been implicated as a parasite of cats (Lowenstine et al., 1979). Prescott (1984) noted five species that have been described on cats: *Bryobia praetiosa*, *Leeuwenhoekia australiensis*, *Leeuwenhoekia adelaidiae*, *Schongastia phillipinensis*, and *Schongastia westraliensis*.

Geographic Distribution

Over 10,000 species of chiggers have been recorded from throughout the world. It is indeed fortunate that not all chiggers produce itch reactions in man and his domestic animals (Harwood and James, 1979). Virtually every continent serves as habitat to chiggers who feed avidly on vertebrate hosts.

Location in Host

In animals other than man, cutaneous lesions tend to be restricted to areas that come in contact with the ground (e.g., the head, ears, limbs, interdigital areas, and ventrum). Other areas on the body of the host may also be infested (Greene et al., 1985). In cats, the external ear is usually involved; an acute inflammatory disease of the ear canal may also occur (Bullmore et al., 1976).

Parasite Identification

The six-legged chigger larva is 200 to 400 μm in diameter. The body of the larval chigger is more or less rounded. The genera of veterinary importance possess a single dorsal scutum and four to six setae (hairs). The palpal tibia has three setae and a terminal claw. The palpal tarsus usually possesses four to seven setae. The palpal tarsus articulates and opposes the tibial claw in a thumb-like manner. The dorsal body setae posterior to the scutum are on the venter between and posterior to the coxae. Each coxa bears at least one plumose seta.

The nonparasitic adult chiggers are about 1 mm long. They may be oval to figure-eight-shaped. They are covered with tiny, dense hairs, giving them a velvet-like appearance. The color of the adult is usually bright red.

Life Cycle

The number of generations per year will vary from species to species and with the local climatic conditions. The eggs of the chigger are spherical. After 1 week, the eggshell splits, revealing the maturing larva or deutovum. The larval chigger is six legged and is the only stage that is parasitic on vertebrates. Larvae are parasitic on a wide variety of vertebrates—animals, birds, reptiles, and humans. The most common hosts are small rodents. The larval mite attaches to the host. Its salivary secretions form a tube (stylostome) through which the larvae suck up liquefied host tissues. Once it is replete, the engorged larva drops off the host and passes into a quiescent prenymphal stage. The nymphal and adult chiggers are eight legged and nonparasitic. The nymph passes into a quiescent preadult stage before molting to the adult. The normal food of the adult chigger is insect eggs and inactive soil invertebrates. Female chiggers are inseminated by males. There is no evidence to support parthenogenesis. One adult female mite often produces many eggs. As a result, the emerging larvae are amassed together in one site in their woodland habitat. Any unwitting mammalian (feline, human, or other) host that enters this site can be parasitized by many mites at a single instance.

Clinical Presentation and Pathogenesis

Chigger larvae do not burrow into the skin as commonly believed (Fig. 5.33). Neither do they feed primarily on blood. Their food consists of the serous components of tissue. A few red blood

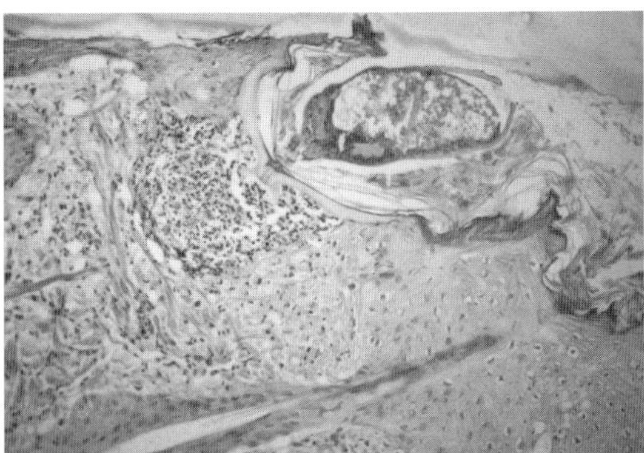

Fig. 5.33. Histologic section of a chigger feeding on the ear of a cat.

cells may be ingested during feeding. Chiggers attach firmly to the definitive host and inject a digestive fluid that produces cellular autolysis. The cytoplasm becomes disorganized and the nuclei fragmented. The host's skin becomes hardened, and a tube called a stylostome forms at the chigger's attachment site. When the mite is satiated, it loosens and falls to the ground. The action of the digestive fluid causes the attachment site to itch after a few hours. The digestive secretions may produce an intense pruritus that may result in self-excoriation (Prescott, 1984).

Bullmore et al. (1976) described a case of chigger infestation in a cat that presented with dry, crusty lesions on the anterior margins of both ears. Chiggers (*Trombicula alfreddugesi*) appeared as multiple orange-red dots within the crusty areas. Lowenstine et al. (1979) presented a similar case of chiggers in a cat that presented with anorexia and reluctance to move. The cat was alert, affectionate, and well nourished but demonstrated a diffuse nodular thickening of the skin. When the cat walked, it would periodically lift one of its hind limbs and shake it as if it had stepped in something. The skin lesions could be readily palpated but could not be observed until the fur was parted or clipped. The skin of the ventrum and the medial aspect of all limbs and the interdigital spaces was nonpliable and thickened. The skin surface was cracked and scaly with moist serous exudate or dried yellow debris. Papules 0.1 to 0.3 cm in diameter were scattered over the sides of the trunk, behind the ears, and around the vulva and anus. Some of the papules were crusted with yellow exudate; all were accompanied by a mild wheal and flare reaction. Indication of self-excoriation was minor. Greene et al. (1985) described trombiculiasis in an 8-year-old domestic shorthair cat with a history of a crusting dermatosis. This cat exhibited multifocal orange crusts on the head and on the base of the external canal of the left ear. Prescott (1984) cited Wilson-Hanson, who reported a case of trombiculosis in a male cat with primary lesions on the ears, the auricular and frontal regions, and the region of the genitalia. Irritation from the chiggers or self-trauma (or both) produce marked edema and urinary retention. A lesion later appeared at the commissure of the lips.

Diagnosis

The diagnosis of trombiculosis is based on the presence of an orange, crusting dermatosis, a history of exposure (roaming the outdoors), identification of the typical six-legged larva on skin scrapings, and histopathologic findings.

In a case described by Lowenstine et al. (1979), microscopic lesions were limited to the epidermis and dermis. This case of trombiculosis is unusual in that the chiggers burrowed deep within the epidermis. The authors were unable to determine if the mites actually burrowed this deeply or whether the skin reactions and proliferation of surface tissue buried them. Epidermal lesions were multifocal, both proliferative and degenerative, and associated with mites located either in tunnels or in regions of inflammation. Some aggregates of hair follicles had undergone acanthosis, loss of hair shafts, near or complete obliteration of follicular lumens by keratinizing epithelium, and fusion of follicles, resulting in epithelial islands that resembled squamous cell carcinoma. Dermal changes were typical of acute allergic dermatitis and were characterized by dilated capillaries, fibrocytes with plump nuclei, and eosinophils and mast cells, which were numerous adjacent to and within edematous regions.

Treatment

Chiggers may be physically removed or removed by application of a 1 percent solution of malathion, or any other acaricide recommended for use on cats. Older remedies include potassium sulphurata and lime sulphur. Rotenone dusting powder has been used to treat for chiggers on cats. Carbaryl powder (5 percent) has been demonstrated to be effective (Prescott, 1984).

Epizootiology

The dermatitis produced by these parasites is usually seen from spring (Prescott, 1984) to late summer and fall (Bullmore et al., 1976). The number of generations per year will vary with the species and local climate.

As mentioned previously, a single adult female mite is capable of producing many eggs. As a result, the emerging larvae are amassed together in one site in their woodland habitat. The natural hosts of the larval chiggers are in most cases small rodents. However, any unwitting mammalian (feline, human, or other) host that enters this habitat may be parasitized by many mites at a single instance.

The larval chiggers typically congregate in a shaded area near the top of a blade of grass or a fallen leaf. Here they remain quiescent until they are stimulated by an air current containing carbon dioxide from an approaching vertebrate host. Some species may remain on the ground.

Hazards to Other Animals

In the wild, chiggers normally feed on mammalian hosts including monotremes, marsupials, insectivores, chiropteres, primates, edentates, lagomorphs, rodents, carnivores, artiodactyls, birds, reptiles, and amphibians and even on nonmammalian hosts such as houseflies, scorpions, and millipedes (Wharton and Fuller, 1952). Larval mites have caused death in chickens from anemia (Prescott, 1984). The chiggers that are causing lesions on the cat will typically not then move onto the pet owner; it is more likely that both the owner and the pet will be infested at the same time.

Hazards to Humans

Human infestations are most commonly acquired by frequenting woodland surroundings (Greene et al., 1985). On humans, chigger larvae attach themselves on the part of the body constricted by clothing. With the exception of the intense pruritus produced, the public health significance of trombiculiasis is minor. The infested pet (cat or dog) rarely acts as a mechanical vector (Greene et al., 1985). Mites in the family Trombiculidae, genus *Leptotrombidium,* are known to be vectors of *Rickettsia tsutsugamushi,* the etiologic agent of scrub typhus.

Control/Prevention

Attack by chiggers can be almost completely prevented by using repellents. Humans often apply repellents to skin and clothing or wear clothing impregnated with repellents (deet, dimethyl phthalate, dimethyl carbate, and ethyl hexanediol). Application of repellents to cats exposed to chigger-infested areas may prove to be impractical. Cats should not be allowed to roam freely (Hendrix and Blagburn, 1983).

A more practical solution to the problem might be the use of sprays or dusts of approved acaricides applied to vegetation around premises. Controlling habitat and natural hosts of chigger mites can also reduce their numbers.

REFERENCES

Bullmore CC, Weiss ME, Phillips JT, Gebhart RN. 1976. Feline trombiculiasis. Feline Pract 6:36.

Greene RT, Scheidt VJ, Moncol DJ. 1985. Trombiculiasis in a cat. J Am Vet Med Assoc 188:1054–1055.

Harwood RF, James MT. 1979. Helminths, Arthropods, and Protozoa of Domesticated Animals. 7th edition. New York, NY: Macmillan. Pp 352–357, 366–370.

Hendrix CM, Blagburn BL. 1983. Common gastrointestinal parasites. Vet Clin N Am 13:627–646.

Lowenstine LJ, Carpenter JL, Oconnor BM. 1979. Trombiculosis in a cat. J Am Vet Med Assoc 175:289–292.

Prescott CW. 1984. Parasitic Diseases of the Cat in Australia. Sydney, Australia: Post-graduate Foundation in Veterinary Science. Pp 68–69.

Wharton GW, Fuller HS. 1952. A Manual of the Chiggers. Washington, DC: Entomological Society of Washington. Pp 1–185.

ASTIGMATA

The astigmatid mites, as suggested by the name, are characterized by a lack of stigmata. These mites tend to be small and to have lightly sclerotized bodies. The third and fourth pairs of legs tend to exit the body some distance behind the first and second pairs of legs. The end of each leg is a tarsal segment that bears the sucker-like feet that support the mite. Some members of Astigmata are free-living mites that feed on organic matter. Other astigmatid mites are external feather mites of birds, live in the quills of feathers, or burrow into the skin of birds; two families are actually internal parasites of birds. The astigmatid mites contain several important parasites of large animals (e.g., *Psoroptes ovis, Chorioptes bovis,* and *Sarcoptes scabiei*).

There are four astigmatid mites that are of importance in feline parasitology: *Otodectes cynotis,* the ear mite of dogs and cats; *Notoedres cati,* the mange mite of cats and rabbits; *Sarcoptes scabiei,* the mange mite of dogs, humans, and other hosts; and *Lynxacarus radovskyi,* the hair-clasping mite of tropical cats. These mites tend to be slow moving and weakly sclerotized. Respiration is integumental (i.e., there are no stigmata). The largest of these mites is *Otodectes;* the smallest is *Notoedres. Otodectes, Sarcoptes,* and *Notoedres* are similar to each other in appearance. These are rather dorsally compressed and round mites that have short legs that terminate in sucker-like feet typical of the astigmatid mites. Although the legs of *Lynxacarus* also terminate in sucker-like feet, the general appearance of this mite is much different than that of the other three found on cats. The body of *Lynxacarus* is elongate and appears laterally compressed. *Otodectes cynotis* is usually found in the ear canal where the mites wander around on the surface of the skin, *Notoedres cati* is found in burrows in the skin (usually on the ears and face), and *Lynxacarus radovskyi* is found clinging to the hairs of the cat (often around the anus and on the tail); *Sarcoptes scabiei* is only rarely found on cats.

Otodectes cynotis (Hering, 1838) Canestrini, 1894

Etymology

Oto = Ear and *dectes* = a beggar, along with *cynotis,* Greek for "of the dog."

Synonyms

The synonyms are listed by Sweatmean (1958): *Sarcoptes cynotis* Hering, 1838; *Sarcoptes auricularum* Lucas and Nicolet, 1849; Sarcoptes *auricularum* var. cati *Lucas* and Nicolet, 1849; *Symbiotes canis* Bendz, 1859; *Symbiotes felis* Huber, 1860; *Chorioptes ecaudatus* Mégnin, 1896; *Choriptes ecaudatus* var. *catotis* Mégnin, 1877; *Choriptes ecaudatus* var. *furonis* Mégnin, 1878; *Psoroptes auricularis* var. *canis* Sewell, 1891; *Symbiotes auricularum* var. *canis* Neumann, 1892; *Symbiotes auricularum* var. *cati* Neumann, 1892; *Symbiotes auricularum* var. *furonis* Neumann, 1892; *Sarcoptes auricularum* var. *canis* Railliet, 1893; *Otodectes furonis* Canestrini, 1894; *Chorioptes cynotis* var. *canis* Neumann, 1914; *Chorioptes cynotis* var. *felis* Neumann, 1914; *Chorioptes cynotis* var. *furonis* Neumann, 1914; *Otodectes cynotis* var. *canis* Neveu-Lemaire, 1938; *Otodectes cynotis* var. *cati* Neveu-Lemaire, 1938; *Otodectes cynotis* var. *furonis* Neveu-Lemaire, 1938. Sweatman felt that there was no difference between the different varieties occurring in the cat, the dog, the ferret, and other hosts.

History

This mite has been long known to occur in the ears of canids, foxes, cats, and ferrets. At times, different species names have been assigned to the forms occurring in different hosts, but there is little evidence that they are separate species. Mites from cats have been transferred to dogs, and the infections have been found to persist for varying lengths of times in the canine host (Railliet and Cadiot, 1892; Sweatman, 1958; Tonn, 1962).

Geographic Distribution

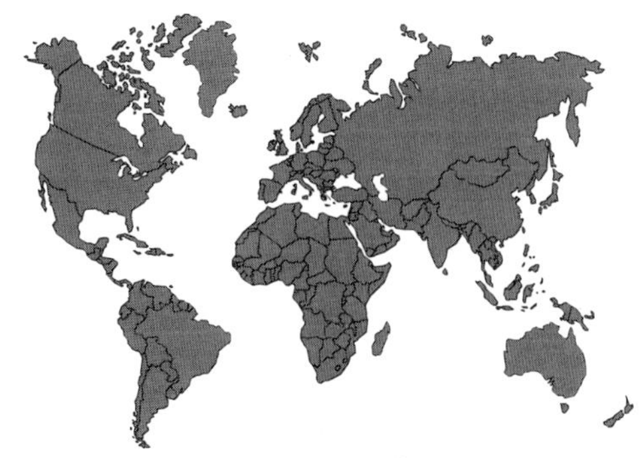

Fig. 5.34.

This mite is found around the world. Reports from different areas include the Americas (Foley, 1991), Europe (Raschka et al., 1994; Trotti et al., 1990), Asia (Fukase et al., 1991, Tacal and Sison, 1969), Middle East (Ismail et al., 1982), and Australia (Coman et al., 1981).

Location in Host

The mites live in the ear canal of the cat. Large numbers of mites (greater than 1,000) can be present in each ear without any apparent mites appearing on the surface of the feline host.

Parasite Identification

Identification is relatively simple. No other nonburrowing mites of this large size are typically found in the ears of the cat. The living mites appear as small white organisms that can be seen moving about within the ears or on swabs of deteritus removed from the ears. The larval mites have a length of 138–224 μm. The adult male is 274 to 362 μm in length. The ovigerous female is between 345 to 451 μm in length (Fig. 5.35). An examination of the distal portions, pretarsi, of the anterior pairs of legs will reveal the "wine-glass-shaped" caruncle on a short pedicel. The male mites have a caruncle on all four pairs of legs, while the third and fourth pairs of legs on the female terminate in long hairs or setae. The posterior of the body of the male also possesses two ventrally situated suckers that are used for the attachment of the male mite to a deutonymph as part of the life cycle (Fig. 5.36). The eggs are white, oval, slightly flattened on one side, and 166 to 206 μm long (Fig. 5.37).

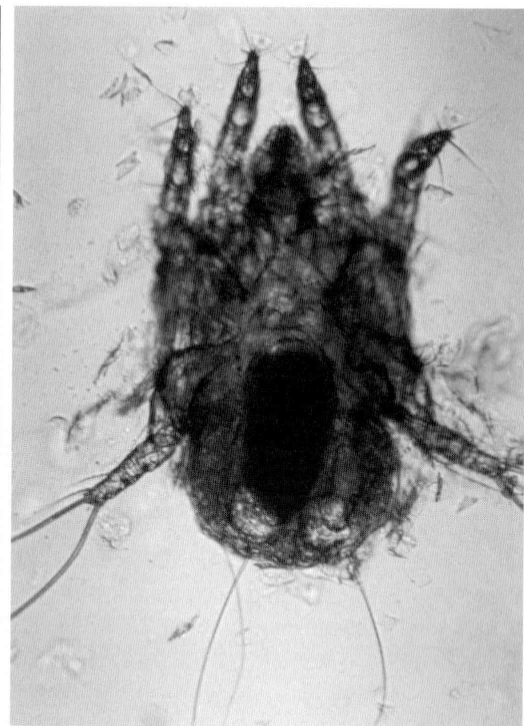

Fig. 5.35. *Otodectes cynotis.* Living adult female. An egg is apparent within the body of this mite.

Life Cycle

Almost all the work on the life cycle was performed by Sweatman (1958). He showed that the eggs laid by the female mites are glued to the ear canal by a secretion from the female mite. The eggs typically required 4 days of incubation prior to hatching. The life cycle includes a larva, a protonymph, and a deutonymph. Each stage takes a minimum of around 3 to 5 days to develop, and the development is followed by a quiescent period of about 24 hours during which time the mites molt and shed their cuticles (ecdyse). As soon as the adult male emerges from a deutonymph cuticle, it will seek out a deutonymph. Sweatman showed that the male mites could not distinguish between male and female deutonymphs and sometimes formed attachments with deutonymphs that developed into males. He also showed that unless the female deutonymphs developed in the presence of a male, the females were infertile and later matings did not occur. Sweatman was under the opinion that copulation occurred at the time when the adult female first shed its deutonymphal exoskeleton. He found that the complete egg-to-egg cycle took approximately 18 to 28 days, or about three weeks. Upon transfer of female mites to cats in Leningrad in August, December, and May, Shustrova (1988) revealed that eggs were laid 2 days and 8 to 10 days after transfer. The larvae hatched in 2 to 4 days in May and August and hatched in 6 to 7 days in December. They felt the full life cycle took 13 to 15 days in the warmer months and 3 weeks in the colder months. They also found that the mites were found at greater depths during colder temperatures.

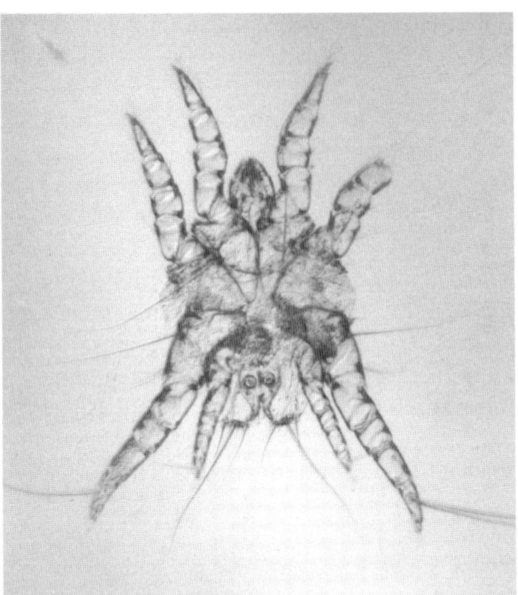

Fig. 5.36. *Otodectes cynotis.* Adult male. The suckers on the posterior end of the body are quite evident in this prepared specimen.

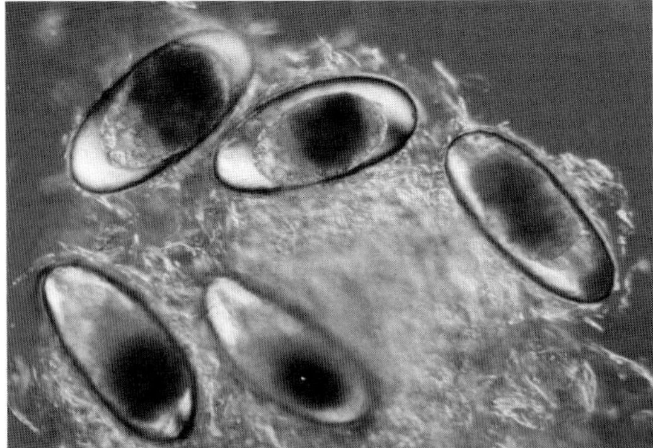

Fig. 5.37. *Otodectes cynotis.* Eggs in detritus removed with a swab from a cat's ear.

Transmission between hosts is probably by direct contact. The mites seem to require a relatively high relative humidity for survival and seem to rapidly desiccate at typical room humidities. Sweatman (1958) found that he could maintain mites for months in vitro by placing them in a 35°C incubator with a relative humidity of 80 percent. Tonn (1962) found by examination of brushings of the hair of the posterior body and flanks of naturally infested cats that the collected material could contain living mites. Thus, it is possible that mites can be found on the surface of their feline host.

Sweatman (1958) fed mites maintained in vitro detritus collected from the ears of dogs and cats, and he was convinced that the mites were basically scavengers not requiring either blood or tissue fluids from the host. The ability to complete the entire cycle in vitro would suggest that there is some validity in this observation. Powell et al. (1980), on the other hand, felt that the presence of feline antigens in mites indicated that the mites were actively feeding on fluids or blood from their feline host.

Clinical Presentation and Pathogenesis

Cats vary remarkably in their abilities to serve as hosts for *Otodectes cynotis*. Observations on a number of cats at necropsy has revealed that some cats can have what appear to be severe lesions with significant quantities of dark cerumen and sometimes even blood present in their ears but only have one or two mites. Other cats will have very clean ear canals, almost devoid of cerumen and detritus, and have 50 to 100 mites present. Still other cats can be host to huge numbers of mites, almost 2,000 per ear, and still will have shown very little in the way of outward signs of infection. Over 8,500 mites have been found at necropsy in a single auditory tube of an infested cat (Preisler, 1985). Ears of cats with very large numbers of mites tend to contain a dry, waxy, parchment-like material that occurs as sheets throughout the ear canal. These sheets will contain mites throughout and consist in part of rafts of eggs that are embedded in the material. These ears tend not to contain large quantities of wax.

Powell et al. (1980) transferred 30 mites into the right ear of each of four laboratory-reared cats. By 7 to 14 days after infestation, an accumulation of red-brown cerumen appeared in the right horizontal ear canal of all four cats. In two cats, red-brown cerumen appeared in the left ear along with mites—in one case 49 days after the infestation of the right ear and in the other case 62 days after the infestation of the right ear. Observations showed that the cats maintained their infestations without spontaneous clearing for at least 9 months and apparently without secondary invasion by bacteria or fungi. These authors also showed that the infested cats developed IgE antibodies to *Otodectes cynotis* by day 14 after infestation. Earlier work by this group (Weisbroth et al., 1974) had shown that there are probably five major histologic components associated with ear mite infestations: (1) the epithelial surface was overlaid with a crusty, waxy, crumbly material; (2) the epithelium had hyperkeratotic and hyperplastic areas; (3) ceruminous and sebaceous glands appeared to have undergone dramatic reactive hyperplasia; (4) inflammatory cells (particularly mast cells and macrophages) were present in greatly increased numbers; and (5) the blood vessels, particularly venules, underlying the dermis were generally dilated.

Lesions on the body due to generalized infestations with *Otodectes cynotis* have been reported in cats and dogs (Kraft et al., 1988). Guaguere (1992) reported on a case of miliary dermatitis in a 4-year-old cat with lesions on the neck and the back. The cat was treated with Amitraz, and the lesions were noted to have significantly regressed and the coexistent ear-mite infestation to have cleared 6 weeks later upon reexamination.

Diagnosis

The mites can be recognized on otoscopic examination by observing movement. Another means of diagnosis is to swab the ear with a cotton-tipped applicator and to place the swab in a glass serum vial with a *small* drop of water. After about an hour, the mites will begin to migrate out of the cerumen and detritus and can be observed walking on the walls of the glass vial or on the applicator stick. Smearing the ear swab onto a glass slide and examining under 40× magnification usually reveals the mites also.

Treatment

The products approved for the treatment of ear mites in cats in the United States of America include pyrethrin-containing compounds (Otomite Allerder/Virbac, Nolvamite® Fort Dodge; Eradimite® Solvay; Aurimite® Schering Plough) and rotenone-containing compounds (Ear Miticide Phoenix; Ear Mite Lotion Durvet; Ear Miticide Vedco). Also, Otomax, a mineral-oil-based otic ointment containing gentamicin sulfate, betamethasone valerate, and clotrimazole, has been shown to have some apparent effect against ear mites in cats (Pappas and Katz, 1995). As part of a trial testing the efficacy of another mineral-oil-based compound, one of the authors this book (Bowman) used 2 ml of mineral oil and 30 seconds of external massage of the base of the ear in the control cats and found that after two treatments 1 week apart there were no mites found in any of the control cats 3 weeks after the second treatment. This large volume of mineral oil tended to leak from the ear, and the hair on the head of the cat would appear oiled for the first day or so after treatment.

Treatment with a phytoaromatic gel, canidor (a mixture of 15 volatile oils), has been examined for its ability to treat ear mite infestations in cats (Mignon and Losson, 1996). This aromatherapy treatment of four cats on days 0, 1, 2, 3, 10, 11, 12, and 13 seemed to be highly effective in removing the mites from the ears of these animals.

Lindane-containing solutions have been examined for their ability to control *Otodectes cynotis* in cats (Gassner et al., 1995). These studies showed that the same preparation with and without lindane was highly effective in removing the mites from the ears of cats, although neither solution was 100 percent effective. The treatments were administered daily to both ears over a 6-day period.

Ivermectin injectable, although not approved for use in cats, has been used to treat feline infestations with *Otodectes cynotis* (Blakstad, 1993; Foley, 1991; Song, 1992). Typical dosages are 0.2 to 0.225 mg/kg injected on one occasion or on two occasions with a 3-week interval between injections. Some cats given over 0.5 mg ivermectin per kilogram body weight have developed signs of ivermectin toxicity (Song, 1992). There have also been reports of toxicity in kittens receiving off-label injections of ivermectin (Frischke and Hunt, 1991; Lewis et al., 1994), and one of these kittens died 7 days after the administration of ivermectin (Lewis et al., 1994). Another approach has been the direct application of the ivermectin into the ear canals of the cats. This method was described by Jeneskog and Falk (1990) as used in the successful elimination of infestations with *Otodectes cynotis* from a laboratory cat breeding colony. Gram et al. (1994) compared subcutaneous administration of 0.3 mg ivermectin per kilogram body weight *versus* the topical application of 0.5 mg of ivermectin into the ear canal. When additional treatments were required, they were given at 1- or 2-week intervals. Cats were otoscopically negative for mites after 2.2 injections or 3.4 topical treatments. To cure cats of their mite infestations (as determined by two consecutive otoscopic examinations 1 to 2 weeks apart), an average of 4.2 subcutaneous treatments were required, while the average for the topical applications was 5.4 treatments. Five of the 14 topically treated cats had an apparent recurrence of their mite infestation during the follow-up period.

More recently, selamectin has been shown to be highly efficacious in the treatment of ear mites in cats (Shanks et al., 2000). Acarexx (Blue Ridge Pharmaceuticals), a liposome formulation containing 0.01 perecent ivermectin, has been approved for the treatment of ear mites in cats.

Epizootiology

As mentioned above, it appears that the cycle may take longer in cold weather than in warm weather (Shustrova, 1988). Grono (1969) surveyed dogs for the presence of ear mites by examination at necropsy. Grono found 22 of 350 dogs in Australia that had mites in one ear and suppurative otitis externa without mites in the other ear. He felt that this was indicative of the mites causing a progression wherein they initiated conditions conducive to otitis externa but then disappeared when the site of infestation was no longer favorable for survival.

It is not known which stage of the mite typically initiates infestations in naturally infested cats. Adults, eggs, and larvae appear to be capable of causing infections under experimental conditions. It is expected, however, that one stage is likely to possess a greater ability to seek out other hosts than the other stages, but this may not actually occur.

Hazards to Other Animals

Otodectes cynotis is transmissible to other household pets, most notably dogs and ferrets. Thus, if these hosts are present in a household, it is necessary to treat all of these animals on the premises.

Hazards to Humans

Two individuals have been found to be infested with mites identified as *Otodectes cynotis*. Herwick (1978) reported on a rather anecdotal case of ear mites biting a Californian lady on the torso and the extremities who recently received a new cocker spaniel that was infested; no mites were actually found on the woman. A second case (Heyning and Thienpont, 1977) reported on otitis in a Belgian farmer's wife. In this case, one adult male, one adult female, and four larvae were recovered from crusts on the eardrum of the right ear.

Control/Prevention

It is very important that all susceptible animals be treated if a case of otodectic mange is diagnosed in a household. Animals with clean ears containing no detritus can harbor mites, and thus, even if no signs of infestation are present, it is important that the animals be treated. When very heavy levels of infestation are present, it may be warranted to try and bathe the infected animals, especially in those cases where topical treatment methods are employed. Monthly treatments with selamectin would be highly efficacious.

REFERENCES

Blakstad E. 1993. Ivermectin in the treatment of ear mites in cats. Norsk Vet 105:621–626.

Coman BJ, Jones EH, Driesen MA. 1981. Helminth parasites and arthropods of feral cats. Aust Vet J 57:324–327.

Foley RH. 1991. Parasitic mites of dogs and cats. Comp Cont Educ Pract Vet 13:783–800.

Frischke H, Hunt L. 1991. Suspected ivermectin toxicity in kittens. Can Vet J 32:245.

Fukase T, Hayashi S, Sugano H, Shikata R, Chinone S, Itagaki H. 1991. Ivermectin treatment of *Otodectes cynotis* infestation of dogs and cats. J Vet Med, Japan 44:160–165.

Gassner G, Albrecht N, Hart S, Johannes B, Keyserlingk-Eberius M. 1995. Prüfung zweier Otitispräparate (lindanhaltic und lindanfrei) zur Behandlung der Otitis externa parasitaria von Hund und Katze. Kleintierpraxis 40:361–372.

Gram D, Payton AJ, Gerig TM, Bevier D. 1994. Treating ear mites in cats: a comparison of subcutaneous and topical ivermectin. Vet Med 89:1122–1125.

Grono LR. 1969. Studies of the ear mite, *Otodectes cynotis*. Vet Rec 85:6–8.

Guaguere E. 1992. Dermatite miliaire a *Otodectes cynotis* chez un chat. Pract Med Chirurg L'Anim Comp 27:705–708.

Herwick RP. 1978. Lesions caused by canine ear mites. Arch Dermatol 114:130.
Heyning JF, Thienpont D. 1977. Otitis externa in man caused by the mite *Otodectes cynotis*. Laryngoscope 87:1938–1941.
Ismail NS, Toor MA, Abdel-Hafez SK. 1982. Prevalence of ectoparasites of cats from northern Jordan. Pak Vet J 2:164–166.
Jeneskog T, Falk K. 1990. The effect of local ivermectin treatment on ear mite infestation in a cat breeding colony. Scand J Lab Anim Sci 17:17–22.
Kraft W, Kraiss-Gothe A, Gothe R. 1988. Die *Otodectes-cynotis*-Infestation von Hund und Katze: Erregerbiologie, Epidemiologie, und Diagnose sowie Fallbeschreibungen generalisierter Räuden bein Hunder. Tierärztl Prax 16:409–415.
Lewis DT, Merchant SR, Neer TM. 1994. Ivermectin toxicosis in a kitten. JAVMA 205:584–586.
Mignon BR, Losson BJ. 1996. Efficacy of a phyto-aromatic gel against auricular mange in rabbits and carnivores. Vet Rec 138:329–332.
Neumann LG. 1897. A Treatise on the Parasites and Parasitic Disease of the Domestic Animals. New York, NY: Williams R. Jenkins.
Pappas C, Katz TL. 1995. Evaluation of a treatment for the ear mite, *Otodectes cynotis,* in kittens. Feline Pract 23:21–24.
Powell MB, Weisbroth SH, Roth L, Wilhelmsen C. 1980. Reaginic hypersensitivity in *Otodectes cynotis* infestation of cats and mode of mite feeding. Am J Vet Res 41:877–882.
Preisler J. 1985. Incidence of ear mites, *Otodectes cynotis,* on some carnivores in the territory of CSR. Folia Parasitol 32:82.
Raschka C, Ribbeck R, Haupt W. 1994. Untersuchungen zum Ektoparasitenbefall bei streuenden Katzen. Mh Vet Med 49:257–261.
Shanks DJ, McTier TL, Rowan TG, Watson P, Thomas CA, Bowman DD, Hair JA, Pengo G, Genchi C, Smothers CD, Smith DG, Jernigan AD. 2000. The efficacy of selamectin in the treatment of naturally acquired aural infestations of *Otodectes cynotis* on dogs and cats. Vet Parasitol 91:283–290.
Shustrova MV. 1988. Experimental study of the biology of the causative organism of ear mange. Ekologo-populyatsionnyi analiz parazito-khozyainnykh otnoshenii 145–151 [cited in CAB Abstracts].
Song MD. 1992. Using ivermectin to treat feline dermatoses caused by external parasites. Vet Med 86: 498–502.
Sweatman GK. 1958. Biology of *Otodectes cynotis,* the ear canker mite of carnivores. Can J Zool 36: 849–862.
Tacal JV, Sison JA. 1969. *Otodectes cynotis:* a study of inapparent infestations in dogs and cats. Philipp J Vet Med 1969:881–891.
Tonn RJ. 1962. Studies on the ear mite *Otodectes cynotis,* including life cycle. Ann Ent Soc Am 54:416–421.
Trotti GC, Corradini L, Visconti S. 1990. Parasitological investigations in a cattery in Ferrara. Parassitologia 32:42–43.
Weisbroth SH, Powell MB, Roth L, Scher S. 1974. Immunopathology of naturally occurring otodectic otoacariasis in the domestic cat. JAVMA 165: 1088–1093.
Wilson-Hanson SL, Prescott CW. 1982. A survey for parasites in cats. Aust Vet J 59:194.

Notoedres cati (Hering, 1838) Railliet, 1893

Etymology

Noto = back and *edres* = seat, referring to the dorsal location of the anus, along with *cati* for the feline host.

Synonyms

Sarcoptes cati Hering, 1838; *Sarcoptes scabiei* var. *cati* (Gerlach, 1857); *Sarcoptes caniculi* of Gerlach, 1857.

History

Notoedres cati has been known as a parasite of cats for several centuries. Early on, it was considered a variety or small form of *Sarcoptes scabiei* of man and the dog. Then in 1893, Railliet defined the genus as *Notoedres.* Fain (1965) placed the species that is found to infest rabbits, *Sarcoptes caniculi,* Gerlach, 1857, in synonymy with *Notoedres cati.* The genus *Notoedres* mainly parasitizes rats and bats; a species has been reported from primates. Carnivores from which specimens of *Notoedres* have been recovered include members of the Felidae and *Nasua nasua,* the coatimundi (Fain, 1965).

Geographic Distribution

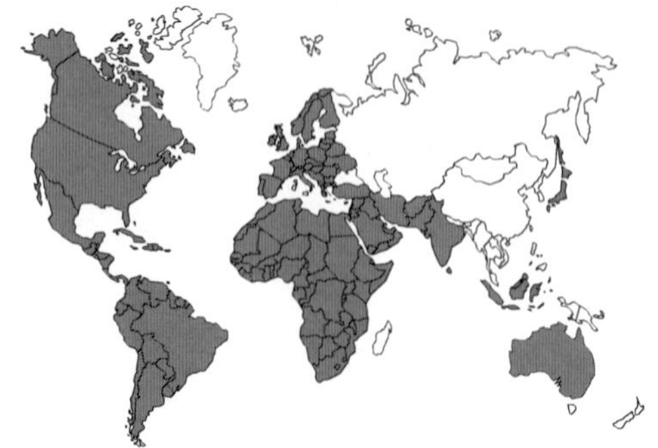

Fig. 5.38.

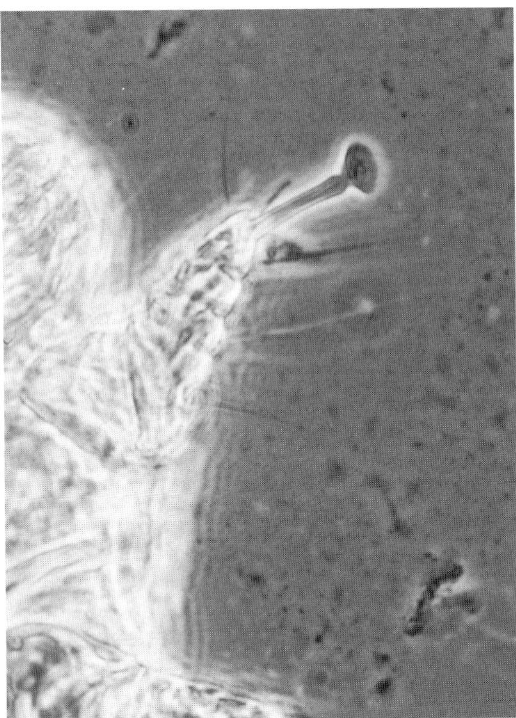

Fig. 5.39. *Notoedres cati.* Sarcoptiform long and unsegmented pretarus.

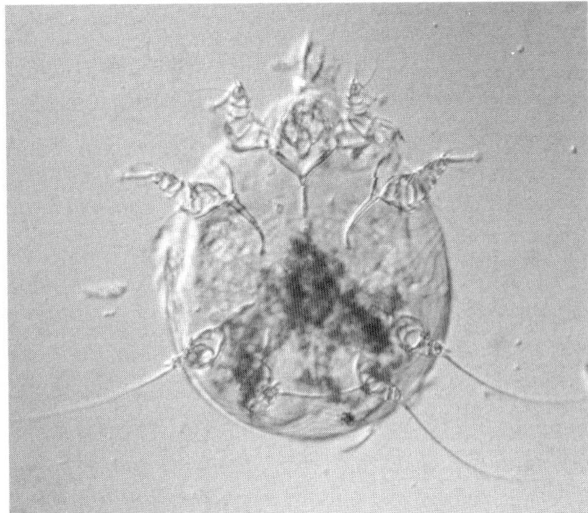

Fig. 5.40. *Notoedres cati.* Adult female ventral view.

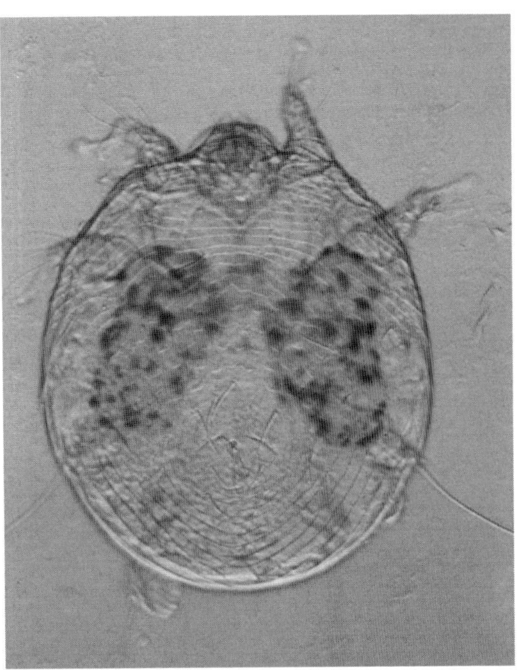

Fig. 5.41. *Notoedres cati.* Dorsal view of adult female showing the dorsally situated anus.

Notoedric mange has been reported in cats in Europe (Bigler et al., 1984; Fabbrini, 1994; Hartmannova and Mouka, 1990; Svalastoga et al., 1980; Tudury and Lorenzoni, 1987), the Middle East (Rak, 1972), India (Yathiraj et al., 1994); Africa (Zumpf, 1961); Japan (Ogata et al., 1980), Indonesia (Sangvaranond, 1979), Australia (Wilson-Hanson and Prescott, 1982), North America (Foley, 1991a), and South America (Larsson, 1989).

Location in Host

The mites live in burrows in the epidermis of the cat; the rather deep burrows are on occasion below the stratum corneum.

Parasite Identification

Notoedres cati can be recognized by its small size and typical sarcoptiform pretarsi with a long, unbranched pedicel (Fig. 5.39). The most characteristic feature is the dorsal anus, which differentiates this mite from *Sarcoptes scabiei* (Figs. 5.40 and 5.41). The adult male has sucker-like feet on the first, second, and fourth pairs of legs; the female has sucker-like feet only on the first two pairs of legs. The adults measure 200 μm by 240 μm and are round with very short legs.

Life Cycle

Notoedres cati produce deep burrows within the dermis of infested cats (Foley, 1991b). The life cycle of *Notoedres cati* is considered to be similar to that of *Sarcoptes scabiei,* but there has been no detailed description of the life cycle of *Notoedres cati.* Schuurmans-Stekhoven and Notokworo (1921) described the morphology of the larva and the adult female of *Notoedres cati.* He noted that the larva only had 6 legs and that only the first two pairs of legs ended in the sucker-like appendages. He gave the length of the larva as between 87 µm and 166 µm with a width of around 80 µm. The measurements for the nymphal stage were 168 µm to 210 µm in length by 130 µm to 183 µm in width. Measurements for two female specimens were 234 µm by 168 µm and 216 µm by 192 µm.

Gordon et al. (1943) examined the life cycle of *Notoedres notoedres* in the white rat. It is expected that the life cycle that occurs with *Notoedres cati* is similar to that which they described for *Notoedres notoedres.* The females of *Notoedres notoedres* lay eggs in burrows in the epidermis; sometimes the female excavates a small cave and lays a small semicircle of eggs. The number of eggs per tunnel may vary from 11 to 25. Females lay three to four eggs each day. The eggs normally hatch 4 to 5 days after oviposition. After the larvae hatch from the eggs, they typically leave the tunnels where they were born and move to the surface of the skin. The larva migrates about on the skin and then prepares a molting burrow (i.e., the larva stops its migration and digs a small burrow in the skin); this takes between 25 minutes to 4.5 hours once it begins digging and crawls inside. Once inside the molting burrow, the larva stays there for 4 to 5 days before it is ready to molt to the first nymphal stage; this molting takes an additional 2 days. About 5 to 7 days are spent as a larva. The nymph leaves the larval molting burrow and wanders off to find another place in which it excavates a second burrow. This burrow is in the stratum corneum and is only just deep enough to cover the mite. In fact, the posterior tip of the nymph often can be seen protruding through the entrance to the burrow. After a couple days in this new burrow, the nymph again undergoes ecdysis to become a second nymphal stage after having spent about 3 to 5 days in the first nymphal stage. After ecdysis, the second nymphal stage goes out and digs a third molting burrow where it molts to the adult stage. About 3 to 5 days are spent in this second nymphal stage. The adult can appear as early as 12 days after the larva hatches from the egg. After molting to adults, the female typically stays in the nymphal molting burrow, but the male tends to leave to look for a female. When the male locates a female, it tunnels down to the female where copulation occurs. The lifespan of the related mite *Sarcoptes scabiei* is thought to be about 2 months. In the case of *Notoedres notoedres,* it is the larvae and nymphs that are typically transferred between hosts.

Clinical Presentation and Pathogenesis

Cats infested with *Notoedres cati* typically present with lichenification of the skin on the ear tips, face, and distal extremities (Foley, 1991a, b; Ribbeck, 1992). The reactions can be severe and in young cats can lead to death (Ribbeck, 1992). Clinical signs include intense pruritis, alopecia, and the formation of crusts on the skin (Fig 5.42). Young and chronically infested cats can become debilitated, and cats can present with leucocytosis and relative and absolute eosinophilia (Foley, 1991a). Foley (1991a) reported that skin biopsy revealed the epidermal penetration of the skin by mites and that the skin was reactive, acanthotic, and hyperkeratotic. Cats may undergo self-mutilation. Foley (1991a) reported that out of 150 cases seen in an epizootic area in the Florida Keys, all cats presented with pruritus and self-mutilation dermatitis and had gray crusts and scale on the skin; weight loss, fever, and alopecia were observed in half the infested cats.

Treatment

Foley (1991a) successfully treated over 500 infested cats with notoedric mange. The treatment typically consisted of the oral or subcutaneous administration of ivermectin (300 µg ivermectin per kilogram body weight). When necessary, cats were also treated with penicillin G benzathine (22,000 U per kilogram body weight) for secondary bacterial infections and with corticosteroids (dexamethasone at 0.33 mg per kilogram body weight) to alleviate self-mutilation and hypersen-

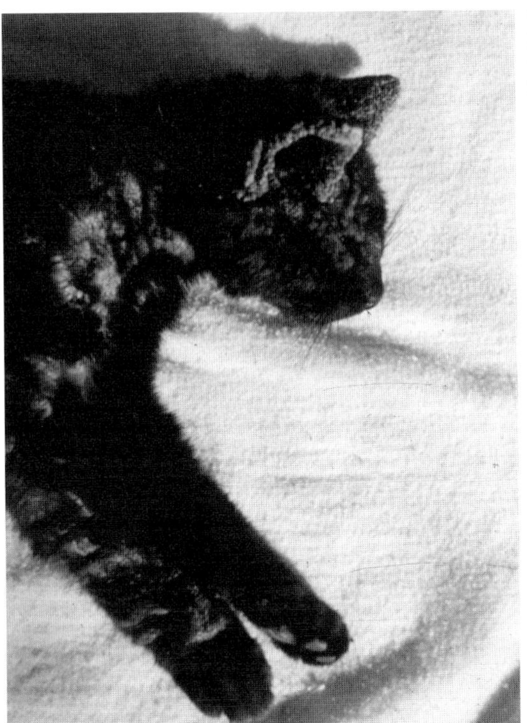

Fig. 5.42. Notoedric mange. Cat with severe crusting lesions due to *Notoedres cati.* (Photograph courtesy of Dr. Robert Foley)

sitivity reactions. Corticosteroids should be given only after treatment of the mite population has been initiated. Pyrethrin shampoos were used to cleanse the cats and soften and remove skin scales. Lime-sulfur dips (2.5 percent) were found to be effective when used weekly for 6 to 8 weeks. Other authors have also reported success with the administration of ivermectin to cats infested with *Notoedres cati;* doses range between 200 µg to 1,000 µg ivermectin per kilogram body weight (Bigler et al., 1984; Fukase et al., 1991; Hartmannova and Mouka, 1990; Olivia and Baldio, 1988; Quintavalla et al., 1985; and Yathiraj et al., 1994); the only side effect noted in these treatments was diarrhea in one cat receiving 1,000 µg ivermectin per kilogram body weight.

Ivermectin toxicity associated with treating notoedric mange has been reported. Tudury and Lorenzoni (1987) treated nine cases of notoedric mange in 60-day-old kittens with 400 µg ivermectin per kilogram body weight administered subcutaneously. Three of the treated kittens had signs of ivermectin toxicity (i.e., motor incoordination, hyperaesthesia, hyperkinesis, mydriasis, and protrusion of the nictitating membrane). These signs disappeared after 36 hours with the affected kittens being treated with a magnesium sulphate cathartic. In all nine treated cases, mites were cleared after treatment.

Selamectin is likely to be highly efficacious against infestations with this mite.

English (1960) had success in treating cats with a 0.5 percent solution of malathion, two times, 7 or 8 days apart. It is important that this be done under veterinary supervision because atropine may have to be administered to some cats that react to the treatment.

Epizootiology

Mites of the genus *Notoedres* are found in cats, rabbits, mice, rats, bats, and one primate (*Galago demidovi pusillus*). Fain (1965) believed that the species reported to cause notoedric mange in rabbits was indistinguishable from that causing disease in cats; thus, Fain synonymized the species from rabbits with that from cats. There has been no published work on the transfer of the mite between rabbits and cats, but it would suggest that cats may acquire their infestations from hunting rabbits. The species in mice and other rodents appear morphologically different from the species that is found on cats and rabbits. Once the organism is in a cat population, it can be highly contagious and spread rapidly between cats and between households (Foley, 1991a).

Hazards to Other Animals

Notoedres cati is likely to be transmitted from infested cats to rabbits. This parasite has also been recorded from *Nasua nasua,* the coatimundi (Fain, 1965). Many members of the Feliudae have been found infested with this parasite: *Felis pardalis,* the ocelot (Pence et al., 1995); *Felis concolor coryi,* the Florida panther (Maehr et al., 1995); *Panthera tigris altaica,* a captive tiger (Malecki and Balcerak, 1988); *Felis rufus,* the bobcat (Pence et al., 1982; Penner and Parke, 1954); *Lynx lynx,* the European lynx (Dobias, 1981); *Uncia uncia,* snow leopards (Fletcher, 1978); and *Acinonyx jubatus,* the cheetah (Young et al., 1972). Thus, it would appear that cats may serve as potential sources of infestation for other feline hosts.

Hazards to Humans

Foley (1991a) reported that clients owning a cat with notoedric mange developed papular and pruritic rash on their arms and forearms that cleared when washed with lime sulfur (the same treatment administered to the cat). Chakrabarti (1986) described an unusual outbreak of notoedric mange in a group of individuals in South Calcutta, India. In this outbreak, 48 individuals lived and worked together in the same building that housed 35 cats. One of the cats was taken to the university veterinary clinic, and the cat was noted to be infested with *Notoedres cati.* It was then decided to examine the household of the owner. It was discovered that 30 of the 35 cats were infested with *Notoedres cati,* 30 of the people living in the building showed signs of notoedric mange, and *Notoedres cati* was recovered from the skin of 15 of these individuals. Most of the lesions appeared on the hands and legs, but lesions were also noted on the face, fingers, and thighs. Feline-associated mange has also been reported from humans in Japan and the former Czechoslovakia (Ito et al., 1968; Nesvadba, 1967). Household outbreaks of feline scabies have also been reported in Germany (Haufe et al., 1966).

Control/Prevention

Control would be by the attempted prevention of the introduction of an already infested cat into an environment where the mite is not present. Similarly, it is possible that cats might become infected by coming into contact with rabbits, either through hunting or through shared living quarters. Thus, attempts must be made to prevent contact with other infected animals. Once a cat is identified as infested, it is important that it be separated from animals that are not infested until it is free of mites. Owners need to be cautioned of the potential spread to other hosts and to themselves.

REFERENCES

Bigler B, Waber S, Pfister K. 1984. Erste erfogversprechende Ergebnisse in der Behandlung von *Notoedres cati* mit Ivermectin. Schweiz Arch Tierheilk 126:365–367.

Chakrabarti A. 1986. Human notoedric scabies from contact with cats infested with *Notoedres cati.* Int J Dermatol 25:646–648.

Dobias J. 1981. Successful treatment of lynx for scabies (*Notoedres cati*). In Verhandlungsberichte des XVI Internationalen Symposiums uber die Erkrankungen der Zootiere 26–30 June 1974, Erfurt, ed R Ippen and HD Schroder. Jena, Germany: Akademie-Verlag.

English PB. 1960. Notoedric mange in cats, with observations on treatment with malathion. Aust Vet J 36:85–88.

Fabbrini F. 1994. Rogna notedrica gerneralizzata in un gatto. Summa 11:61–62.

Fain A. 1965. Notes sur le genre *Notoedres* Tailliet, 1893 (Sarcoptidae: Sarcoptiformes). Acarologia 7:321–342.

Fletcher KC. 1978. Notoedric mange in a litter of snow leopards. JAVMA 173:1231–1232.

Foley RH. 1991a. A notoedric mange epizootic in an island's cat population. Feline Pract 19:8–10.

Foley RH. 1991b. Parasitic mites of dogs and cats. Comp Cont Educ Pract Vet 13:783–800.

Fukase T, Kajiwara T, Sugano H, Shikata R, Chinone S, Itagaki H. 1991. Ivermectin treatment of *Notoedres cati* infestations in cats. J Vet Med Japan 44:41–45.

Gordon RM, Unsworth K, Seaton DR. 1943. The development and transmission of scabies as studied in rodent infections. Ann Trop Med Parasitol 37:174–194.

Hartmannova B, Mouka J. 1990. Lécení králíku, kocek, nutrií a lisek postizenych invazemi nematodu a zákozek ivermectinem. Verterinarstvi 40:122–123.

Haufe U, Meyer D, Hhafe F. 1966. Katzen scabies bein Menschen hervorgerufen durch eine an Sarcoptesräude und Trichophyte erkrankte Katze. Dermatol Wochenschr 152:977–980.

Ito K, Ito Y, Kondo S, Otani N. 1968. Animal scabies in humans. Bull Pharmacol Res Inst 77:1–3.

Larsson CE. 1989. Dermatologia veterinaria. I. Dermatites parasitarias dos carnivoros domesticos: sartnas sarcxoptrica, notoedrica e otoacariase. Com Cine Fac Med Vet Zootec Univ Sao Paulo 13:7–17.

Maehr DS, Greiner EC, Lanier JE, Murphy D. 1995. Notoedric mange in the Florida panther (*Felis concolor coryi*). J Wildl Dis 31:251–254.

Malecki G, Balcerak J. 1988. Use of ivomec in Felidae in a zoological garden. Med Wet 44:466–467.

Nesvadba J. 1967. Notoedric mange as a parasitological, public health and economic problem. Acta Univ Agric Brno, Fac Vetr 36:521–526.

Ogata M, Suzuki T, Itagaki H, Ishida F, Nakai T. 1980. Two feline cases of *Notoedres cati* infestation. J Jap Vet Med Assoc 33:276–279.

Olivia G, Baldio L. 1988. Impiego dell'ivermectina in alcune endo ed ectoparassitosi del gatto. Acta Med Vet 34:471–477.

Pence DB, Mathews FD, Windberg LA. 1982. Notoedric mange in the bobcat, *Felis rufus,* from south Texas. J Wildl Dis 18:47–50.

Pence DB, Tewes ME, Shindle DB, Dunn DM. 1995. Notoedric mange in an ocelot (*Felis pardalis*) from southern Texas. J Wildl Dis 31:558–561.

Penner LG, Parke WN. 1954. Notoedric mange in the bobcat, *Lynx rufus.* J Mamm 35:458.

Quintavalla F, Carnevali G, Iotto G. 1985. L'impiego della ivermectina nella rogna notoedrica del gatto. Obvit Doc Vet 4(4):85–86.

Railliet A. 1893. Traité de zoologie médicale et Africole. Paris: Asselin and Houzeau.
Rak H. 1972. Ectoparasites of dogs and cats in Iran. Entomol Monthly Mag 108:189.
Ribbeck R. 1992. Parasitosen. In Krankheiten der Katze, ed V Schmidt and MC Horzinek, pp 384–473. Jena, Germany: Gustav Fischer Verlag.
Sangvaranond A. 1979. Mange infestation in domestic animals (Acarina: Sarcoptidae, Psorptidae and Demodicidae) in Bogor and vicinity, West Java, Indonesia. BIOTROP Special Publication 6:45.
Schuurmans-Stekhoven JH, Notokworo RM. 1921. Zur Biologie der Kätzmilben. Verh Konink Akad Wetensch Amsterdam 21(2):1–152.
Svalastoga E, Mølbak I, Kristensen S, Grymer J. 1980. *Notoedres cati:* et memento. Dansk Veterinaert 63:699–701.
Tudury EA, Lorenzoni OD. 1987. Efeitos adversos do ivermectin em tres gatinhos Siamese com sarna notedrica. Riv Cent Cien Rrurais, Univ Fed Santa Maria 17:275–281.
Wilson-Hanson SL, Prescott CW. 1982. A survey for parasites in cats. Aust Vet J 59:194.
Yathiraj S, Thimmappa Rai M, Jayagopala Reddy NR, Muralidhara A. 1994. Treatment of scabies in a cat with ivermectin—a case report. Ind Vet J 71:596–597.
Young E, Zumpf F, Whyte IJ. 1972. *Notoedres cati* (Hering, 1838) infestation of the cheetah: preliminary report. J S Afr Vet Med Assoc 43:205.
Zumpf F. 1961. The arthropod parasites of vertebrates in Africa south of the Sahara (Ethiopian region). Vol 1. Chelicerata. Publ S Afr Inst Med Res 9:1–457.

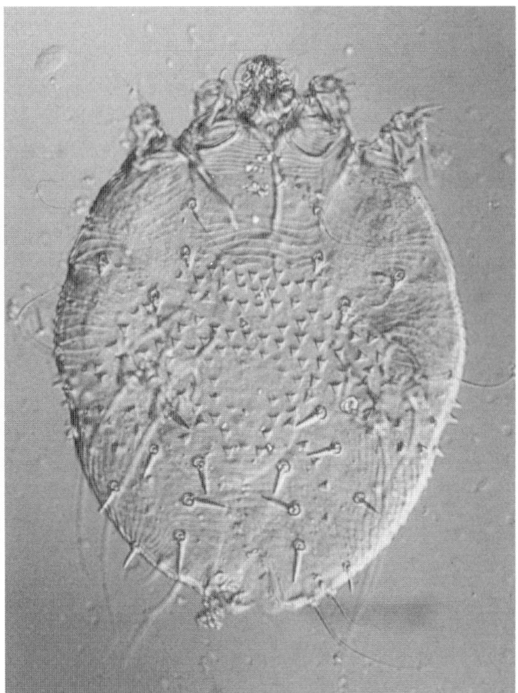

Fig. 5.43. *Sarcoptes scabiei.* Dorsal view of an adult female showing the large triangular spines that appear on the body.

Sarcoptes scabiei (Linnaeus, 1758) Latreille, 1802

Sarcoptes scabiei is not commonly reported from cats. The adults of *Sarcoptes* are larger than those of *Notoedres,* and the female has large triangular spines on the surface of its body (Fig. 5.43). Work by Arlian et al. (1988) has reinforced the long-held belief that the isolates of this species from different hosts tend to be host specific. Others have suggested that hosts that are natural hosts to a species of *Notoedres* tend to be refractory to infection with species of *Sarcoptes.* There have been three reports of sarcoptic mange in cats.

Linquist and Cash (1973) reported that an 8- to 10-week-old kitten had extensive hair loss over the ears, head, neck, abdomen, and tail, with the skin on the abdomen being thickened, scaly, and wrinkled. The kitten had been owned by two families. The first family (husband, wife, and two visiting daughters) kept the kitten a week and then gave it to a second family (a father and daughter). The second family noticed the hair loss and brought the kitten to the veterinary clinic. Four of the six family members in contact with the cats developed lesions. The father in the second family developed scabby lesions on his back and on the bridge of his nose; the kitten would sometimes curl up on his bare back while he was sleeping on the sofa. He treated himself with an over-the-counter ectoparasiticid preparation (pyrethrins and piperonyl butoxide). The daughter developed similar lesions on her abdomen (where the kitten would sometimes rest while she read), and she also was treated with the same over-the-counter product. The two daughters in the first family also developed skin lesions 2 weeks after having the kitten; the lesions were treated with either 1 percent benzene hexachloride or a pyrethrin and piperonyl butoxide preparation. Infections with *Sarcoptes scabiei* were never actually identified in any family member, and the two dogs owned by the first family showed no evidence of scabies.

Bussieras (1984) reported on skin lesions in a 15-month-old Persian cat with a history of pruriginous dermatitis. Examination of the cat revealed *Microsporum canis* and numerous mites identified as *Sarcoptes scabiei.* Again, lesions were also noted on the owner. The cat was treated by the weekly application of 0.025 percent amitraz for 5 weeks and with griseofulvin and enilconazole for the *Microsporum canis.* It was suspected that the cat had an underlying abnormal susceptibility to dermatologic pathogens that remained undiagnosed.

Hawkins et al. (1987) reported on a case of *Sarcoptes scabiei* infestation in an adult cat that had lived in a household for 6 years after being taken in as a stray. The owner had seven other cats, several of which had been diagnosed as positive for feline leukemia virus. The cat when admitted for examination was recumbent, unresponsive, 8 percent to 10 percent dehydrated, and emaciated. The lesions consisted of a 1 cm thick, tightly adhering, yellowish gray, exudative crust on the tail, caudal aspect of the thighs, and all feet. Paronychia and dystrophic nails were also observed. The lesions had worsened over a 12-month period, but the depression was of acute onset. This cat was found to be negative for feline leukemia virus, and no mites were discovered in an examination of a single skin scraping. The cat was then placed on a regimen of oral prednisolone (2 mg per kilogram of body weight every 12 hours). Within a few days of the cat's discharge, a veterinary student and a technician who had handled the cat developed pruritic cutaneous papules that lasted for 10 to 14 days. The owner was then questioned, and it was found that he also had had pruritic skin lesions for an extended period. The cat was then readmitted, and additional skin scrapings revealed numerous mites identified as *Sarcoptes scabiei.* A skin biopsy taken at this time revealed orthokeratotic and parakeratotic hyperkeratosis and irregular epidermal hyperplasia, and mites were observed in the biopsy. The administration of prednisolone was discontinued; however, after a second traumatic lime-sulfur dip, the cat was readmitted again severely distressed and unfortunately this time it did not respond to supportive therapy and died.

Currently, ivermectin (200 μg per kilogram body weight) would probably be the treatment of choice for sarcoptic mange in cats. There is every reason to believe from the success of this compound in treating scabies in other hosts and in treating notoedric mange that it would be highly efficacious in the treatment of feline scabies. It is important to note that in all three cases of feline infestations with *Sarcoptes scabiei* there was apparent transmission of the mite to humans who came in contact with the infested cat. Thus, it appears much more important to confine cats that are infested with *Sarcoptes scabiei* after treatment than would be needed in cases of notoedric mange. It would also suggest that when cases of suspected notoedric mange are found transmitted to owners or other individuals who have handled the cats, the identification of the species of mite involved is important because of the much greater risk of contamination that accompanies infestation with *Sarcoptes scabiei* in the feline host.

Treating cats with selamectin would probably be a very successful therapy and preventative for this infestation.

REFERENCES

Arlian LG, Vyszenski-Mohert DL, Cordova D. 1988. Host specificity of *S. scabiei* var. *canis* (Acari: Sarcoptidae) and the role of host odor. J Med Entomol 25:52–56.

Bussieras J. 1984. Un cas exceptionnel de gale sarcoptique chez le chat. Prat Med Chir Anim Comp 19:375–377.

Hawkins JA, McDonald RK, Woody BJ. 1987. *Sarcoptes scabiei* infestation in a cat. JAVMA 190:1572–1573.

Linquist WD, Cash WC. 1973. Sarcoptic mange in a cat. JAVMA 162:639–640.

Lynxacarus radovskyi Tenorio, 1974

Etymology

Lynx for the host from which the first species in the genus was described and *acarus* for mite, along with *radovskyi* for Dr. Radovsky of the Bishop Museum, Honolulu, Hawaii.

Synonyms

Felistrophorus radovskyi (Tenorio, 1974) Fox, 1977.

History

The genus *Lynxacarus* was originally described by Radord (1951) for specimens collected from a lynx in Georgia. The species typically collected from cats was described as a new species by Tenorio (1974) using specimens that she examined that had been collected from cats in Hawaii.

Geographic Distribution

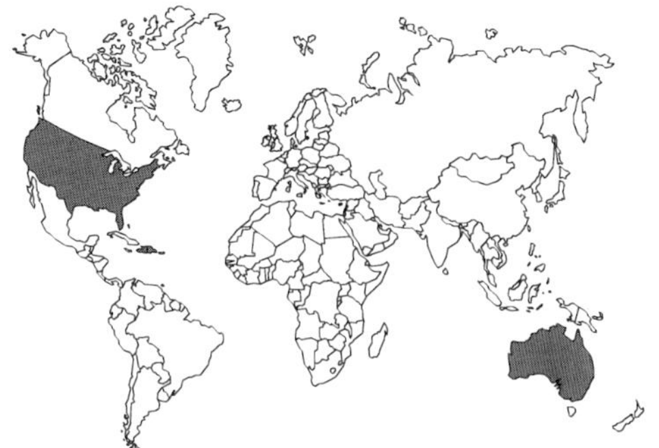

Fig. 5.44.

Infestations with *Lynxacarus radovskyi* have been reported in the United States in cats from southern Texas (Craig et al., 1993), southern Florida (Greve and Gerrish, 1981), and the Florida Keys (Foley, 1991a), as well as in Puerto Rico (Fox, 1977). The mite has also been reported from Hawaii (Tenorio, 1974), Fiji (Munro and Munro, 1979), and Australia (Bowman and Domrow, 1978).

Location in Host

This hair-clasping mite is found clinging to the hair of the cat (Fig. 5.45). The large eggs are attached to the hair of the cat. The larvae, nymphs, and adults are equipped with sternal plates that encircle the hair, and the first two sets of legs "monorail" the mites along the hair shaft (Foley, 1991a).

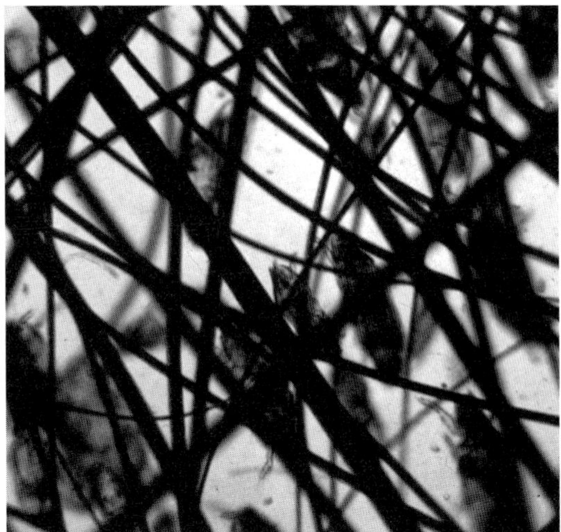

Fig. 5.45. *Lynxacarus radovskyi.* Hairs from a naturally infested cat with many mites present. (Photograph courtesy of Dr. Robert Foley)

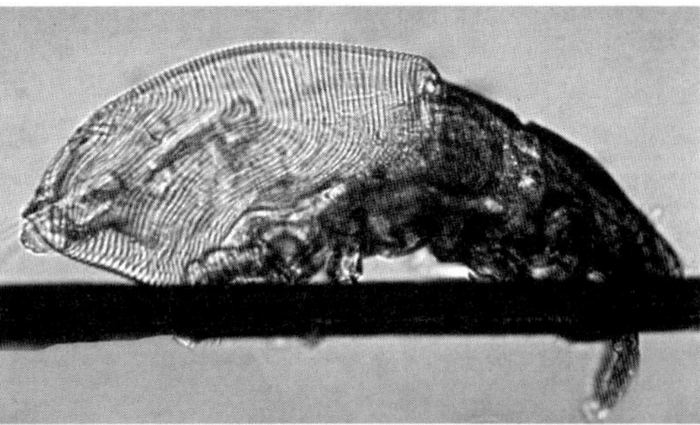

Fig. 5.46. *Lynxacarus radovskyi.* Adult mite clinging to the hair of a cat.

Parasite Identification

The tan mites, which are less than 0.5 mm in length, can be identified by their typical laterally compressed shape and by being found clinging to the hairs of the host (Fig. 5.46). The male mites have a greatly enlarged fourth pair of legs. The adult mites can be specifically identified as *Lynxacarus radovskyi* by the observation of the anteriorly directed bridge on the propodosomal plate that contacts the head plate of the mite; this is lacking on the other species that has been reported from felines, *Lynxacarus morlani* from the bobcat (Greve and Gerrish, 1981). The species that *Lynxacarus radovskyi* most resembles is *Lynxacarus mustelae* recovered from the least weasel (*Mustela nivalis*), and to be distinguished from this species, a careful examination of the shape and position of the dorsal plates must be performed (Tenorio, 1974).

Life Cycle

The life cycle is very poorly described. The large eggs (about 200 μm in length) produce a six-legged larval stage. The next stage in the life cycle is a nymph, which lacks the characteristic bridge on the propodosomal plate. The adult males and females are found clinging to the hairs. Foley (1991a) found that the mites were most commonly found on the tail head, tail tip, and perineal area and that heavily parasitized cats had whole body involvement with a haircoat that appeared "peppered" and that felt granular. There has been no work examining the amount of time required for adult mites to develop from eggs. It is assumed that transmission occurs by direct contact.

Clinical Presentation and Pathogenesis

Foley (1991a) described a large number of signs associated with infestation with this parasite. Most commonly seen was a dry, dull, and rust-colored haircoat. The next most common signs were gastrointestinal disturbances, including vomiting, constipation, rectal irritation or prolapse, and hairballs, which he felt was due to the excess grooming induced by the infestation. Also noted were gingivitis, anorexia, restlessness, fever, and weight loss.

Diagnosis

The mites can be visualized on the skin using a head loupe or magnifying glass. Microscopic examination will reveal the typical morphology of the mites, usually found attached to hairs.

Treatment

Craig et al. (1993) reported that two treatments with a pyrethrin-based miticidal shampoo appeared to eliminate the infestation but that the cat in this case was treated four times at weekly intervals. Foley (1991a) reported that pyrethrin products and lime-sulfur dips were both capable of clearing infestations. Foley (1991a) also noted that ivermectin at 300 μg/kg administered subcutaneously was highly efficacious when it was administered to the cats for other purposes.

Epizootiology

Foley (1991a) reported on an epizootic of lynxacariasis in cats in the Florida Keys where over 300 mites were treated in a single year. Most other reports have dealt with one or two cases from isolated island cat populations—Fox (1977) reported that the infestation was common in cats in Puerto Rico. It is assumed that the parasite is transmitted between cats by direct transmission, although Craig et al. (1993) reported that the cat that they observed in southern Texas had been sleeping in packing material that had accompanied a package that the owners had received from Hawaii.

Hazards to Other Animals

It is not known that the species in cats is restricted to the feline host, but as of this time *Lynxacarus radovskyi* has not been reported from other hosts.

Hazards to Humans

Foley (1991b) reported that one client with a heavily parasitized cat developed a papular forearm rash that cleared after the infestation of the cat was treated.

Control/Prevention

It is necessary to separate infested cats in order to prevent further spread of the infestation to other cats in the household. When owners take pets on vacations to areas where this parasite is common, it needs to be considered as part of the differential if any dermatological problems are noted in these animals.

REFERENCES

Bowman WL, Domrow R. 1978. The cat fur-mite (*Lynxacarus radovskyi*) in Australia. Aust Vet J 54:403–404.

Craig TM, Teel PD, Dubuisson LM, Dubuisson RK. 1993. *Lynxacarus radovskyi* infestation in a cat. J Am Vet Med Assoc 202:613–614.

Foley RH. 1991a. An epizootic of a rare fur mite in an island's cat population. Feline Pract 19:17–19.

Foley RH. 1991b. Parasitic mites of dogs and cats. Comp Cont Educ Pract Vet 13:783–800.

Fox I. 1977. *Felistrophorus,* a new genus of mites on cats in Puerto Rico (Acarina: Listrophoridae). Proc Entomol Soc Wash 79:242–244.

Greve JH, Gerrish RR. 1981. Fur mites (*Lynxacarus*) from cats in Florida. Feline Pract 11:28–30.

Munro R, Munro HMC. 1979. *Lynxacarus* on cats in Fiji. Aust Vet J 55:90.

Radford CD. 1951. Two new genera of parasitic mites (Acarina: Laelaptidae and Listrophoridae). Parasitology 41:102–104.

Tenorio JM. 1974. A new species of *Lynxacarus* (Acarina: Astigmata: Listrophoridae) from *Felis catus* in the Hawaiian Islands. J Med Entomol 11:599–604.

PENTASTOMIDA

The pentastomids comprise a small group of organisms that have worm-like adults and a larval stage within the eggshell that appears to be mite-like. It appears that they are probably related in some way to the parasitic crustacea and have developed in a manner that allows them to live within the respiratory tract of vertebrates. Typically, the final host is a carnivorous vertebrate that becomes infected by eating an intermediate host that has larvae encysted in its viscera. Cats can become infected either by the ingestion of eggs, when they will serve as intermediate hosts supporting the larval stage internally, or by eating an intermediate host, and then if the correct species of pentastomid is involved, they will develop infections of the upper respiratory system.

The adult pentastome has a mouth surrounded by four hooks; these were described initially as five mouths and hence the parasite's name. In veterinary medicine, pentastomes are most commonly seen in the air sacs of snakes (the location in the host is often misidentified as the body cavity because the air sacs are transparent and thin) and encysted as larvae in the viscera of primates. The adults in snakes and the larvae in primates can be quite large, several inches or more in length, so their discovery can be highly disconcerting.

The reports of pentastomiasis in cats have described the infection of the cats with the larval stage. These reports have come from Central Africa (Graber et al., 1973; Moens and Tshamala, 1986; Mohammed, 1972), India (Gretillat and Thiery, 1960), and Malaysia (Chooi et al., 1982). The cases have all dealt with infections of larval *Armillifer armillatus*. The adults of this pentastome are found in the lungs and air sacs of large snakes.

The cases in cats have either been incidental findings or cats that have presented with signs of abdominal disease (e.g., vomiting, anorexia, depression, and cachexia). The nymphs that are recovered tend to be yellowish white and are about 1 to 2 cm long. The larvae have a thick, stocky body that has pseudosegmentation that gives them a maggot-like appearance. The larvae are usually found in a coiled body position, looking like a C or a circle that is firmly attached to the omentum or the surfaces of various abdominal organs such as the liver, spleen, or kidney. To date, there has been no treatment attempted other than the surgical removal of the larvae.

REFERENCES

Chooi KF, Omar AR, Lee JYS. 1982. Melioidosis in a domestic cat, with concurrent infestation by nymphs of the cat pentastome, *Armillifer moniliformis*. Kajian Veterinar 14:41–43.

Graber M, Troncy PM, Thal J. 1973. Présence de larves d'*Armillifer armillatus* Wyman, 1847 chez divers mammifères domestiques et sauvages d'Afrique Centrale. Bull Soc Pathol Exot 66:183–191.

Gretillat S, Thiery G. 1960. Porocephalose a *Nettorhynchus* (*Armillifer*) *armillatus* (Wyman 1845) chez un cat. Rev Elev Med Vet Pays Trop 13: 305–308.

Moens Y, Tshamala M. 1986. Nymphal pentastomiasis in a cat. Vet Rec 119:44.

Mohammed AN. 1972. A note on the occurrence of *Armillifer armillatus* (Wyman, 1845) (Phylum: Pentastomida, Order Porocephalida) in a cat. Niger J Sci 6:139–142.

INSECTS

Insects differ from arachnids in that they typically have a distinct head, thorax, and abdomen. Most insects have a pair of wings that originate from the thorax, but these may be lost in some groups (the Siphonaptera or Phthiraptera) or reduced to a single pair, as in the Diptera (although in the Diptera, there are halteres, which are wings developed for specialized functions). Some groups, such as the lice, undergo simple metamorphosis (i.e., the larval stage that comes out of the egg looks very similar to the adult except for the lack of sexual characters). Other groups, such as the flies and the fleas, have a worm-like larva that leaves the egg. This larva will undergo complete metamorphosis in a cocoon or pupal case to ultimately develop into an adult that looks very little like its worm-like larva.

HEMIPTERA

Members of the Hemiptera are the "true" bugs of entomology. The Hemiptera is a large group of insects that contains over 50,000 species, most of which are parasites of plants. There are some species that are predatory and that can inflict painful bites if handled. There are two groups that have developed a true parasitic form of existence: the Cimicidae (bedbugs) and the subfamily Triatominae (kissing bugs) of the family Reduviidae.

Members of the Cimicidae have dorsoventrally flattened bodies and hide in cracks and crevices of households or nests. They lay their eggs in the cracks and molt five times with one blood meal for each molt. The bugs can undergo starvation for several months.

The reduviid subfamily Triatominae contains the genera *Triatoma, Rhodnius,* and *Panstrongylus,* which transmits *Trypanosoma cruzi* and *Trypanosoma rangeli.*

Cimicidae

The bedbugs, most commonly represented by *Cimex lectularis,* are a group of wingless, blood-feeding bugs that live in cracks and crevices in human habitations. Other species feed on bats, rodents, and birds and are found living in caves and nesting areas. The bugs feed while the host is in the nest. *Cimex lectularis* is active at night, rapidly filling to repletion on the blood of its host. There are five nymphal stages, as is the case with the triatomin bugs, and all stages will take at least one blood meal. The female glues the eggs in cracks and crevices where she lives. The bugs will feed on many different hosts if they share the same environment, and it is suspected that they would feed on cats. They are not known to transmit any diseases between cats.

Reduviidae

The Reduviidae contains a subfamily Triatominae, which contains the genera of blood-sucking insects responsible for the transmission of *Trypanosoma cruzi;* there are some 111 species in this subfamily. Most of the other members of the Reduviidae are predatory bugs that are called assassin bugs. The triatomin bugs have a bite that is relatively painless while that of the assassin bugs is painful. The triatomins, like the bedbugs, hide in various locations in nests and houses and feed on their hosts typically at night. Triatomins are mainly found in the American tropics, but some species are found in the areas of the Nearctic. One species, *Triatoma rubrofasciata,* has been carried by humans to various port cities around the world, including Asia and Africa. There are rare representatives that are indigenous to parts of the Orient and northeastern Australia.

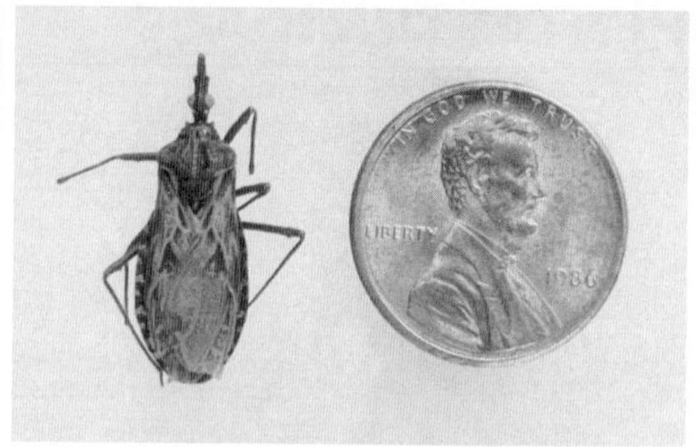

Fig. 5.47. *Triatoma protractor* adult shown next to a U.S. penny for scale.

The triatomins are large insects that as adults are often over an inch in length (Fig. 5.47). The bug has a large anteriorly protruding head that bears two large forward-projecting antennae and large eyes. The long, piercing mouthparts are folded back under the head of the bug (Fig. 5.48). The adults have well-developed wings. Often the bugs have brightly colored red, yellow, orange, and black borders on the lateral edges of the abdomen and on the anterior portion of the wing covers.

The triatomins undergo simple metamorphosis, and the nymphs resemble the adults, except that they lack wings and sexual structures. All stages require a blood meal, and the adults will feed repeatedly. The bugs are capable of long periods of starvation. The blood meal is required for egg production, and the eggs are laid often in cracks but without any glutinous material being secreted

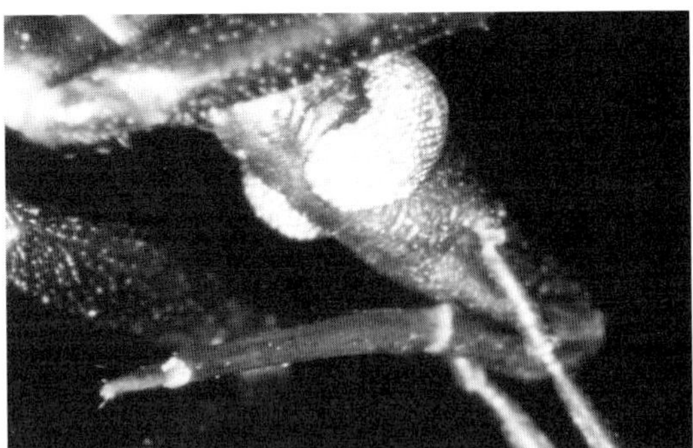

Fig. 5.48. Mouthparts of a triatomin bug folded back under the head.

as in the Cimicidae. Some bugs (e.g., *Rhodnius prolixus*) have a tendency to defecate sooner than other bugs examined; this defecation removes excess water from the blood meal to reduce its weight. This rapid defecation, which often occurs on the host, is one reason why some bugs may be better vectors of a posterior station parasite such as *Trypanosoma cruzi,* which is passed in the feces of the bug. Another aspect that determines how well certain bugs serve as vectors is how easily they enter human habitations. Some bugs, especially those in Mexico and Central and South America, are primarily domestic.

Triatomin bugs will feed on cats, and cats have been implicated as reservoirs of *Trypanosoma cruzi*. There has been very little work done on the presentation of the disease in cats. Gurtler et al. (1993) examined the role of cats and dogs in the transmission of *Trypanosoma cruzi* in Argentina. Of cats in 31 households, 39.3 percent were infected with this trypanosome, and bug infection rates in the vector *Triatoma infestans* were significantly associated with the presence of infected cats. A study in Oaxaca, Mexico, revealed that 13 percent of *Triatoma barberi* collected from village houses had fed on cats, 70 percent had fed on rodents, 36 percent had fed on humans, and multiple feedings were found in 48 percent of the bugs; 72 percent of the bugs were infected with *Trypanosoma cruzi* (Zarate et al., 1980). *Panstrongylus megistus* has been shown in the Santa Catarina Island of Brazil to feed on the feline hosts by the examination of blood meals by precipitin tests (Stendel et al., 1994).

REFERENCES

Gurtler RE, Cecere MC, Petersen RM, Rubel DN, Schweigmann NJ. 1993. Chagas disease in northwest Argentina: association between *Trypanosoma cruzi* parasitaemia in dogs and cats and infection rates in domestic *Triatoma infestans.* Trans Roy Soc Trop Med Hyg 87:12–15.

Stendel M, Toma HK, Carvalho-Pinto CJ, Grisard EC, Schlemper BR. 1994. Colonizacao de ecotopos artificiais pelo *Panstrongylus megistus* na Ilha de Santa Catarina, Florianopolis, Santa Catarina, Brasil. Rev Inst Med Trop Sao Paulo 36:43–50.

Zarate LG, Zaratc RJ, Tempelis CH, Goldsmith RS. 1980. The biology and behavior of *Triatoma barberi* (Hemiptera: Reduviidae) in Mexico. I. Blood meal sources and infection with *Trypanosoma cruzi.* J Med Entomol 17:103–116.

PHTHIRAPTERA

Lice are dorsoventrally flattened, wingless insects that live in close contact with the skin, hair, and feathers of their vertebrate hosts. They develop with simple metamorphosis (i.e., each stage is very similar to the next). There are two major groups of lice. One group, the Mallophaga, is also called the chewing lice. The mallophagan lice have broad heads and strongly chitinized jaws that are used for feeding on feathers, hairs, and epidermal scales. The mallophagan lice are found on birds and mammals. The second group, the Anoplura, is composed of the sucking lice. These lice have narrow heads and mouthparts that are adapted for sucking the host's blood and cutaneous fluids. The anopluran lice are exclusively parasites of mammals.

Cats are host to only a single louse, a mallophagan, *Felicola subrostratus.* Cats are occasionally blamed for infesting the human members of their households with the human louse *Pediculus humanus capitis* (the head louse, Fig. 5.49) and *Pthirus pubis* (the pubic louse, Fig 5.50), but humans, almost without exception, acquire these infestations from other humans. If one of these human lice is found on the cat, then the cat's human family must be led to understand that the cat is a victim of and not the source of the family's infestation.

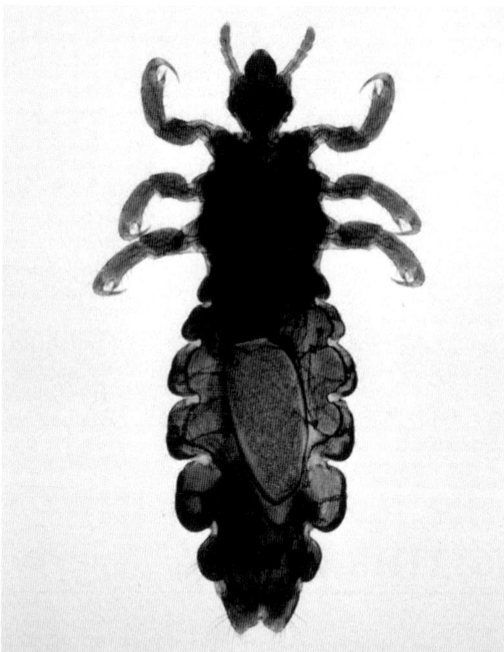

Fig. 5.49. *Pediculus humanus capitis.* An adult female head louse removed from the head of a child in Ithaca, New York, USA.

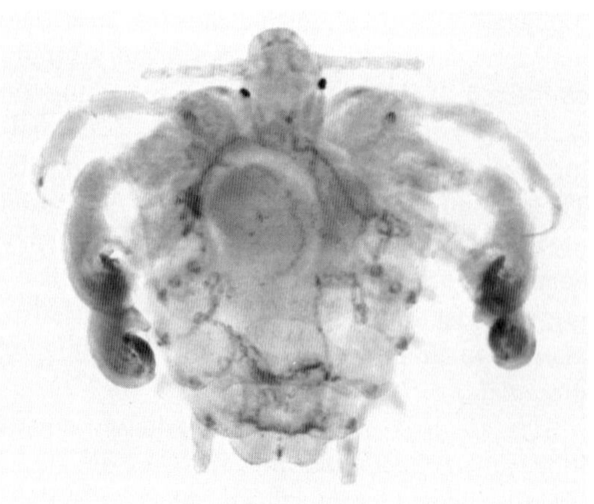

Fig. 5.50. *Pthirus pubis.* The pubic louse.

Felicola subrostratus (Burmeister, 1839) Ewing, 1929

Etymology

Feli = cat and *cola* = tiller, along with *subrostratus* = under beak.

Synonyms

Trichodectes subrostratus Burmeister, 1839; *Felicina subrostratus* (Burmeister, 1939) Bedford (1929); *Bedfordia helogale* (Bedford, 1932) Kéler (1939).

History

This louse has long been known to occur on cats. Lyal (1985) divided the genus *Felicola* into two genera: *Felicola* (containing the subgenera *Felicola* and *Suricatoecus*) and *Loriscola* (containing the subgenera *Loriscola* and *Paradoxuroecus*). Timm and Price (1994) felt that the characters separating *Felicola* and *Loriscola* were not sufficient for the differentiation of genera and considered all four subgenera within the single genus *Felicola.* There are 55 species within the genus *Felicola,* and within the four subgenera, *Felicola, Suricatoecus, Loriscola,* and *Paradoxuroecus,* are 18, 11, 13, and 13 species, respectively. Of these 55 species, 48 are from hosts of the families Felidae, Herpestidae, and Viverridae, 6 are from the Canidae, and 1 is from the Lorisidae (primates).

Geographic Distribution

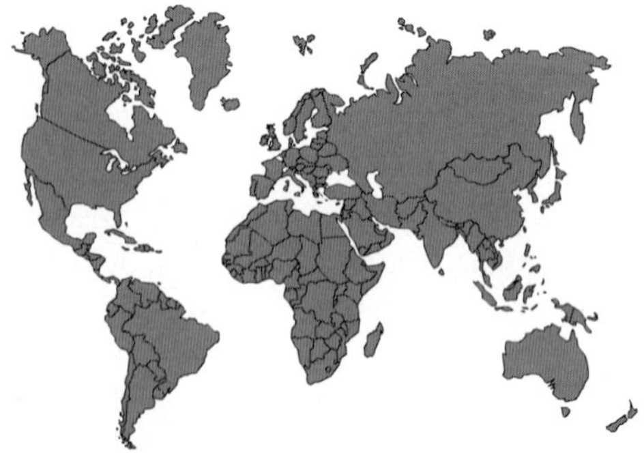

Fig. 5.51.

Felicola subrostratus is within the subgenus *Felicola.* Interestingly, the other 11 species of the genus *Felicola* reported from the family Felidae, many of which are from the Americas, are in the subgenus *Loriscola.* It is believed that as the domestic cat was transported out of northern Africa where it originated, taken along with the cat was the *Felicola subrostratus* associated with it. Thus, *Felicola subrostratus* is found throughout the world. Infections with this louse are not

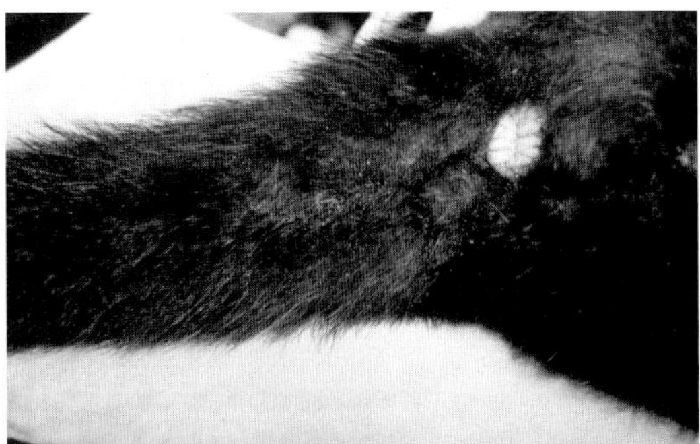

Fig. 5.52. *Felicola subrostratus.* Tail of a cat that initially appeared to have dandruff.

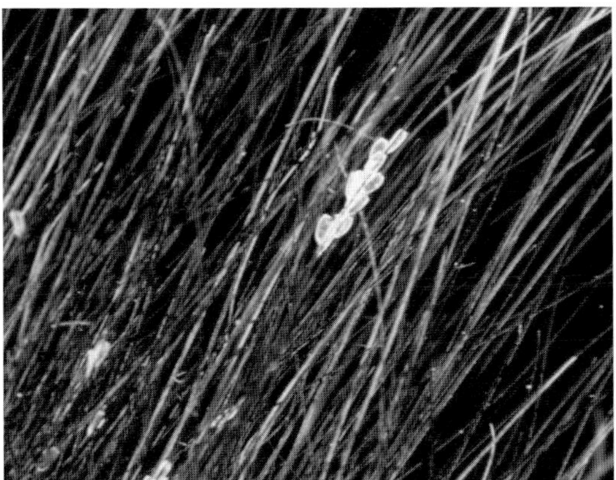

Fig. 5.53. *Felicola subrostratus.* Eggs glued to hair of an infested cat.

common in cats but are present in the cat population. Infested cats have been observed in Europe (Trotti et al., 1990), Asia (Shanta et al., 1980), the Philippines (Eduardo et al., 1977), Australia (Coman et al., 1981), South America (Santa Cruz and Lombardero, 1987), and North America.

Location in Host

The lice live on the fur of the cat (Fig 5.52). The eggs or nits are glued by the female to the hair shaft (Fig 5.53).

Parasite Identification

Felicola subrostratus on cats is readily identified by the shape of the head (Figs. 5.54 and 5.55). As described by Ewing (1929) in his designation of the genus: "In this genus the forehead is triangular, the sides converging in a straight line from the bases of the antennae to the borders of the very narrow hair-groove at the apex." If one is collecting lice from a nondomestic felid, it is highly likely that the species involved is not *Felicola subrostratus,* and reference should be made to the

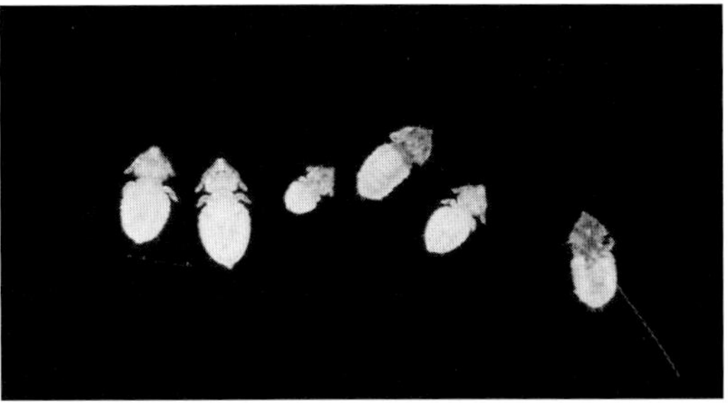

Fig. 5.54. *Felicola subrostratus.* Several adult lice recovered from an infested cat; the triangular-shaped head is obvious.

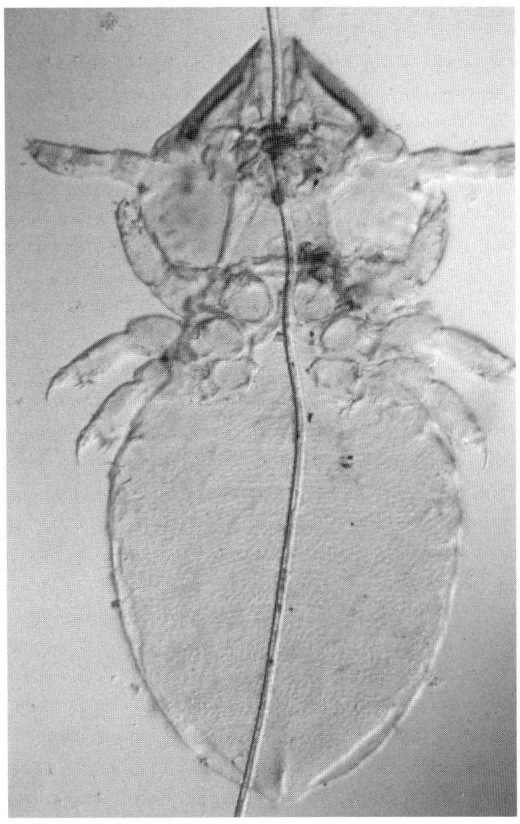

Fig. 5.55. *Felicola subrostratus.* An adult clinging to the hair of a cat by its chelicerae. The mouthparts and the legs are exquisitely shaped for moving along the hair shaft.

key of Emerson and Price (1983) for *Felicola* species from the Americas and to Timm and Price (1994). Pérez-Jiménez et al. (1990) reviewed some of the *Felicola* from European hosts.

Life Cycle

The biology of *Felicola subrostratus* is very poorly known. The female glues her operculate eggs to the hair of her feline host. After several hours to days, the eggs hatch, giving birth to nymphal lice that feed and molt in several days. After probably 2 to 3 weeks, the adults will again be present, and a couple of days after insemination, the female will again lay eggs. It is not known how long the adults will live. The adult lice hold onto the hair with their mandibles and are capable of rapid movement along the hair shaft using their legs for propulsion. It is presumed that their only significant source of food is epidermal debris. Only two members of the Mallophaga are known to ingest blood: *Trichodectes canis* of the dog (Bouvier, 1945) and *Fulica americana,* a louse of birds (Bartlett and Anderson, 1989).

Clinical Presentation and Pathogenesis.

Few clinical signs have been described in cats with infestations of *Felicola subrostratus.* Debilitated cats can develop large numbers of lice if they lose the ability to groom.

Diagnosis

The lice and nits are easily visible on the fur of the cat. For certain identification, the louse can be placed on a microscope slide and the triangular head observed. If only the eggs are present, they will be conspicuously operculate when examined under the microscope.

With lice, fleas, and mites in cats, it is not uncommon to find the cuticular remains of the arthropod in the feces of the feline host. As the cat grooms, it ingests the arthropod, and the cuticle is not digested. Thus, the infestation with one of these ectoparasites is often actually detected by the performance of a fecal flotation, especially when a centrifugal sugar flotation method is used.

Treatment

Lice on cats are easily treated with most pyrethrin-based powders, sprays, or foams. Fipronil and imidacloprid both would also work well.

Epizootiology

Very little is known about the epizootiology of this parasite. It is suspected that the infestation will be more common in the winter than in the summer, but this may be an unwarranted supposition.

Hazards to Other Animals

The species of *Felicola* seem highly host specific (Timm and Price, 1994). Thus, it is expected that the many species on wild Felidae will not be found on the domestic cat. It is possible that *Felicola subrostratus* can infest other felines, but how commonly this occurs is not known.

Hazards to Humans

It does not appear that these lice will bite humans.

Control/Prevention

Control and prevention are achieved mainly by prevention of contact with infested cats. It is also important that cats be isolated for a period of time and treated with an ectoparasiticide before they are admitted to a cattery. Cats on fipronil or imidacloprid monthly treatments should not be affected.

REFERENCES

Bartlett CM, Anderson RC. 1989. Mallophaga vectors and the avian filaroids: new subspecies of *Pelecitus fulicaeatrae* (Nematoda: Filaroidea) in sympatric North American hosts, with development, epizootiology, and pathogenesis of the parasite in *Fulica americana.* Can J Zool 67:2821–2833.

Bouvier G. 1945. Die l'hématologie de quelques Mallophages des animaux domestiques. Schweiz Arch Tierheilk 87:429–434.

Coman BJ, Jones EH, Driesen MA. 1981. Helminth parasites and arthropods of feral cats. Aust Vet J 57:324–327.

Eduardo SL, Celo EM, Tongson MS, Manuel MF. 1977. *Felicola subrostratus* (Nitzsch) (Mallophaga: Trichodectidae) from a native cat—a Philippine record. Philipp J Vet Med 16:69–71.

Emerson KC, Price RD. 1983. A review of the *Felicola felis* complex (Mallophaga: Trichodectidae) found on New World cats (Carnivora: Felidae). Proc Entomol Soc Wash 85:1–9.

Ewing HE. 1929. A Manual of External Parasites. Springfield, Ill: CC Thomas. Pp 120–123.
Lyal CHC. 1985. A cladistic analysis and classification of trichodectid mammal lice (Phthiraptera: Ischnocera). Bull Br Mus (Nat Hist) 51:187–346.
Pérez-Jiménez JM, Diaz-Lopez M, Palomares-Fernandez F, Delihes de Castro M. 1990. Phthiraptera from some wild carnivores in Spain. Sytem Parasitol 15:107–117.
Santa Cruz AM, Lombardero OJ. 1987. Resultatos parasitologicos de 50 necropsias de gatos de la ciudad de Corrientes. Vet Arg 4:735–739.
Shanta CS, Wan SP, Kwong KH. 1980. A survey of the endo- and ectoparasites of cats in and around Ipoh, West Malaysia. Malay Vet J 7:17–27.
Timm RM, Price RD. 1994. A new species of *Felicola* (Phthiraptera: Trichodectidae) from a Costa Rican jaguar, *Panterha onca* (Carnivora: Felidae). Proc Biol Soc Wash 107:114–118.
Trotti GC, Corradini L, Visconti S. 1990. Parasitological investigation in a cattery in Ferrara. Parassitologia 32:42–43.

DIPTERA

The diptera (*di* = two and *ptera* = wings) are flies bearing one pair of wings. The second set of wings is represented by a structure called the haltere, which resembles a lollipop. The wings supply motion, and the halteres act as stabilizers. Flies, unlike bugs and lice, undergo complete metamorphosis (i.e., there is a pupal stage in which the fly is transformed from a wingless maggot-like stage into the winged adult). The sexes are separate. Most female flies are ovoviviparous (i.e., they produce eggs), but some produce larvae (e.g., the blowflies), and some even produce a third-stage larva that is ready to pupate (e.g., the tsetse). Many of the species of flies are of importance because they require a blood meal as adults or because the larval stages are parasitic. The Diptera can also serve as important vectors of blood-borne diseases.

There are three major groups of flies: the Nematocera, which includes the gnats and mosquitoes; the Brachycera, the deer- and horseflies; and the Cyclorrhapha, the botflies and the house-, blow-, and flesh flies. In the Nematocera and Brachycera, the fly escapes from the pupal case through a T-shaped opening in the back of the pupal case; in the Cyclorrhapha, the fly escapes through a round opening in the front of the pupal case. The important Nematocera and Brachycera are those in which the adult female requires a blood meal in order to produce eggs. Some of the Cyclorrhapha are important because the adult flies suck blood, and others are important because their larval stages are parasitic.

NEMATOCERA

The Nematocera (*nemato* = thread and *cera* = horns; referring to the long, segmented antennae that are typical of this suborder) represents a group of flies that are important, for the most part, in feline medicine as the vectors of disease. These flies tend to be small and delicate. Only the females of this group require blood or tissue fluids from a vertebrate host; the males feed on nectar. The eggs are typically laid in water or semiaquatic habitats. The larvae undergo several molts and then pupate. The adult fly emerges from a longitudinal slit along the dorsal surface of the pupal case in the area overlying the thorax. The families that are important in feline medicine include the Culicidae (the mosquitoes), the Psychodidae (the sand flies), the Ceratopogonidae (no-see-ums), and the Simuliidae (the blackflies).

Culicidae

Mosquitoes are well-known pests of humans and animals (Fig. 5.56). This group is divided into three subfamilies: the Culicinae, the Anophelinae, and the Toxorhynchitinae. Only the Culicinae and the Anophelinae are important as parasites; the Toxorhynchitinae has predatory larvae, and the adults feed on plant fluids. The distinction between culicine and anopheline mosquitoes is especially important in human medicine and in mosquito control operations because the anopheline mosquitoes are vectors of the *Plasmodium* species, which cause malaria in humans. In feline medicine, mosquitoes are important as vectors of heartworms and as the cause of hypersensitivity.

In the life cycle of a mosquito, the female lays eggs in or near water or in areas that are likely to have water when the water level rises. Culicine

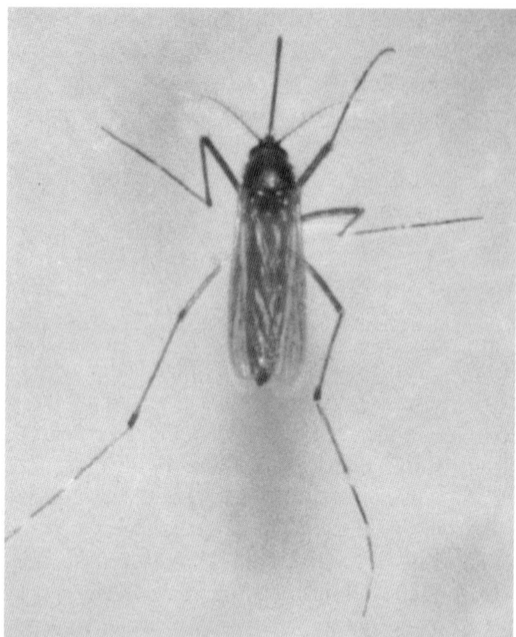

Fig. 5.56. *Aedes aegypti.* Adult mosquito probing on a human arm for a feeding site. This mosquito is missing one of its legs.

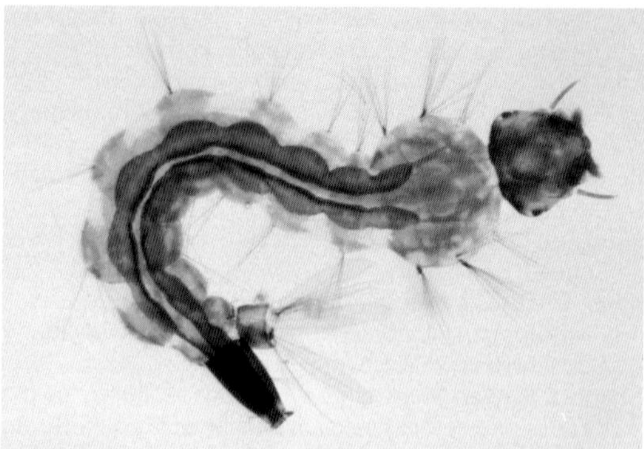

Fig. 5.57. *Aedes aegypti.* Larval stage that is found in water.

mosquitoes often lay their eggs in rafts, and the eggs of anopheline mosquitoes often bear lateral projections or wings that add buoyancy, causing the eggs to float better. From the eggs, a larval stage hatches. The larvae of the culicine mosquitoes have a posterior breathing tube on the end of the body (Fig. 5.57); this breathing tube is lacking in anopheline larvae. The larvae tend to be filter feeders: culicine larvae tend to hang from the surface film of the water from the breathing tube, while the anopheline lies parallel to the surface film with the aid of palmate hairs that are present on the latero-ventral surfaces of the body segments. The larvae undergo four instars before pupation. The pupa is comma shaped and has a pair of breathing tubes on the dorsal surface from which it hangs in calm water. If disturbed, the pupa will use its tail with terminal paddles to again force its way to the surface. After about 1 to 5 days as a pupa, the adult is ready to emerge. A split appears along the midline of the dorsal surface of the pupa, and the adult head and thorax emerge, next the wings come out and unfold, and finally, the legs are freed and stretch out. The adult is ready to fly in just a few minutes after emergence is complete. Males swarm, and the females fly into the swarms where they pair with a male and copulate, typically 1 to 2 days after emergence. Female mosquitoes tend to mate only once during their lives, and the males tend to live only for a few days, dying soon after copulation. Some females live for weeks to months in nature, and a few are capable of overwintering in cold or dry weather.

For female mosquitoes to be successful vectors of a pathogen, they must either take more than one blood meal as adults or be infected transovarily with a pathogen that was ingested by their mother. In feline medicine, the parasites that are transmitted by mosquitoes are those that are obtained from a prior blood meal.

Many different genera and species of mosquito are capable of serving as vectors of heartworms, *Dirofilaria immitis.* One important vector of *Dirofilaria immitis* is *Culex pipiens,* which is worldwide in distribution. *Culex pipiens* breeds around human habitation, is willing to enter houses, and feeds at night. The mosquito vectors of canine dirofilariasis include species of *Culex, Aedes,* and *Anopheles.* There have been approximately 70 species of mosquito incriminated as potential vectors of canine dirofilariasis although not all are considered to be principal vectors in nature (Otto and Jachowski, 1981). At the same time, it is not clear how many of these mosquitoes that are potential or principal vectors of canine heartworm are willing or prefer to feed on cats.

Work by Genchi et al. (1992) revealed that in northern Italy *Culex pipiens* was found to feed on cats at night while both *Aedes caspius* and *Culex pipiens* fed on dogs. Fewer total mosquitoes were recovered each night from cats than from dogs. This is obviously a field that requires more study in order to understand the dynamics of feline dirofilariasis transmission.

A direct pathogenic effect of mosquitoes to the feline host is manifested as eosinophilic dermatitis (Mason and Evans, 1991). This condition was first described by workers in Australia as a seasonal and intermittent condition that usually resolved in the winter (Wilkinson and Bate, 1984). The disease has also been observed in the United States. The condition presents as papular eruptions, erosions, and depigmentation of the skin over the bridge of the nose; papular eruptions on the pinnae of the ears; and sometimes lesions on the pads of the paws. These cats will sometimes have positive skin tests to extracts of mosquito antigens (Mason and Evans, 1991). *Culex orbostiensis* and *Aedes multiplex* have been collected from affected cats in Australia (Mason and Evans, 1991), and potential causes in New Zealand include *Aedes notoscriptus* and *Culex pervigilans* (Johnstone et al., 1992).

REFERENCES

Genchi C, Sacco BD, Cancrini G. 1992. Epizootiology of canine and feline heartworm infection in northern Italy: possible mosquito vectors. Proc Heartworm Symp '92, Austin, Tex, 39–46.

Johnstone AC, Graham DG, Andersen HJ. 1992. A seasonal eosinophilic dermatitis in cats. N Z Vet J 40:168–172.

Mason KV, Evans AG. 1991. Mosquito bite-caused eosinophilic dermatitis in cats. JAVMA 198: 2086–2088.

Otto GF, Jachowski LA. 1981. Mosquitoes and canine heartworm disease. Proc Am Heartworm Symp '80, Dallas, Tex, 17–32.

Wilkinson GT, Bate MJ. 1984. A possible further clinical manifestation of the feline eosinophilic granuloma complex. J Am Anim Hosp Assoc 20:325–331.

Ceratopogonidae

This group is also known by the common name of biting gnats or sand flies. The bite of the fly produces a lesion with a wheal that may be 1 to 2 cm in diameter. The flies have mouthparts that unlike the mosquito tear a small hole in the skin from which they lap up blood and tissue fluids. There are a number of genera in this group, but only *Culicoides, Leptoconops, Forcipomyia,* and *Austroconops* are considered as regularly feeding on mammals; most of the other species feed on reptiles and amphibia.

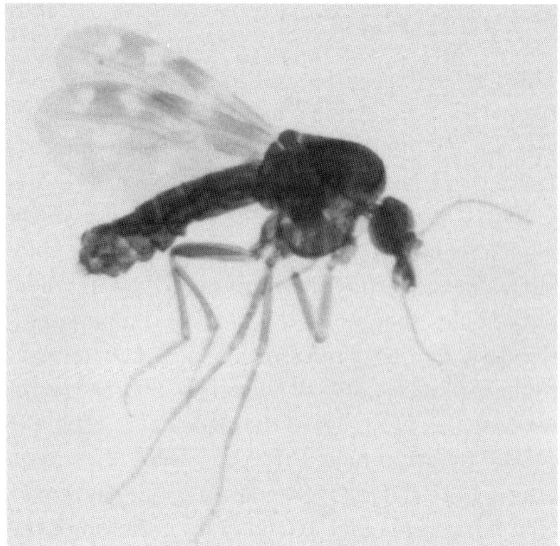

Fig. 5.58. *Culicoides* species. Note the short and stocky mouthparts and the mottled wings.

The fly is characterized by being small (less than a millimeter long) and dark with long delicate antennae. The wings tend to be narrow and are folded flat over the body when the fly is feeding. The wings often appear spotted when examined closely (Fig. 5.58).

Eggs are laid in tree holes, decaying vegetation in water, the surface of wet sand, manure, aquatic plants, or leaf mold. Some prefer salt water. The larvae are maggot-like. The pupa is elongate and has a pair of long thoracic breathing trumpets.

Cats are apt to be affected by bites of these flies in a way similar to humans, but there seem to be no descriptions of the effects of these bites on cats. The bite of a *Culicoides* has been associated with the transmission of a filarid nematode parasite of the raccoon, *Tetrapetalonema llewellyni,* which was discovered in the microfilarial stage in the blood of a cat in Switzerland (Gafner and Hörning, 1988).

REFERENCES

Gafner F, Hörning B. 1988. Mikrofilarien bein einer Katze. Schweiz Arch Tierheilk 130:651–654.

Psychodidae

The Psychodidae is composed of two groups of flies: the Psychodinae and the Phlebotominae. The Psychodinae is a group of free-living flies that are nuisance pests that develop in dirty water such as that found around sewage treatment plants, manure lagoons, and cesspools. The phlebotomine sand flies are a group of flies in which the females require a blood meal. The genera of flies of importance are *Lutzomyia,* which is found in the Americas, and *Phlebotomus* and *Sergentomyia,* which are found in Eurasia and Africa.

The phlebotomine flies are small flies with long antennae, long legs, and wings that have parallel wing veins that extend from the base of the wing to the wingtip (Fig. 5.59). The mouthparts of the female are designed for the rasping of a small hole in the skin from which she drinks blood and tissue fluids. The female lays long, ovoid eggs in crevices, hollows, animal burrows, and cracks in soil that may or may not contain organic debris but are dark and have a high humidity. The small maggot-like larvae go through four instars and then pupate. The period from egg to adult is about 2 months. Most adults tend to fly relatively short distances, feeding near the breeding sites, although some are capable of extended flight.

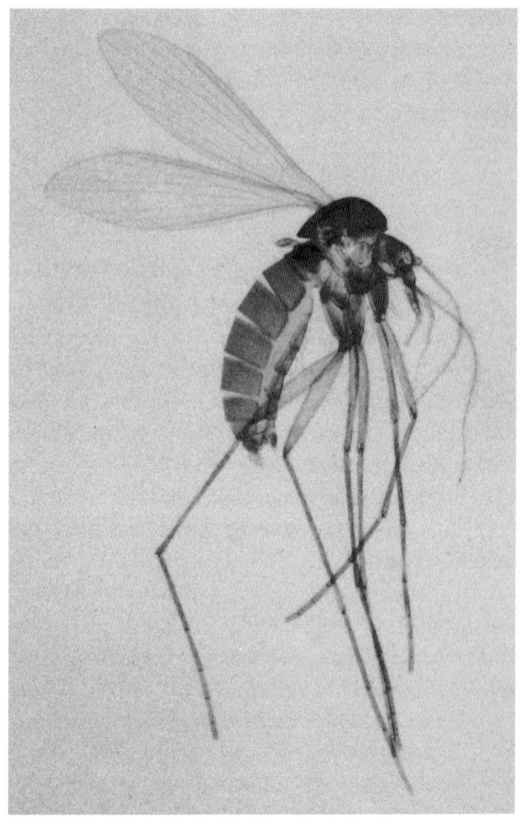

Fig. 5.59. *Phlebotomus* species. Note the short mouthparts and the parallel venation on the wings.

Although there have been no studies on the transmission of leishmaniasis between cats by phlebotomine sand flies, blood meals of flies have been identified as coming from cats. In Peru, for the flies *Lutzomyia peruensis* and *Lutzomyia verrucarum,* cats were identified as the major source of blood meals after humans and cattle, with 10.8 percent of the flies having fed on cats (Ogusuku et al., 1994); these species have been incriminated as vectors of *Leishmania peruviana* and *Leishmania braziliensis. Lutzomyia shannoni* and *Lutzomyia diabolica* are species in the United States that feed on humans and that have been shown to experimentally transmit *Leishmania mexicana.* In Kenya, vector preference studies using various hosts as bait have shown that cats were almost as attractive to *Phlebotomus guggisbergi* as sheep and goats, which were the most attractive hosts (Johnson et al., 1993); *Phlebotomus guggisbergi* serves as a vector of *Leishmania tropica.* In Spain, *Phlebotomus perniciosus,* a vector of *Leishmania donovani,* has been shown to feed on the cats, and 2 percent to 25 percent of flies that were sampled from five different locations contained feline blood meals (Colmenares et al., 1995). In Egypt, two vectors of *Leishmania donovani, Phlebotomus papatasi* and *Phlebotomus langeroni,* did not significantly feed on cats, preferring human hosts to the exclusion of almost all others (El Sawaf et al., 1989).

REFERENCES

Colmenares MD, Portus M, Botet J, Dobano C, Gallego M, Wolff M, Segui G. 1995. Identification of blood meals of *Phlebotomus perniciosus* (Diptera: Psychodidae) in Spain by a competitive enzyme-linked immunosorbent assay biotin/avidin method. J Med Entomol 32:229–233.

El Sawaf BM, Mansour NS, El Said SM, Daba S, Youssef FG, Kenawy MA, Beier JC. 1989. Feeding patterns of *Phlebotomus papatasi* and *Phlebotomus langeroni* (Diptera: Psychodidae) in El Agamy, Egypt. J Med Entomol 26:497–498.

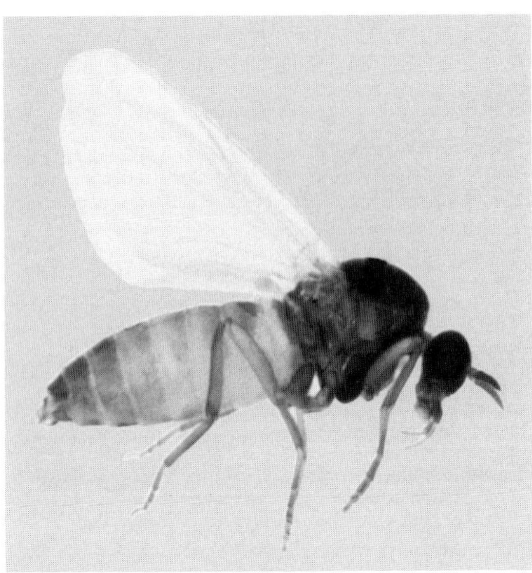

Fig. 5.60. *Simulium* species. Note the short mouthparts and the shape of the antennae.

Johnson RN, Ngumbi PM, Mwanyumba JP, Roberts CR. 1993. Host feeding preference of *Phlebotomus guggisbergi* a vector of *Leishmania tropica* in Kenya. Med Vet Entomol 7:216–218.

Ogusuku E, Perez JE, Paz L, Nieto E, Monje J, Guerra H. 1994. Identification of bloodmeal sources of *Lutzomyia* spp. in Peru. Ann Trop Med Parasitol 88:329–335.

Simuliidae

The Simuliidae, blackflies, are small flies whose females require a blood meal for egg production (Fig. 5.60). These flies are found throughout the world, but they are more common in cooler climates. Larval development occurs in running water. The larvae are attached to the bottom of the stream by a silken strand and are filter feeders. There are six or seven larval instars, then the larvae pupate. The adult emerges from the puparium and then rapidly bobs to the surface. The cycle takes 1 or 2 weeks from egg to adult. Important genera include *Simulium* and *Prosimulium.*

Blackflies are vicious biters, and the fly's scraping mouthparts rasp small holes in the skin from which the fly feeds. The flies are significant pests of humans and livestock, and they can be devastating when present in large numbers. Some humans react quite severely to the bite of these flies, although many have no reaction or only small wheals at the feeding site. There is every reason to believe that cats also fall prey to the bites of these flies, but there have been no significant reports on the effects of these dipterans on the feline host.

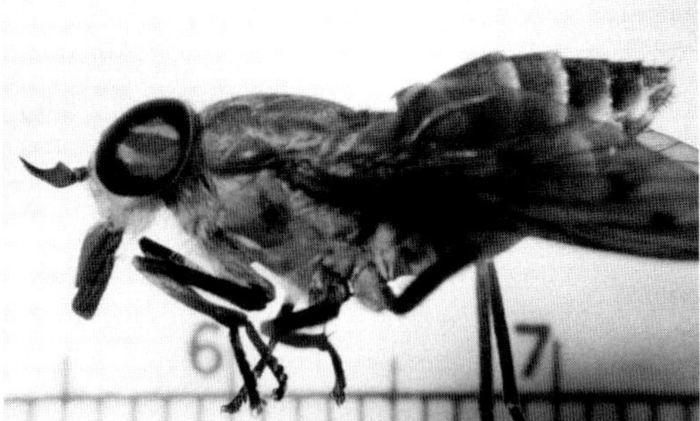

Fig. 5.61. *Tabanus* species. Lateral view of an adult; note the shape of the antennae.

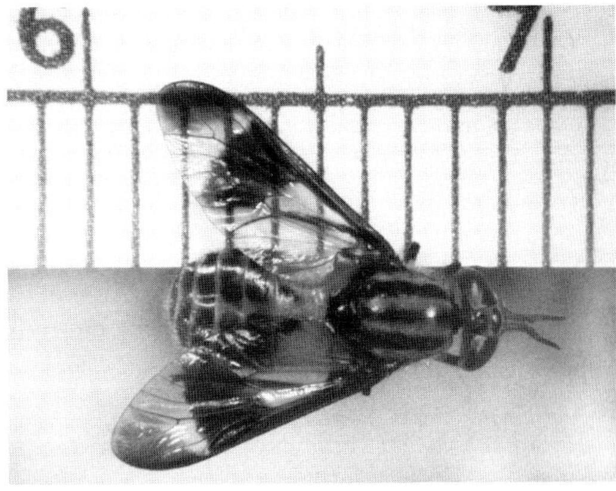

Fig. 5.62. *Chrysops* species. Dorsal view of an adult female; note the mottled appearance to the wings and the triangular shape of flies of this genus due to the way the wings are held when at rest.

BRACHYCERA

The Brachycera, horseflies and deerflies, are large and vicious daytime biters that are found throughout the world. Genera include *Tabanus* (Fig. 5.61), *Haemtopota, Silvius, Hybomitra, Diachlorus,* and *Chrysops* (Fig. 5.62). Like the Nematocera, only the female fly feeds on blood.

The female lays eggs near foliage overhanging water or at the water's edge. The larva enters the water where, in some species, it feeds on organic debris and, in others, it is a predator. Larvae may remain active a year before they pupate. The pupa occurs in drier soil, and after 1 to 2 weeks the adult fly emerges. The adult flies are large, up to 5 cm in length, and cause significant lesions at the site of the bite. The major biting activity is likely to occur during the heat of midday. Some humans react significantly to the bites and develop large swellings that may be up to 10 cm or more in diameter. It is to be expected that cats are also plagued by the bites of these flies, but specific cases have not been described.

CYCLORRHAPHA

The Cyclorrhapha is composed of those flies where the adult escapes from the pupal case through a circular opening in the anterior end. These flies are characterized by the possession of three-segmented antennae where the last segment bears an arista or style. The suborder Cyclorrhapha has historically represented one of three suborders of the Diptera, along with the Nematocera and Brachycera. Recently, it has been proposed that the Brachycera and Cyclorrhapha be combined in an infraorder called the Muscomorpha (Crosskey, 1993).

The Cyclorrhapha contains many adult flies that are free-living and many flies that are true parasites of vertebrates as larval stages. Within this group are the filth flies (Muscidae), the flesh flies (Sarcophagidae), the blowflies (Calliphoridae), and the tsetse (Glossinidae). Some of these flies are parasitic as larvae, causing myiasis that may be obligatory or that can be facultative. One last family of these flies, the Cuteribridae, causes significant disease in cats through the migration of the large bot-like larval stage that is usually found in rodents or lagomorphs.

REFERENCES

Crosskey RW. 1993. Introduction to the Diptera. In Medical Insects and Arachnids, ed RP Lane and RP Crosskey, pp 389–428. London: Chapman and Hall.

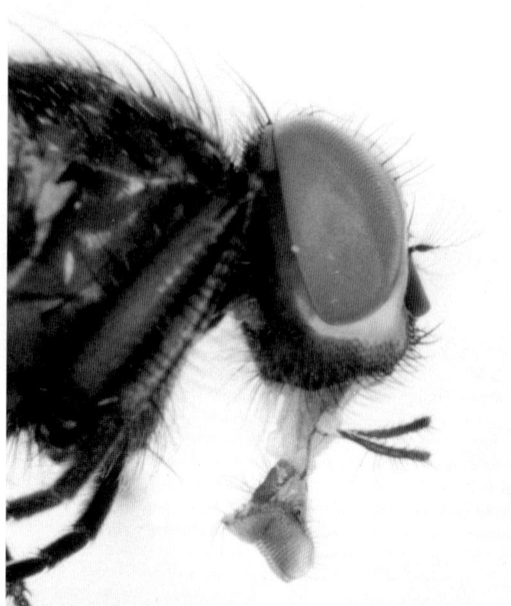

Fig. 5.63. *Musca* species. Head of the adult fly.

Muscidae

The dull-colored flies of Muscidae are best known by the common representative the housefly, *Musca domestica.* These flies are very similar in appearance as adults to the adults of the Sarcophagidae and the Calliphoridae. The family contains two groups of flies, species of *Musca* and *Stomoxys,* that are of importance in feline medicine only because they probably typically bother cats in a fashion similar to how they bother humans and other animals.

Musca Species

The genus *Musca* is most commonly represented by the housefly, *Musca domestica.* The adult fly feeds on various foodstuffs through the use of its sponging mouthparts (Fig. 5.63), and it will just as readily feed on feces and garbage as upon food consumed by cats or their owners. The larval stage, the maggot, is commonly seen developing in garbage, feces, and other decaying animal and vegetable material. The pupal stage is found in slightly drier areas around the site of larval feeding. The feeding process of the fly, whereby there is regurgitation of recently imbibed food along with saliva that aids in the liquefaction of the surface of the material being ingested, makes the fly an excellent means of transferring microorganisms from one site to another.

The fact that the nematode *Thelazia* has been reported from the eyes of cats would indicate that *Musca* or *Musca*-like flies (e.g., *Fannia* or *Phortica* species) are feeding around the eyes of cats. In this case the larval stage leaves the mouthpart of the fly while the fly is feeding on lachrymal fluids. Gardiner et al. (1983) reported on a case of visceral myiasis that they believed due to *Musca domestica;* it is possible, however, that they were dealing with small larvae of a *Cuterebra* species.

REFERENCES

Gardiner CH, James VS, Valentine BA. 1983. Visceral myiasis caused by *Musca domestica* in a cat. J Am Vet Med Assoc 182:68–69.

Stomoxys Species

Stomoxys is composed of several species of flies that resemble *Musca domestica* generally, but the mouthparts are designed for piercing the skin and feeding upon blood. Both the male and female flies take blood meals. The female fly lays eggs in decaying vegetable matter, and the larvae hatch, feed, and pupate in these locations. The adult flies are vicious daytime feeders.

There have been no reports of these flies specifically bothering cats, although they have been found to cause cutaneous lesions at the site of feeding in dogs (White and Bourdeau, 1995). There is every reason to believe that these flies are capable of feeding on cats, and it is likely that there would be reactions at the feeding site.

REFERENCES

White SD, Bourdeau P. 1995. Hypersensibilitès aux piqûres de diptères chez les carnivores. Point Vet 27:203–206.

Glossinidae

The Glossinidae is represented by a single genus, *Glossina,* which is the tsetse of Africa (Fig. 5.64).

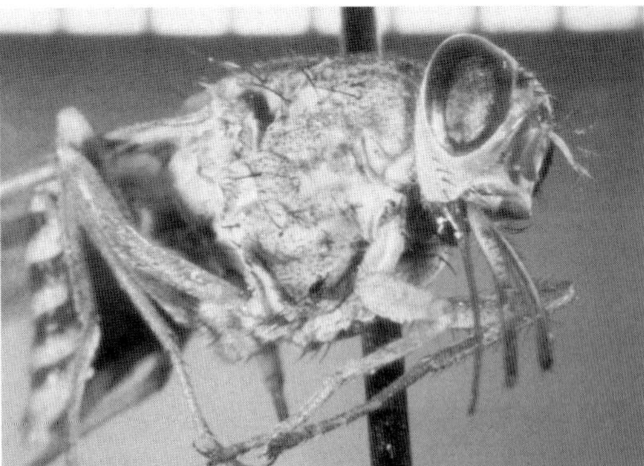

Fig. 5.64. *Glossina* species. The tsetse.

Tsetse flies are the vectors of African trypanosomiasis, which is passed through their bite. Cats, like other vertebrates, are bitten by this fly.

Facultative and Primary Muscoid Fly Myiasis

"Myiasis" is the term that describes the infestation of organs or tissues of humans or animals by fly maggots that, at least for a period of time, feed upon living, necrotic, or dead tissues or upon ingested food of the host. Many species of *Musca*-like fly larvae that normally breed in decaying meat or carrion may infest traumatic skin wounds of cats and produce a condition known as facultative myiasis. Facultative myiasis resulting from infestation by flies of the *Musca, Calliphora, Phaenicia, Lucilia, Phormia,* and *Sarcophaga* genera should be distinguished from obligatory myiasis resulting from primary myiasis–producing species.

Facultative myiasis is one of the oldest recorded diseases affecting man and domestic animals. Many human skin diseases in ancient times, although different in their cutaneous manifestations and etiologies, were grouped together under the catch-all term "leprosy." Such was not the case for the presence of fly larvae (maggots) in the tissues or wounds of man or domestic animals. The presence of live maggots in a wound or their escape from a living being's body is a condition that could not be confused with any other syndrome. As early as 520 B.C., Herodotus described a case of facultative myiasis in a woman. "No sooner had she returned to Egypt, than she died a horrible death, her body seething with maggots while she was still alive." The Bible alludes several times to maggots infesting human flesh. In Job 7:5, the afflicted Job stated, "My flesh is clothed with maggots and clods of dust, my skin rotted and fouled afresh." In Acts 12:23, it was recorded that King Herod died 5 days after being smitten with gangrene, during which time maggots bred in the gangrenous mass. Historical descriptions, however, are not restricted to man. In the *Hortus Sanitatis* published in Antwerp, Belgium, in 1521, there are woodcuts that imply that the authors were aware of the life cycle of flies; flies swarm on maggot-infested meat and attack a dead or dying animal (Greenberg, 1973). Reports of this syndrome in cats are rare, although facultative myiasis probably does occur frequently.

Facultative myiasis is often a condition of the skin. It is most commonly found around the perineal region or along the dorsal midline. Lesions appear as "punched out" ulcers. These ulcers frequently merge to produce larger ulcers with scalloped edges. Sections of skin may be undermined, and the movement of large numbers of active larvae may be observed and felt (Prescott, 1984).

Adult *Calliphora* species, *Phaenicia* species, *Lucilia* species, and *Phormia* species, often referred to as blowflies or bottle flies, are metallic blue, green, or black. Adult *Sarcophaga* species, often referred to as flesh flies, have a gray longitudinal striped thorax with a checkerboard-patterned abdomen. Keys are available for the first and second larval stages of the facultative myiasis–producing flies (Zumpt, 1965). The third-stage larva of the facultative myiasis–producing flies is pointed anteriorly and possesses a broad, flattened posterior end. It may either have a smooth surface or be "hairy," possessing thorn-like, fleshy projections over most of its surface. The larva is approximately 10 to 14 mm long and pale yellow to grayish white, but it may possess a slight pink tinge. The anterior end bears a pair of oral hooks that are connected to the internal, chitinous, cephalopharyngeal skeleton. The posterior end of the larva exhibits one pair of stigmatic, stigmal, or spiracular plates. Each plate consists of 3 long, slender, parallel slits located within the spiracle. The different species of myiasis-producing flies may be differentiated by the cephalopharyngeal skeleton and by the shape of the spiracular plates. Of these two features, the structure of the larva's spiracular plate is the more important diagnostic characteristic.

As soon as a tentative diagnosis of facultative myiasis is rendered, the veterinarian must rule out the possibility of obligatory myiasis due to one of the primary screwworm maggots. In contrast to the facultative myiasis–producing flies, flies that induce primary myiasis will not breed in carrion but lay their eggs at the edge of fresh, uncontaminated wounds of various warm-blooded animals. Within the wound, the larvae penetrate into, feed on, and rapidly devour fresh, live host tissue. The larvae of the primary screwworms basically require a living host. Because of the obligatory nature with regard to breeding in fresh wounds and the fear of introduction of screwworms from one continent to another, the practitioner should report infestations with primary screwworms to the proper control authorities in countries where the screwworms are not autochthonous.

Life Cycle

The mouthparts of the adult flies are of a sponging type and are never used to lacerate tissues; rather they are used for imbibing liquid food. Solid food, feces, or necrotic tissue must be made fluid before being sucked up by the fly. The fly disgorges saliva and crop contents; this mixture serves to liquefy the solid matter. The fly then sponges up the liquefied digestate using its mouthparts.

It is the larval stage that is important in facultative myiasis because it is this stage that resides within the tissues of the host. Adult female flies lay clusters of light-colored eggs in feces, carcasses, wounds, or soiled hair. While the female fly is selecting a suitable spot to lay her eggs, she feeds on the moist matter that may be present. If the female fly chooses feces or carrion as a feeding/egg-laying site, her offspring will develop in a non-parasitic lifestyle. However, if the female fly chooses a cat's contaminated wounds or soiled, matted hair as an egg-laying site, her offspring could develop into parasites.

The female flies are attracted to material containing protein, which is necessary for ovarian development. She will lay from 50 to 150 eggs in one batch and, in her lifespan, will produce from 1,000 to 3,000 eggs. The newly laid eggs are about 1 mm long. The first-stage larvae hatch from these eggs in 8 to 72 hours and begin to feed on the moist food in the contaminated wound. First-stage larvae have underdeveloped mouthparts and must feed on liquid protein, which may be found in wound exudate. Without liquid protein, they cannot develop to second-stage larvae. Second-stage larvae demonstrate well-developed mouthparts capable of scratching the skin; they then feed on the protein-rich fluid that exudes. This begins the pathologic sequence of events. The larvae grow rapidly to fully developed, third-stage larvae. The larval developmental rate is dependent upon the amount and suitability of food, the temperature, and the degree of competition among the larvae present. Development from the egg to the third larval stage takes from a few days to a couple of weeks.

When the larva is ready to pupate, it usually drops off the host, crawls over or through the soil, and pupates beneath the soil surface. In some instances, however, the larvae of facultative myiasis–producing flies may pupate in the haircoat of the live animal. Under conditions of cold weather, pupation may become delayed, and the larva may hibernate in the soil until warm weather prevails. At pupation, the larva loosens its skin, and the skin turns brown and rigid. The resulting developmental stage is the pupa or puparium. During the summer months the pupal stage lasts from 3 to 7 days while hibernation usually occurs over the winter months. The adult fly emerges from the end of the puparium by alternately inflating and deflating the ptilinal sac within its head. It also uses this technique to move through the soil to the surface. As an adult, the female fly again has the choice of laying her eggs in feces, carcasses, wounds, or soiled, matted hair.

Clinical Presentation and Pathogenesis

For facultative myiasis to develop in any warm-blooded animal, some inciting lesion must be present in the animal's skin or haircoat. In many instances, the lesion is either in an area of fecal soiling, a neglected wound or other traumatic area, or where there is an ocular discharge (Wilkinson, 1985). The common characteristic of these situations is sustained, moist conditions within the haircoat. A study of fleece rot and fly strike in sheep revealed that oviposition by flies was found to be markedly affected by the availability of protein and by bacterial activity, especially that of *Pseudomonas* species. Odors emanating from culture plates containing wool and these bacteria played an important role in fly attraction and oviposition (Merritt and Watts, 1978).

In time, the eggs hatch, and the larvae emerge. It must be remembered that the first-stage larvae have underdeveloped mouthparts and must feed on liquid protein. These mouthparts of first-stage larvae do little to physically damage the skin. Second- and third-stage larvae have mouthparts capable of rasping the skin and inflicting considerable damage (Monzu, 1978). Throughout the infestation process, the later larval stages of facultative myiasis–producing flies move independently about the wound surface. The larvae of these flies ingest dead cells, exudates, secretions, and debris, but not live tissues. They irritate, injure, and kill successive layers of cells and provoke exudation. Large numbers of maggots rapidly consume dead cells and exudates. In time, the maggots tunnel through the thinned epidermis into the subcutis where they continue to feed upon dead cells and exudative debris. This erosive process forms tissue cavities up to several centimeters in diameter. Unless this process is halted by appropriate therapy, the infested animal may die from shock, intoxication, histolysis, or infection (Kimberling, 1988).

Close examination of the early lesions reveals a moist dermatitis, varying numbers of small maggots, and a peculiar, distinct, pungent odor. The epidermis is thin, and the skin is inflamed and appears reddened and tender. Advanced lesions may contain thousands of maggots, some of which have produced cavitations in the subcutaneous tissues. The lesion can become quite large and the tissue destruction quite extensive. Fly larvae may even destroy portions of musculature and invade body cavities. By this time, infested animals are usually depressed, febrile, and usually prostrate (Hendrix, 1991).

Diagnosis

The diagnosis of maggot infestation in cats can be easily made by a layperson because maggots can be observed in an existing wound or among soiled, matted hairs. As mentioned in above, people have been doing this for centuries. A history of traumatic injury or surgical intervention may alert the owner or veterinarian. Most cases of facultative myiasis in small animals occur in geriatric patients with fecal or urinary incontinence that result in soiling of the haircoat. In those breeds of cats with long, thick haircoats that become matted or soiled by feces or urine, the diagnosis may not be made in an early stage of infestation; the infested animal may become depressed, febrile, and prostrate before the problem is recognized. In such cases, the peculiar, distinct, pungent odor characteristic of facultative myiasis will also be present.

Cats infested with larvae of the facultative myiasis–producing flies may often ingest these larvae during the grooming process. Fly larvae have been known to pass through the gastrointestinal tract in an undigested state; owners or veterinarians might therefore suspect facultative myiasis, although diagnosis by this method is a rare occurrence. Such larval passing may occur because of pseudomyiasis, which occurs when a free-roaming cat ingests carrion that contains maggots and the maggots then pass via the feces in an undigested state.

Treatment

The literature on treatment and control measures for facultative myiasis in sheep is voluminous, but such is not the case for the condition in cats (Prescott, 1984; Hendrix, 1991). Should the larvae of facultative myiasis–producing flies be detected in small animals, immediate therapy is necessary. The extent of the lesion is determined by clipping the animal's haircoat, thus removing many larvae that are present in the hair. However, removal of the maggots from existing deep tissue pockets may prove to be difficult. Sedation or anesthetizing may be required to allow physical extraction of the larvae from subcutaneous locations. The practitioner should examine the lesions for the presence of fly larvae on successive days; it must be remembered that adult flies lay eggs in the wounds at different times and that hatching of larvae may not be synchronous. Dead tissues should be debrided and pockets exposed or adequately drained.

Depressed, febrile, and prostrate patients should be treated symptomatically (intravenous fluids, nutritional support, etc.). Ideally, culture and sensitivity examinations should be performed on wounds. If secondary bacterial or fungal infections are present, they must be treated. Administration of broad-spectrum antibiotics would be a wise decision.

Various insecticides have been used to kill the adult flies and their larvae within wounds in sheep. These include the chlorinated hydrocarbons and the organophosphates including chlorfenvinphos, diazinon, and bromophos ethyl. More recently, the synthetic pyrethroids (permethrin, cypermethrin, and cyprothrin) have been demonstrated to be safe, effective insecticides for use in sheep dips. Analogous insecticides may be used to treat the larvae of facultative myiasis–producing flies in small animals.

Epizootiology

Facultative myiasis is usually observed in weakened or grossly ignored cats. It usually occurs during hot weather and is always associated with neglected wounds or with haircoats that have become matted and stained with urine or feces. There is no age or sex predilection; however, this condition does tend to occur more commonly in long-haired cats (Prescott, 1984).

Hazards to Other Animals

Facultative myiasis may develop in any warm-blooded animal. A prerequisite is some inciting lesion in the animal's skin or haircoat (Wilkinson, 1985).

Hazards to Humans

Likewise, neglected lesions in humans may be subjected to infestation by the myiasis-producing flies (Miller et al., 1990). There is an additional hazard to humans—the repulsion when one observes or smells a maggot-infested wound.

Control/Prevention

The best control techniques against the facultative myiasis–producing flies are always preventive (Zumpt, 1965). The veterinarian should educate the client concerning the immediate treatment of all skin wounds. The client must be aware that the animal must be confined in a fly-free area. The cat's haircoat has to be kept clean of urine or feces and should not be allowed to become matted. Contaminated wounds and matted haircoats soaked in urine or feces rapidly attract the adult myiasis-producing flies. Recognition of this fact can help the client protect the animal from attack by myiasis-producing flies (Hendrix, 1991).

REFERENCES

Greenberg B. 1973. In Flies and Disease, vol II, 1st ed, pp 11-18. Princeton, NJ: Princeton University Press.

Harwood RF , James MT. 1979. In Entomology in Human and Animal Health, 7th ed, pp 37–38, 248–251, 255–266, 296–318. New York, NY: Macmillan.

Hendrix CM. 1991. Facultative myiasis in dogs and cats. Comp Cont Educ Pract Vet 13:86–96.

Kimberling CV. 1988. In Jensen and Swift's Diseases of Sheep, pp 308–312. Philadelphia, Pa: Lea and Febiger.

Merritt GC, Watts JE. 1978. An in-vitro technique for studying fleece-rot and fly strike in sheep. Aust Vet J 54:513–516.

Miller KB, Hribar LJ, Sanders LJ. 1990. Human myiasis caused by *Phormia regina* in Pennsylvania. J Am Pod Med Assoc 80:600–602.

Monzu N. 1978. Some basic facts about primary blowflies. J Agric, W Aust 19:93–95.

Prescott CW. 1984. In Parasitic Diseases of the Cat in Australia, 2nd ed, p 76. Sydney: University of Sydney, Post-Graduate Foundation in Veterinary Science.

Wilkinson, GT. 1985. In Color Atlas of Small Animal Dermatology, p 64. Baltimore, Md: Williams and Wilkins.

Zumpt F. 1965. In Myiasis in Man and Animals in the Old World, pp 1–267. London: Butterworths.

Calliphorid Myiasis

The Calliphoridae (blowfly) is similar in general appearance to the common housefly, but it usually displays metallic bodies of brilliant hues with colors such as blue, green, copper, and black (Fig. 5.65). The flies are called blowflies because the females hover over decaying flesh while they oviposit or larviposit ("blow") eggs or larvae on the meat. Like the sarcophagid flies, the calliphorid flies are usually nonpathogenic species, most of which are important in that they feed on decaying animal tissue, but some species are important as facultative or primary myiasis producers.

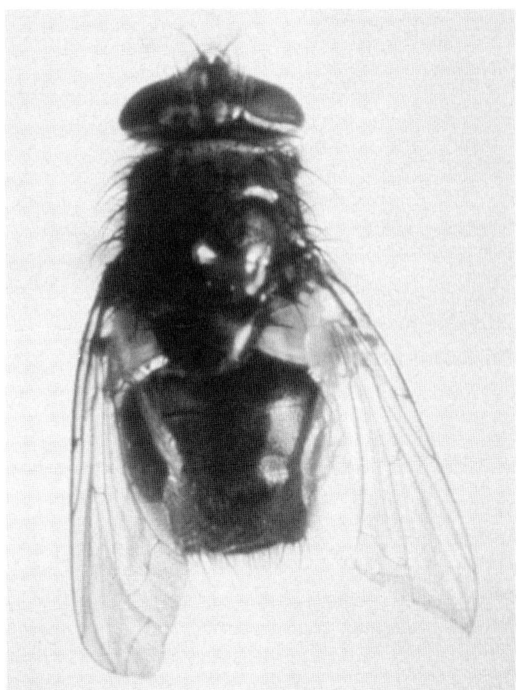

Fig. 5.65. A calliphorid fly with the typical metallic body.

Phaenicia (*Lucilia*) *sericata* (Meigen)

The green blowfly *Phaenicia sericata* causes cases of myiasis around the world. Green blowflies commonly breed on carrion, but they can be attracted to sores or to soiled hair. These are a common cause of myiasis in sheep in certain parts of the world where sheep are raised, and human cases of infestation have occurred. Thus, species in Asia are thought to be highly dangerous pests in that they are quite comfortable with living hosts, whereas in North America, the flies seem to prefer carrion, and these have been the maggots most commonly used in wound therapy. The eggs are deposited on the wound or soiled hair, and the larvae (Fig. 5.66) feed for 2 to 10 days before they drop to the ground where pupation occurs.

Cats have been reported parasitized by these facultative myiasis producers in Europe and the Americas. Dermal lesions were reported from a cat in Germany (Ribbeck et al., 1979), and two cases of dermal myiasis have been described from

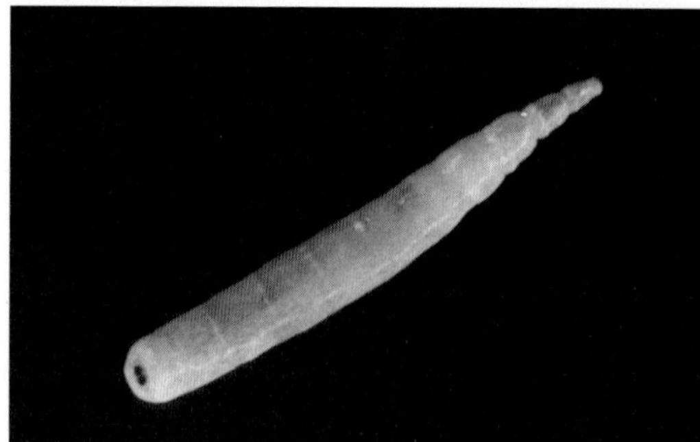

Fig. 5.66. The larva (maggot) of *Lucilia.*

Austria (Hinaidy and Frey, 1984). One other case of myiasis from Austria was perineal myiasis following diarrhea due to infectious peritonitis, while another case was preputial myiasis (Hinaidy and Frey, 1984). A cat from Missouri was described as having a vaginal myiasis shortly after parturition (Hall, 1979). Vignau and Arias (1997) and Mariluis et al. (1994) presented cases of dermal myiasis due to *Phaenicia sericata* from cats in Argentina.

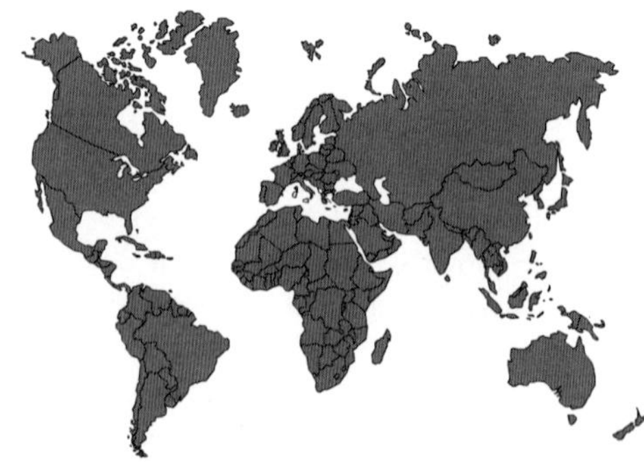

Fig. 5.67.

REFERENCES

Hall R-D. 1979. The blowflies of Missouri: an annotated checklist (Diptera: Calliphoridae). Trans Mo Acad Sci 13:33–36.

Hinaidy HK, Frey H. 1984. Weitere Fakultativmyiasis-Falle bei Wirbeltieren in Osterreich. Wien Tierarztl Monatschr 71:237–238.

Mariluis J-C, Schnack J-A, Cerverizzo I, Quintana C. 1994. *Cochliomyia hominivorax* (Coquerel, 1858) and *Phaenicia sericata (*Meigen, 1826) parasitizing domestic animals in Buenos Aires and vicinities (Diptera, Calliphoridae). Mem Inst Oswaldo Cruz 89:139.

Ribbeck R, Schroder E, and Schumann H. 1979. Lucilia sericata-Larven als Ereger von Wundmyiasis bei Hund und Katze. Veterinarmedizin 34:383–384.

Vignau ML, Arias DO. 1997. Myiasis cutaneoulcerosas en pequenos animales. Parasitologia al Dia 21:36–39.

Phaenicia (*Lucilia*) *caesar* (Linnaeus)

This bluish green blowfly is restricted to Europe, North Africa, and Asia. Typically, the larvae develop in decaying meat, but it has been occasionally reported from animals and humans in Europe. Supperer and Hinaidy reported an infestation of a cat in Austria (1986).

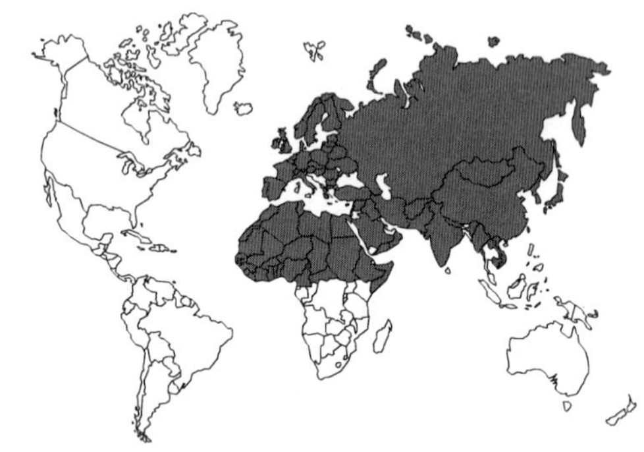

Fig. 5.68.

REFERENCES

Supperer R, Hinaidy HK. 1986. Ein Beitrag zum Parasitenbefall der Hunde und Katzen in Osterreich. Deutsch Tierarztl Wochenschr 93:383–386.

Cochliomyia hominivorax (Coquerel, 1858)

Cochliomyia hominivorax, the New World screwworm, is indiscriminant in its choice of hosts, and this fly will infest cats. The female lays batches of eggs in rows on the edge of any small wound in the skin, and after about a half to 1 day, the eggs hatch, and the larvae crawl into the wound site. The larvae feed on the wounds for about a week and then fall to the ground where they burrow into the soil prior to pupation. The lesions produced can be severe and can attract other species of flies that will secondarily establish in the wound. Such lesions can be very debilitating and can become life threatening. The screwworm maggots can be identified by their very black tracheae that are present in the posterior of the body and that are easy to observe upon dissection. Fortunately, due to a successful control program that involves the release of irradiation-sterilized males, *Cochliomyia hominivorax* only occurs in the Americas south of Mexico.

Cats have been infested with this parasite. Vignau and Arias (1997) observed cases in nine cats in Argentina during January through May. Santa Cruz and Lombardero (1987) found it in 1 of 50 cats examined in Correintes City, Argentina.

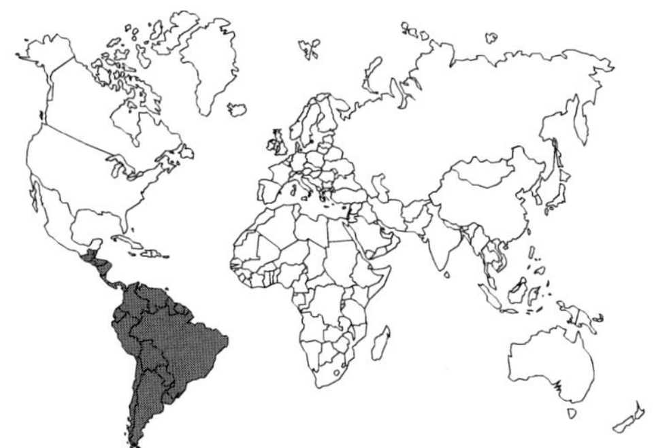

Fig. 5.69.

REFERENCES

Santa Cruz AM, Lombardero OJ. 1987. Resultados parasitologicos de 50 necropsias de gatos de la ciudad de Corrientes. Vet Argent 4:735–739.

Vignau ML, Arias DO. 1997. Myiasis cutaneo-ulcerosas en pequenos animales. Parasitologia al Dia 21:36–39.

Chrysomyia bezziana Villeneuve

Etymology

Chryso = gold + *myia* = fly; along with *bezziana* for Dr. Bezzi.

History

In 1910, Dr. Rovere described several cases of traumatic myiasis in cattle from the Congo. He sent some of the adults he reared to a Professor Bezzi in Turin, Italy, who incorrectly identified them as *Chrysomyia megacephala.* Also in 1910, Gedoelst reported similar findings from the Congo and also referred to the larvae as *Chrysomyia megacephala.* Roubaud and Bouet studied this fly again in West Africa and found its behavior different from other species of *Chrysomyia* in this area. They also believed erroneously that they were dealing with *Chrysomyia megacephala.* Villeneuve reexamined the type specimen, which had an incorrect locality designation, and found it conspecific with *Chrysomyia dux* from the Orient. The species that Roubaud and the others were dealing with had to be renamed, so Villeneuve did so in honor of Professor Bezzi, who had already noted that this fly was different from *Chrysomyia dux* (Zumpt, 1965).

Geographic Distribution

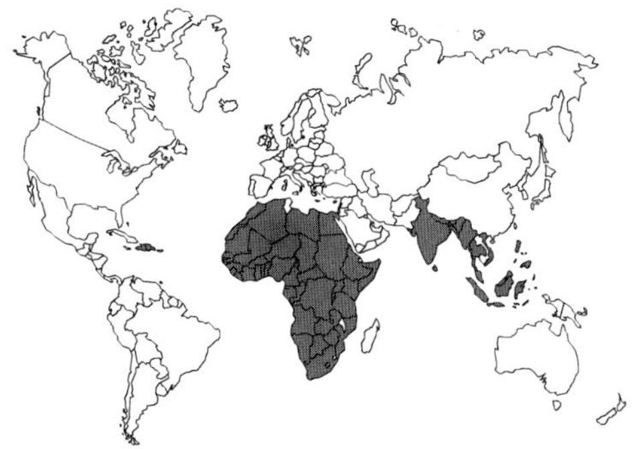

Fig. 5.70.

Chrysomyia bezziana, the Old World screwworm, is a primary myiasis-producing fly that attacks a wide range of warm-blooded animals throughout Africa, the Indian subcontinent, and Southeast Asia from Taiwan in the north to Papua New Guinea in the south. The only continent with a tropical zone still free of primary screwworm is Australia (Davidson, 1992; Spradbery, 1992). There are secondary myiasis-producing flies in Australia that can be of significant importance, such as *Chrysomyia rufifacies* (Figs. 5.71 and 5.72).

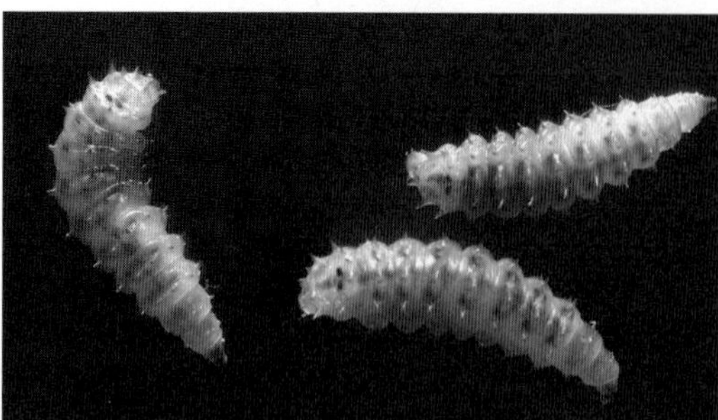

Fig. 5.71. The larvae of *Chrysomyia rufifacies* from Australia.

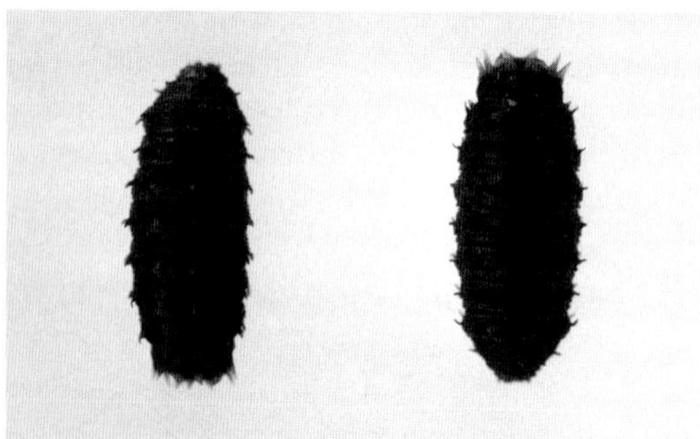

Fig. 5.72. Two pupal cases of *Chrysomyia rufifacies* from Australia.

Location in Host

The larvae of *Chrysomyia bezziana* are obligatory wound parasites and never develop in carcasses or other decomposing matter. The female flies are attracted to the open wounds of humans and domesticated animals. Any slight, bleeding wound, even the smallest sore caused by a feeding tick, inflicted accidentally on domestic animals is subject to infestation.

Parasite Identification

Adult *Chrysomyia bezziana* are nonparasitic and as a result will not be observed by the client or the veterinarian. The adults are rarely found in the field. They are never found feeding on food in open air markets (Patton and Evans, 1929). This fly possesses a dark metallic green or blue body with abdominal segments with narrow dark bands along the posterior margins. The legs are black or partially dark brown; the face is orange-yellow.

The first larval stage will probably go unnoticed due to its small size, up to 3 mm at the time of its molt to the second stage. The second stage is quite similar to the third but is from 4 to 9 mm in length. The third stage larva is a large larva, up to 18 mm in length. The body is composed of 12 segments that have broad encircling bands of spinules. All three stages are "maggot-like" in their appearance and exhibit cephalopharyngeal sclerites and posterior spiracles that are unique to the species (Zumpt, 1965). The posterior end of the larva has its spiracular plate located in a deep cleft at the end of the eighth abdominal segment. The spiracular plates are large and well separated. The peritreme is wide with a break in its inferointernal border. The button is situated in the break in the peritreme. The three breathing slits are very wide (Patton and Evans, 1929).

The second- and third-stage larval *Chrysomyia bezziana* are the stages that will be usually observed in the skin of an infested cat by either the owner or the veterinarian. These stages can probably be best identified by an entomologist. Extensive descriptions of these morphologic stages do exist (Patton and Evans, 1929; Zumpt, 1965).

Life Cycle

Chrysomyia bezziana has been described as a fly that produces a "particularly vile" myiasis (Davidson, 1985). Female flies lay their eggs in masses of 150 to 500 at the edge of wounds (Harwood and James, 1979) or near body orifices (Davidson, 1985). Larvae develop to the third stage about 2 days following hatching. They burrow deep into the wound to such a depth that only their caudal ends are observable. The entire larval stage lasts 5 to 6 days. Under tropical conditions, the pupal stage lasts 7 to 9 days; however, this time will increase in cooler ecosystems (Harwood and James, 1979). The adult flies merge later to mate, locate a new host, and continue the cycle. The female flies mate only once during their lifetime. Under favorable conditions, there may be eight or more generations per year (Zumpt, 1965).

Clinical Presentation and Pathogenesis

Myiasis due to *Chrysomyia bezziana* is extremely rare in cats. A single described case of infestation occurred in a Persian cat from Port Moresby,

Papua New Guinea. Secondary infestation with the facultative myiasis-producing flies may complicate treatment and control of the infestation (Davidson, 1985).

The larvae of *Chrysomyia bezziana* are obligatory wound parasites, developing only in live tissue. The female flies are attracted to open wounds of humans and domesticated and wild animals. Occasionally eggs are deposited on the unbroken, soft skin of various parts of the body, especially if it is contaminated by blood or mucous discharge. When the larvae hatch, they burrow into the flesh of the host, using their hooked mouthparts to scrape away at the tissues and lacerate the fine blood vessels. Larvae actively feed on the host's blood. During the blood-sucking phase, only the caudal ends of the maggots with their blackish peritremes remain visible at the surface of the lesion, enabling the larvae to breathe. As many as 3,000 maggots have been observed in some wounds (Davidson, 1985). In untreated wounds, the destructive activity of the larvae may lead to the death of the animals within a very short period of time.

Treatment

Treatment of screwworm infestation involves killing the larvae in the lesions, promoting healing, and preventing secondary reinfestation with larvae of the facultative myiasis-producing flies. The extent of the lesions is determined by clipping the haircoat and removing as many larvae as possible. The larvae that are removed should be killed to prevent them from pupating and developing into adults. The larvae located deep within tissues must be extracted. The dressing should be bland and nontoxic to the cat and should promote healing.

Ivermectin at dosages of 50, 100, and 200 μg per kilogram administered to infested cattle resulted in 100 percent larval *Chrysomyia bezziana* mortality for at least 6, 12, and 14 days, respectively. Depending upon their age, larvae survived in established strikes following treatment at 200 μg per kilogram. Larvae up to 2 days old demonstrated 100 percent mortality, while older larvae showed greater resistance. At this dosage, residual protection lasted 16 to 20 days, two to three times that produced by most insecticide smears. These mortality rates were very conservative; many of the larvae that survived ivermectin therapy failed to develop to the adult stage (Spradbery et al., 1985). The product should not be given to kittens (O'Dair and Shaw, 1991). Treating cats monthly with imidacloprid, fipronil, or selamectin may prevent infestations of cats.

Epizootiology

The effects of infestation with *Chrysomyia bezziana* are particularly devastating. Strike on naturally occurring wounds (e.g., tick bites) and on external body openings can be quite serious. Fly strike also has the ability to follow elective feline surgical procedures (e.g., spays or castrations).

Hazards to Other Animals

All warm-blooded animals are subject to infestation by *Chrysomyia bezziana.* The animals most commonly infested are cattle. Other known hosts include sheep, goats, buffalo, pigs, chickens, dogs and horses (Patton, 1920; Davidson, 1985). Reports of infestations on wild animals are rare. A survey of the records of the Malaysian National Zoo revealed 91 cases of myiasis in 21 host species during the period 1965 to 1980. Those animals included the honey bear, polar bear, camel, fallow deer, hog deer, red deer, sambar deer, donkey, Asian elephant, gnu, Sumatran horse, striped hyena, red kangaroo, African lion, Asian lion, slow loris, puma, rhinoceros, sheep, Malay tapir, and agile wallaby (Spradbery and Vanniasingham, 1980).

Hazards to Humans

Infestations of humans with the larvae of *Chrysomyia bezziana* are very common in India and other parts of Asia (Patton, 1920). This parasite has been reported to occur in humans in Africa (Zumpt, 1965). Children are often subject to infestation in scalp wounds (Davidson, 1985).

Control/Prevention

All wounds on domesticated animals should be properly dressed. All elective surgical procedures should be avoided during the fly season.

REFERENCES

Davidson S. 1985. Screw-worm fly: meeting the threat. Rural Res 129:4–10.

Davidson S. 1992. Screw-worm stowaways—assessing the risk. Rural Res 146:29–31.
Harwood RF, James MT. 1979. In *Entomology in Human and Animal Health,* 7th ed, pp 37–38, 248–251, 255–266, 296–318. New York, NY: Macmillan.
O'Dair HA, Shaw SE. 1991. Mite treatment of cats. Vet Rec 129:272.
Paradis M, Scott D, Villeneuve A. 1990. Efficacy of ivermectin against *Cheyletiella blakei* infestation in cats. J Am Anim Hosp Assoc 26:125–128.
Patton WS. 1920. Some notes on Indian Calliphorinae. Part I. *Chrysomyia bezziana* Villeneuve, the common Indian calliphorine whose larvae cause cutaneous myiasis in man and animals. Ind J Med Res 8:17–29.
Patton WS, Evans AM. 1929. In *Insects, Ticks, Mites and Venomous Animals,* pp 408, 421–424, 455, 464–466, 734. Croydon: HR Grubb.
Spradbery JP. 1992. Screw-worm fly: an Australian perspective. Aust Vet J 69:88.
Spradbery JP, Vanniasingham JA. 1980. Incidence of the screw-worm fly, *Chrysomyia bezziana,* at the Zoo Negara, Malaysia. Malays Vet J 7:28–32.
Spradbery JP, Tozer RS, Drewett N, Lindsey MJ. 1985. The efficacy of ivermectin against screw-worm fly (*Chrysomyia bezziana*) in vitro and in cattle. Aust Vet J 62:311–314.
Zumpt F. 1965. In *Myiasis in Man and Animals in the Old World,* pp 99–102. London: Butterworths.

Cordylobia anthropophaga

History

The larvae of the African tumbu fly, *Cordylobia anthropophaga,* were first discovered by Coquerel and Mondière in 1862 in Senegal in both humans and dogs. The adult fly was unknown to them (Zumpt, 1965). It was not until 1893 that Blanchard described the adult and gave it the name *Ochromyia anthropophaga.* In 1903, Grunberg placed the fly in a new genus, *Cordylobia* (Rice and Gleason, 1972).

Geographic Distribution

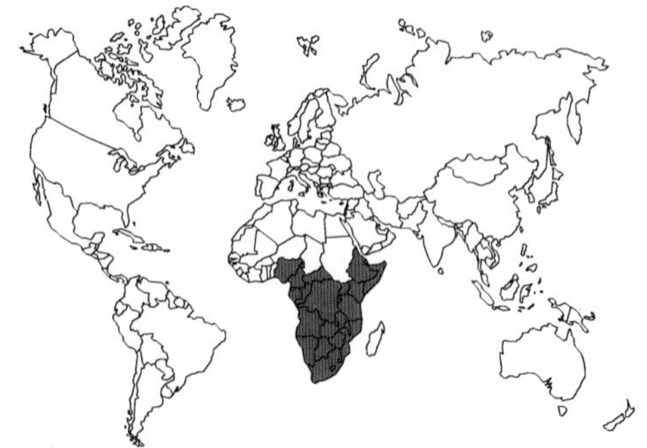

Fig. 5.73.

This parasite is responsible for cutaneous myiasis in the sub-Saharan region of Africa (Zumpt, 1965). However, with the extensive travel patterns of today's "air mobile" world citizen, the parasite has been diagnosed in travelers (Rice and Gleason, 1972; Laurence and Herman, 1973; Scholten and Hicks, 1973; Kozminska-Kubarska, 1981; Ockenhouse et al., 1990; Veraldi et al., 1993) and their accompanying pets (Idowu and Olote, 1976; Roberts et al., 1982; Fox et al., 1992) in geographic areas where the parasite does not exist.

Location in Host

The parasite produces a painful boil-like (furuncular) swelling in the skin in both man and animals (Idowu and Olote, 1976). The lesions caused by the developing larvae are localized to the skin or subcutaneous tissue (Ockenhouse et al., 1990). In animals, the chief sites of infestation are the feet, genitals, tail, and axillary region; however, in heavy infestations any area of the body may be affected, including the nose (Zumpt, 1965).

Parasite Identification

Adult *Cordylobia anthropophaga* are nonparasitic and as a result will not be observed by the client or the veterinarian. They are stout, compact flies, averaging about 9.5 mm long. Their general color is light brown, with diffuse blue-gray patches on the thorax and a dark gray color on the posterior part of the abdomen. The face and legs are yellow. The body length of the adult fly is variable, between 6 and 12 mm (Zumpt, 1965). It is very difficult to recognize the adult fly if it has not been reared from a larva extracted from the host.

The second- and third-stage larvae of *Cordylobia anthropophaga* are the stages that will be usually observed in the skin of an infested cat. The second-stage larva is slightly club shaped and exhibits large, black, posteriorly directed cuticular spines irregularly distributed over the third to the eighth segments. Segments nine to 11 are almost bare when compared with the preceding segments. The segments have a few rows of small, pale spines posteriorly. Segment 12 is densely covered with these spinules. Segment 13 is indistinctly demarcated, lacking spines but possessing two pair of short processes. Each tracheal tube opens through two slightly bent slits. The cephaloskeleton is strongly sclerotized and armed with two hook-shaped labial sclerites. The early second-stage larva is from 2.5 to 4 mm in length. Great variation is seen in the size of the advanced second-stage larva.

Great variation is also seen in the size of the third-stage larva; the fully mature larva is from 1.3 to 1.5 cm in length. The body is cylindrical with 12 identifiable segments. The two hook-shaped labial sclerites are projected. On either side of the sclerites is a ridge of yellow sclerotized integument. Posteriorly directed curved spines are densely arranged at least up to segment seven; the last five segments may be either partially covered or densely covered with spines. The posterior spiracles open through three sinuous slits located on a weakly schlerotized peritreme (Zumpt, 1965). The presence of a dermal swelling with a central opening may lead to a tentative diagnosis of myiasis due to *Cordylobia anthropophaga.* A definitive diagnosis can be made only after extraction and identification of the typical larva.

Diagnosis is often made by a history of either residence in or travel to an area endemic for *Cordylobia anthropophaga.* There are other flies from different areas throughout the world that might produce a lesion similar to *Cordylobia anthropophaga.* These should also be considered in a differential diagnosis. These myiasis-producing flies include *Dermatobia hominis,* the South American tórsalo fly; *Wohlfahrtia vigil,* the gray flesh fly; *Chrysomyia bezziana,* the Oriental fly; *Cochliomyia hominivorax,* the New World primary screwworm; and *Cuterebra* species, the rabbit botflies. These obligatory myiasis-producing flies should be considered in the differential diagnosis in cats with an appropriate residence or travel history.

Life Cycle

The adult flies are rarely observed during the daytime but instead rest on the ceilings of huts and open porches. They are active from seven to nine in the early morning and from four to six in the late afternoon. The adults feed on the juices of plants (bananas, pineapples), decomposing animal tissues, and excreta. For egg laying, the female is attracted to dry sand contaminated with urine or feces. A cat's litter box (either clean or soiled) may be a prime medium for egg laying. If the sand is too moist, the eggs are not laid there but are deposited nearby on a dry spot. The flies never lay their eggs on the exposed skin or attach them to hairs.

Fertilization and oviposition continue all year-round. The female fly lives for about 2 weeks and produces 300 to 500 eggs, deposited in two batches of 100 to 300 eggs each. The larvae hatch after 1 to 3 days and remain alive without food for about 9 days. Some may persist for as long as 15 days. The larvae remain just below the surface of the sand, in anticipation of a passing host. If the surface of the sand is disturbed, the larvae quickly crawl out. They adhere to grains of sand and by means of their posterior ends, raise their bodies, and wave about actively, seeking a host to which they can attach. Once the larva attaches to the skin of the host, it immediately begins to penetrate. The time required for penetration depends on the thickness of the host's skin. At the end of the invasion process, the larva is covered by a thin layer of skin. Its last segment protrudes slightly through the aperture, but it can be withdrawn if touched. The first larval stage molts to the second after 2 to 4 days. The molt to the next stage takes place on the fifth or sixth day after invasion. In the rat, maturity is reached on or about the eighth day. The larva then leaves the boil, drops to the ground, and pupates within 24 hours. At room temperature, the fly hatches after 10 to 11 days. At lower temperatures, the pupal stage lasts longer (Zumpt, 1965).

Clinical Presentation and Pathogenesis

Penetration of the skin by the first-stage larva may not be noticed by the owner. A small red pimple forms at the penetration site. The reaction caused by the entrance of the larva is said to be palpable for the first 2 days. The symptoms then subside, and the infected area may be overlooked. Serous fluid exudes from the opening made by the larva for breathing. The skin becomes inflamed, and there is tenderness on pressure. The lesion now resembles a small boil. There may be multiple sites of infestation (Patton and Evans, 1929). As mentioned previously, the lesions caused by the developing larvae are localized to the skin or subcutaneous tissue (Ockenhouse et al., 1990).

With the increase in size of the furuncular lesion and the surrounding inflammation of the tissues, more serious symptoms develop. The tissues surrounding the swelling, now large, are hardened and erythematous. During this period, the larva is very active and can cause great pain. The larva can be observed moving in the swelling as it attempts to enlarge the cavity and the respiratory opening as it grows. For this process, the larva produces a lytic reaction. The secretions from the opening now contain more and more larval feces (Gunther, 1971).

One or two larvae normally do not produce conspicuous stress, but when they are numerous, considerable irritation and restlessness may arise, resulting from septic absorption. Where larvae are close together, swelling and edema occur. The tissues may become gangrenous. The larvae may invade deeper tissues and may cause severe destruction leading to the death of the host (Zumpt, 1965).

Furuncular myiasis due to *Cordylobia anthropophaga* is characterized by the simultaneous finding of four clinical signs: (1) occurrence of boil-like lesions, (2) the indolence of the lesions, (3) a small opening in which lies the caudal end of the larva with its spiracular plate, and (4) the secretion of a serous fluid, sometimes stained with blood or larval feces (Gunther, 1971).

Treatment

As with all subcutaneous tissue–dwelling flies, treatment is based on the fact that the larvae need communication with outside air for respiration. Air exchange is accomplished via the larva's posterior spiracles. The airway may be occluded using heavy oil, liquid paraffin, sticking plaster, pork fat, or petroleum jelly (Ockenhouse et al., 1990).

Surgical intervention involves the injection of lidocaine hydrochloride into the furuncular lesion, producing local anesthesia for the cat and also anesthetizing the larva, allowing it to be manually extracted using thumb forceps. Antibiotics should be prescribed. Ockenhouse et al. (1990) stated that surgical excision is usually unnecessary and unwarranted while the larvae are alive but is used to remove dead or decaying larvae.

Great care should be taken during the extraction process to avoid rupturing the larva in situ, although no mention is made of anaphylaxis as occurs when larvae of *Cuterebra* species are ruptured during extraction. In suspect cases, the extracted larva should be submitted to an entomologist for definitive diagnosis. Parasitologists (and veterinarians) not well acquainted with the taxonomy of these myiasis-producing flies should always contact an expert when correct identification is needed.

Epizootiology

In the tropics, cordylobiasis occasionally spreads during the flies' breeding season and during the period of animal migration, especially among rats during floods occurring in the rainy season (Gunther, 1971). Young animals are much more susceptible than older ones and are more heavily infested (Patton and Evans, 1929).

Hazards to Other Animals

Of domestic animals, the dog is primarily affected and must be regarded as an important reservoir host; the rat is the most important wild reservoir host (Gunther, 1971). In addition to cats, other domesticated animals naturally infected are the goat, pig, rabbit, guinea pig, and chicken. Wild animals infected include mice, monkeys, mongooses, squirrels, leopards, boars, and antelopes. Reptiles and amphibians are never infected (Veraldi et al., 1993).

Hazards to Humans

The larvae are capable of penetrating any part of the skin surface of humans. Young children may demonstrate involvement of the scalp and the face. Children are more frequently infected than adults due to the thinness of their skin. Thin skin facilitates penetration of the larvae (Veraldi et al., 1993). The lesions in humans are often found on covered parts of the body, such as the waist, buttocks, arms, armpits, and sometimes the legs, suggesting that the larvae may have become fixed to some article of clothing (Patton and Evans, 1929).

Control/Prevention

Adult flies should be killed if observed indoors. Larvae should be removed from animals entering the house and destroyed. All rats should be killed and burned. Clothes should not be left lying out; they should be ironed and put away (Patton and Evans, 1929).

In Africa south of the Sahara Desert, *Cordylobia anthropophaga* is a common parasite of dogs and rabbits. Prevention of an infestation depends on cleanliness and regular disinfection of the animal's sleeping quarters. In the case of valuable animals (e.g., Angora rabbits), protection can be provided by keeping flies out of rabbit pens using gauze wire.

With regard to cats in an area endemic for the tumbu fly, feces should not be allowed to accumulate in litter boxes.

REFERENCES

Fox MT, Jacobs DE, Hall MJR, Bennett MP. 1992. Tumbu fly (*Cordylobia anthropophaga*) myiasis in a quarantined dog in England. Vet Rec 130:100–101.

Gunther S. 1971. Clinical and epidemiological aspects of the dermal tumbu-fly-myiasis in equatorial-Africa. Br J Dermatol 85:226–231.

Idowu L, Olote O. 1976. Furuncular myiasis caused by the larvae of *Cordylobia anthropophaga* in an Alsatian bitch and her owners in Apapa, Nigeria. Trans Roy Soc Trop Med Hyg 70:262.

Kozminska-Kubarska A. 1981. *Cordylobia anthropophaga* infestation. Int J Dermatol 20:495–496.

Laurence BR, Herman FG. 1973. Tumbu fly (*Cordylobia*) infection outside Africa. Trans Roy Soc Trop Med Hyg 67:888.

Ockenhouse CF, Samlaska CP, Benson PM, Roberts LW, Eliasson A, Malane S, Menich MD. 1990. Cutaneous myiasis caused by the African tumbu fly (*Cordylobia anthropophaga*). Arch Dermatol 126:199–202.

Patton WS, Evans AM. 1929. In *Insects, Ticks, Mites, and Venomous Animals,* Part I–Medical, pp 410, 453–454. Croydon: H.R. Grubb.

Rice PL, Gleason N. 1972. Two cases of myiasis in the United States by the African tumbu fly, *Cordylobia anthropophaga* (Diptera, Calliphoridae). Am J Trop Med Hyg 21:62–65.

Roberts LW, Boyce WL, Lyerly WH. 1982. *Cordylobia anthropophaga* (Diptera, Calliphoridae) myiasis in an infant and a dog and a technique for larval rearing. J Med Entomol 19:350–351.

Scholten TH, Hicks RJ. 1973. Myiasis by *Cordylobia rodhaini* contracted in Africa and diagnosed in Canada. Can J Pub Health 64:488–489.

Veraldi S, Brusasco A, Suss L. 1993. Cutaneous myiasis caused by larvae of *Cordylobia anthropophaga* (Blanchard). Int J Dermatol 32:184–187.

Zumpt F. 1965. In *Myiasis in Man and Animals in the Old World,* pp 70–77. London: Butterworths.

Sarcophagid Myiasis

Sarcophagid flies, flesh flies, resemble large houseflies. Very typically, the adults have gray longitudinal stripes on their backs and gray and black checkered abdomens. The larvae of many species are parasites of invertebrates, but others are carrion feeders, or parasites of vertebrates in which the larvae develop in cutaneous lesions. Some are important as facultative myiasis producers (e.g., *Sarcophaga hemorrhoidalis*), while others cause primary myiasis: *Wohlfahrtia magnifica* in Europe and North Africa, *Wohlfahrtia vigil* in Canada and the northern United States, and *Wohlfahrtia opaca* in the western United States.

The general life cycle involves larvae that are produced by larviparous females. The larvae invade wounds, or in the case of the primary myiasis producers, unbroken skin. The larvae then develop through three instars. The larvae can be recognized by the deep pit at the posterior end that contains the posterior spiracles. The spiracular plates are characteristic in that the inner slit of each spiracle is directed down and away from the median line. The pupa is dark brown and has a posterior pit at the base that houses the spiracles.

Wohlfahrtia vigil Walker

Etymology

Wohlfahrtia for Dr. Wohlfahrt and *vigil* = keeping vigil about the host.

Synonyms

Paraphyto chittendeni Coquillett.

History

Walker (1920, 1922, 1931) reported the first and subsequent cases of *Wohlfahrtia vigil* in children; Brady (1923) and Chown (1924) reported additional cases in infants. Johannsen (1926) reported this parasite in rabbits near Ithaca, New York, while Kingscote (1931) reported the disease in a silver fox puppy. The first documentation of this parasite in domestic cats was in a report by Kingscote (1935), who recorded it in four cats; he also recorded the parasite in mink, humans, dogs, ferrets, rabbits, and foxes. *Wohlfahrtia vigil* produces an extremely rare cutaneous myiasis in cats. Only one case report of *Wohlfahrtia vigil* in cats, a case from the Veterinary Teaching Hospital at Colorado State University, could be documented using the Veterinary Medical Data Base (Purdue University, West Lafayette, Indiana).

Geographic Distribution

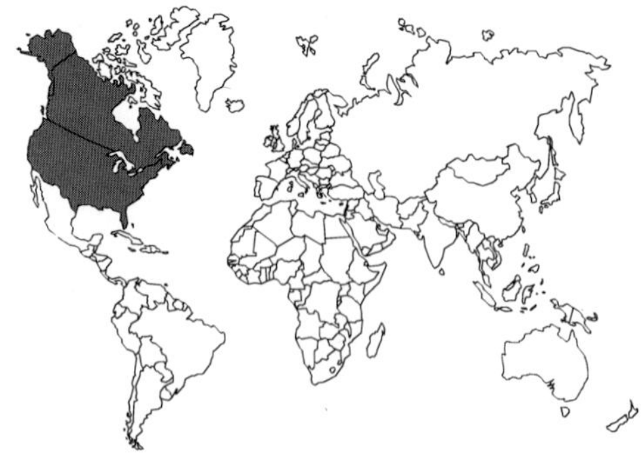

Fig. 5.74.

This parasite is responsible for cutaneous myiasis in North America, particularly in southern Canada and the northern part of the United States (James, 1947). The adult flies have been recorded from the New England states to Alaska (Walker, 1931), but most records of myiasis produced by their larvae are from eastern sections of Canada and the neighboring northeastern parts of the United States. The area in which most cases have been recorded extends roughly from the 43rd parallel of latitude to the 50th and from the 74th to the 104th parallels of longitude. The most southern record is from Erie, Pennsylvania; the northern from Winnipeg, Manitoba; the eastern from Montreal, Quebec; and the western from the Dakotas (Kingscote, 1935). A case of *Wohlfahrtia* has been reported in a cat from the Veterinary Teaching Hospital, Colorado State University (personal communication, Nancy Hampel, DVM, 1994).

Location in Host

Many members of the family Sarcophagidae, the flesh flies, deposit their eggs or larvae in carrion, others in purulent wounds or sores, and others in feces. *Wohlfahrtia vigil* is the only species for which all reports of infection are in the skin of healthy animals (Walker, 1931). Infection follows the deposition of fly larvae on the unbroken skin of young animals. The lesions in cats have been predominantly located on the head, often between the eyes (Kingscote, 1935).

Parasite Identification

Adult *Wohlfahrtia vigil* are nonparasitic and as a result will probably not be observed by the client or the veterinarian. They are large, grayish flies (approximately 13 mm in length), about twice the size of the housefly, *Musca domestica.* The dorsal surface of the thorax is marked with three longitudinal bands, while the dorsal surface of the abdomen exhibits three, well-defined rows of oval black spots that are confluent with one another (Kingscote, 1935).

The first larval stage will probably go unnoticed due to its small size, from 1.5 mm at its hatching to 3.5 mm at the time of its molt to the second stage. The third stage is from 7 to 16.5 mm in length. The second stage fills in the size gaps. All three stages are “maggot-like” in their appearance and exhibit cephalopharyngeal sclerites and posterior spiracles that are unique to the species (Walker, 1931). The third-stage larva is a large larva. Its posterior end is narrow, and its integument is covered with many irregular rows of small, dark, pointed, posteriorly directed spines that are larger than those of the members of the genus *Sarcophaga.* This larva is better adapted to maintain an attachment to living tissues. The oral hooks are strongly developed, and the cephalopharyngeal skeleton is like that of the larva of *Sarcophaga.* The posterior end of the larva has its spiracular plate located in a deep pit formed by the margins of the segment. The posterior spiracles have slits that are wider and a peritreme that is stronger and wider than those of *Sarcophaga* species (Kingscote, 1935; Walker, 1937).

The second- and third-stage larval *Wohlfahrtia vigil* are the stages that will usually be observed in the skin of an infested cat by either the owner or the veterinarian. These stages can probably be best identified by an entomologist. Extensive descriptions and dichotomous keys for these larval stages are available (Johannsen, 1921; Walker, 1937; James and Gassner, 1947).

Life Cycle

This flesh fly is larviparous; it deposits larvae instead of eggs on healthy and uninjured skin of suitable hosts (Eschle and DeFoliart, 1965). The larva penetrates the unbroken skin and forms a boil-like (furuncular) swelling through which the posterior end of the larva may be seen. Here the larva develops to the third larval stage. The larval development is usually completed in 9 to 14 days (Kingscote, 1935). The parasite then leaves the host tissue, drops to the ground, and pupates. The pupation period usually lasts from 11 to 18 days; this variation corresponds with the season of the year and the temperature. When cold weather approaches, the pupation period is greatly prolonged. Under laboratory conditions, it has been observed to last 7 months. The parasite survives the winter in the pupal form. The adults emerge from pupae and about 3 or 4 days later mate. About a week later, the female flies commence larviposition, depositing 6 to 16 larvae at a time. The female flies live from 35 to 40 days. The males seldom survive more than 3 weeks (Kingscote, 1935). Details of the life cycle of *Wohlfahrtia vigil* have been defined in the laboratory (Ford, 1932, 1936; Eschle and DeFoliart, 1965).

Clinical Presentation and Pathogenesis

The female *Wohlfahrtia vigil* deposits active larvae in the neighborhood of a suitable host or directly on the host itself. The larva penetrates the unbroken skin and forms a boil-like (furuncular) swelling through which the posterior end of the larva may be seen. In small animals, penetration may go deeper than the dermal tissue, even into the coelomic cavity.

The first indication that an animal is infected is an exudation of serum and matting of haircoat over the site of penetration. In light-skinned animals, a small inflammatory area is noticeable in the center or to one side in which a tiny opening is at times visible. As the lesions develop, they may be palpated. On the third or fourth day, the larvae are 1.5 to 2 cm in length and produce abscess-like lesions resembling a warble of *Hypoderma* species in cattle. These lesions vary in size, shape, position, and the number of larvae they may contain. The haircoat often becomes parted over the summit of the lesions and reveals an opening generally 2 to 3 mm in diameter. The posterior aspects of the larvae are presented to these openings through which they breathe. These openings are circular and well defined. If several larvae are present in a single lesion, the shape of the aperture is quite variable. Small animals infected with five or more larvae for several days become emaciated, and the skin becomes dry and loses its luster.

The penetration of the skin by the larvae, their development in the subcutaneous tissues, and the secondary bacterial infection produce intense irritation and inflammation of the tissues. Attempts by the cat to remove the larvae or relieve the irritation tend to aggravate the condition. There is fever, loss of appetite and rest, and progressive emaciation. Young animals may die from exhaustion. It has also been suggested that the larvae may produce toxic secretions (Kingscote, 1935).

Diagnosis

The presence of a dermal swelling with a central opening may lead to a tentative diagnosis of myiasis due to *Wohlfahrtia vigil.* A definitive diagnosis can be made only after extraction and identification of a typical larva. Extensive descriptions and dichotomous keys for the three larval stages are available (Johannsen, 1921; Walker, 1937; James and Gassner, 1947).

A tentative diagnosis may often be made by a history of either residence in or travel to a geographic area endemic for *Wohlfahrtia vigil.* There are other flies from different areas throughout the world that might produce a lesion similar to *Wohlfahrtia vigil.* These should also be considered in a differential diagnosis. These myiasis-producing flies include *Cordylobia anthropophaga,* the African tumbu fly; *Dermatobia hominis,* the South American tórsalo fly; *Chrysomyia bezziana,* the Oriental fly; *Cochliomyia hominivorax,* the primary screwworm; and *Cuterebra* species, the rabbit and rodent botflies. The obligatory myiasis-producing flies should be considered in the differential diagnosis in cats with an appropriate residence or travel history.

Treatment

The larva must be extracted from the skin of the feline host. As with all flies that localize in subcutaneous tissues, treatment is based on the requirement of the larvae for communication with the outside environment. Air exchange is accomplished via the larva's posterior spiracles. The airway may be occluded using heavy oil, liquid paraffin, pork fat, or petroleum jelly.

Surgical intervention involves the injection of lidocaine hydrochloride into the furuncular lesion. This anesthetizes both the cat and the larva, allowing the larva to be manually extracted using thumb forceps. Antibiotics should be prescribed.

Great care should be taken during the extraction process to avoid rupturing the larva in situ, although no mention is made in the literature of anaphylaxis as occurs when larvae of *Cuterebra* species are ruptured during the extraction process. In suspect cases, the extracted larva should be submitted to an entomologist for definitive diagnosis.

Epizootiology

There is evidence that adult rabbits and rodents may be implicated in maintaining populations of the fly other than in the whelping season of the carnivore host. It appears that the combination most conducive to a severe outbreak of myiasis in mink is warm temperatures in May and June following a winter with good snow cover and a decline in the rabbit population (Eschle and DeFoliart, 1965). Children and young mink, ferrets, dogs, cats, foxes, and rabbits may become infected from the beginning of June until the end of September. Adult animals are seldom affected (Kingscote, 1935).

Hazards to Other Animals

Wohlfahrtia vigil is a pest of fox and mink ranches in parts of the United States and Canada. Young, newborn animals are attacked, usually fatally. Dogs, rodents, and rabbits may be attacked (Kingscote, 1935). Craine and Boonstra (1986) described myiasis by *Wohlfahrtia vigil* in nesting *Microtus pennsylvanicus.* Although birds, mice, and other small mammals may be suitable hosts for *Wohlfahrtia,* it has been observed that the cottontail rabbit, *Sylvilagus floridanus mearnsii,* is an especially suitable host and perhaps the major host (Johannsen, 1926; Eschle and DeFoliart, 1965).

Hazards to Humans

Wohlfahrtia vigil has been recovered from the skin of young children, particularly infants.

REFERENCES

Brady MJ. 1923. Cutaneous myiasis in an infant-*Wohlfahrtia vigil* (Walker) infection. Arch Pediatr 40:638–640.

Chown G. 1924. Report of a case of cutaneous myiasis in an infant. *Wohlfahrtia vigil* (Walker) Infect 14:967–968.

Craine ITM, Boonstra R. 1986. Myiasis by *Wohlfahrtia vigil* in nestling *Microtus pennsylvanicus.* J Wildl Dis 22:587–589.

Eschle JL, DeFoliart GR. 1965. Rearing and biology of *Wohlfahrtia vigil* (Diptera; Sarcophagidae). Ann Entomol Soc Am 58:849–855.

Ford N. 1932. Observations on the behaviour of the sarcophagid fly, *Wohlfahrtia vigil* (Walker). J Parasitol 19:106–111.

Ford N. 1936. Further observations on the behaviour of *Wohlfahrtia vigil* (Walk.). With notes on the collecting and rearing of the flies J Parasitol 22:309–328.

Holmes PR, Kell M. 1922. Some cases of cutaneous myiasis, with notes on the larvae of *Wohlfahrtia vigil* (Walker). J Parasitol 9:1–5.

James MT. 1947. The flies that cause myiasis in man. USDA Misc Publ no. 631. 175 pp.

James MT, Gassner FX. 1947. The immature stages of the fox maggot, *Wohlfahrtia opaca* Cog. J Parasitol 33:241–252.

Johannsen OA. 1921. The first instar of *Wohlfahrtia vigil* (Walker). J Parasitol 7:154–155.

Johannsen OA. 1926. *Wohlfahrtia vigil* a parasite upon rabbits. J Parasitol 13:156.

Kingscote AA. 1931. A case of myiasis in silver black fox produced by *Wohlfahrtia vigil* (Walker). Ont Vet Coll, pp 38–39.

Kingscote AA. 1935. Myiasis in man and animals due to infection with the larvae of *Wohlfahrtia vigil* (Walker). Ontario Vet Coll Rep 51–69.

Walker EM. 1920. *Wohlfahrtia vigil* (Walker) as a human parasite (Diptera-Sarcophagidae). J Parasitol 7:1–77

Walker EM. 1922. Some cases of cutaneous myiasis with notes on the larvae of *Wohlfahrtia vigil* (Walker). J Parasitol 9:1–5.

Walker EM. 1931. Cutaneous myiasis in Canada. Can Publ Health J 22:504–508.

Walker EM. 1937. The larval stages of *Wohlfahrtia vigil* Walker. J Parasitol 23:163–174.

Cuteribridae

This is a family of flies that occurs only in the Americas. All species of this group are obligate primary myiasis producers that have maggot stages that make extensive migrations through the tissues of the intermediate host. These larvae appear most similar to the large bots of cattle (e.g., species of *Hypoderma*).

Cuterebra Species

Etymology

Cutis = skin and *terebro* = to bore.

History

The genus *Cuterebra* was first described by Bracy Clark in 1815; however, the first published record is that of John Lawson (1709) in his book *A New Voyage to Carolina* (both cited in Sabrosky, 1986). The North American species of *Cuterebra* were described in detail by Sabrosky (1986), who provided an in-depth taxonomic description of each species that he considered valid. In this work, Sabrosky divided the genus *Cuterebra* into two subgenera: *Cuterebra* and *Trypoderma*. *Cuterebra Cuterebra* species are parasites of lagomorphs while *Cuterebra Trypoderma* species are parasites of rodents.

Geographic Distribution

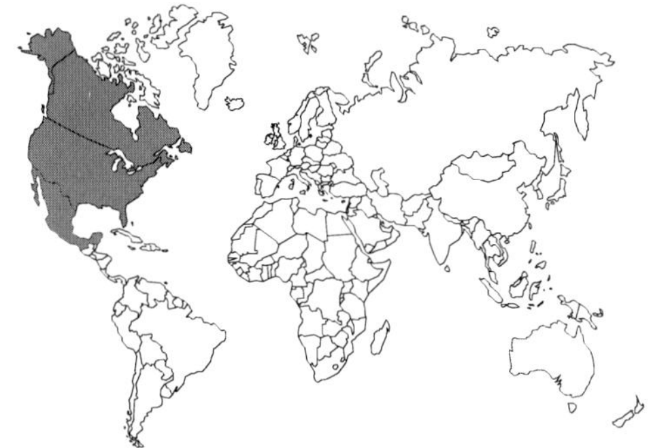

Fig. 5.75.

It is found in the Western Hemisphere, throughout the Americas. Fossils of *Cuterebra* sixty million years old have been recovered in North America (Townsend, 1942). There are maps showing collection sites of each North American species of *Cuterebra* in Sabrosky (1986).

According to Sabrosky (1986) there are 34 species of *Cuterebra* in North America. There are 12 species in the subgenus *Cuterebra* and 22 species in the subgenus *Trypoderma*. Of the 12 members of the *Cuterebra* subgenus parasitic on rodents, three species, *Cuterebra Cuterebra emasculator, Cuterebra Cuterebra fontinella,* and *Cuterebra Cuterebra americana,* are found in the eastern United States, with the latter being more southern in distribution. Of the 22 species in the subgenus *Trypoderma* parasitic on lagomorphs, two species, *Cuterebra Trypoderma abdominalis* and *Cuterebra Trypoderma buccata,* are distributed throughout the eastern United States; one species, *Cuterebra Trypoderma cuniculi,* is restricted to the southeastern coastal areas; and one species, *Cuterebra Trypoderma maculosa,* is restricted to Panama and Guatemala. The remaining 27 species of *Cuterebra* are found in the western United States and in Mexico and Central America.

There are related genera, *Metacuterebra, Pseudogametes, Rogenhofera,* and *Andinocuterebra,* that parasitize rodents in South America. Also, the genus *Alouattamyia* is found in the necks of howler monkeys, *Alouatta* species, and has been reported on several occasions from humans (Fraiha et al., 1984). None of these genera have been reported from cats.

Location in Host

The larval stages of this parasite are commonly found in furuncular lesions in the skin of the rodent host. In the cat, these furuncular lesions may appear on the cheek, neck, top of the head, or the thorax (Fischer, 1983). Larvae have also been reported from the nasal pharynx (Thirloway, 1982; Wolf, 1979), from the pharyngeal area (Kazacos et al., 1980), and from the orbit (Fischer, 1983) and anterior chamber of the eye (Johnson et al., 1988). Intracranial myiasis due to larval *Cuterebra* has been reported in cats on several occasions (Hendrix et al., 1989).

Parasite Identification

The adults are about the size and shape of bumblebees (Fig. 5.76). If one wants to identify the adult fly from a bot recovered from a warble, it will be necessary to allow the bot to pupate in some soil in a jar covered with a bit of screen or mesh; however, it has been found that bots from aberrant hosts often do not successfully pupate to the adult stage even under the best of conditions (Catts, 1982). The mature larvae are characterized by their large size (about 3 cm) and the large spines on the segments (Fig. 5.77). These larvae also have spiracles that are distinctive of the genus, with three serpentine openings forming what appears as three pie slice–shaped tracts within each spiracular opening (Fig. 5.78). The spines on the anterior and posterior bands can be used to determine whether or not the larva is of the "rodent" or "lagomorph" subgenera (Sabrosky, 1986). The "rodent" bots have somewhat flattened, plate-like spines, occasionally somewhat conical, usually bifid to many-pointed in the anterior and posterior bands of spines on

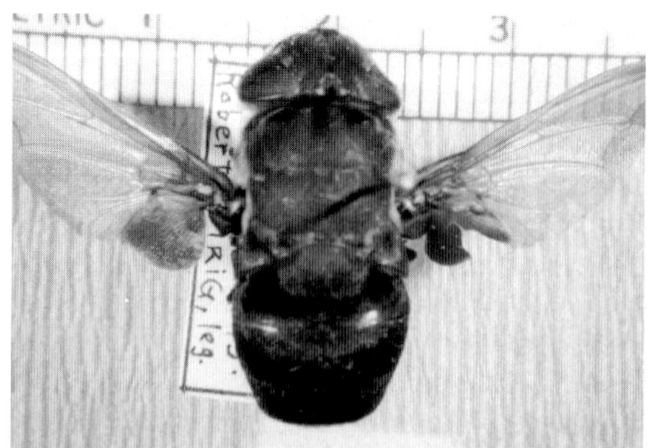

Fig. 5.76. Adult *Cuterebra* species. Typically, the living fly holds its wings along the body when at rest.

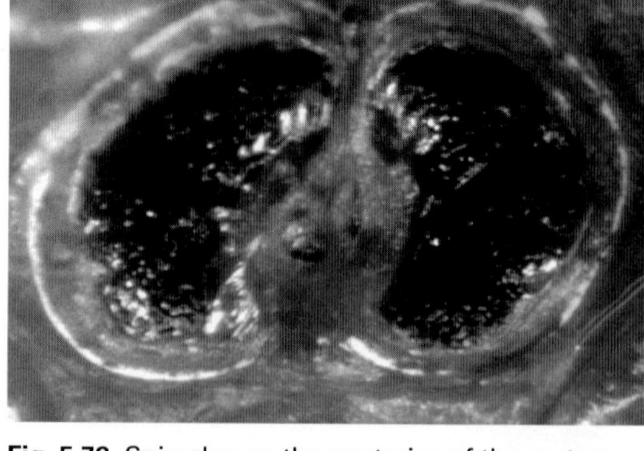

Fig. 5.78. Spiracles on the posterior of the mature *Cuterebra* species removed from a cat.

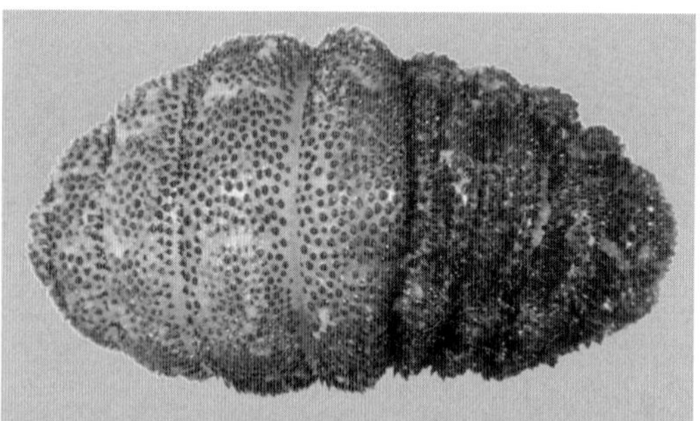

Fig. 5.77. Third-stage larva of a *Cuterebra* species removed from a cat. This larva is about 3 cm in length.

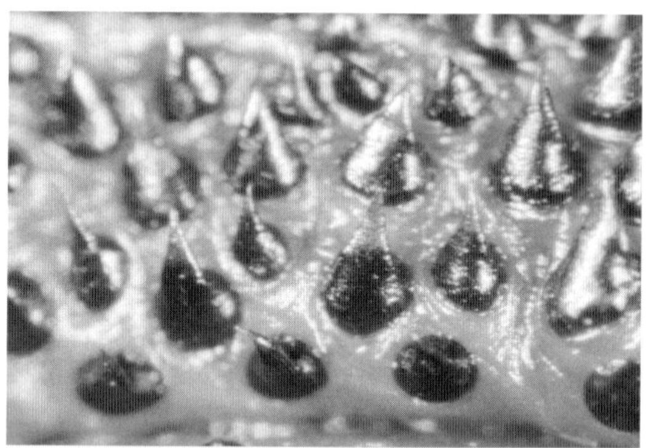

Fig. 5.79. Spines on the body of a third-stage larva of *Cuterebra* recovered from a rabbit. They are conical with single points.

each segment. The mature larvae of the "rabbit" bots have conical, single-pointed spines, especially in the anterior and posterior bands on most segments (Fig. 5.79). The first- and second-instar larvae of the rodent and rabbit bots can be recognized by the large bands of dark spines that are present on the body segments (Fig. 5.80). These larvae have spiracles that are different from the mature third instar (Fig. 5.81).

In histological sections, the larvae of *Cuterebra* can be recognized by their large size and the spines on the surface of the body. Baird et al. (1989) described the features that can be used to distinguish between the genera *Cuterebra, Dermatobia,* and *Cordylobia* in tissue sections.

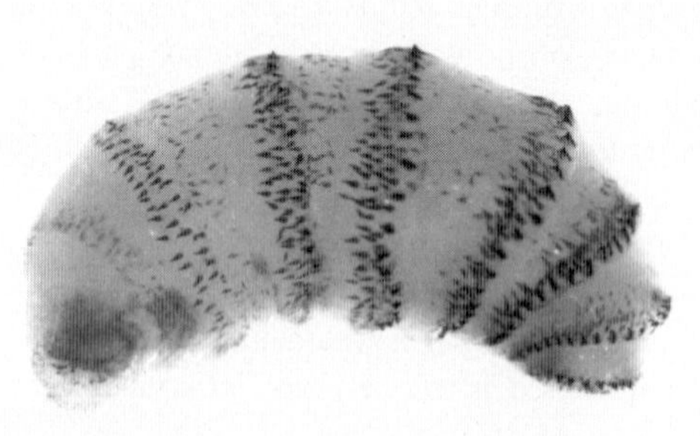

Fig. 5.80. Second-instar larva of *Cuterebra* surgically removed from a subcutaneous lesion on a cat.

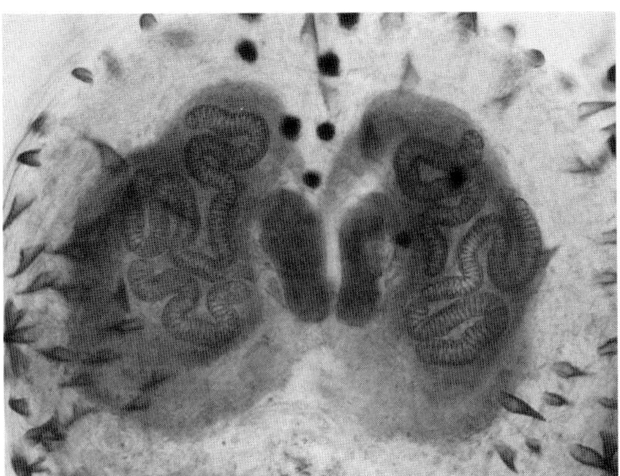

Fig. 5.81. Spiracles of a second-instar larval *Cuterebra* recovered from a cat.

Life Cycle

Adult botflies live only a few weeks, during which they mate and lay eggs (Figs. 5.82 and 5.83). Each day, male rodent botflies find and defend lek territories within botfly aggregation sites (Catts, 1994). When virgin females enter the area of congregation, they become conspicuous by making multiple flights over the summit. They are then chased by a male who will grab the female in midair with copulation being completed on land. Once the female has mated, she then goes off to lay her eggs. The female botfly lays her eggs in different locations depending on the species. The typical female will lay one to several thousand eggs, in groups of around 5–15 per site. Some species lay the eggs on grass stems, wood chips, and bark along narrow trails or rodent runs near the opening to the rodent burrow (similar methods are employed by the horse bots, *Gasterophilus* species, when they attach eggs to the hairs of the face and legs of the horse), while other species actually enter the rodent burrow and lay their eggs within it.

Eggs of these bots hatch in response to sudden rises in temperature. The newly hatched larvae are moist and stick to the fur coats of passing rodents and lagomorphs. Hosts typically become infected by larvae entering some natural body opening (e.g., mouth, nose, eyes, or anus). It had been reported that larvae can enter through unbroken skin (Beamer and Penner, 1942; Penner, 1958), but this could not be repeated by other workers (Catts, 1982). Once within the rodent host, the larvae remain as first stages within the nasopharyngeal region for 6 to 8 days (Baird, 1975; Catts, 1967), where the small, transparent larvae are found at the posterior end of the soft palate in the nasal passages of experimentally infected house mice and woodrats (*Neotoma fuscipes*). In these mice, the larvae remain quite small and transparent, being only two to three times larger than the larvae that hatch from eggs. Work with other species of bots has shown that there may be a migration to the area of the trachea, migration through the tracheal wall into the thoracic cavity, followed by migration through the diaphragm into the abdominal cavity prior to movement to their subcutaneous positions in the inguinal and thoracic areas (Gingrich, 1981). Once within the subcutaneous site, the larvae molt to the second instar and continue to grow within the developing warble. The molt to the third stage occurs around 17 to 19 days after infection in the case of *Cuterebra latifrans* (actually occurring about 2 days earlier in the house mouse). During the last 4 or 5 days of development, the larva enlarges the pore of the warble to make exit possible. It takes about 10 hours for the active larva to back out of the warble once the segments posterior to the spiracles are exposed. The time of larval maturation, from infection to when the larva leaves the warble, ranges from slightly less than 3 to over 8 weeks. The maturation time of the rodent bots seems to be on the average more rapid than that of the rabbit bots; the rodent bots tend to develop in 3 to 4 weeks, while the rabbit bots tend to require 4 to 6 weeks.

Once the fully developed third-stage larva leaves the host, it burrows into the soil, where pupation occurs. It may be anywhere from a month to several years before the adult fly emerges from the pupal case. Also, if larvae have developed in less than adequate hosts, there is a good chance that adult flies will not develop from the mature larvae, even after pupation (Catts, 1982).

The seasonality of infection is due to the timing of adult emergence in the late spring. Then, after 1 to 2 weeks for mating, the eggs are laid by the fertilized females. It then typically takes approximately 3 to 4 weeks for the warbles to become apparent. In the cooler climates, there is typically

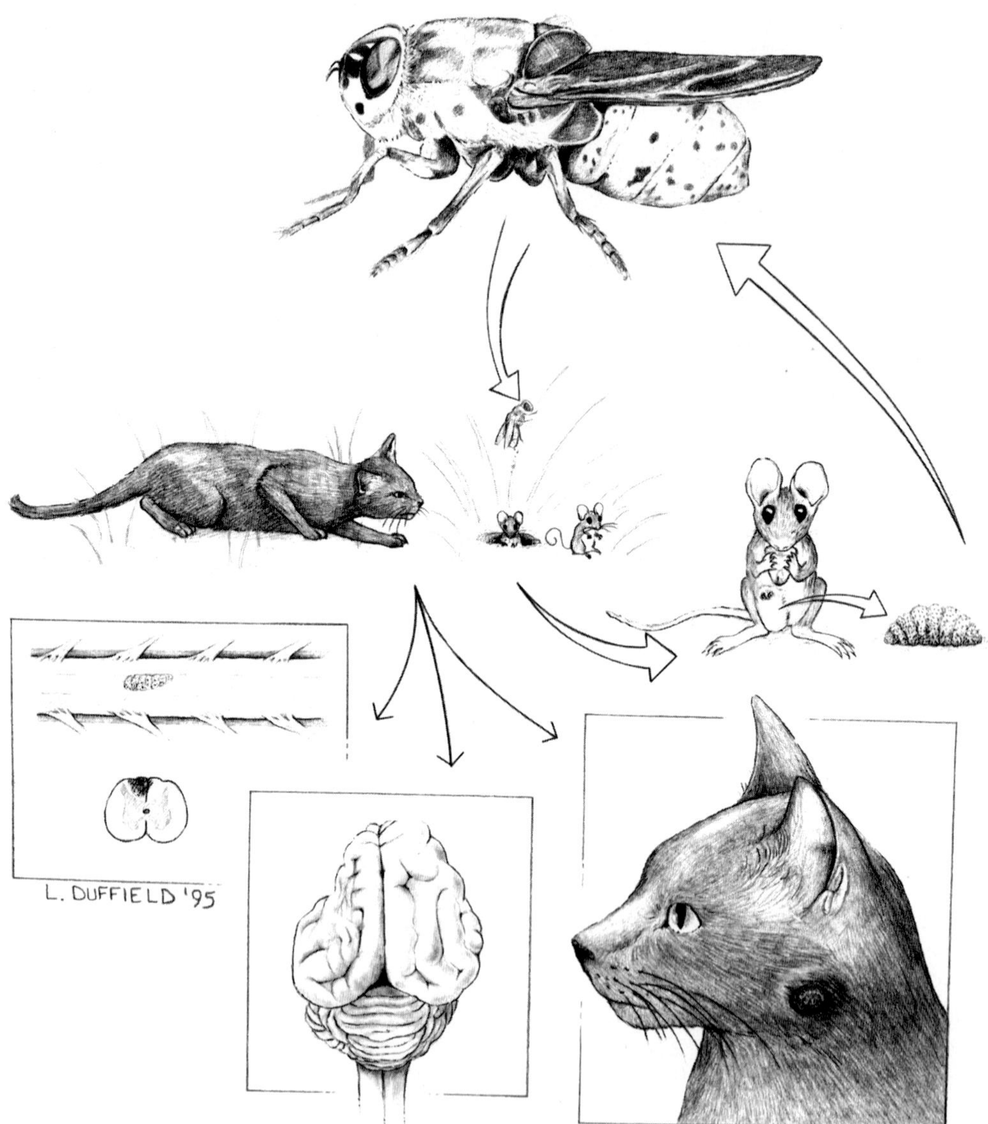

Fig. 5.82. Diagram of the life cycle and pathology caused by *Cuterebra* species in cats. The adult female fly lays its eggs on grass, plant stems, bark, or wood chips around the entrance to a rodent burrow. After several days, the larvae have matured and hatch from eggshells in response to increases in temperature; some larvae can persist within the eggs for months. The hatched larvae attach to a passing host and then enter the body of the host through an opening such as the mouth or nose. In the rodent and rabbit hosts, the larvae migrate first to areas associated with the lungs or pharynx and then migrate to the subcutaneous site where the larvae mature within the warble. Once the larvae have matured, they drop to the ground where they wriggle into the soil to pupate. Typically, the pupal stage is the stage in which the flies overwinter, with the adults emerging from pupal cases in the spring. The most common presentation in the cat is to have the larvae developing in a warble much like they do in the rodent or rabbit, with the posterior end of the bot with its large paired spiracles protruding from the opening in the warble. In the cat, neurologic manifestations of infection can be caused by early stage larvae migrating into the spinal cord or brain and producing lesions similar to those seen in feline ischemic encephalopathy with appreciable asymmetry of the cerebral hemispheres.

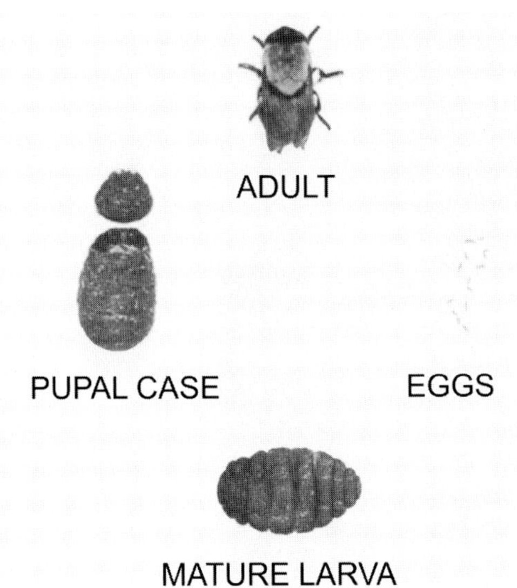

Fig. 5.83. The major life stages of *Cuterebra cuniculi.*

only one hatching of adults each year; however, in warmer climates, there is likely to be less ordered hatching of adult flies (Catts, 1982). There may be an occasional infection observed in winter in colder climates due most likely to eggs maintained within some protected location within the environment.

Cats probably become infected as they prowl in areas frequented by rodents and rabbits. It is possible for very young kittens to be infected with larvae crawling about on the queen's fur. It is not known how the larvae enter the cat, but it would be assumed that they enter through the mouth, nose, or anus as they do in the rodent and lagomorph hosts.

Clinical Presentation and Pathogenesis

Clinical signs depend largely on where the larvae have migrated. Cases tend to be more common during the midsummer to fall months. The most common presentation is that of a subcutaneous warble (a 2 to 4 mm opening with well-defined margins through the skin with a serosanguineous discharge). In these cases, the mature third-stage larva with its pair of large spiracles can be observed moving within the pore of the warble (Fig. 5.84). Most warbles occur around the face or neck; rarely, larvae may enter the globe of the eye causing chemosis, blepharospasm, serous occular discharge, and exudative uveitis with blindness. The larvae may be observed within the anterior chamber of the eye (Johnson et al., 1988; Fischer, 1983). Some owners may observe the warble earlier in its development when the larva is smaller and often white to light cream colored. On this larva, the dark body spines are clearly visible (Fig. 5.80). When extracted, the larva is found to be several centimeters long and often quite dark (Figs. 5.77 and 5.85). Typically, there are no signs of disease or distress in cats.

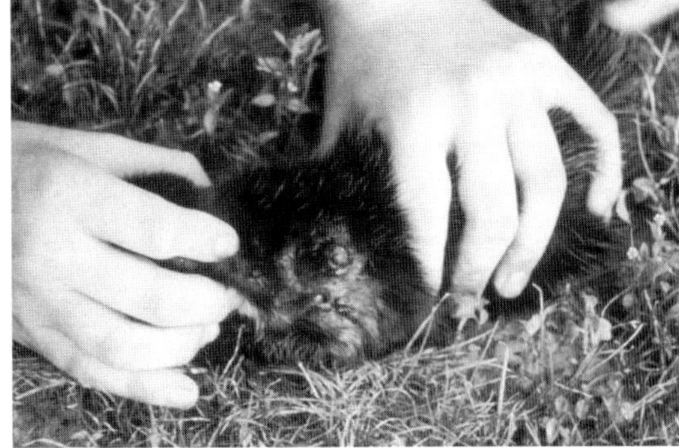

Fig. 5.84. A warble in the back of a cat with a mature third-instar larva.

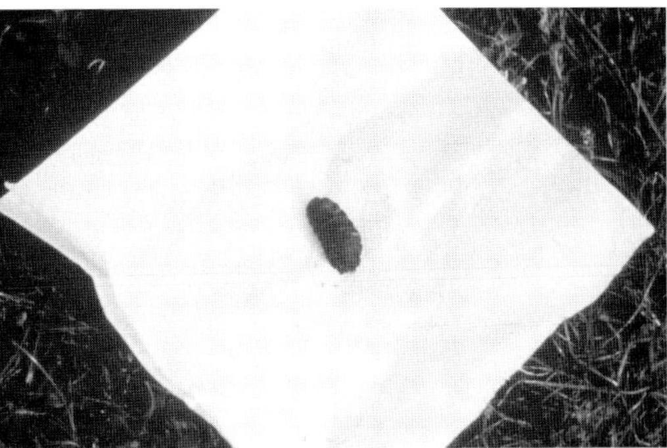

Fig. 5.85. The larva removed from the warble in the back of the cat in Fig. 5.84.

Those cats in which larvae migrate through the brain develop neurologic disease, the clinical signs of which depend on the migratory path of the larva. Clinical signs vary from acute onset of status epilepticus with no recovery, to multiple signs (head tilt, unilateral or bilateral central

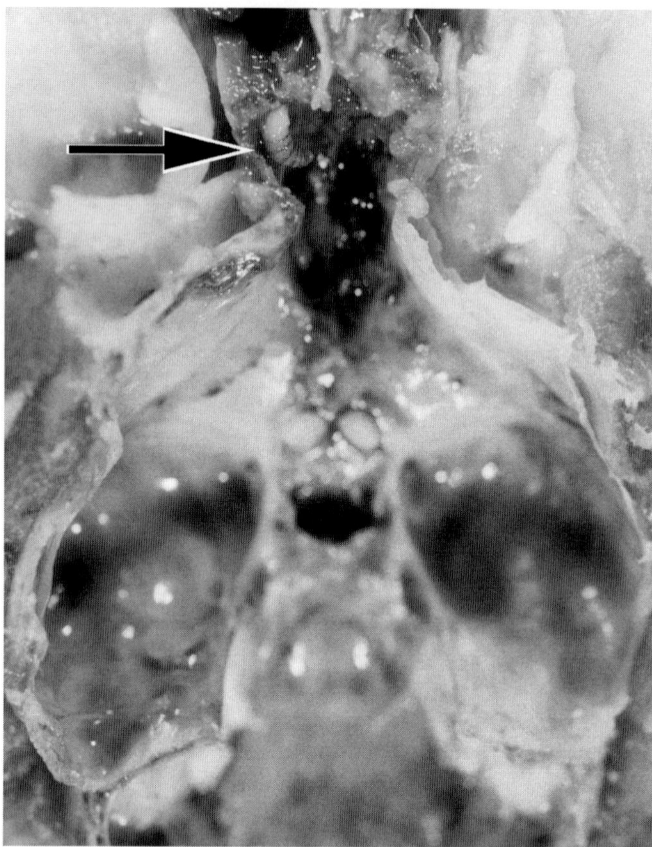

Fig. 5.86. Exposed larva (arrow) within a cat that was euthanatized with severe neurologic signs. (Photo courtesy of Dr. A. de Lahunta)

blindness, head pressing, dementia, continuous vocalization, abnormal pacing reflexes, circling) designating multifocal CNS lesions, to only severe depressed mutation (Hendrix et al., 1989; McKenzie et al., 1978; Bennett et al., 1985; Cook et al., 1985). Many cats present in states of dementia, disorientation, and inappropriate responses to external stimuli (Glass et al., 1998). After an acute onset, signs are usually rapidly progressive with a fatal outcome; more rarely, some cases may linger for weeks or months. Some cases bear a striking similarity to the syndrome of feline ischemic encephalopathy (Cook et al., 1985; Summers et al., 1995). Although reported, it is uncommon for cats that develop neurologic disease to initially present with the cutaneous manifestations (warble) of infection (Hendrix et al., 1989). At necropsy, larvae may be observed intracranially (Fig. 5.86) or within the spinal cord (Figs. 5.87 and 5.88).

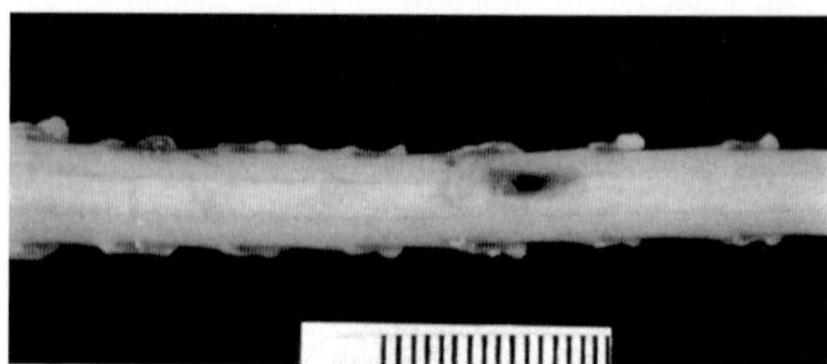

Fig. 5.87. The spinal cord of a cat showing a *Cuterebra* species.

Some cats, after an acute onset of cerebral signs, recover and are left with residual signs of abnormal behavior (e.g., constant pacing or circling, abnormal mentation, or seizures). Occasionally spontaneous recovery appears to be complete.

Another typical presentation in cats can be signs of respiratory distress or upper respiratory disease. Some present with a history of sneezing and nasal discharge (sometimes for up to a weeks

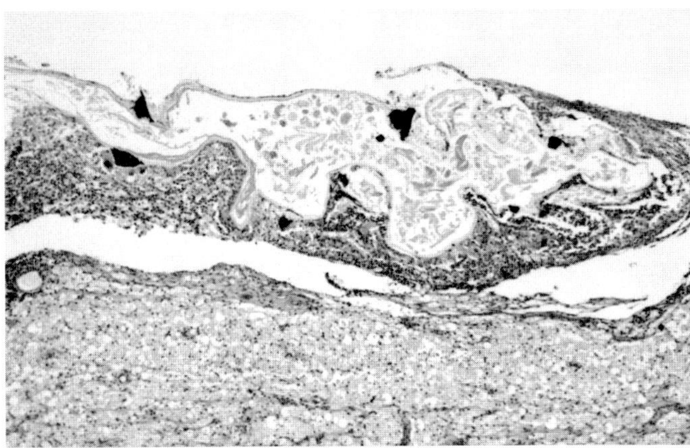

Fig. 5.88. A histological section of a spinal cord of a cat showing the aposition of the *Cuterebra* larva to the cord material. The larva can be recognized by the large black triangles that represent sections through the large body spines present on the developing bot's surface.

duration), unilateral facial swellings especially over the nose, extreme respiratory dyspnea sometimes with a bloody nasal discharge, and soft palate and pharyngeal swelling (Kazacos et al., 1980; Thirloway, 1982; Wolf, 1979). Laryngeal edema resulting in laryngeal obstruction and respiratory arrest due to migration of larvae in the cervical neck has been reported in a snow leopard (Ryan et al., 1990). Unlike cutaneous lesions, respiratory signs more often precede the development of neurologic signs (Cook et al., 1985; personal communication, S.C. Barr and A. de Lahunta). Typically, if neurologic signs develop, they do so 1 to 2 weeks after respiratory signs, although respiratory signs may occur as long as 4 to 10 weeks before the onset of neurologic disease (Cook et al., 1985).

There seems to be a good indication that cerebrospinal cuterebriasis in cats is associated with or the cause of feline ischemic encephalopathy (Williams et al., 1998). This disease is not known to occur in areas where *Cuterebra* is not present, and it occurs most commonly at the same time of the year as cases of cuterebriasis. It is postulated that the vascular spasm associated with feline ischemic syndrome may be due to some toxin elaborated by the circulating fly larva.

Diagnosis

Infections with *Cuterebra* in cats are typically observed in the late summer and early fall in those parts of North America that have cold enough winters to prevent year-round fly activity on a regular basis. A *Cuterebra* bot in a warble in the back of a cat is distinctive and diagnostic. Larvae migrating to cause neurologic or respiratory signs represent more of a challenge. The clinician should be suspicious of *Cuterebra* infection in cats developing severe upper respiratory disease (especially with unilateral signs of nasal discharge or nasal/facial swellings) during the late summer or fall months. Acute onset of neurologic disease sometimes preceded by upper respiratory signs 1 to 2 weeks previously should provide strong suspicion of intracranial cuterebral myiasis. In some cats with upper respiratory signs, a leukocytosis with eosinophilia is present on peripheral hemograms. However, hematology and serum biochemistry findings are usually nonspecific but might help to rule out other diseases. If neurologic signs are present, cerebrospinal fluid analysis may show an elevation in protein, as well as pleocytosis with neutrophils, mononuclear cells, or eosinophils. A CAT scan of an affected cat revealed a mottled appearance to the brain consistent with encephalitis, but no conclusive evidence of infection. Magnetic resonance imaging to reveal larvae or their migration tracks in the brain of affected animals appears to show promise, but as of yet images have not yet been published or the details of the observed lesions described (de Lahunta, personal communication). In cases presenting with upper respiratory disease, examination of the pharynx, larynx, and nasal passages under general anesthesia may reveal a larva.

Treatment

Treatment of cuterebriasis currently requires the surgical extraction of the bot or bots. When mature bots are present within a warble, they are probably going to extract themselves very shortly, but they can be assisted in their leaving of the warble by the expansion of the pore and extraction with forceps, using care not to crush the bot. Squashing the larvae within the warble may result in a severe tissue reaction resulting from a Type I hypersensitivity-like reaction. Smaller and less-developed larvae within the skin will require removal by careful dissection. Similarly, larvae within the soft tissues of the mouth, nasal sinus, larynx, or eye will require surgical extraction.

When larvae are present intracranially or within the spinal cord, the treatment of choice is likely to remain the extraction of the larvae. As methods or radiographic imaging are improving, it may become possible to localize the developing larva and extract it. As of this time, however, no such success has been reported.

Ivermectin has been shown to be effective against *Cuterebra* species at 0.1 mg/kg, and is well tolerated when given at 0.3 mg/kg. Ivermectin (0.3 mg/kg subcutaneously on alternate days for three treatments) in association with corticosteroids has been reportedly used to treat two cats with neurologic signs; in both cats the eventual outcome of the infection was not improved, although the larvae in one case at necropsy was decomposing (Hendrix et al., 1989).

At Cornell Veterinary College, a limited number of cats with the upper respiratory syndrome during late summer and fall have responded to the above regimen of ivermectin treatment (but given orally) combined with prednisone (1 mg/kg, PO, every 12 h for 3 weeks, then 1 mg/kg, PO, every 24 h for 3 weeks). Although the diagnosis has been presumptive, these cases improve, and none to date have developed neurologic disease.

The monthly administration of fipronil, imidacloprid, or selamectin to cats is likely to prevent infections with this parasite. In areas where infections occur, this disease may warrant putting cats on these monthly products. Also, Heartgard (ivermectin) for cats given monthly may contain sufficient ivermectin to also prevent these larvae from developing.

Epizootiology

In the northern United States, most cases are observed in late summer and early fall; this is due to the univoltine life cycle of flies in these latitudes (i.e., flies only mate and lay eggs once a year). Thus, most rodents, rabbits, and cats are being infected at about the same time in the summer. Work at an aggregation site in Marin County, California, revealed that most of the males of *Cuterebra latifrons* were present at the site around the end of August, although males were present from the beginning of June through the end of October (Catts, 1967). At an aggregation site in Pennsylvania, the most males of *Cuterebra fontinella* were present in the first half of August, with males being present from mid to late June through the first half of September (Shiffer, 1983). The appearance of warbles in the late summer and early fall would coincide with the 3 to 6 weeks required for the larvae to reach the stage where they are ready to leave the host and pupate. In climates where the flies are multivoltine, there is the likely possibility that the seasonality of bot appearance would be less dramatic than in the cooler climes.

Hazards to Other Animals

The larva in the back of the cat is no hazard to either the handler or the other animals that may share the hospital areas.

Hazards to Humans

The larva in the cat is not a hazard to humans. There have been reports, however, of the recovery of larvae of *Cuterebra* from humans who have become infected in much the same manner as cats (Baird et al., 1989; Schiff, 1993). Most human cases have been reported in the northeastern United States within late August and early September. In humans most larvae have been recovered from the head, neck, shoulders, and chest. There have been rare cases of ocular and upper respiratory involvement. It does not appear that central nervous system disease happens in humans as it does in cats.

Control/Prevention

Owners could be advised of the life cycle, but it would be difficult to prevent a cat with a desire to hunt from visiting potential sites of egg deposition. Thus, it is important to make owners in areas where the neurologic disease occurs to be aware that the signs of respiratory infection in late summer and early fall would warrant a veterinary consultation and the potential need for careful monitoring. Again, monthly treatment with or application of ivermectin, selamectin, fipronil, or imidacloprid is likely to prevent these infections.

REFERENCES

Baird CR. 1975. Larval development of the rodent bot fly, *Cuterebra tenebrosa*, in bushy-tailed wood rats and its relationship to pupal diapause. Can J Zool 53:1788–1798.
Baird JK, Baird CR, Sabrosky CW. 1989. North American cuterebrid myiasis; report of seventeen new infections of human beings and review of the disease. J Am Acad Dermatol 21:763–772.
Beamer RH, Penner LR. 1942. Observation on the life history of a rabbit cuterebrid, the larvae of which may penetrate the human skin. J Parasitol 28(suppl):25.
Bennett RA, Lowrie CT, Bell TG. 1985. An intracranial *Cuterebra* sp. larva in a cat. Calif Vet 39:13–14, 49.
Catts EP. 1967. Biology of a California rodent bot fly *Cuterebra latifrons* Coquillett (Diptera: Cuterebridae). J Med Entomol 4:87–101.
Catts EP. 1982. Biology of new world bot flies: Cuterebridae. Ann Rev Entomol 27:313–338.
Catts EP. 1994. Sex and the bachelor bot (Diptera: Oiestridae). Am Entomol Fall:153–160.
Cook JR, Levesque DC, Nuehring LP. 1985. Intracranial cuterebral myiasis causing acute lateralizing meningoencephalitis in two cats. JAAHA 21:279–284.
Fischer K. 1983. *Cuterebra* larvae in domestic cats. Vet Med, Sm Anim Clin 78:1231–1233.
Fraiha H, Chaves LCL, Burges IC, de Freitas RB. 1984. Miiases humanas na Amozonia—III: miiase pulmonary por Alouattamyia baeri (Shannon and Greene, 1926)(Diptera: Cuteribridae). Rev Fundacao SESP 290:63–68.
Gingrich RE. 1981. Migratory kinetics of *Cuterebra fontinella* (Diptera: Cuterebridae) in the white-footed mouse, *Peromyscus leucopus*. J Parasitol 67:398–402.
Glass EN, Cornetta AM, de Lahunta A, Center SA, Kent M. 1998. Clinical and clinicopathologic features in 11 cats with *Cuterebra* larvae myiasis of the central nervous system. J Vet Int Med 12: 365–368.
Hendrix CM, Cox NR, Clemons-Chevis CL, DiPinto MN, Sartin EA. 1989. Aberrant intracranial myiasis caused by larval *Cuterebra* infection. Comp Cont Ed Pract Vet 11:550–559.
Johnson BW, Helper LC, Szajerski ME. 1988. Intraocular *Cuterebra* in a cat. JAVMA 193:829–830.
Kazacos KR, Bright RM, Johnson KE, Anderson KL, Cantwell HD. 1980. *Cuterebra* sp. as a cause of pharyngeal myiasis in cats. JAAHA 16:773–776.
McKenzie BE, Lyles DI, Clinkscales JA. 1978. Intracerebral migration of *Cuterebra* larva in a kitten. JAVMA 172:173–175.
Penner LR. 1958. Concerning a rabbit cuterebrid, the larvae of which may penetrate the human skin (Diptera, Cuterebridae). J Kans Entomol Soc 31:67–71.
Ryan JA, Roudebush P, Shores JA. 1990. Laryngeal obstruction associated with cuterebrosis in a snow leopard (*Felis uncia*). J Zoo Wild Med 21: 351–352.
Sabrosky CW. 1986. North American Species of Cuterebra: The Rabbit and Rodent Bot Flies (Diptera: Cuterebridae). Thomas Say Monograph. College Park, Md: Entomol Soc Am. 240 pp.
Schiff TA. 1993. Furuncular cutaneous myiasis caused by *Cuterebra* larva. J Am Acad Dermatol 28:261–263.
Shiffer CN. 1983. Aggregation behaviour of adult *Cuterebra fontinella* (Diptera: Cuterebridae) in Pennsylvania. J Med Entomol 20:365–370.
Summers BA, Cummings JF, de Lahunta A. 1995. Feline ischemic encephalopathy. In Chapter 5, Degenerative diseases of the central nervous system, Veterinary Neuropathology, pp 242–244. St. Louis Mo: Mosby.
Thirloway L. 1982. Aberrant migration of a *Cuterebra* larva in a cat. Vet Med/Sm Anim Clin 77:619–620.
Townsend CHT. 1942. Manual of Myiology, part 12. Sao Paulo, Brazil.
Williams KJ, Summers BA, de Lahunta A. 1998. Cerebrospinal cuterebriasis in cats and its association with feline ischemic encephalopathy. Vet Pathol 35:330–343.
Wolf AM. 1979. *Cuterebra* larva in the nasal passage of a kitten. Feline Pract 9:25–26.

Dermatobia hominis (Linnaeus, 1781)

Etymology

Dermato = skin + *obia* = way of living and *hominis* for the choice of human hosts. Common names include the human botfly, tropical warble fly, beef worm, bekuru, bikuru, berne, borro, colmoyte, forcel, gusano macaco, gusano de monte, gusano de mosquito, gusano de zancudo, gusano peludo, kturn, kitudn, ikitugn, mberuaró, mirunta, moyocuil, muskietenworm, nuche, nunche, suglacuru, suylacuru, torsel, tórsalo, tupe, ura, and ver macacque.

Synonyms

Oestrus hominis, Oestrus humanus, Oestrus guildingii, Cuterebra cyaniventris, Cuterebra noxialis, Dermatobia noxialis, and *Dermatobia cyaniventris* (Guimaraes and Papavero, 1966).

History

Records of early exploration in Panama reveal that *Dermatobia hominis* has been known as a human parasite in Panama for almost a century and a half. If earlier records were available, they would probably show that this fly had been known by indigenous Americans for centuries (Dunn, 1934). The natives of Central and South America have long known animals to be infected with larvae of *Dermatobia* species. The ancient Mayans referred to this parasite as "saglacuru" and believed that it owed its existence to the bite of some kind of mosquito (Hoeppli, 1959). It is strange how close to the truth these ancient peoples were. The ancient Mayans extracted the larva of *Dermatobia* by covering its breathing pore with heavy oil (Ockenhouse et al., 1990). In the earliest report of feline infestation by *Dermatobia hominis,* Dunn (1934) reported that "three half-grown larvae were found in a vagrant cat."

Geographic Distribution

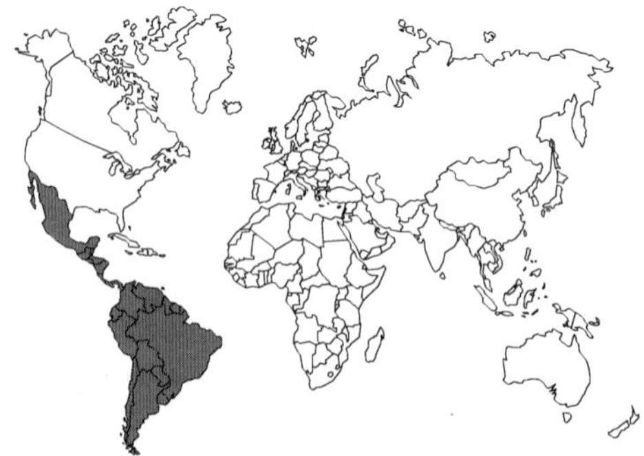

Fig. 5.89.

This botfly occurs in Mexico, Central America, and South America (File et al., 1985).

Location in Host

The larval *Dermatobia hominis* penetrates the skin of the definitive host, producing a cutaneous furunculoid (boil-like) myiasis (Pallai et al., 1992).

Parasite Identification

The adult *Dermatobia hominis* is about 1.5 to 1.8 cm in length, approximately the size of a bumblebee. It has a blue-gray thorax, a metallic blue abdomen, and yellow-orange legs (Pallai et al., 1992). The adult has no functional mouthparts and takes no nourishment (Rossi and Zucoloto, 1973). Food stored during the larval stage provides the adults with nourishment (Prasad and Beck, 1969).

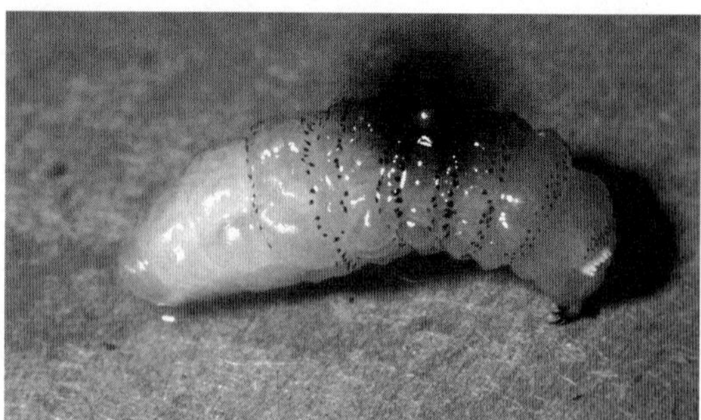

Fig. 5.90. *Dermatobia hominis.* Larva recovered from the arm of a human that had been working in South America.

The mature larva at 2 to 3 months of age is 1.8 to 2.4 cm in length (Fig. 5.90). It has a definite club shape and can be identified by rows of posteriorly directed spines on its anterior segments. The larval stage also possesses caudal spiracles that protrude through the host's skin to the exterior to guarantee an adequate air supply (File et al., 1985).

The larva of *Dermatobia hominis* is narrow and tubular at its posterior extremity and somewhat flask shaped anteriorly (Patton and Evans, 1929). The presence of the superficially positioned swelling with a central opening may lead to a tentative diagnosis of myiasis due to *Dermatobia hominis.* A definitive diagnosis can be made only after extraction and identification of the typical larva.

Diagnosis of infestation with *Dermatobia hominis* may often be made if the patient has a history of residence in or travel to an endemic area (Prasad and Beck, 1969; Rossi and Zucoloto, 1973; Iannini et al., 1975; Kleeman, 1983; Kenney and Baker, 1984; File et al., 1985; Pallai et al., 1992). However, there are other flies from different geographic areas that might produce a similar lesion. These should also be considered in a differential diagnosis. These myiasis-producing flies include *Cordylobia anthropophaga,* the African tumbu fly; *Wohlfahrtia vigil,* the gray flesh fly; *Chrysomyia bezziana,* the Oriental fly; *Cochliomyia hominivorax,* the primary screwworm; and *Cuterebra* species, the rabbit and rodent botflies. These obligatory myiasis-producing flies should be considered in the differential diagnosis in cats with an appropriate residence or travel history.

Life Cycle

This dipteran fly has a most unusual life cycle. The adult fly inhabits the forests of Mexico, Central America and South America. Unlike many of the obligatory myiasis-producing dipterans (with the exception of *Cuterebra* species), the female fly does not deposit her eggs directly on the host. Instead, she captures another dipteran fly, usually a bloodsucker, or a tick and, using a quick-drying adhesive, cements the eggs to one side of the carrier's body. The eggs are attached to the carrier in such a manner that when contact is made with the prospective definitive host, the anterior end of the egg is directed downward. An operculum forms on this end of the egg, through which the larva emerges. The larva penetrates the skin of the host to the subcutaneous tissues and produces a warble (swelling) at the point of contact. *Dermatobia hominis* does not meander through the subcutis. The tórsalo matures to its most advanced larval stage in the body of the host (Harwood and James, 1979). Development in the host requires 35 to 70 days. The larva then drops to the ground where it enters the soil for pupation. The entire life cycle takes 90 to 120 days (Harwood and James, 1979).

Clinical Presentation and Pathogenesis

Although often not reported, cats are host to infestation with this parasite (Silva Junior et al., 1998). Clinically, the initial lesion is a small, often pruritic, nodule resembling a common insect bite. As the larva matures, the lesion enlarges around it to form a malodorous, purulent, furuncular lesion. It may be 1 to 2 cm in diameter and 0.5 to 1 cm in height. A serosanguineous fluid begins to exude from the lesion during the second week. Purulent discharge may result from excretions from the larva or from secondary bacterial infection. Each nodule contains a central pore that denotes the presence of the larva (Pallai et al., 1992). Close examination of the larva in situ may reveal the up-and-down respiratory movements of the larva (Kenney and Baker, 1984) or actual visualization of the larval spiracles. It is possible to palpate the larva within the nodule (Pallai et al., 1992).

Treatment

The goal of treatment is to remove the larva. In man, several methods have been reported for extraction of larval *Dermatobia hominis* from the skin. These techniques should also apply to the feline definitive host. The simplest method (although somewhat time-consuming) is the application of a viscous, occlusive substance (e.g., petroleum jelly) over the hole through which the larva breathes. This cuts off the larva's air supply and stimulates premature extrusion. Manual extraction of the dead larva may be necessary using this technique. Hot compresses may be used to make the lesion more pliable and reduce discomfort.

Topical application of 5 percent chloroform in olive oil to produce a sublethal hypoxia of *Dermatobia hominis,* followed by manual extraction, has been used successfully in man.

Surgical intervention involves the injection of lidocaine hydrochloride into the furuncular lesion. This anesthetizes both the cat and the larva, allowing the larva to be manually extracted through a linear incision using thumb forceps. The wound should be irrigated, debrided, and packed open to provide adequate drainage. A disadvantage of surgical removal is that remains of the larval bodies may be accidentally left in the lesion. Careful inspection of the extracted larva and irrigation of the wound should reduce complications (Pallai et al., 1992).

Epizootiology

Since this parasite is spread by both zoophilous and anthropophilous mosquitoes (and other blood-feeding arthropods), it may be found in a wide variety of definitive hosts. Host selection is performed by "porter" species—mosquitoes and flies. *Dermatobia hominis* females oviposit on these arthropods and depend on them to carry their eggs to mammalian species.

Hazards to Other Animals

Because *Dermatobia hominis* is the human botfly and because it may be transmitted to a wide variety of domesticated and wild animals, it is considered to be a zooanthroponosis. In addition to cats, suitable hosts include cattle, swine, dogs, horses, mules, sheep, goats, monkeys, and certain wild mammals. Birds (toucans and ant birds) are known to harbor it (Harwood and James, 1979). *Dermatobia hominis* is a serious pest of livestock in many parts of Latin America (Thomas, 1988).

Hazards to Humans

Dermatobia hominis is also known as the human botfly. Its larval forms have been extracted from various parts of the human body, primarily the head, arms, back, abdomen, buttocks, genitalia, thighs, and axilla (Prasad and Beck, 1969; Rossi and Zucoloto, 1973; Iannini et al., 1975; Kleeman, 1983; Kenney and Baker, 1984; File et al., 1985; Pallai et al., 1992).

Control/Prevention

Perhaps the best method of controlling this parasite depends on controlling *Dermatobia hominis* in cattle, its major definitive host in Latin America. Ivermectin in both topical application and in slow-release bolus forms has been demonstrated to be effective in controlling this parasite in cattle (McMullin et al., 1989; Uribe et al., 1989). Mosquitoes and other blood-feeding flies that can serve as phoretic hosts of this fly should be restricted from indoor environments.

REFERENCES

Chitwood M, Lichtenfels JR. 1972. Identification of parasitic metazoa in tissue sections. Exp Parasitol 32:404–519.

Dunn LH. 1934. Prevalence and importance of the tropical warble fly, *Dermatobia hominis* Linn., in Panama. J Parasitol 20:219–226.

Elgart ML. 1990. Flies and myiasis. Dermatol Clin 8:237–244.

File TM, Thomson RB, Tan JS. 1985. *Dermatobia hominis* dermal myiasis. Arch Dermatol 121: 1195–1196.

Guimaraes JH, Papavero N. 1966. A tentative annotated bibliography of *Dermatobia hominis* (Linnaeus Jr., 1781) (Diptera, Cuterebridae). Arq Zool 14:223–294.

Harwood RF, James MT. 1979. In Entomology in Human and Animal Health, 7th ed, pp 313–315.New York, NY: Macmillan.

Hoeppli R. 1959. In Parasites and Parasitic Infections in Early Medicine and Science, p 158. Singapore: University of Malaya Press.

Iannini PB, Brandt D, LaForce FM. 1975. Furuncular myiasis. J Am Med Assoc 233:1375–1376.

Kenney RL, Baker FJ. 1984. Botfly (*Dermatobia hominis*) myiasis. Int J Dermatol 23:676–677.

Kleeman FJ. 1983. *Dermatobia hominis* comes to Boston. N Engl J Med 308:847–848.

McMullin PF, Cramer LG, Benz G, Jeromel PC, Gross SJ. 1989. Control of *Dermatobia hominis* infestation in cattle using an ivermectin slow-release bolus. Vet Rec 124:465.

Ockenhouse CF, Samlaska CP, Benson PM, Roberts LW, Eliasson A, Malane S, Menich MD. 1990. Cutaneous myiasis caused by the African tumbu fly (*Cordylobia anthropophaga*). Arch Dermatol 126:199–202.

Pallai L, Hodge J, Fishman SJ, Millikan LE, Phelps RG. 1992. Case report: Myiasis—the botfly boil. Am J Med Sci 303:245–248.

Patton W, Evans AM. 1929. In Insects, Ticks, Mites, and Venomous Animals, Part I—Medical, p 435. Croydon: H.R. Grubb.

Prasad C, Beck AR. 1969. Myiasis of the scalp from *Dermatobia hominis*. J Am Med Assoc 210:133.

Rossi M, Zucoloto S. 1973. Fatal cerebral myiasis caused by the tropical warble fly, *Dermatobia hominis*. Am J Trop Med Hyg 22:267–269.

Silva Junior VP da, Leandro AS, Borja GEM. 1998. Ocorrencia do berne, Dermatobia hominis (Diptera: Cuterebridae) em varios hospedeiros, no Rio de Janeiro, Brasil. Parasitologia al Dia 22:97–101.

Thomas DB, Jr. 1988. The pattern of *Dermatobia* (Diptera: Cuterebridae) myiasis in cattle in tropical Mexico. J Med Entomol 25:131–135.

Uribe LF, McMullin PF, Cramer LG, Amaral NK. 1989. Topically applied ivermectin: Efficacy against torsalo (Diptera: Cuterebridae). J Econ Entomol 82:847–849.

SIPHONAPTERA

Fleas are laterally compressed insects that have been the bane of humans and their animal companions for eons. Fleas suck blood from their feline hosts and are capable of taking enough blood to cause severe anemia that in kittens can induce cardiomegaly (King, 1997; Yaphe et al., 1993). The major flea of importance to the cat is the species *Ctenocephalides felis*. Several species and several subspecies of these fleas will bother the cat around the world (*Ctenocephalides felis strongylus* in Africa and *Ctenocephalides orientis* in the Orient and Oceania), but by far the most important parasite of the cat is *Ctenocephalides felis felis*. Cats will sometimes fall prey to infestation with fleas from other hosts such as rabbits or rodents (e.g., infestations with *Cediopsylla* or *Spilopsyllus*), but typically cats are host mainly to the cat flea. On rare occasions, cats will also become infested with *Echidnophaga gallinacea,* the stick tight flea of poultry.

Ctenocephalides felis

The biology of the cat flea, *Ctenocephalides felis,* has been reviewed in detail in recent years as more new information has been brought together on its biology (Rust and Dryden, 1997). Georgi and Georgi (1992) did an excellent job of presenting images that allow the easy recognition of the species and subspecies of importance. The adult fleas in this genus have both genal (cheek) and pronotal (neck) combs (i.e., thick bristles that give the flea the appearance of having a very thick mustache) (Fig. 5.91). Adult fleas (Fig. 5.92) remain on their feline host if at all possible. However, some cats are excellent groomers and can easily remove 50 to 100 fleas in a 24-hour period. While on the cat, the adult fleas suck blood. A large portion of the blood imbibed by the fleas seems to pass directly through their system. Female fleas make helixes, and males make small spheres. In both cases, the blood passed through the flea will dry and along with other detritus forms the basis of "flea dirt" that is found on a cat or under where an infested cat will usually rest. It appears that what the adult fleas are actually doing is in part providing a dietary supplement for their offspring who will develop and feed in the material dropped where the host usually rests.

Two days after a male and female flea take up residence on a host, the female flea produces about 15 ovoid white and waxy eggs each day that do not stick to the haircoat but fall to the ground (Figs. 5.93 and 5.94). About 2 days after an egg gets to the ground, a first-stage caterpillar-like larva hatches by cutting through the eggshell with a structure that is analogous to the egg tooth of birds and reptiles. The larva then eats and grows, and as long as the humidity does not get too low or the temperature too cold, development will proceed (Fig. 5.95). The dark intestinal tract of the larva can often be viewed through the cuticle, the dark appearance of the gut being due to the ingested flea feces that have been produced by the adults still on the host. After a period of about a week, the flea larva will have molted twice to become a third-stage larva. This stage will then spin a silken cocoon that attracts bits of sand particles and other detritus that serve to protect it and conceal it within the environment. About 15 days after the eggs were laid, the adult fleas will begin emerging from their cocoons and be in search of a host. Adult fleas will emerge spontaneously from the pupal cases, but they can also be induced to eclose by the application of warmth and increased humidity, created, for example, by the resting of a cat upon a blanket.

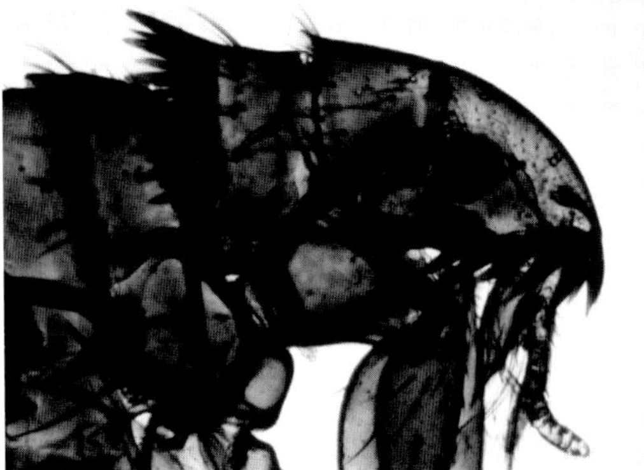

Fig. 5.91. *Ctenocephalides felis.* Anterior end showing the genal and pronotal combs.

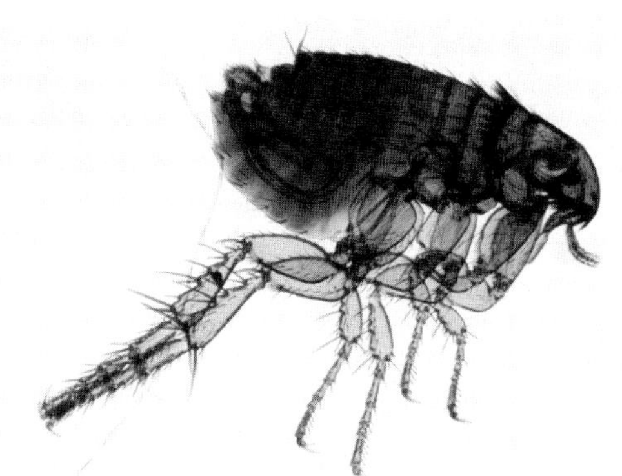

Fig. 5.92. *Ctenocephalides felis.* Adult male.

During the past few years the development of new flea control products (e.g., lufenuron, fipronil, imidacloprid, and selamectin) have given the veterinarian, pet, and client a major respite from flea problems. These products all work to provide the pet with long-term protection that is

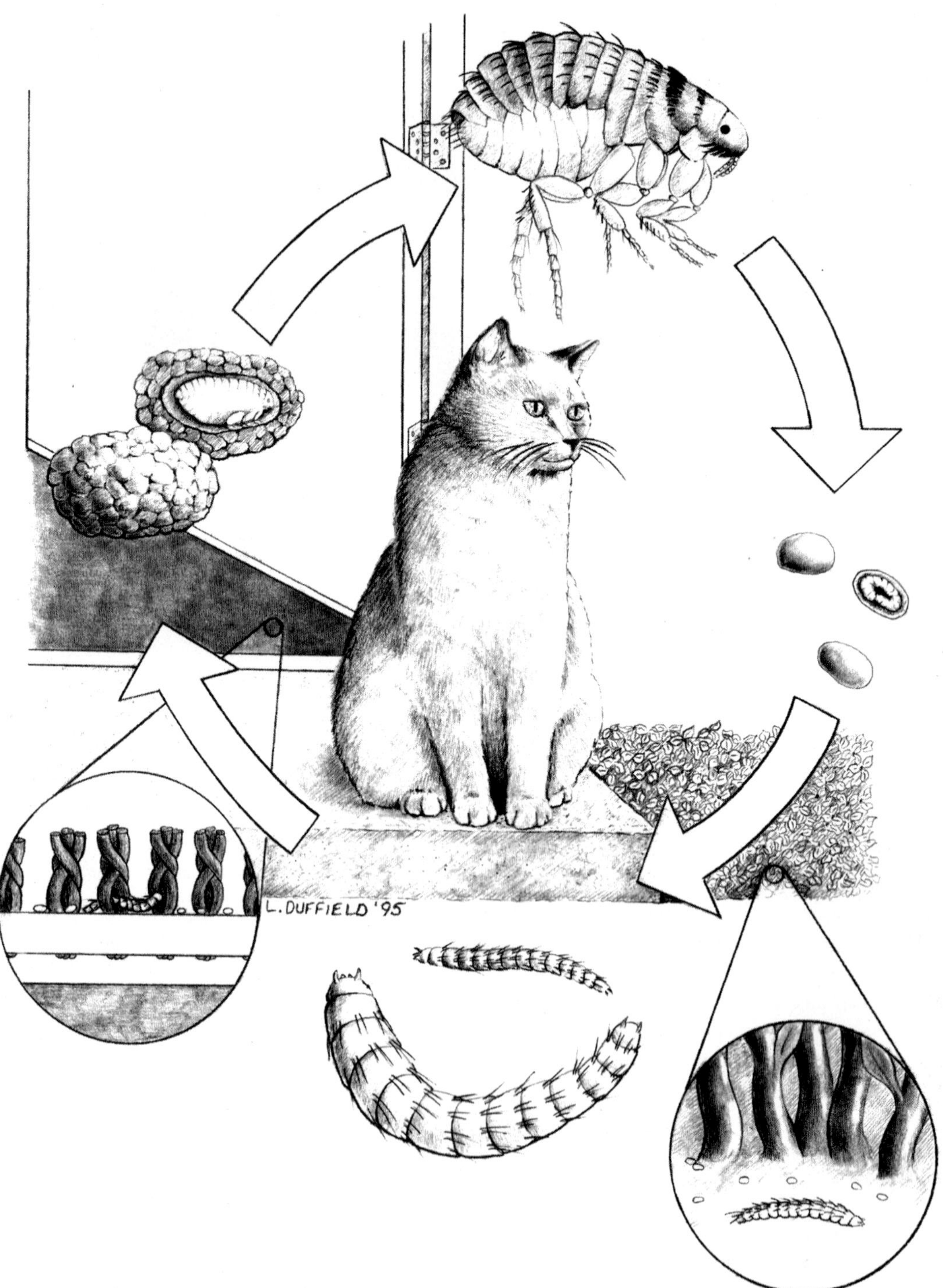

Fig. 5.93. Diagram of the life cycle of the cat flea. The adult fleas live on the cat and produce eggs that fall to the carpet or the soil. The eggs hatch and produce larvae. The larva crawls about in this environment and feeds. The larva undergoes two molts while growing, and it is the third-stage larva that ultimately spins a silken cocoon. The cocoon is sticky and will incorporate fibers and particles from the surrounding environment. The fibers and particles serve to help hold the cocoon in place and to camouflage the pupal case. The flea can remain in the pupal case for an extended period after it has developed to the adult stage. The flea in the pupal case is able to sense changes in the external environment, and adult fleas will eclose when they sense the presence of an appropriate host.

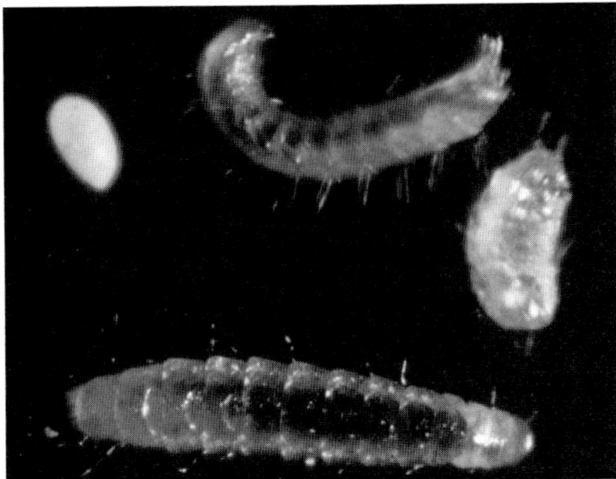

Fig. 5.94. *Ctenocephalides felis* life stages. In this image are the white ovoid egg, two third-stage larvae, and a pupa that does not have any attached fibers or particles.

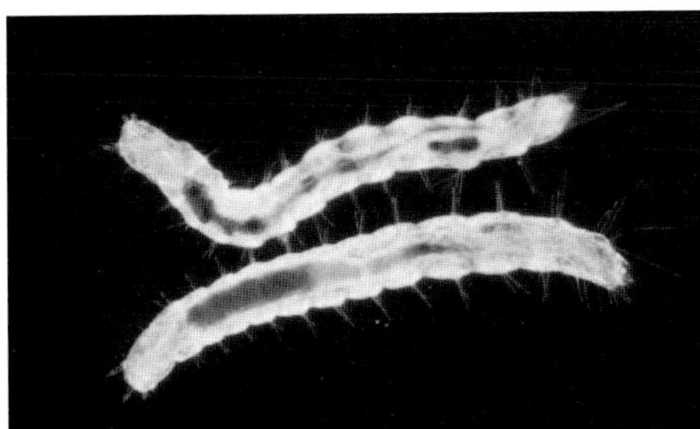

Fig. 5.95. *Ctenocephalides felis.* Two larvae that have dark intestinal tracts visible through their body walls. The dark color is due to the ingested blood that is shed in the form of feces by the feeding adult male and female fleas.

very safe. They differ in their method of application and in the mode of action as to how the fleas are killed, and this allows for designing flea-control programs that fit the lifestyle and needs of certain pets and owners. A major concern is that resistance to these products will develop that will make them less efficacious in years to come. Only time will tell, but it argues that people should not forget to work to maintain an environment where fleas do not thrive (i.e., it should be dry and regularly cleaned with a vacuum).

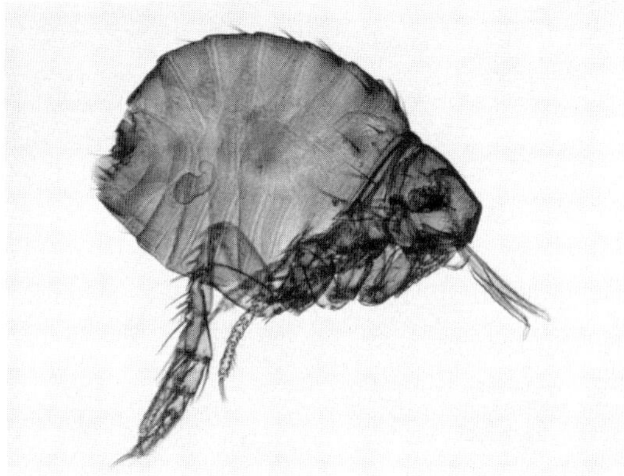

Fig. 5.96. *Echinophaga gallinacea.* Adult female.

REFERENCES

Georgi JR, Georgi ME. 1992. Canine Clinical Parasitology. Philadelphia, Pa.: Lea and Febiger. 227 pp.

King JM. 1997. Anemia caused by flea infestation in a cat. Vet Med 92:692.

Rust MK, Dryden MW. 1997. The biology, ecology, and management of the cat flea. Ann Rev Entomol 42:451–473.

Yaphe W, Giovengo S, Moise NS. 1993. Severe cardiomegaly secondary to anemia in a kitten. JAVMA 202:961–964.

Echinophaga gallinacea

This flea has been recovered from cats on more than a few occasions (Georgi and Georgi, 1992; Coman et al., 1981). The flea differs from the regular "cat" flea in that the adult embeds its head into the skin of the host while it feeds. The adult fleas differ from *Ctenocephalides* in that there are no combs, and the dorsally compressed thorax gives the flea a humped up appearance (Fig. 5.96). These fleas are found mainly in the tropics and subtropics. The pathology associated with these fleas is not so much loss of blood and anemia; rather it is the reaction to the site of attachment.

REFERENCES

Coman BJ, Jones EH, Driesen MA. 1981. Helminth parasites and arthropods of feral cats. Aust Vet J 57:324–327.

Georgi JR, Georgi ME. 1992. Canine Clinical Parasitology. Philadelphia, Pa.: Lea and Febiger. 227 pp.

INDEX

ISBN 0-8138-0333-0